Endoscopic Retrograde Cholangiopancreatography

Technique, Diagnosis, and Therapy

Endoscopic Retrograde Cholangiopancreatography

Technique, Diagnosis, and Therapy

Jerome H. Siegel, M.D., F.A.C.P., F.A.C.G.

Chief of Endoscopy
Beth Israel Hospital North
New York, New York

with a contribution by J. Delmont and A. G. Harris

Raven Press New York

Raven Press, 1185 Avenue of the Americas, New York, New York 10036

Made in the United States of America

Library of Congress Cataloging-in-Publication Data

Siegel, Jerome H., 1932–
Endoscopic retrograde cholangiopancreatography : technique, diagnosis, and therapy / by Jerome H. Siegel ; with a contribution by Jean Delmont and Alan G. Harris ; foreword by Charles A. Flood.
p. cm.
Includes bibliographical references and index.
ISBN 0-88167-815-5
1. Endoscopic retrograde cholangiopancreatography. I. Delmont, J. II. Harris, Alan G. III. Title.
[DNLM: 1. Biliary Tract Diseases—diagnosis. 2. Biliary Tract Diseases—therapy. 3. Pancreatic Diseases—diagnosis. 4. Pancreatic Diseases—therapy. WI 750 S571e]
RC847.5.E53S54 1991
616.3'650757—dc20
DNLM/DLC
for Library of Congress 91-18631
CIP

The material contained in this volume was submitted as previously unpublished material, except in the instances in which some of the illustrative material was derived.

Great care has been taken to maintain the accuracy of the information contained in the volume. However, neither Raven Press nor the editors can be held responsible for errors or for any consequences arising from the use of the information contained herein.

The enormous effort required to complete this book is shared by my wife, Beverly. It is with great admiration, respect, and love that I dedicate this book to a strong, courageous, and wonderful woman—she is truly the "wind beneath my wings."

Contents

Foreword

Over the last 20 years, we have witnessed major changes in the diagnostic approach to disorders of the pancreas and biliary tract. New ultrasound techniques, computerized axial tomography, improvements in the technique of percutaneous cholangiography, and endoscopic retrograde cholangiopancreatography (ERCP) have increased the accuracy of diagnosis immeasurably. ERCP, the subject of this book, has also helped increase the variety of therapeutic options.

Gastrointestinal diagnosis depends to a major extent on radiologic and endoscopic techniques. ERCP has become a feasible technique through combined efforts of endoscopists and radiologists. Several Japanese workers were the first to establish the procedure on a firm basis, using specially modified endoscopes; the reports of their procedures appeared about 1970.

Before 1970, the diagnosis of lesions of the biliary tree depended chiefly on the oral cholecystogram and the intravenous cholangiogram. The pancreatic duct could not be seen, except during surgery.

Radiologic imaging of the biliary tract dates back to 1924. In that year Graham and Cole reported x-ray visualization of the gallbladder. They took advantage of the fact that phthaleins are secreted by the liver into bile. They injected the calcium salt of tetrabromophenolphthalein intravenously and opacified the gallbladder and common bile duct. The presence of a halogen in the compound rendered it radiopaque (1).

Others modified the contrast medium, which resulted in a preparation that, when administered orally, yielded excellent x-ray pictures of the gallbladder (2). The oral cholecystogram became a routine diagnostic method. Intravenous contrast media, however, did not yield high quality x-rays of the common duct. Moreover, vascular collapse occurred occasionally during the procedure, so intravenous cholangiography was performed infrequently.

It was found that high quality images of the biliary tree could be obtained in the operating room. In 1932, Mirizzi of Argentina introduced the practice of intraoperative cholangiography. Excellent pictures of the common duct resulted when a contrast medium was injected directly into the cystic duct during surgery (3). Intraoperative and postoperative T-tube cholangiography soon became routine. Later, Royer and colleagues, also from Argentina, were able to obtain excellent radiologic pictures of the gallbladder and biliary tree during laparoscopy (4), but this technique was not widely adopted.

Modifications in the chemical structure of the contrast medium used for intravenous cholangiography that caused fewer side effects were sought, and in 1953 in Germany, biligrafin (cholegrafin) was introduced. Although its use spread rapidly to other countries (5), serious adverse reactions continued to occur.

In the meantime, yet another approach to the problem of visualizing the biliary duct system was evolving. The first percutaneous transhepatic cholangiogram was reported by workers from Indochina who happened to obtain bile while aspirating for a liver abscess. They injected Lipiodol for the purpose of visualizing the cause of the apparent biliary obstruction (6).

Shortly before and during World War II, clinicians began to acquire experience in needle aspiration of the liver. Improvements in the design of needles used for biopsy of the liver contributed to the use of biopsy as a standard procedure. It became feasible to obtain x-ray images of the biliary tree by the percutaneous route, and the percutaneous method was used increasingly in the 1950s (7,8). It was especially useful in the study of patients who appeared to present a clinical picture of obstructive jaundice. However, serious complications—namely, hemorrhage or biliary leakage—occasionally occurred.

Percutaneous transhepatic cholangiography finally became a safer and more useful technique with the introduction of the Chiba needle in 1969 (9,10). This so-called skinny needle has a length of 15 cm and an outer diameter of 1.7 mm. It became available about the same time as the ERCP.

The pancreatic duct, in contrast to the biliary tract, remained inaccessible to the radiologist and endoscopist for many years. In 1947, Doubilet et al. began to perform pancreatography during operations. They reported the results of their studies in 1955 (11).

Nonoperative attempts to fill the pancreatic duct with a radiopaque medium by other workers were unrewarding. A number of authors reported such attempts (12,13). The theory that acute pancreatitis results from the reflux of duodenal contents into the pancreatic duct impelled workers to devise techniques that might cause such reflux. Long tubes were passed by mouth into the duodenum. Two balloons were attached near the distal tip of the tube at levels that corresponded approximately to the first part of the duodenum and to the ligament of Treitz. After positioning and inflating of the balloons, contrast medium was injected into the second portion of the duodenum. Reflux into the pancreatic duct usually did not occur. The simultaneous administration of various substances to relax the sphincter of Oddi had no effect on the occurrence of reflux. The obliquity of the course of the distal ducts through the duodenal wall was thought to be an obstacle to the reflux of duodenal contents. It was of interest that reflux might occur in patients in whom the sphincter of Oddi had been divided during previous surgery.

Experiments attempting to cause reflux of duodenal contents into the pancreatic duct in animals met with more success. A tube with double balloon attachments was inserted into the duodenum of anesthetized dogs, and contrast material was injected under pressure. No reflux took place without additional measures. When the local anesthetic, Xylocaine, was also introduced into the duodenal lumen and Aminophylline was administered intravenously, reflux occurred, and images of the pancreatic duct could be obtained (14).

Success in visualizing the pancreatic duct was likewise reported in experiments using anesthetized Rhesus monkeys. At operation, a closed loop obstruction of the duodenum was produced with tapes encircling the organ. If secretin and cholecystokinin were then administered, reflux into the pancreatic duct occurred. Most animals also developed pancreatitis (15).

While such experimental work was in progress, successful endoscopic cannulation of the pancreatic and common ducts in humans was reported by Japanese workers.

The history of upper gastrointestinal endoscopy dates back to the late nineteenth century. The rigid metal instruments that were available at the time only permitted visualization of the esophagus and, to a small extent, the stomach. The creation of the flexirigid gastroscope by Schindler and Wolf in 1932 was a landmark event. With this instrument the examiner was able to inspect most of the stomach. The distal half of this gastroscope was flexible. The image of the gastric mucosa was transmitted back through a large series of accurately juxtaposed lenses (16). Various improvements soon extended the usefulness of gastroscopy, but the procedure remained difficult and was not completely accepted by the medical community until the creation of the fiberscope.

The fiberscope, created by Hirschowitz and coworkers in 1958, made it possible to see the duodenum (17). The fiberscope contains bundles of glass rods that transmit light. The fibers are of hair thickness and are coated. The coating causes internal reflection of light, resulting in transmission of an image. The fibers permit complete flexibility of the instrument without distortion of the image.

By 1968 McCune et al. were able to visualize and cannulate the papilla of Vater and to obtain x-ray pictures of the pancreatic and bile ducts (18). They used an American instrument, the Eder fiberoptic duodenoscope, with a balloon attachment placed just above the lens in order to help distend the duodenum. They were successful in about one-fourth of their attempts.

During the next two years, Japanese workers reported success in cannulating the papilla of Vater in the majority of their patients who underwent ERCP (19–22). These researchers used side-viewing instruments with special manual dexterity. The procedure then spread quickly to Europe and United States.

A new modality was thus available to aid in the diagnosis and management of diseases of the pancreas and biliary tract. Soon a number of experts were available at various centers to perform ERCP and to instruct others in the technique. Jerome Siegel, the author of the present volume, joined this group. He is a devoted teacher who has made numerous important contributions to the literature, especially on papillotomy and the treatment of retained common duct stones and on the palliative relief of obstructive jaundice.

This volume is an up-to-date review of the procedure of ERCP. It will be most useful to those who are acquiring this technique and will also be of great value to any physician in assessing the indications, value, and the scope of ERCP in the management of patients with gastrointestinal disorders.

REFERENCES

1. Graham EA, Cole WH, Copher GH. Roentgenologic examination of the gallbladder. *JAMA* 1924;82:613–4.
2. Meness TO, Robinson HC. Oral administration of sodium tetrabromphenolphthalein. *Am J Roentgen* 1925;13:368–9.
3. Mirizzi PI. La colangiografía durante las operaciones de las vias biliares. *Bol Trab Soc Cir* 1932;16:1133–61.
4. Royer M, Mazure P, Kohan S. Biliary dyskinesia studied by means of peritoneoscopic cholangiography. *Gastroenterology* 1950;16:83–90.
5. Püschel C. Clinical and roentgenological experiences with the new intravenous bile contrast medium "Biligrafin." *Dtsch Med Wochenschr* 1953;48:1327–9.
6. Huaed P, Do-Xuan-Hop. La ponción transhépatique des canaux biliares. *Bull Soc Med Chir Indocine* 1937;1090–1100.
7. Carter RF, Saypol GM. Transabdominal cholangiography. *JAMA* 1952;148:253–5.
8. Remolar J, Katz S, Rypak B, Pellizari O. Percutaneous transhepatic cholangiography. *Gastroenterology* 1956;31:39–46.
9. Tsuchiya Y. A new safer method of percutaneous transhepatic cholangiography *Jpn J Gastroenterol* 1969;66:438–55.
10. Okuda K, Tanikawa K, Emura T, et al. Nonsurgical percutaneous transhepatic cholangiography—diagnostic significance in medical problems of the liver. *Am J Dig Dis* 1974;19:21–36.
11. Doubilet H, Poppel MH, Mulholland GH. Pancreatography. *Radiology* 1955;64:325–39.
12. Gaylis H, Gunn K. Transduodenal cholangiography. *Surg Gynecol Obstet* 1955;100:249–53.
13. Greenfield H, Siegel LH, De Francis N. Attempted visualization of the pancreatic ducts by ampullary reflux. *Gastroenterology* 1955;29:280–84.
14. Waldron RL II, Bragg DG, Daly WJ, Seaman WB. Experimental reflux pancreatography and cholangiography. *Radiology* 1967;88:357–60.
15. Doppman J, Johnson RH. Reflux pancreatography. *Invest Radiol* 1967;2:113–8.
16. Schindler R. Gastroscopy. The Endoscopic Study of Gastric Pathology. Chicago: University of Chicago Press, 1937; 62–4.
17. Hirschowitz BI, Curtiss LE, Peters CW, Pollard HM. Demonstration of a new gastroscope, the fiberscope. *Gastroenterology* 1958;35:50–3.
18. McCune WS, Shorb PE, Moscovitz H. Endoscopic cannulation of the ampulla of Vater. *Ann Surg* 1968;167:752–6.
19. Oi I. Endoscopic pancreatography by fiberduodenoscope (F.D.S.-L.b). *Jpn J Gastroenterol* 1969;66:880–3.
20. Oi I. Fiberduodenoscopy and endoscopic pancreaticocholangiography. *Gastrointest Endosc* 1970;17:59–62.
21. Takagi K, Ikeda S, Nakagawa Y, et al. Retrograde pancreatography and cholangiography by fiberduedenoscope. *Gastroenterology* 1970;59:445–52.
22. Okuda K, Someya M, Goto A, et al. Endoscopic pancreatocholangiography. A preliminary report on technique and diagnostic significance. *Am J Roentgen* 1973;117:437–45.

Charles A. Flood, M.D.

Preface

Since the introduction of endoscopic retrograde cholangiopancreatography (ERCP) in 1968, no other endoscopic procedure has developed as rapidly, attracted as much interest, attention and scientific inquiry, or made as great an impact on the management of diseases of the gastrointestinal tract. Keeping current with new developments in this ever-expanding field is a major challenge, not only to the practitioner but to the teacher. Although postgraduate courses and contributed texts, specific in scope, are available to the student and practitioner, there was no comprehensive state-of-the-art reference text on ERCP available. This book was conceived and written to fill that void.

In order to become accomplished in ERCP, an endoscopist must be equally versed in endoscopy and radiology. This book brings together these disciplines by presenting endoscopic techniques and findings along with a compendium of radiographs that contain the key elements of interpretation. This approach should assist the reader in understanding the pathophysiologic elements affecting these organ systems while enhancing the technical and interpretive skills necessary for providing a diagnosis and prudent and appropriate management.

A team approach is essential to the management scheme of pancreaticobiliary disorders. This book should serve as a valuable tool to all members of this diagnostic-therapeutic team—gastroenterologists, hepatologists, pancreatologists, endoscopists, as well as radiologists, surgeons, and primary care physicians.

I am sure that today's endoscopists will continue the extraordinary discovery and development of our distinguished predecessors and that our current achievements will inspire and challenge future generations of endoscopists.

Jerome H. Siegel, M.D.

Acknowledgments

I am especially grateful to Dr. Charles Flood, the ultimate diagnostician and clinician, for his continued support and interest in my career. It is especially meaningful that Dr. Flood, my teacher and a founding member of The American Gastroscopic Club, contributed the important *Foreword* to my book.

A special thanks is extended to Dr. Henry Colcher whose energetic and inquisitive nature pervaded his teaching. He taught me the high art of advanced endoscopic techniques and interpretation. Dr. Julius Wolf, my residency program director, presented me with a firm grounding in gastroenterology through his fully developed training program. Working with my friend and colleague, Dr. Laszlo Safrany, provided the opportunity to refine my skills and techniques for endoscopic sphincterotomy which proved to be invaluable. The two years I spent with Professor Dame Sheila Sherlock at the Royal Free Hospital in London, England, as a Research Fellow influenced my career immeasurably. Professor Sherlock's energy, productivity, and creative understanding of science and medicine have left an indelible mark.

I thank my colleagues who boosted my career as well as my patients. Professor Jean Delmont of Hospital Cimiez, Nice, France, deserves special recognition for contributing Chapter 8, which addresses practical approaches to sphincter of Oddi dysfunction. More than 200 students, Fellows, and practitioners have worked, studied and participated in my clinical research and deserve special recognition for their contributions and scientific inquiry which affected this work positively. Their enthusiasm permeated our environment and promulgated published reports—a difficult accomplishment especially since many of these clinicians were engaged in private practice.

I want to give special thanks to Tamika Jeter, who singlehandedly typed the entire manuscript with extraordinary skill, and Kathy Hoey, who efficiently organized my practice schedule allowing time for work on the manuscript. Lynne Cooper, Medical Illustrator, Beth Israel Medical Center, deserves special thanks for her outstanding ability to translate my thoughts into the clear and meaningful illustrations seen throughout the book. I thank Antoinette Drago, head librarian, Beth Israel Hospital North, for her timely accession of reference material essential to the completion of this book. I have been fortunate to work with two dedicated assistants, Ruth Fregon, RN, and Alma Mattison, without whom the complicated and delicate therapeutic endoscopic procedures described in this book could not have been completed. I want to extend a special thanks to John Molyneux, an extraordinary editor, whose persuasive but gentle efforts extracted essential material from me and helped put it into final form. And of course, Raven Press is to be thanked for asking me to write this book. To all of the above, I extend my deepest appreciation.

PART I

Technique

CHAPTER 1

Introduction and Development

Although endoscopic retrograde cholangiopancreatography (ERCP) has been part of our diagnostic and therapeutic armamentarium for about two decades, its impact on the management of biliary and pancreatic disorders is incalculable. Prior to its introduction in 1970 (1,2), many inquisitive physicians and surgeons thought that opacification of the biliary tree and pancreas could be accomplished endoscopically through a transpapillary route (3,4), which was considerably less invasive than the methods then available, such as surgery or percutaneous cholangiography. The earlier technique of percutaneous cholangiography was performed using a 17-gauge or 18-gauge needle and was associated with a high morbidity rate (5,6). The procedure was usually performed in the radiology suite immediately prior to surgery, providing the surgeon with an appropriate cholangiogram and definition of the anatomy. By its temporal performance—immediately prior to surgery, for example—it reduced a potentially higher morbidity rate because of planned, early surgical intervention. On the positive side, the experience gained by performing this large-needle cholangiogram later enabled the therapeutic radiologist to employ similar techniques in providing biliary decompression. Because of its high morbidity, large-needle cholangiography was used less frequently and fell into disrepute. As ERCP was developed, however, radiologists again became interested in invasive procedures, especially because many of them were employing more invasive techniques, such as angiography, and were skilled and adept with these procedures (7,8). The field of percutaneous cholangiography was revolutionized by Okuda of Chiba University in Japan (9) when he and his colleagues introduced the technique of "skinny needle" cholangiography in 1974. Thus, the radiologists were beginning to move forward by providing both a diagnostic and a therapeutic maneuver in the same setting (10–12).

McCune et al. are credited with first using a semirigid endoscope for performing ERCP in 1968 (4). Their report of the technique and their follow-up data reveal that they entered the duodenum in only 50% of the patients in whom they attempted the procedure and that their rate of success for cannulating the papilla was only about 25%. This success was achieved, however, using an earlier model panendoscope and not the duodenoscope that was ultimately developed for selective cannulation of the papilla. McCune and his colleagues led the way for the development of a specialized field placing both diagnostic and therapeutic endoscopy into proper perspective. Their approach to the papilla of Vater was innovative and creative.

Although others have been credited for introduction and development of ERCP, Dr. R. Hansen, a New York surgeon deserves recognition for performing an ERCP as early as 1945. Figure 1.1, which was provided by Dr. Lee Gillette, shows a cholangiogram and cholecystogram obtained during a postmortem study of a patient with gallstones. This radiograph was obtained by cannulating the papilla using a semirigid or semiflexible gastroscope, which was the only type of endoscope available at that time. This study was not published, and, to my knowledge, no other similar reports were made during that period in history, but the side-viewing instrument (which was the usual configuration of endoscopes prior to the ACMI-Lopresti endoscopes of 1965) used by Hansen was subsequently refined and developed into the flexible fiberoptic duodenoscope used today. Those with previous gastroscopy experience who, for the first time, entered the duodenum in the late 1960s using the forward-viewing fiberscopes appreciated the periampullary structures, but from a tangential perspective rather than the appropriate orientation provided by the enface image obtained using a proper duodenoscope (Fig. 1.2). After endoscopists acquired experience with the appropriate duodenoscope, the rest, as they say, is history.

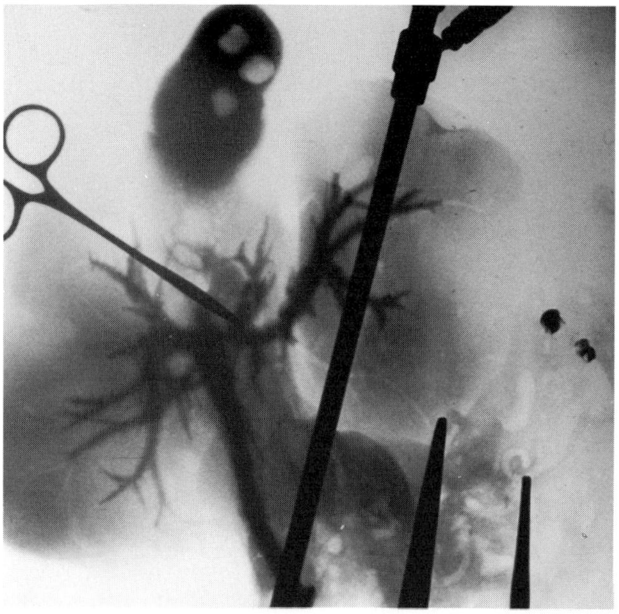

FIG. 1.1. A negative of an x-ray of the first known ERCP. The long instrument crossing the picture diagonally is a rigid endoscope. A catheter is seen exiting the tip of the endoscope and is inserted into the bile duct. The biliary tree is opacified, and the gallbladder is noted in the upper left of the picture containing three stones.

The advances achieved by ERCP are dutifully recorded in the literature and reflect the enormous progress achieved in only a few years (11). Table 1.1 lists the accomplishments achieved with ERCP and its therapeutic applications in the diagnosis and treatment of pancreaticobiliary disorders. This book attempts to put into perspective the development of ERCP and its therapeutic counterparts that have assumed a prominent position in this rapidly developing field; it is not a review of the ERCP literature in its entirety nor a thorough comparison of ERCP and other modalities.

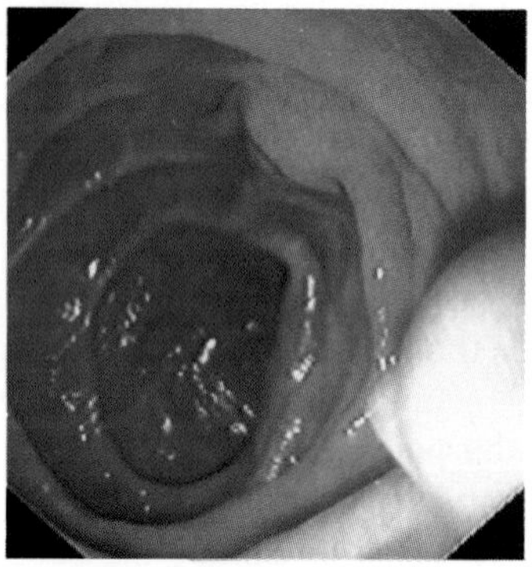

FIG. 1.2. The second portion of duodenum visualized with a forward-viewing videoendoscope. The minor papilla is in the foreground (*lower right corner*), and the major papilla is seen at 2:00. Obviously, cannulation is not possible because the papilla is not enface.

TABLE 1.1. *Endoscopic diagnosis and treatment of pancreaticobiliary disorders*

ERCP
Sphincterotomy
Stone extraction
Balloon
Basket
Lithotripsy
Mechanical
Electrohydraulic
Pulsed-dye lasers
Peroral cholangioscopy
Intubation of enterostomy
Mother-daughter system
Percutaneous
T-tube tract
Stones—PEERS[a]
Strictures
De novo and fistula
Stones—PEERS
Strictures
Perfusion techniques (nasobiliary tube)
Dilatation techniques
Catheters
Balloons
Drains
Nasobiliary
Endoprostheses
Intraluminal irradiation
Primary
Metastatic

[a] Percutaneous endoscopic extraction of retained stones

This great task of review and comparison has been achieved in recent publications and texts and continues to challenge researchers (13,14). This book does, however, present my experience and cite specific references for data comparison.

With the introduction of ERCP, pancreatography became a routine procedure accomplished for the first time outside the operating field (15–20). Atlases of cholangiography were available prior to the development of ERCP; pancreatography, however, could be obtained *in vivo* only during surgery or at necropsy. Pancreatography was therefore relatively new and unfamiliar to most gastroenterologists and endoscopists. Subsequent to the development of pancreatography, atlases describing the normal and pathologic appearances of the pancreatic duct were published, elucidating the morphology; these publications have ultimately become the standards for comparison (19–22).

This book is divided into three general sections with emphasis on technique, diagnosis, and therapy. Many endoscopists need and request the basics, so I have made an effort to describe the performance of ERCP from start to finish, providing tricks, illustrations, and descriptions of the methods I use to complete an examination and study successfully.

TABLE 1.2. *ERCP specificity in 7,487 examinations*

	Attempted	Cannulation	% success
Pancreatic disease	2,547	2,471	97
Biliary disease	4,940	4,693	95
Single duct cannulated		873	
Both ducts cannulated		6,161	86
Total		7,164	95.7
Duct of intention		6,748	94.2

The second section describes and illustrates what is accepted to be the normal configuration and morphology of both the biliary and the pancreatic ductal systems. Variations of these structures, which are normal and are not associated with disease, are illustrated.

Separate parts illustrate diseases affecting both duct systems. These disease states are discussed in detail and distinguish the normal variations, which may or may not be associated with symptoms and should not be construed as abnormal. The latter examples are intended to be used for reference (and as an atlas) because many have not been described previously.

Most of the data contained in the book come from my personal experience, accumulated over the past 15 years. During that time, I have performed nearly 7,500 ERCPs and more than 5,000 sphincterotomies (Chapter 10) and therapeutic procedures. Data from this large series are presented for comparison to other diagnostic and therapeutic modalities, especially when determining cost analyses and comparing procedure-related morbidity/mortality occurrence data. The specificity of ERCP accounts for the important role this procedure has assumed in the diagnoses and management of pancreaticobiliary disorders (Table 1.2).

Finally, I will attempt to look into the future and have included a chapter on new horizons. Since I initially prepared the outline for this book 4 years ago, some of these new ideas and procedures have become standards, such as needle knife sphincterotomies,

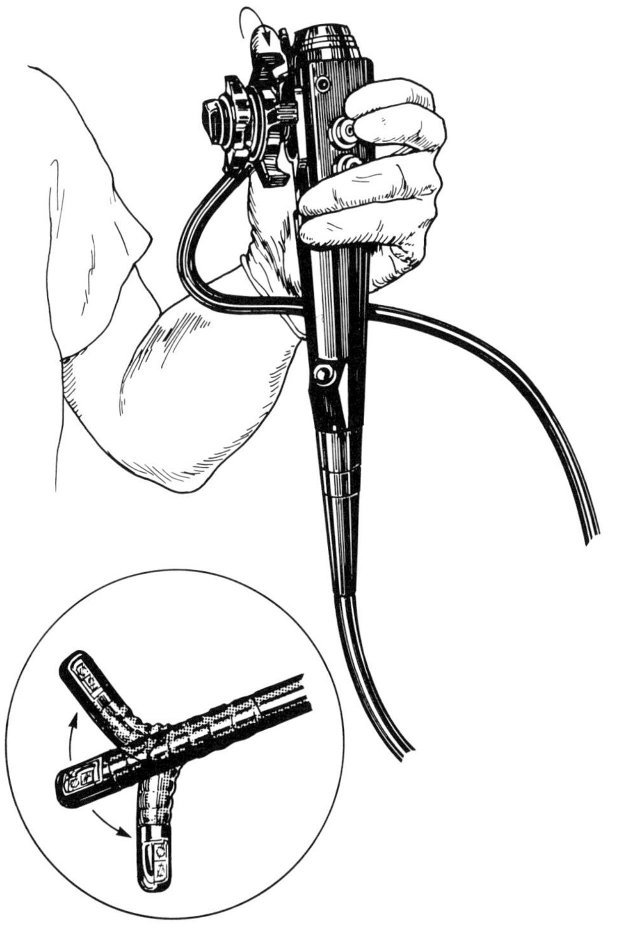

FIG. 1.3. A videoduodenoscope, demonstrating the proximal control section and showing the endoscopist's thumb manipulating the up-down control. The inset demonstrates the flexibility of the distal or optical end of the endoscope when the up-down control is manipulated.

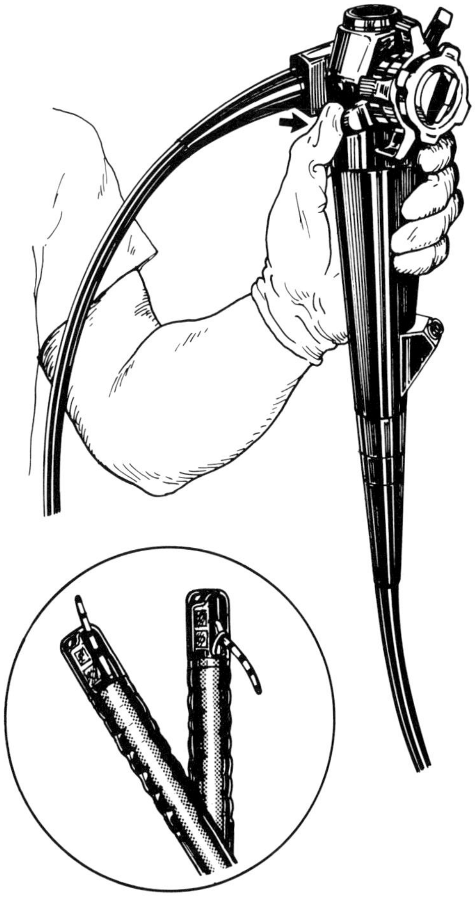

FIG. 1.4. The endoscopist's thumb moving the elevator control on the proximal end of the videoendoscope. The inset shows movement of the elevator at the distal end of the endoscope, with the cannula in both the relaxed and the flexed positions.

wire-guided systems, and electronic endoscopes. Many procedures under development, however, are never introduced or, by virtue of their degree of difficulty or lack of success, are never accepted. This section will be used to describe procedures that are used infrequently or by only a few endoscopists; appropriately, this last chapter will include my experience with choledochoscopy.

Certainly, most of the success in this field is attributed to the improvement and development of the endoscope. Standardization of endoscopes and improvements in the quality of the fiber bundles, which provide improved resolution and resistance to the damaging effects of x-rays, have permitted us to advance far beyond our earliest predictions. The introduction of electronic endoscopes, which I employ routinely in my practice, has also enabled us to make technologic advances far beyond our expectations (Figs. 1.3, 1.4). It is therefore difficult to gaze into a crystal ball and predict what the future holds for the field of ERCP because the crystal ball is held by the instrument manufacturers. Manufacturers have instruments and systems on the drawing boards and in prototype form that will soon make our present equipment obsolete.

REFERENCES

1. Oi I, Takemoto T, Kondo T. Fiberduodenoscope: direct observation of the papilla of Vater. *Endoscopy* 1970;17:59–62.
2. Takagi K, Ikeda S, Nakagawa Y, et al. Retrograde pancreatography and cholangiography by fiberduodenoscope. *Gastroenterology* 1970;59:445–52.
3. Watson WC. Direct vision of the ampulla of Vater with the gastroduodenal fiberscope. *Lancet* 1966;1:902–3.
4. McCune WS, Short PE, Moscovitz H. Endoscopic cannulation of the ampulla of Vater. *Ann Surg* 1968;167:752–6.
5. Fuente RD, Patillo C, Koch W, Mallet-Guy P. Exploration des voies uiliaires un moyen de la cholangiographie trans-abdominale. *Lyon Chir* 1954;49:959.
6. Glenn F. Percutaneous transhepatic cholangiography. *Ann Surg* 1962;156:451.
7. Tsuchiya Y. A new safer method of percutaneous transhepatic cholangiography. *Jpn J Gastroenterol* 1969;66:438–52.
8. Kaude JV, Weidenheimer CH, Agee OF. Decompression of bile ducts with the percutaneous transhepatic technic. *Radiology* 1969;93:69–71.
9. Okuda K, Tanikawa K, Emura T, et al. Non-surgical percutaneous transhepatic cholangiography: diagnostic significance in medical problems of the liver. *Am J Dig Dis* 1974;19:21–36.
10. Nakayama T, Ikeda A, Okuda K. Percutaneous transhepatic drainage of the biliary tract: technique and results in 104 cases. *Gastroenterology* 1978;74:554–59.
11. Ring EJ, Oleaga JA, Freiman DB, Husted JW, Lunderquist A. Therapeutic applications of catheter cholangiography. *Radiology* 1978;128:333–8.
12. Hoevels J, Lunderquist A, Ihse I: Percutaneous transhepatic intubation of bile ducts for combined internal-external drainage in preoperative and palliative treatment of obstructive jaundice. *Gastrointest Radiol* 1978;3:23–31.
13. Jacobson IM. *ERCP: diagnostic and therapeutic applications.* New York: Elsevier Scientific Publishers, 1989.
14. Cotton PB, Tytgat GNJ, Williams CB. *Annual of gastrointestinal endoscopy*. London: Current Science, 1990.
15. Cotton PB, Salmon PR, Beales JSM, Burwood RJ. Endoscopic trans-papillary radiographs of pancreatic and bile ducts. *Gastrointest Endosc* 1972;19:60–2.
16. Cotton PB. Cannulation of the papilla of Vater by endoscopy and retrograde cholangiopancreatography (ERCP). *Gut* 1972;13:1014–25.
17. Dickinson PB, Belsito AA, Cramer GG. Diagnostic value of endoscopic cholangiopancreatography. *JAMA* 1973;225:994–8.
18. Cotton PB. Progress report. ERCP. *Gut* 1977;18:316–41.
19. Stewart ET, Vennes JA, Geenen JE. *Atlas of endoscopic retrograde cholangiography*. St. Louis: CV Mosby, 1977.
20. Siegel JH. Endoscopic retrograde cholangiopancreatography (ERCP): present position, and papillotomy. *NY State J Med* 1978;78:538–91.
21. Siegel JH, Yatto RP, Vender RJ. Anomalous pancreatic ducts causing "Pseudomass" of the pancreas. *J Clin Gastroenterol* 1983;5:33–6.
22. Yatto RP, Siegel JH. Variant pancreatography. *Am J Gastroenterol* 1983;78:115–8.

CHAPTER 2

Indications, Contraindications, and Preparation

By now, most physicians and surgeons should be familiar with the indications and contraindications for ERCP listed in Table 2.1. Emphasis *must* be placed on the importance of early but appropriate utilization of ERCP in suspected disease of the biliary tree and pancreas. Prolonged hospitalization of a patient and delay in arriving at a diagnosis is usually attributable to the reticence of the referring physician in requesting a consultation from either the surgeon or the gastroenterologist/endoscopist. The primary care physician, in his or her quest for establishing a diagnosis without the aid of a consultant, usually orders unnecessary tests or tests that may interfere with the performance of a cholangiogram or CT scan, such as upper GI series or other barium contrast studies in which barium is eliminated from the gastrointestinal tract too slowly and obscures the essential structures that should be opacified. This pedantic approach delays the utilization of other procedures. If the presenting cholestatic syndrome is associated with nausea and vomiting and gastric outlet obstruction is suspected, an upper gastrointestinal series is usually indicated and may be performed. One must bear in mind that nausea is an accompanying symptom of pancreatic cancer and biliary tract obstruction and that it may not be pathognomonic of gastric outlet obstruction. Endoscopy, however, may obviate the need for barium contrast studies. For example, during the performance of ERCP, the endoscopist confirms outlet obstruction when visually encountering retained gastric secretions and partially digested food and when experiencing difficulty or an inability to traverse the pylorus (Fig. 2.1). Gastric outlet obstruction determines whether nonsurgical procedures should be performed because its presence favors surgical decompression of both the biliary tree and stomach.

To facilitate the evaluation of a patient presenting with biliary tract or pancreatic disorders, I suggest following an algorithim (Table 2.2), which will assist the primary care physician and consultant in providing an expedient but safe and cost-effective workup (1,2). Clinicians should adhere to this type of workup plan because it expedites the diagnostic evaluation leading to early therapeutic maneuvers and avoids unnecessary delays.

Initially, most patients should be evaluated as outpatients undergoing a careful and thorough history and physical examination, a chemical profile, and noninvasive diagnostic studies that provide a high yield. The suspicion of intrahepatic biliary disease is amplified further by knowledge of the patient's medical history; drug and medication history; prior surgical procedures; medical history, including a history of hepatitis or other liver diseases; and a history of alcohol and/ or substance abuse. Even though a history is available, the preliminary workup may remain equivocal, and an ERCP or cholangiogram would be indicated to determine intrahepatic cholestasis.

The choice of either ERCP or percutaneous cholangiography for definition of the anatomy in patients presenting with cholestasis depends on the institution and the experience of the endoscopist or radiologist. In

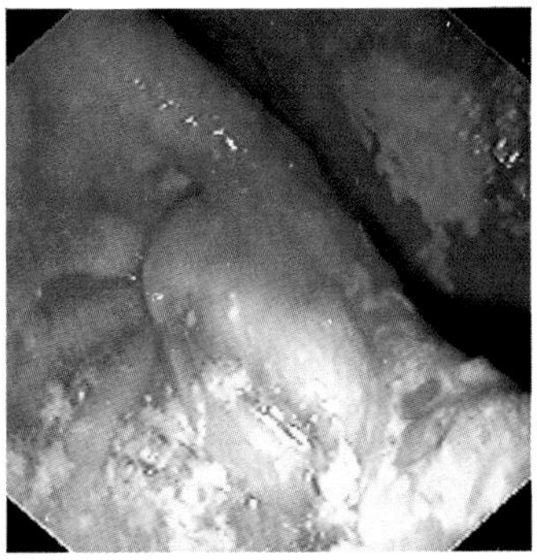

FIG. 2.1. Endoscopic appearance of an obstructed pylorus. Note the edematous and radiating-convergent gastric folds at the closed pylorus. Note also the retained food near the pylorus and in the fundus, which is seen above the angularis.

TABLE 2.1. *Indications and contraindications for ERCP*

Indications

- Jaundice
  - Intrahepatic
    - Hepatocellular (virus, drug, alcohol)
    - Cirrhosis
    - Tumor
    - Abscess
  - Extrahepatic
    - Choledocholithiasis
      - Cholangitis
      - Pancreatitis
  - Tumor
    - Primary
    - Periampullary
    - Metastatic
    - Pancreatic disease
    - Paraneoplastic
- Pancreatic disease
  - Recurrent acute
    - Subacute
    - Subclinical
  - Chronic relapsing
  - Pseudocyst
  - Abscess
  - Tumor
- Gallbladder disease
- Pre- and postoperative evaluation of biliary tract and pancreatic duct
- Abdominal pain of unknown cause
- Other applications of ERCP
  - Collection of pancreatic secretions for cytology, CEA, chemistries
  - Biopsy
  - Research
- Therapeutic applications of ERCP
  - Sphincterotomy
  - Stone removal
  - Lithotripsy
  - Drains and stents
  - Balloon dilatation
  - Irradiation

Contraindications

- Acute pancreatitis, idiopathic
- Comorbid life-threatening conditions

In experienced hands, ERCP and its therapeutic counterparts, sphincterotomy and stent insertion, are certainly more comfortable procedures and are better tolerated than percutaneous transhepatic cholangiography and insertion of drains. If ERCP fails, however, percutaneous cholangiography should be requested before undertaking an exploratory laparotomy. Note that in this algorithm (Table 2.2) the definitive treatment for biliary obstruction is *decompression,* which can be provided by percutaneous, endoscopic, or surgical techniques. It is not my intention to be critical of other techniques (i.e., radiologic or surgical); I firmly believe in cooperation among the disciplines because the patient is the ultimate beneficiary. Therefore, it is inappropriate and egotistical for any *providers* to advocate only their own procedures or techniques and to rule out other modalities or to be critical of other disciplines. Each patient must be evaluated and treated as an individual because no one procedure or discipline is effective all the time. Most physicians rely on their radiologic and surgical colleagues for assistance, and vice versa, so the patient and the health care delivery system deserve an expeditious but safe workup and evaluation that includes the early utilization of services provided by other disciplines.

The indications and contraindications for ERCP are clearly stated in Table 2.1. In earlier reports and texts (7,8), pancreatitis and cholangitis were considered contraindications for ERCP. Since the introduction of some institutions, radiologists have developed enormous skill and experience with both diagnostic and therapeutic procedures, and the endoscopist may have less experience in ERCP. In this example, the endoscopist has little opportunity to develop his or her skills and should work in a cooperative effort with the radiologist. In other institutions, where the endoscopists have led the development of diagnostic and therapeutic procedures, the radiologist should be called to assist in difficult procedures, such as Bilroth II gastrectomy or other postsurgical alterations or variant anatomy, including periampillary diverticula and neoplasia (3–6).

TABLE 2.2. *Workup of cholestasis*

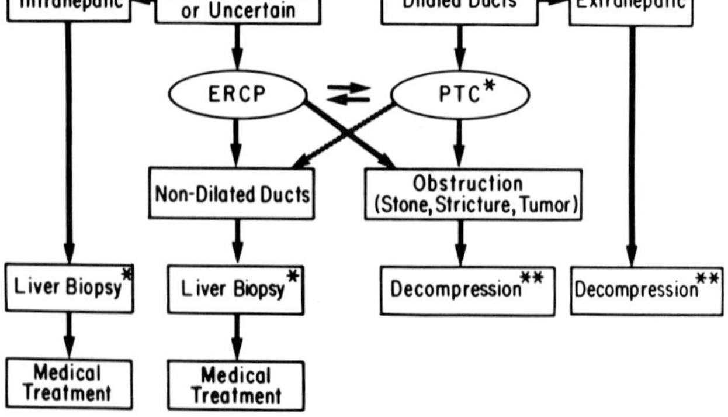

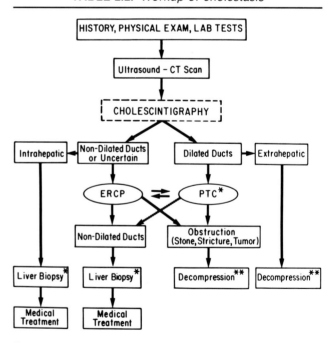

* Normal Coagulation

** Percutaneous Drainage, Duodenoscopic Sphincterotomy Transpapillary Drainage, Surgery sphincterotomy and endoscopic decompression techniques, however, most physicians today have made an exception to these contraindications and include gallstone pancreatitis and cholangitis as clear indications for early utilization of ERCP and sphincterotomy (9–11). Hesitation in providing this expeditious approach may lead to a dismal outcome. As will be discussed in chapters 9, 10, 11, and 12, the accumulated experience in the endoscopic management of gallstone pancreatitis and cholangitis supports the premise that ERCP should be employed early in the presentation of these illnesses.

Research is another important indication for ERCP. Without the inquisitive nature of resourceful endoscopists, this field would not have progressed to its present level. Collection of specimens, including pancreatic juice and bile, is useful for studying drug metabolism and pharmacokinetics, and special assays currently under investigation may ultimately offer information regarding the development of neoplasms of these organ systems.

The contraindications to the performance of ERCP are few and are usually the same as those for any endoscopic procedure. However, idiopathic pancreatitis and pancreatitis of known cause (e.g., alcohol) but exclusive of gallstones are considered contraindications for ERCP. Patients with recent cardiac injury would be at greater risk to undergo an endoscopic procedure, and, therefore, unless faced with a life-threatening situation, the endoscopist should delay ERCP until the patient has been cleared by the cardiologist. There are times, however, when ERCP is clearly necessary despite the recent history of cardiac injury. The performance of ERCP and sphincterotomy in this latter example would be associated with a lower morbidity rate than surgery.

Relative contraindications to ERCP include severe *cardiopulmonary disease*. I have, on occasion, out of necessity, performed ERCP in these patients with an anesthesiologist and appropriate monitoring equipment as standby. Sometimes keeping the patient in a more upright position, as in the case of severe chronic obstructive pulmonary disease, is important for maintaining adequate tidal volume. Although altering the patient's position may make the performance of ERCP more difficult for the endoscopist, I have successfully completed the examination and treatment of compromised patients in unorthodox positions, and these patients endured the procedure with little anxiety and apprehension.

PATIENT PREPARATION

Preparation for the performance of ERCP is simple. Patients should be fasting and NPO (nothing by mouth) for at least four hours prior to the procedure. It is my routine in performing ERCP in the morning to have the patient NPO after midnight. If the procedure is performed in the afternoon, I permit clear liquids early, then NPO after 8:30 A.M. I do permit patients to take medications if they take them within two hours of the procedure. Because I perform the procedure using intravenous analgesia, I prefer to start an infusion at the bedside in the patient's room before having the patient brought to the endoscopic suite to conserve time. An appropriate intravenous solution is tailored for the patient, which considers his or her cardiac and pulmonary status and other metabolic conditions, such as diabetes mellitus. This not only facilitates the administration of medication but also prevents a delay in beginning the procedure by having to start the infusion in the endoscopic suite. As part of my regimen, I have incorporated the administration of intramuscular sedation prior to transporting the patient from his or her room to the endoscopic suite. I find that, as with sedation prior to surgery, the patient is more relaxed, less anxious, and more cooperative. As a bonus, requirements for intravenous sedation are decreased.

If the patient has undergone recent barium radiographic contrast studies, I routinely obtain a flat film of the abdomen the day before the procedure to determine if the barium has been eliminated. If barium is seen on the radiograph in this sequence, administering appropriate laxatives the evening before the procedure ensures an unobscured radiologic field.

PATIENT POSITION (Fig. 2.2)

When the patient is brought into the endoscopic/radiology suite, he or she is placed onto the table in the left lateral recumbent position. This attitude allows for a partial oblique position of the patient with the right hip slightly elevated. The position is held by bending the patient's right leg so that the hip is positioned slightly off the table. This position, in general, appears to place the liver, pancreas, and bile duct more optimally for radiography, and it also permits the endoscopist to advance the endoscope directly into the duodenum with little manipulation or changes of the patient's position. Before the availability of wide-angled endoscopes, insertion of the duodenoscope was made with the patient in the left lateral position, similar to positioning for routine endoscopy. This position theoretically permitted an easier introduction through the pylorus into the duodenum. After entering the duodenum, the patient is rolled into a more prone or partial oblique attitude for cannulation. This latter maneuver requires assistance because the patient is sedated, and it remains the usual practice in most institutions. Even though I do not routinely position the

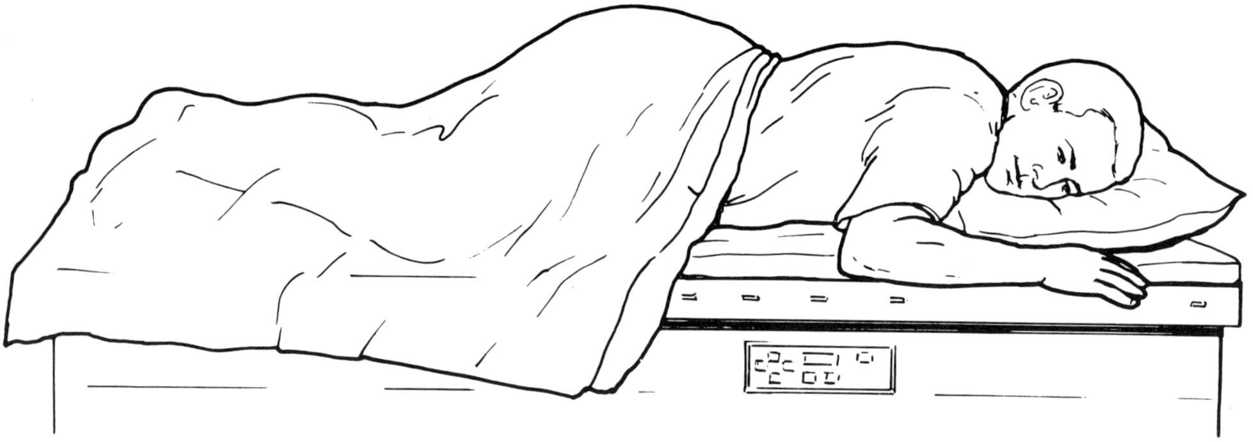

FIG. 2.2. The position of the patient on the fluoroscope table.

patient in the left lateral attitude, this position may facilitate the passage of the duodenoscope for the less experienced endoscopist. I rarely have to adjust the patient's position to enter the duodenum when I begin with the patient in the left lateral recumbent position as described.

CONSCIOUS SEDATION, ANTIPERISTALSIS

I have not altered my preferred types of analgesic or antiperistaltic agents for several years. Although several agents are available, I routinely use meperidine and midazolam. These drugs are titrated to the level of conscious sedation desired for total patient cooperation. If there is a reported sensitivity to meperidine, I use morphine or a suitable substitute or a synthetic narcotic agonist-antagonist such as nalbuphine or butorphanol. Since incorporating midazolam into my protocol, I have experienced few problems with respiratory depression and few, if any, problems of phlebitis or cellulitis at the injection site. For example, at the beginning of the procedure, I usually inject 50 mg of meperidine and 1 mg to 1.5 mg of midazolam. If the procedure lasts longer than 30 minutes, it may be necessary to add one or both drugs in small increments. Careful visual monitoring of the patient may be combined with electronic types of monitoring—i.e., blood pressure, cardiac monitoring, and pulse oximetry (Nellcor)—which are important but not yet essential for safely performing ERCP. Close monitoring is advantageous, especially in compromised patients, and I usually have an anesthesiologist standing by when ERCP is performed in patients at risk. Pulse oximetry is not currently mandatory, but it can be very helpful in monitoring the vital signs of the patient and preventing potential problems. I routinely use the Nellcor unit, which provides the necessary electronic data I need for monitoring all patients. Monitors, however, are not a substitute for quality visual monitoring. Nasal oxygen has become more routine in our unit and helps to maintain a satisfactory oxygen saturation, especially in the elderly patient. Being familiar with drug pharmacology is helpful in avoiding problems, and antidotes, which are available to reverse the maximum effect of the sedatives, should be available for use should a problem arise.

Glucagon has long been the standard for antiperistalsis. Because the pharmacologic effect of glucagon is predictable (approximately 15 minutes), I have found that a dose smaller than 1 mg produces the same effect as the 1 mg dose. Therefore, my assistant or I administer this agent in 0.25 mg increments (¼cc). The procedure can usually be performed in its entirety using no more than 0.5 mg.

After entering the duodenum, my assistant or I usually administer 0.25 mg of glucagon as an I.V. push. Increments of 0.25 mg are administered throughout the procedure. Additionally, atropine may be necessary in patients with a more active but less responsive duodenum.

All these drugs may have an adverse effect on the patient's blood pressure; meperidine lowers the pressure. Therefore, I prefer to monitor the patient's vital signs during the procedure using an automatic device. I have incorporated blood pressure, cardiac, and pulse oximetry monitoring into my protocol and recommend monitoring these vital functions in all patients and especially in elderly patients, because lying prone for long periods of time may lead to hypoxia. Hypoxia is manifested by restlessness, and, unless recognized and treated with oxygen, the patient may be given more sedative medication to suppress the restlessness, compounding the clinical picture.

We have only recently begun to recognize some of the potential hazards of I.V. analgesia in patients undergoing endoscopic procedures (12–14), mostly in the elderly, and I strongly advise readers to consider incorporating electronic monitoring equipment into their protocols to avoid potential complications and misadventures. Although these additional monitoring devices are not part of the standard requirements for the performance of endoscopy or ERCP, I strongly recommend their utilization because many therapeutic procedures are performed in elderly patients placed in a prone or near-prone position for long periods. Careful patient monitoring, adherence to strict indications for the performance of the procedure, adequate preparation of the patient, and a complete check of all equipment—monitoring, endoscopic, and cautery—before starting the procedure enable the endoscopist to direct his or her attention to the performance and successful completion of the procedure.

REFERENCES

1. Siegel JH, Yatto RP. Approach to cholestasis—an update. *Arch Intern Med* 1982;142:1877–9.
2. Siegel JH, Schapiro M, Hughes RW Jr. Endoscopy, obstructive jaundice, and DRG's: the buck stops in the hospital bank account. *Am J Gastroenterol* 1986;82:173–4.
3. Brams HJ, Billmann P, Pausch J, Hostege A, Salm R. Nonsurgical biliary drainage: endoscopic conversion of percutaneous transhepatic into endoprosthetic drainage. *Endoscopy* 1986;18:52–4.
4. Tsang T, Crampton AR, Bernstein JR, Ramos SR, Wieland JM. Percutaneous endoscopic biliary stent placement—a preliminary report. *Ann Intern Med* 1987;106:389–92.
5. Shorvon PJ, Cotton PB, Mason RR, Siegel JH, Hatfield ARW. Percutaneous transhepatic assistance for duodenoscopic sphincterotomy. *Gut* 1985;26:1373–6.
6. Dowsett JF, Vaira D, Hatfield ARW, et al. Endoscopic biliary therapy using the combined percutaneous and endoscopic technique. *Gastroenterology* 1989;96:1180–6.
7. Siegel JH. Endoscopic retrograde cholangiopancreatography (ERCP): present position and papillotomy. *NY State J Med* 1978;78:583–91.
8. Siegel JH. Newer diagnostic and therapeutic approaches to the bile ducts and pancreas: ERCP. *Famous teachings in modern medicine*. Med Com, 1978.
9. Leese T, Neoptolemos JP, Baker AR, Carr-Locke DL. The management of acute cholangitis and the impact of endoscopic sphincterotomy. *Br J Surg* 1986;73:988–92.
10. Neoptolemos JP, Carr-Locke DL. ERCP in acute cholangitis and pancreatitis. In: Jacobson IM, ed. *ERCP: diagnostic and therapeutic application*. New York: Elsevier Scientific Publishing, 1989.
11. Neoptolemos JP, Carr-Locke DL, London NJ, et al. Controlled trial of urgent endoscopic retrograde cholangiopancreatography and endoscopic sphincterotomy versus conservative treatment for acute pancreatitis due to gallstones. *Lancet* 1988;2:979–83.
12. Fleischer D. Monitoring the patient receiving conscious sedation for gastrointestinal endoscopy: issues and guidelines. *Gastrointest Endosc* 1989;35:262–6.
13. Woods SDS, Chung SCS, Leung JWC, Chan ACW, Li AKC. Hypoxia and tachycardia during endoscopic retrograde cholangiopancreatography: detection by pulse oximetry. *Gastrointest Endosc* 1989;35:523–5.
14. Dark DS, Campbell DR, Wesselius LJ. Arterial oxygen desaturation during gastrointestinal endoscopy. *Am J Gastroenterol* 1990;85:1317–21.

CHAPTER 3

Endoscopic Technique

PATIENT POSITION

As I described in the preceding chapter, I perform ERCP with the patient in the left lateral or right oblique position. The right hip is slightly elevated off the table, and the right leg is slightly bent at the knee to support the elevation of the hip. The patient's head is turned right, and the left arm is placed alongside the patient's body. Occasionally, the patient's left arm may be flexed parallel to the head (Fig. 3.1). Other endoscopists may prefer placing the patient in the left lateral position—that is, the left side down and right side up—similar to the position used for routine upper endoscopy. The latter position was used routinely before the introduction of wide-angled instruments. Thus, the patient is in position for esophagogastroduodenoscopy (EGD). If the patient is in the left lateral position, after negotiating the pylorus, he or she is rolled into a more prone position facilitating not only orientation and cannulation of the papilla but also radiography of both the biliary tree and pancreas.

Prior to placing the patient in the position for introduction of the endoscope, I apply the blood pressure cuff (which is part of an automatic system such as Dinamap) to the arm that does not contain the intravenous line. This is usually the left arm, because I prefer placement of the intravenous line in the right arm to facilitate the administration of medications (closer to the assistant and endoscopist). The blood pressure is monitored every five minutes during the procedure, and the cardiac monitor and oxygen saturation (pulse oximeter) record continuously. Having the line closer to the physician and assistant eliminates the need to stretch over the patient to search for the I.V. line, which may be under the fluoroscope.

Before placing the patient on the fluoroscopy table, I typically spray the patient's throat with a topical anesthetic agent or give him or her a topical anesthetic agent to gargle. The patient is then rolled from the stretcher onto the table and into position. I have found through experience that this step eliminates a clumsy attempt at having the patient roll into the prone position from the supine position while lying on the fluoroscope table. The patient is usually wrapped in sheets and lying on a cushion, and the sheets usually become entangled while attempting to change the patient's position. Therefore, I prefer rolling the patient, who is in the supine position, from the stretcher onto the fluoroscope table and into the prone position.

Once the patient is in position, monitors are connected and operational, and the I.V. is running satisfactorily, the initial dose of medication is slowly administered while observing the patient's response to the analgesia. While the patient is being given the medication and is still conscious, the bite block can be placed between the teeth. I prefer a bite block for all patients, even those who are edentulous, because patients without teeth can apply pressure on the endoscope using their gums and jaws. Without a bite block I have found that the edentulous patient's lips may entrap the endoscope, producing a drag effect. As the patient is sedated, the room lights can be dimmed to the appropriate illumination to permit an adequate view through the endoscope or to allow a clear view of the television monitor of the video endoscope system.

INSERTION OF ENDOSCOPE

When the patient is sedated adequately, his or her head is bent forward or flexed toward the chest to permit easy insertion of the endoscope. Most patients can be intubated directly with the endoscope without the endoscopist having to place his or her fingers into the oropharynx to assist guidance. The instrument is directed over the patient's tongue, and the distal tip is flexed downward to accommodate the curve of the tongue into the oropharynx; with the patient's head and neck properly flexed, the endoscope can then be

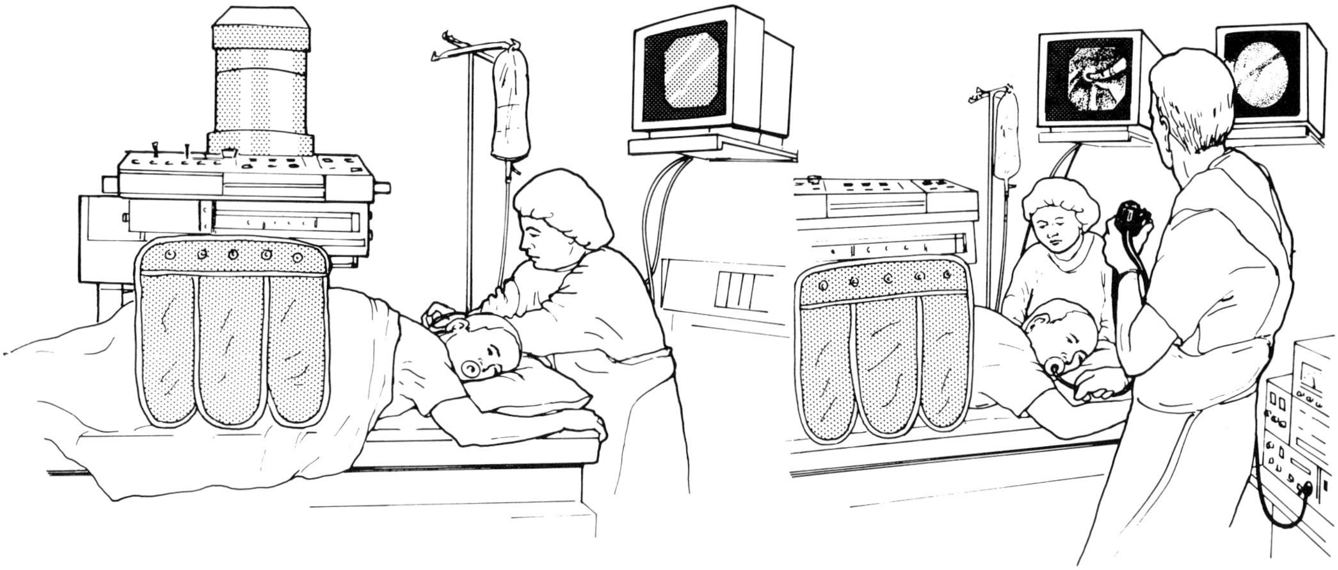

FIG. 3.1. Left: The patient is in position on the x-ray table with the fluoroscope in place. The nurse is at the head of the table working over the patient. **Right:** This ERCP is being performed by an endoscopist using a videoduodenoscope. The video and fluoroscope monitors display images during the procedure.

easily advanced into the esophagus with or without a swallow.

Occasionally, it may be necessary to place the patient in the left lateral position, and, with the assistant's help, the head and neck may be flexed sufficiently to eliminate extrinsic compression by osteophytes. I have had very little difficulty in introducing any endoscope using this technique, even with patients who have severe cervical osteoarthritis and osteophytes. Even the larger caliber endoscopes, the 4.2 and 5.5 channel scopes, have been introduced into nearly all patients using this technique.

Alternative Methods of Insertion

Sometimes, a patient with a congenital or acquired variation of the oropharynx and cricopharyngeus is encountered and may be difficult to intubate. More typically this is a result of rigidity or stiffness of the neck secondary to osteoarthritis and to the presence of osteophytes. I have employed two techniques for intubating patients with deformities of the neck and internal structures. The first is placing a guidewire, which has been preloaded into an endoscope, through the oropharyngeus and into the esophagus. This can be accomplished in several ways: The patient may be placed in the left lateral position and the guidewire introduced as one would introduce the endoscope, or, while the patient is sitting, he or she can assist in passing the wire by voluntarily swallowing to permit its passage into the esophagus. Once the wire has been advanced deeply into the esophagus or stomach, it can be used as the guide over which the endoscope can be advanced. If this technique should fail, I employ the tried and true technique of intubation to which we were accustomed using the rigid or semirigid endoscopes. In this situation, the patient's neck is hyperextended (similar to intubation using an endotracheal tube); the endoscope is advanced into the oropharynx; and, while the patient swallows, the endoscope is advanced gently. With these two techniques, I have been able to intubate every patient but one and complete the diagnostic procedure.

ENDOSCOPIC EXAMINATION

Esophagus

The newer endoscopes provide an adequate view of the lower two-thirds of the esophagus. Even with the lateral-viewing endoscope, the distal esophagus and gastroesophageal junction (Figs. 3.2, 3.3) can be appreciated. If the endoscopist angles the distal tip downward while the endoscope is in the esophagus, the lumen of the esophagus can be appreciated, especially as the instrument is inserted more deeply; I make a special effort to examine the distal esophagus, especially in patients with chronic liver disease or jaundice, to appreciate evidence of portal hypertension such as esophageal varices. Certainly, an adequate examination of the upper gastrointestinal tract can be carried out with the lateral-viewing instrument, but, if one is

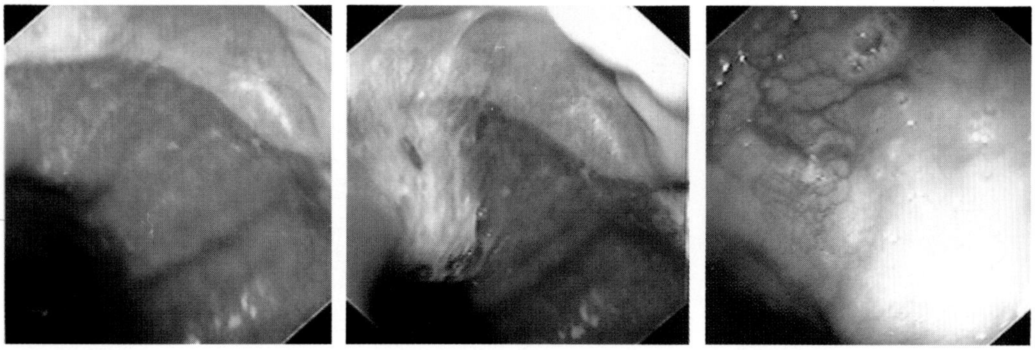

FIG. 3.2. Left: The mucosa of the distal esophagus. Note the normal vascular pattern provided by the high resolution of the videoduodenoscope. The "Z" line is appreciated. **Middle:** The gastroesophageal junction. Note the varix at 2:00. **Right:** 1+-2+ esophageal varices in this patient with primary sclerosing cholangitis.

using the standard, forward-viewing endoscope prior to the introduction of the cannulating endoscope, a more complete endoscopic examination can be performed before attempting an ERCP.

Stomach

After entering the stomach, the endoscope is directed toward the longitudinal axis of the stomach, which leads to the body and antrum. This position is facilitated by rotating the instrument slightly to the right by a torquing maneuver. Adequate views of the body and antrum of the stomach are achieved, and, if the endoscopist is so inclined, a complete examination can be conducted (Fig. 3.3). Usually, when the endoscope enters the body of the stomach, retained gastric secretions are encountered. I take this opportunity to aspirate these secretions, which will eliminate any possible interference during or after the procedure such as regurgitation or vomiting and aspiration.

If the endoscope is lined up in the longitudinal axis while in the stomach, the endoscopist can appreciate the wide angle of view provided by the instrument (Figs. 3.4–3.6). By deflecting the tip of the endoscope downward, the endoscopist can localize the pylorus, which is usually straight ahead, and, if the distal tip is deflected upward, he or she can easily retroflex the endoscope, which is visualized at the gastroesophageal junction. With this maneuver, an examination of the gastric fundus can be completed. Following the preceding orientation of the endoscope in the stomach will allow the endoscopist to feel secure about having performed a more than adequate gastroscopy.

Entering The Duodenum

After examining the stomach, the endoscopist advances the endoscope toward the pylorus. One appreciates the axial orientation of the pylorus to the gastroesophageal junction during retroflexion of the endoscope when deflecting the distal tip upward and downward, identifying both structures. Positioning the endoscope along the longitudinal axis allows entry into the duodenum through the pylorus. The endoscopist advances the endoscope up to the pylorus, which is

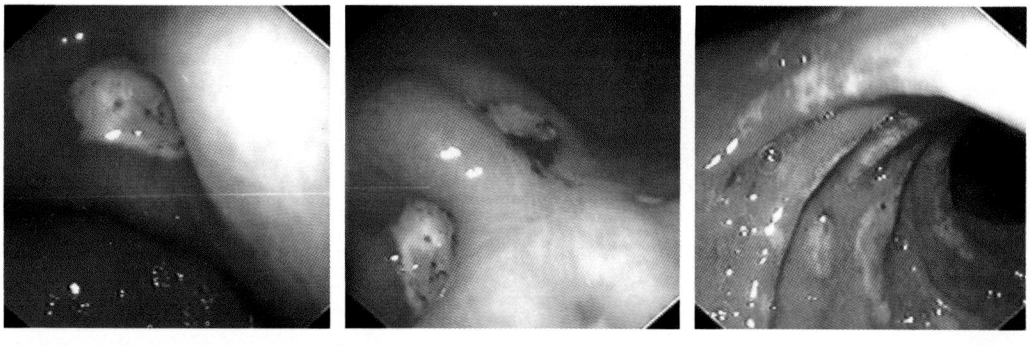

FIG. 3.3. Left: A gastric ulcer on the lesser curvature of the stomach visualized with a videoduodenoscope. **Center:** An index gastric ulcer. Several others are seen with the videoduodenoscope. **Right:** Several superficial ulcers are appreciated in the proximal duodenum in this patient presenting with obstructive jaundice.

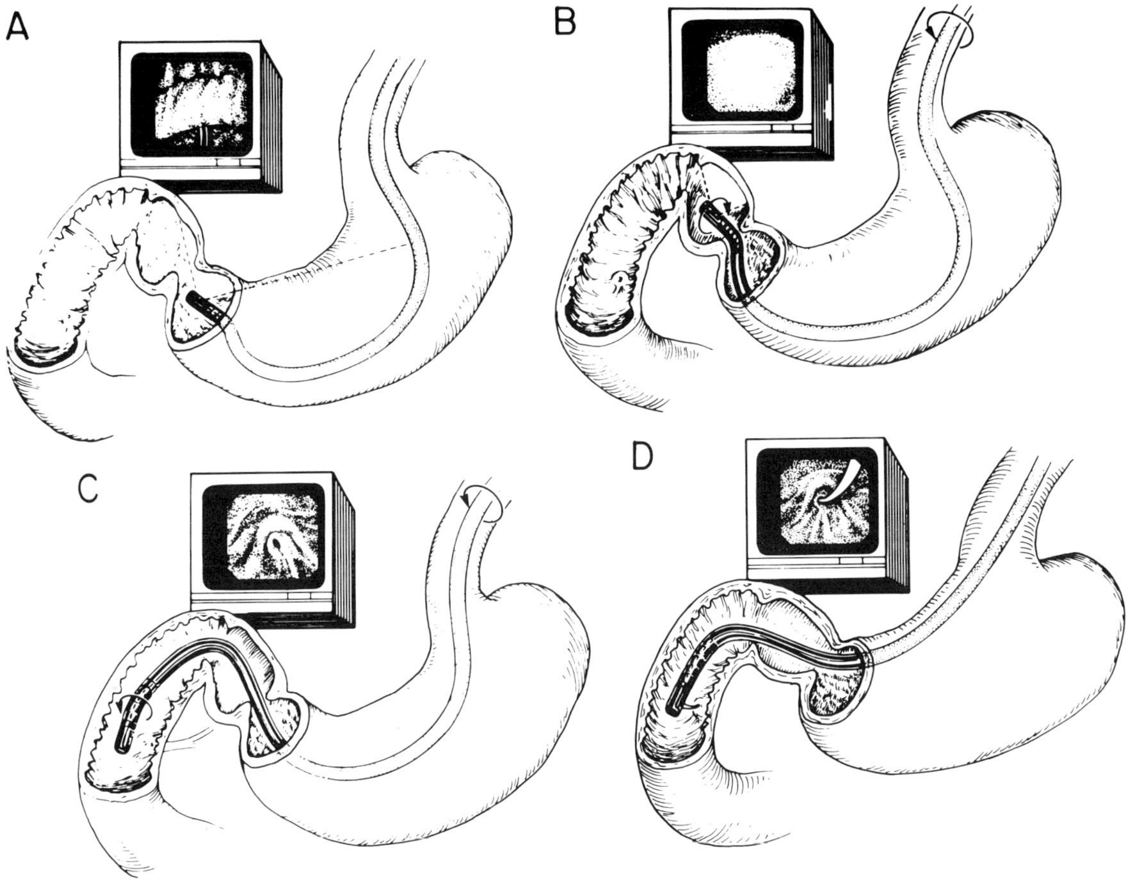

FIG. 3.4. A: The position of the duodenoscope in the gastric antrum approaching the pylorus. Because of the wide angle of view of the duodenoscope, the fundus of the stomach can be appreciated by flexing the distal tip; the pylorus can be seen by extending the distal tip. The TV monitor shows the radiating gastric folds of the angularis, and the insertion tube of the endoscope is seen. **B:** After negotiating the pylorus and bulb, the endoscope is turned clockwise. The videoimage is obscured at this point because of close mucosal contact with the lens system. **C:** The endoscope is turned in a clockwise fashion and advanced distally. The distal tip is turned right using the hand controls and is deflected downward and locked. The papilla is appreciated in this position and is seen enface on the video screen. The endoscope is in the long position. **D:** After the endoscopist pulls back and straightens the endoscope, the papilla is cannulated, as seen on the video screen.

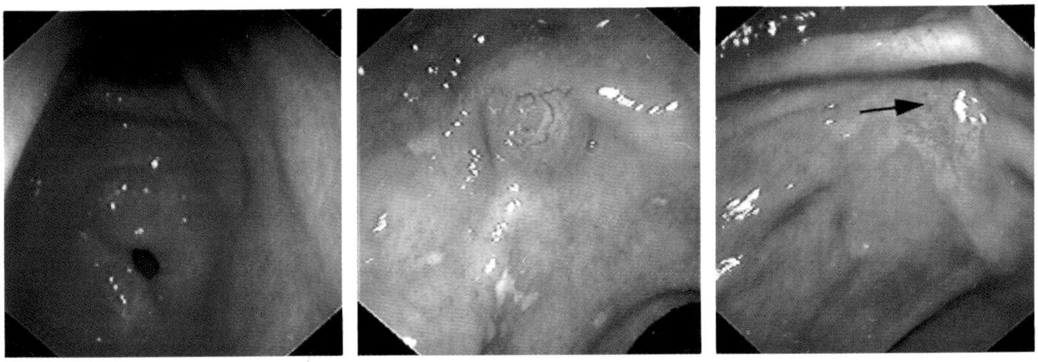

FIG. 3.5. Left: The pylorus is visualized by the videoendoscope. Note the wide angle of view as the fundus is visualized simultaneously. **Center:** After negotiating the pylorus, rotating the endoscope, and straightening it, the endoscopist places the papilla into the optimal cannulating position enface. The papilla is not always as obvious as in this case. Note the vascular pattern of this papilla. **Right:** This papilla is not obvious. Note the longitudinal fold leading to it, with the opening inferior to the horizontal fold (*arrow*).

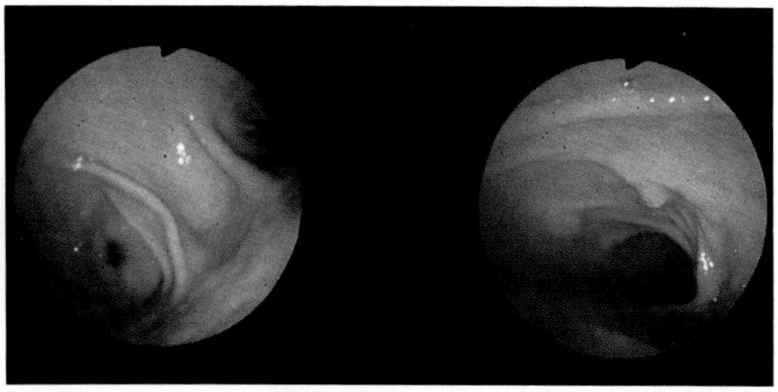

FIG. 3.6. Left: A fiberscope image of the pylorus and fundus, illustrating the wide angle of view. **Right:** A fiberscope image of the second portion of the duodenum. The minor papilla is in the foreground, and the major papilla is seen in the distance.

kept in view by deflecting the distal tip of the endoscope downward. As the pylorus becomes larger and closer to the endoscope, the distal tip of the endoscope is flexed upward or flexed into a neutral position in order to traverse the pylorus (Fig. 3.4). (If the distal tip of the endoscope is held in a downward, fixed, and flexed configuration, the endoscope cannot be advanced through the pylorus.) After deflecting the distal tip slightly upward or keeping it in neutral, however, the endoscope can be passed easily through the pylorus into the duodenal bulb.

Because a large loop is formed along the greater curvature of the stomach as the endoscope is advanced toward the pylorus, the endoscope may advance spontaneously into the duodenum after it traverses the pylorus because of the pressure created along the longitudinal axis of the endoscope. Therefore, after entering the duodenal bulb, I deflect the distal tip of the endoscope downward and to the right using the hand controls (Fig. 3.4). With this maneuver, the endoscope advances more deeply into the duodenum without requiring a push. The duodenum is located inferiorly and posteriorly in the abdomen. Therefore, deflecting the distal tip downward and to the right facilitates the passage of the endoscope into the second portion of the duodenum, which lies posteriorly. After deflecting the distal tip to the right, I lock this control. Usually, by this time, the major papilla has been visualized. With the right control locked and the endoscope tip deflected downward, keeping the papilla in view, I begin to withdraw or straighten the endoscope by pulling back while keeping the controls locked. The locked controls anchor the endoscope in the second portion of duodenum, and, while I straighten the instrument, the papilla is actually closer to the endoscope and enface. With the endoscope maximally straightened, it exits from the patient's mouth between 60 centimeters and 70 centimeters (Fig. 3.4).

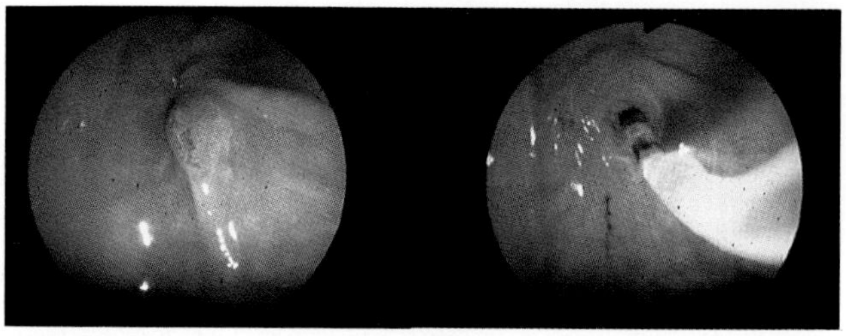

FIG. 3.7. Left: A fiberscope image of the papilla seen enface. **Right:** The cannula is being inserted into the papilla.

DUODENOSCOPY—CANNULATION

With the endoscope close to the papilla, manipulation of the cannula is minimal and accurate. In this position it is easier to control the cannula for fine tuning and selective cannulation. The papilla is examined carefully for the possible location of an orifice of a ductal system. In general, the pancreatic orifice is located centrally on the papilla and is more perpendicular in orientation, whereas the bile duct orifice is usually located near the top of the papilla at approximately 11:00 and is more parallel to the duodenal wall (Fig. 3.7). Selective cannulation of the bile duct is usually accomplished by extending the cannula upward (Fig. 3.8).

CANNULATING THE PANCREAS

If opacification of the pancreatic duct is desired, the cannula can be inserted into the middle of the papilla; if more than one of the marks on the cannula disappear into the orifice, an injection of contrast material should opacify the pancreatic duct system. Care is exercised regarding the pressure and volume of injection to avoid submucosal injection and edema. In order to confirm the presence of a stricture rather than assuming its presence, however, an adequate volume of contrast

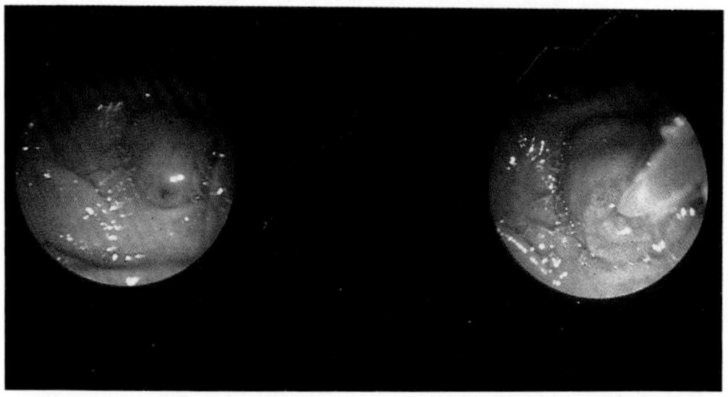

FIG. 3.8. Left: A fiberscope image of a prominent, bulging papilla. **Right:** The cannula is placed deeply into the papilla.

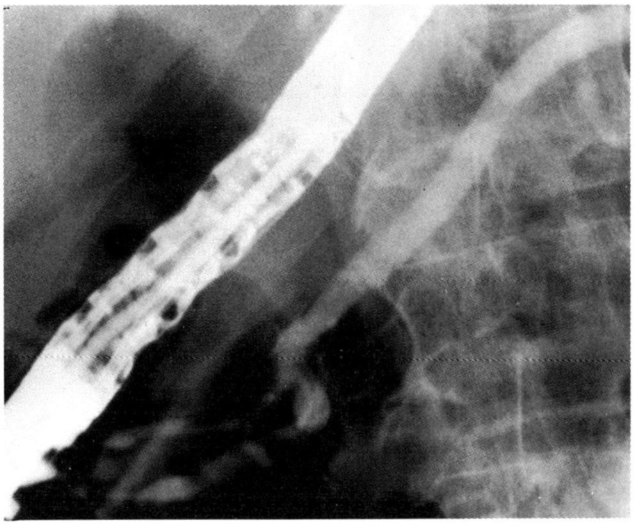

FIG. 3.9. There is evidence of pancreatitis on this pancreatogram, as confirmed by changes seen in the accessory duct. Dilatation of the main pancreatic duct is noted.

material should be injected to opacify the duct system completely (Fig. 3.9). Filling the main pancreatic duct to the tail is essential in ruling out intrinsic disease such as strictures and cysts (1–5). Overfilling the pancreatic duct can result in acinarization, such as extravasation of contrast into the parenchyma of the gland, which may increase the incidence of pancreatitis following ERCP. Also, overfilling the pancreatic duct results in absorption of contrast material, and one may appreciate a pyelogram if enough contrast is absorbed (Figs. 3.10, 3.11). Fortunately, the blood concentrations of meglumine diatrazoate do not approach those when contrast is injected intravenously, such as for intravenous pyelography, and, according to an earlier study (6), these levels are not significant enough to produce a sensitivity reaction. Because of this report, sensitivity to the contrast should not be considered an absolute contraindication to ERCP but, rather, a relative con-

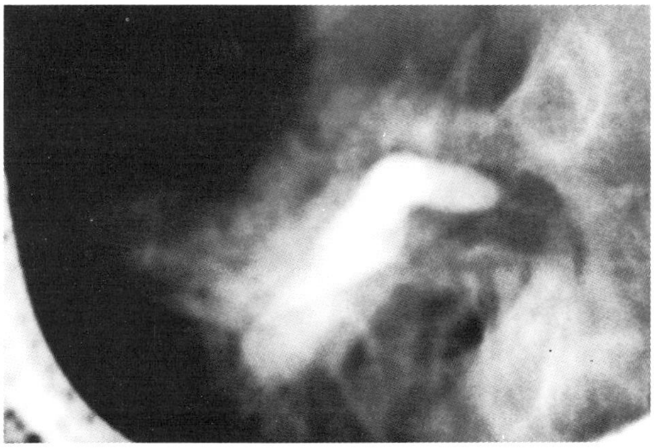

FIG. 3.10. This radiograph shows complete obstruction of the pancreatic duct proximal (toward tail) to the genu of the duct in a patient with a history of alcohol abuse and clinical features of chronic pancreatitis and/or neoplasm. Note extravasation of contrast into the head of the gland, resulting from obstruction to retrograde flow of contrast.

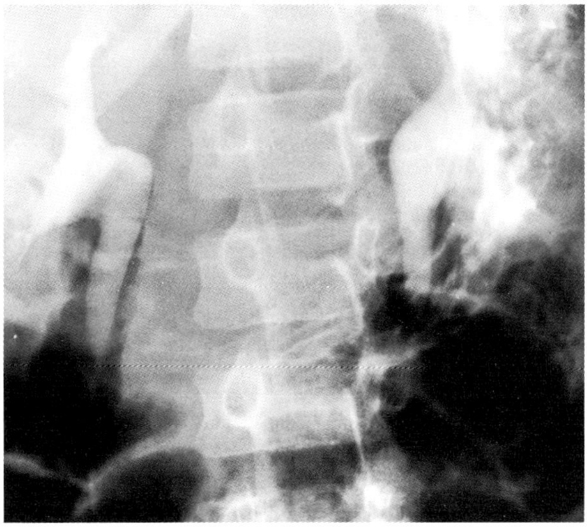

FIG. 3.11. This radiograph was taken after completing an ERCP and demonstrates a bilateral pyelogram resulting from overinjection of contrast medium into the pancreatic duct, resulting in absorption into the systemic circulation and clearance through the kidneys.

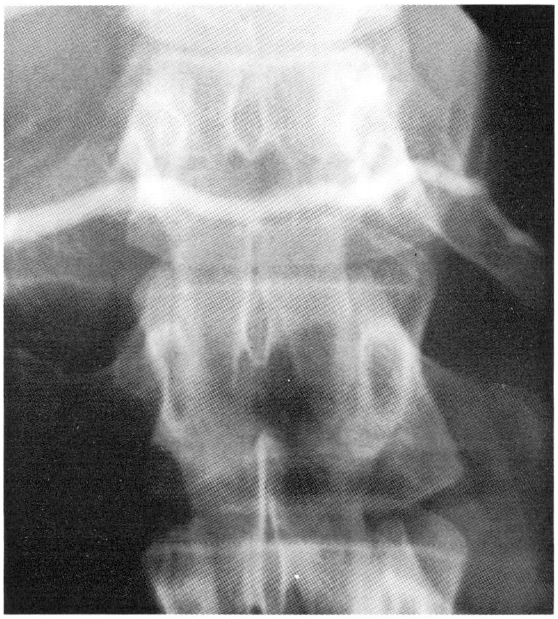

FIG. 3.12. Filling of the accessory and uncinate branches and secondary radicals in the head of the gland suggests resistance to retrograde flow of contrast. If corroborated with the clinical history and biochemical abnormalities, these findings are compatible with pancreatitis.

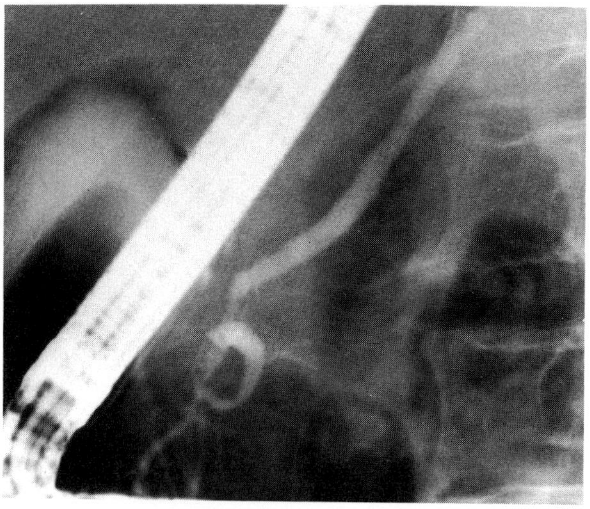

FIG. 3.13. A loop variation in the head of the pancreas with filling of the accessory and uncinate branches. Note narrowing proximal (toward tail) to the loop with resultant dilatation of the proximal duct. These findings support the clinical features of pancreatitis with partial obstruction secondary to a loop variation.

traindication. If one is concerned about contrast sensitivity, especially if the patient reports a severe reaction to intravenous contrast medium (iodine sensitivity), one may desensitize the patient or use Benadryl, 50 mg I.V., and Solu-Cortef, 100 mg I.V., before and after ERCP. Newer contrast compounds for intravenous administration are safer to use than *meglumine diatrazoate* but are not necessary for ERCP.

Filling of the accessory duct, uncinate radicals, and/or secondary radicals in the head of the gland before filling of the main pancreatic duct, body, and tail may represent confirmatory evidence of a partial obstruction or definite stricture (5,7) (Figs. 3.12, 3.13). Filling of secondary branches downstream occurs because a stricture prohibits retrograde flow of contrast through it, thus allowing filling of the systems with less resistance (i.e., accessory duct, uncinate radicals, and the secondary radicals of the main pancreatic duct). A stricture, or obstruction to retrograde flow, is thus confirmed if the secondary and tertiary radicals are opacified before filling of the duct in the body and tail is completed. Additionally, early filling of these minor structures occurs when the main pancreatic duct is obstructed by a stone or mucous plug (Fig. 3.14).

Once adequate radiographs of the pancreatic duct have been obtained, and if a cholangiogram is desired, the endoscopist must approach the papilla at a different angle in order to cannulate the bile duct selectively and to avoid overfilling or manipulation of the pancreatic duct, which may ultimately lead to pancreatitis.

CANNULATING THE BILE DUCT

As previously mentioned, the bile duct is usually located near the uppermost portion of the papilla between the 11:00 and 12:00 positions. The cannula should be directed underneath the papilla, parallel to the duodenal wall, in order to enter the bile duct. A septum may be present, separating the pancreatic duct and bile duct when they share a common channel. Lifting up on the cannula while gently advancing it may permit entry into the bile duct as the septum is negotiated. This approach should be tried several times at different angles before attempting to use other ac-

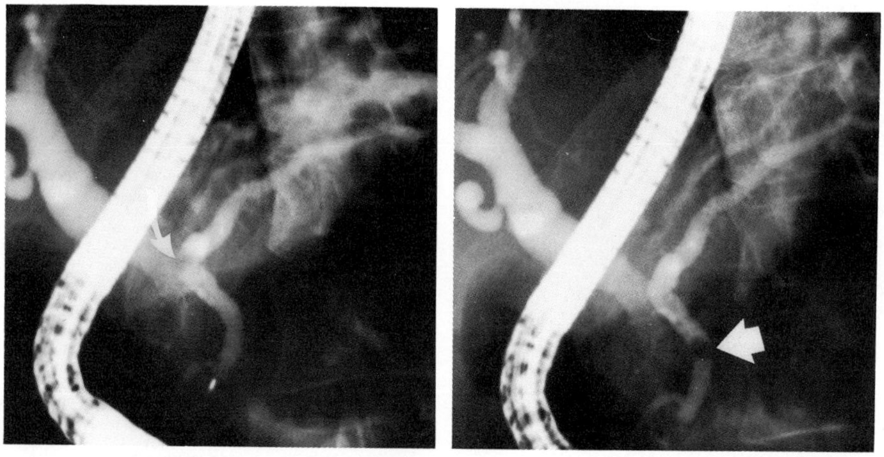

FIG. 3.14. Left: This ERCP shows a dilated pancreatic duct with parenchymal filling of the gland resulting from obstruction of the duct at the genu by a stone (*arrow*). **Right:** The stone is better seen (*arrow*) after it was moved by the injection of contrast.

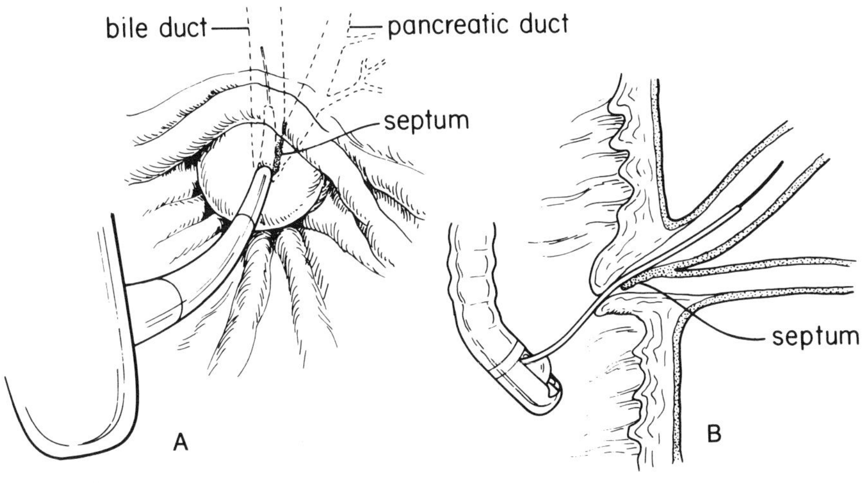

FIG. 3.15. A: Selective cannulation of the bile duct. The cannula contains a guidewire, which is directed superiorly on the papilla over the septum and into the bile duct. **B:** A side view of the papilla, illustrating the septum and the catheter with a guidewire entering the bile duct.

cessories to access the bile duct. Another technique for opacifying the bile duct is bowing or angulating the cannula after impacting it into the orifice. This maneuver places the cannula tip in a more optimal position for entry into the bile duct but, more specifically, allows for the passage or flow of contrast material into the duct to provide opacification. If the pancreatic duct predominates the channel and the bile duct arises proximally off this channel, cannulation of the bile duct may not be possible without using a guidewire or opening the ampulla with a sphincterotome (precut) (8–10) (Figs. 3.15, 3.16).

With these techniques, opacification of the bile duct may be possible, although selective deep insertion of the cannula is unlikely. Again, care should be taken in injecting contrast material to avoid a submucosal injection, which will obscure the papilla because of the associated swelling and edema. Use of a tapered catheter or needle catheter may permit opacification of the bile duct. Once again, however, there is an increased risk of producing a submucosal injection, subsequent edema, and an incomplete study (8).

Catheter Guidewire Technique

My next approach for selective cannulation, when other techniques have failed, is to employ the catheter-guidewire assembly technique that was described previously (Fig. 3.17) (8). With this technique, a 7 French Van Andel tapered-tip dilating catheter is preloaded with a 0.035″ flexible tip guidewire. This guidewire is the standard guidewire produced by Cook & Company and distributed by Wilson Cook, Inc. Microvasive, Inc., and Olympus Corporation also produce and distribute similar guidewires and catheter systems (Bilitrac 35, Microvasive, Inc). With the papilla enface, the catheter-guidewire assembly is introduced into the

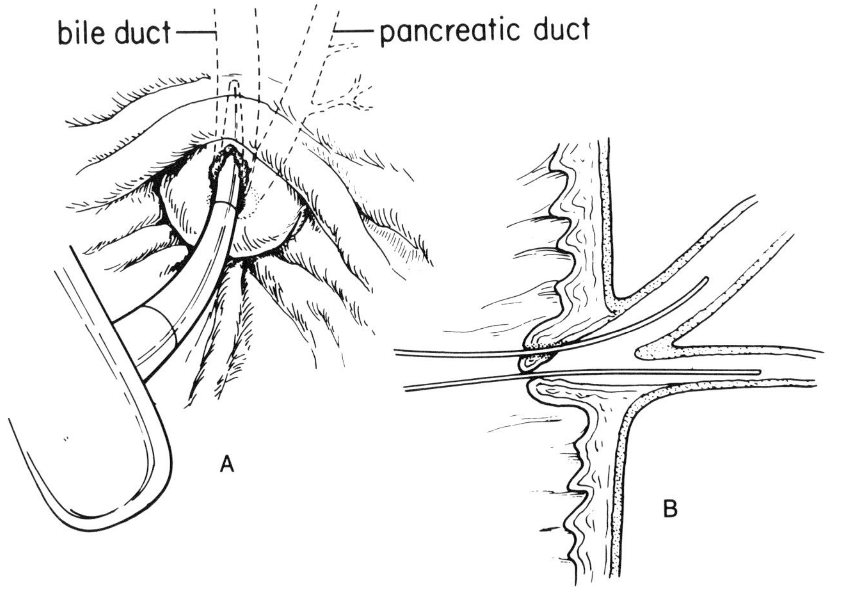

FIG. 3.16. A: A precut has been performed using a sphincterotome, which is placed high on the papilla to enter the bile duct selectively. The bile duct could not be cannulated selectively without a precut. **B:** This side view of the papilla shows how a precut incision will permit a guidewire to enter the bile duct. Without an incision, the wire goes directly into the pancreatic duct.

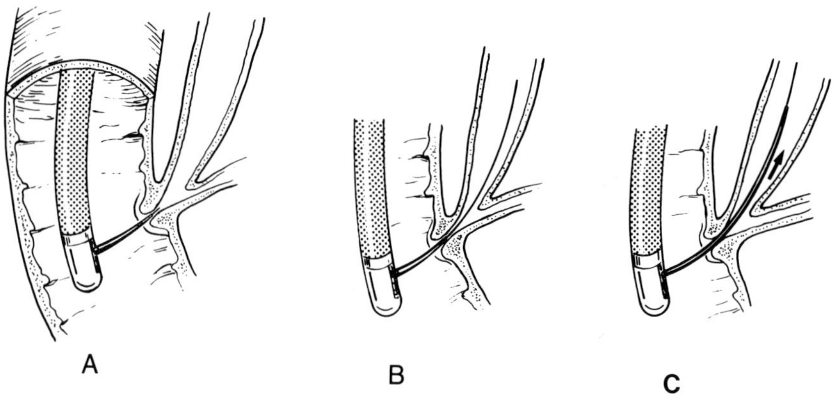

FIG. 3.17. This is a technique the author routinely uses for selectively cannulating the bile duct, which utilizes a 7 French Van Andel catheter and a 0.035″ guidewire. **A:** With the wire extending 2 mm to 3 mm from the tip of the catheter, the endoscopist probes the papilla. The assistant advances the guidewire while the endoscopist pushes the catheter. **B:** The guidewire has been advanced into the bile duct. **C:** The catheter is then advanced over the guidewire into the bile duct. (From ref. 8, with permission.)

11:00 position with the guidewire extending from the catheter approximately 2 mm. As the guidewire engages the tissue anchoring itself, the assistant gently attempts to advance the guidewire while the endoscopist holds the catheter firmly (Fig. 3.17A). If no orifice is entered and pressure is applied to the guidewire, the guidewire will push the catheter into the duodenum; at this point the endoscopist instructs the assistant to withdraw the wire unless the assistant sees this on the video monitor, if an electronic endoscope system is being used, and withdraws the wire automatically. After several attempts directed at the upper portion of the papilla at approximately the 11:00 position, the guidewire may enter the bile duct without resistance. Entry is appreciated immediately by the assistant, who reports that the guidewire is advancing freely, without resistance (Fig. 3.17B). At this point, the endoscopist refers to the fluoroscope while the assistant begins to advance the dilating catheter or cannula. The catheter can be easily advanced more deeply into the bile duct if the assistant applies gentle traction to the guidewire by holding the guidewire alone with tension and permitting a friction-free advance of the catheter (Fig. 3.17C). The guidewire is appreciated easily on the fluoroscope screen because of its opaque nature, and the direction of passage will be indicative of the duct system entered (e.g., vertical–bile duct: vertical short distance and then a 45° to 90° turn toward the spine–pancreatic duct).

The catheter-guidewire assembly can be primed with contrast material prior to its introduction by placing a special guidewire adaptor onto the luer-lock of the catheter (Fig. 3.18). This fitting is first attached to the catheter before introducing the guidewire, which is then manipulated by the assistant by holding onto the fitting. When contrast is injected through the special fitting, the fitting is tightened onto a gasket, preventing leakage of contrast during injection. Contrast is injected through the catheter-guidewire assembly, filling the desired duct. The reason for priming the catheter prior to insertion into the bile duct is to decrease the probability of air bubbles, which will produce a false positive study. Once the guidewire is set in place, the endoscopist can utilize the options provided by this accessory, such as advancing a dilating balloon or using a special double-lumen or wire-guided sphincterotome for performing a sphincterotomy.

Other Cannulating Techniques—Sphincterotome

Some endoscopists advocate using a standard sphincterotome for performance of cholangiography when other options have been exhausted because a sphincterotome can be flexed to provide more acute angulation to access entry into the bile duct. The sphincterotome can be introduced into the papillary orifice, flexed, and selectively introduced into the bile duct. Using a sphincterotome for cholangiography requires that the sphincterotome be deeply inserted into the bile duct beyond the most proximal insertion of the cutting wire because the cutting wire exits the cannula through an opening in the catheter; if this opening is not in the bile duct, contrast material will flow out of the hole into the duodenum and not fill the bile duct. If manipulation of the distal tip of the sphincterotome provides access into the bile duct, cholangiography can be accomplished, followed by a sphincterotomy, without exchanging accessories. In fact, some endoscopists, anticipating that a sphincterotomy will be performed, begin the procedure with a sphincterotome to save time and the extra step of using a cannula. This, of course, requires experience and the confidence that comes with experience.

Other, more invasive techniques for entering the bile duct, such as precut sphincterotomy and fistulotomy, will be discussed in Chapter 10.

In summary, experience is necessary in comfortably performing an adequate endoscopic examination of the stomach and duodenum using the lateral-viewing duo-

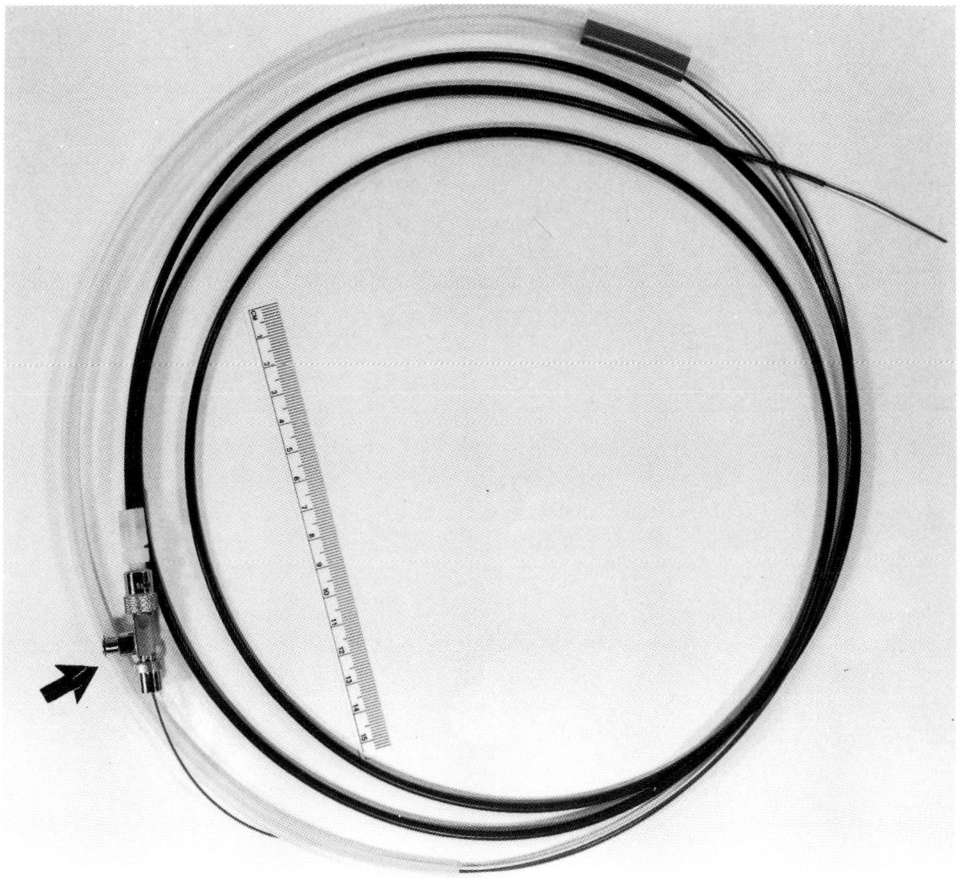

FIG. 3.18. An adapter (*arrow*) attached to a Van Andel dilating catheter, which allows the guidewire to pass through it. At the same time, contrast can be injected to prime the catheter, eliminating air from the catheter. A rubber gasket permits a tight fit around the guidewire to prevent leakage.

denoscope. Successful completion of an ERCP and opacification of both the biliary tree and the pancreatic duct (or, more specifically, the duct of intention) requires much more experience, probably between 300 and 500 examinations, before the endoscopist is comfortable with ERCP. More experience leads to better success in completing the diagnostic and therapeutic procedures. An endoscopist who has little experience but good eye-hand coordination and who has mastered some of the other therapeutic endoscopic procedures that require experience in manipulating accessories, such as PEG or polypectomy, should study with an ERCP expert or with someone who has vast experience with both diagnostic and therapeutic ERCP. The novice endoscopist should review the literature and study videotapes in great detail before embarking on therapeutic ERCP. Most endoscopists should have experience using electrocautery generators and should become familiar with the principles of electrocautery, eventually mastering these techniques. Not every endoscopist will succeed, however, and an endoscopist should not continue with ERCP if his or her success rate is less than 85% for selective cannulation. If the examination is not completed successfully in a reasonable time (45 minutes), and if the procedure is an ordeal for both the endoscopist and the patient, the endoscopist should not persevere but, for patient safety and cost effectiveness, refer the patient to someone who has greater experience and a proven record. An experienced endoscopist should know when to discontinue a procedure and when to stop pursuing an impossible task.

REFERENCES

1. Cotton PB. Cannulation of the papilla of Vater by endoscopy and retrograde cholangiopancreatography (ERCP). *Gut* 1972;13:1014–25.
2. Kasugai T, Kuno N, Kizu M, Kobayashi S, Hattori I. Endoscopic pancreatocholangiogram. *Gastroenterology* 1972;63:227–34.

3. Dickinson PB, Belsito AA, Cramer GG. Diagnostic value of endoscopic cholangiography. *JAMA* 1973;225:944–8.
4. Salmon PR. Endoscopic retrograde choledochopancreatography in the diagnosis of pancreatic disease. *Gut* 1975;16:653–63.
5. Siegel JH. Endoscopic retrograde cholangiopancreatography (ERCP): present position and papillotomy. *NY State J Med* 1978;78:583–91.
6. Sable RA, Rosenthal WS, Siegel JH, Ho R, Jankowski RH. Absorption of contrast medium during ERCP. *Dig Dis Sci* 1983;28:801–6.
7. Siegel JH. Endoscopy and papillotomy in diseases of the biliary tract and pancreas. *J Clin Gastenterol* 1980;2:337–47.
8. Siegel JH, Pullano W. Two new methods for selective bile duct cannulation and sphincterotomy. *Gastrointest Endosc* 1987;33:438–40.
9. Siegel JH. Precut papillotomy: a method to improve success of ERCP and papillotomy. *Endoscopy* 1980;12:130–3.
10. Siegel JH, Ben-Zvi JS, Pullano W. The needleknife: a valuable tool in diagnostic and therapeutic ERCP. *Gastrointest Endosc* 1989;35:499–503.

PART II

Diagnosis

CHAPTER 4

Radiologic Interpretation: Normal Biliary System and Variations; Normal Pancreatic Duct and Variations

Most gastroenterologists, surgeons, and endoscopists have become familiar with the normal anatomy of the biliary system owing to the many atlases and textbooks published in the radiologic, surgical, and endoscopic literature (1–3). It is not my intention to describe the embryology of the liver and bile ducts and their ultimate formation but to present radiographs and illustrations of the biliary tree that are considered normal or variations of normal and which demonstrate the diagnostic differences between the normal and the pathologic.

Attention is first directed to the extrahepatic biliary tree and its usual configuration and diameter because these ducts are initially filled on retrograde injection. The diameter of the bile duct in a person with an intact gallbladder, when measured at cholangiography, should not exceed 1 cm (Fig. 4.1). More often, it is approximately 5 mm to 8 mm in normal situations. This baseline diameter may be less when measured by ultrasound (US) and computerized tomography (CT) scan because, with these studies, no contrast is injected retrograde into the duct system to dilate it. Without exception, the diameter of the common bile duct or common hepatic duct should not exceed 1.3 cm after cholecystectomy (Fig. 4.2) (4,5). A wider bile duct connotes stenosis; obstruction; or a paraneoplastic state, a newly described entity (6). After cholecystectomy, the extrahepatic biliary tree may distend with pressure of injection during cholangiography (Fig. 4.3), allowing for the slightly wider duct in this situation when compared to less-invasive measurements provided by US and CT scans. This finding, wider bile duct, which is a false-positive finding, is attributed to the loss of the

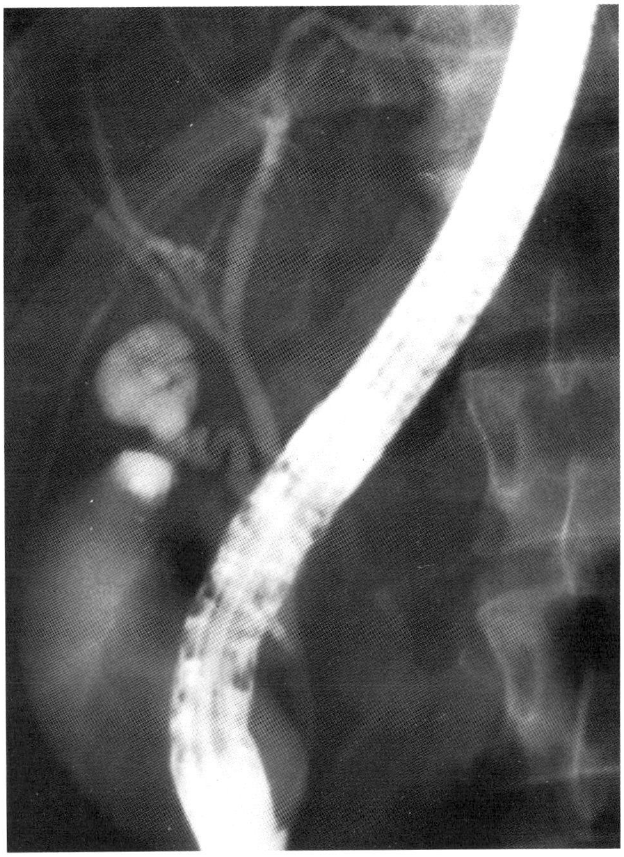

FIG. 4.1. Cholangiogram demonstrating filling of both the biliary and the pancreatic systems (pancreatic duct faintly opacified as contrast has drained from it). The gallbladder is completely filled, and most biliary radicals are filled. The bile duct is approximately 4 mm in diameter, and the biliary radicals arborize normally and extend to the periphery of the liver.

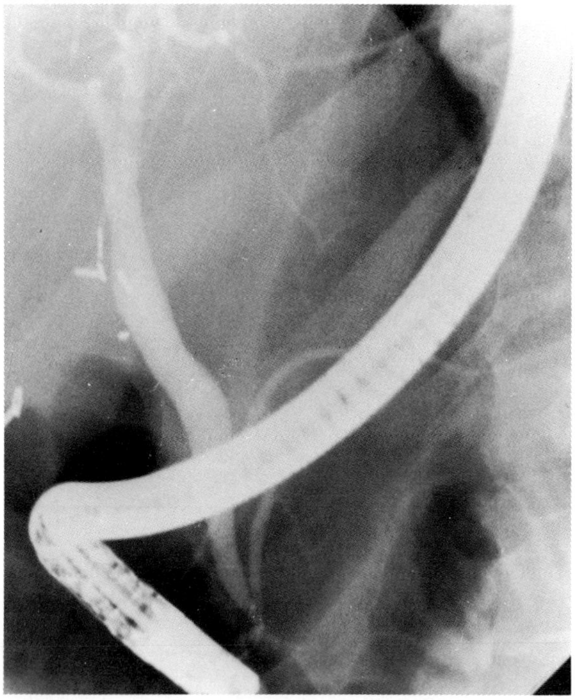

FIG. 4.2. Cholangiopancreatogram obtained in a patient post cholecystectomy (note surgical clips in the lower left quadrant). Without the presence of a gallbladder, complete filling of all biliary radicals is accomplished. Normal arborization of the biliary radicals extending to the periphery of the liver is present . The common bile duct measures 8 mm when distended with contrast. The pancreatic duct is normal in caliber, measuring 3 mm in head, 2 mm in neck, and 1 mm in body.

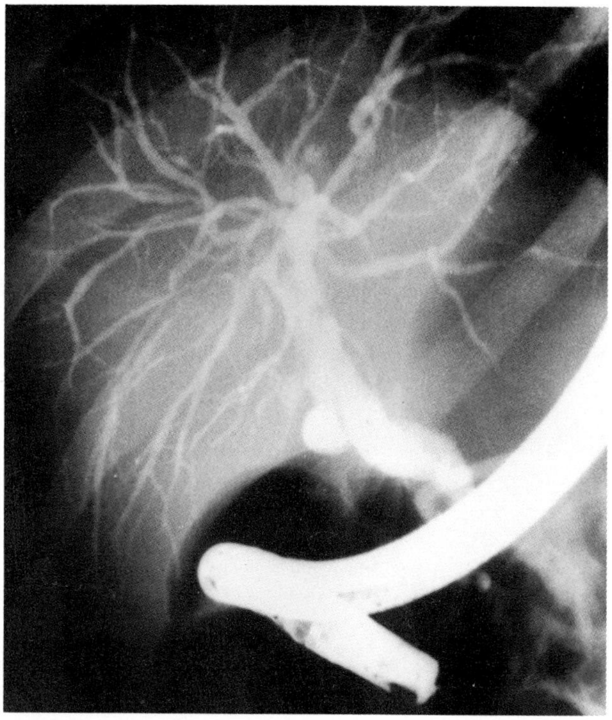

FIG. 4.3. Cholangiogram obtained in a patient post cholecystectomy. Note the distended biliary tree. The radials are completely filled to the periphery of the liver. The common bile duct is also distended, measuring approximately 9 mm (the endoscope, used for comparison, measures 11 mm).

gallbladder, which functions physiologically as a reservoir; the bile duct then compensates as a storage structure by distending to accommodate the volume of bile produced by the liver. Unless pathologic findings of strictures or stenoses affecting the extrahepatic system are present (stricture, stenosis, paraneoplastic), the preceding criteria will be used for normal (acceptable) diameters as baseline for interpretation of the appropriate radiographs throughout this book.

TABLE 4.1. *Causes of incomplete filling of the biliary tree*

Position of patient
Filling of gallbladder—cannula impacted in distal duct
Stricture common bile duct or common hepatic duct
Benign
Iatrogenic
Acquired
Malignant
Ligation of duct
Enteric-biliary anastamosis or fistula
Benign disease, intrahepatic
Fibrosis
Cirrhosis
Sclerosing cholangitis
Malignant disease, intrahepatic
Primary
Metastatic

RADIOLOGIC INTERPRETATION: BILIARY TREE

Filling of the right hepatic system may be delayed or incomplete because of the patient's position on the fluoroscopic table (left lateral recumbent), because filling of that system is affected by gravity. However, one must rule out true disease by completing the study, which is the object of the exercise, and opacifying the duct systems. Table 4.1 lists the true- and false-positive causes for failure to opacify the biliary tree, and Table 4.2 lists the methods to facilitate completion of the study. Usually, with the technique I employ (see Chapter 2), the patient's right side is slightly elevated off the table during the cannulation attempt. Therefore,

TABLE 4.2. *Methods to facilitate filling of biliary tree*

Rotate patient, inject
Insert cannula deeply into duct, inject
Insert balloon catheter, inflate, inject
Insert dilating catheter or cannula with guidewire, inject

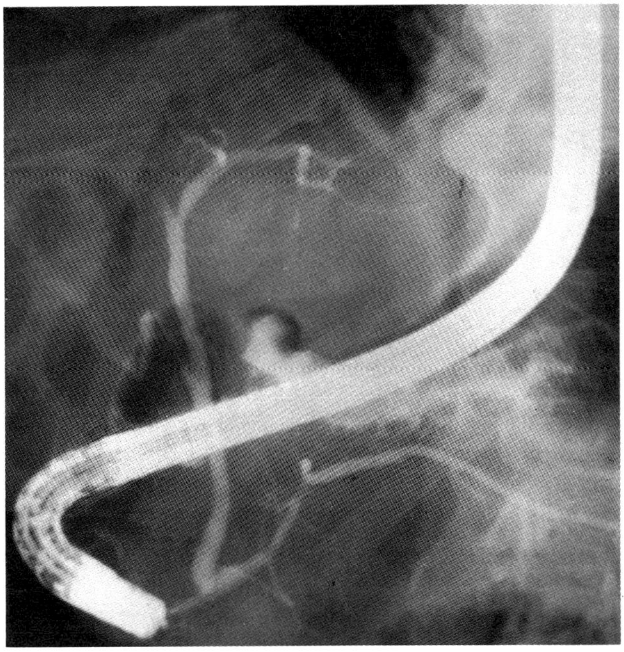

FIG. 4.4. Contrast has been injected into both the pancreas and the biliary tree. The pancreas is normal, with filling of the uncinate and secondary branches in the head. Note the small loop at the genu in the head and slight dilatation of the duct proximal to the loop. The duct measures 4 mm at the sphincter zone and head, 2 mm at the genu, and 3 mm in the proximal body. Filling of the left hepatic duct system is incomplete in this study, but no filling of the right hepatic duct is seen. Note filling of the cystic duct and flow of contrast toward the gallbladder, which is not shown on this view. Because of filling of the gallbladder, the biliary tree has not filled yet.

when contrast material is injected into the biliary tree, it will flow more readily into the left hepatic system, partially filling the right side or not filling it at all (Fig. 4.4) until a large volume of contrast is injected or the gallbladder is filled (see the following). This is a false-positive result and should not be considered abnormal or consistent with obstruction or intrahepatic disease unless the patient's position is altered, an adequate volume of contrast is injected, the gallbladder has completely filled, the cannula is advanced more deeply into the right system, or an occlusion balloon is being used and filling remains incomplete. It may be necessary to rotate the patient to a more prone position, a left oblique position or supine position, to facilitate filling of the right hepatic duct system. If a cannula, catheter, or occlusion balloon is selectively inserted into the unfilled duct and contrast is injected, filling usually occurs unless true obstruction is present (Fig. 4.5).

Incomplete filling of the biliary tree can result from early filling of the gallbladder, which delays filling of the tree. This scenario usually occurs when the cannula is impacted into the papilla or is not deeply inserted, allowing for filling of the less-resistant flow system, the gallbladder. If a proximal obstruction of the bile duct is present (proximal to the cystic duct) (Figs. 4.6, 4.7) and the cannula is not deeply inserted into the duct, the gallbladder will fill initially because it offers less resistance to retrograde flow. Again, if the cannula can be passed proximal to the cystic duct, intrahepatic filling will occur if the bile duct is not obstructed. If there is still no filling of the intrahepatic duct, a balloon

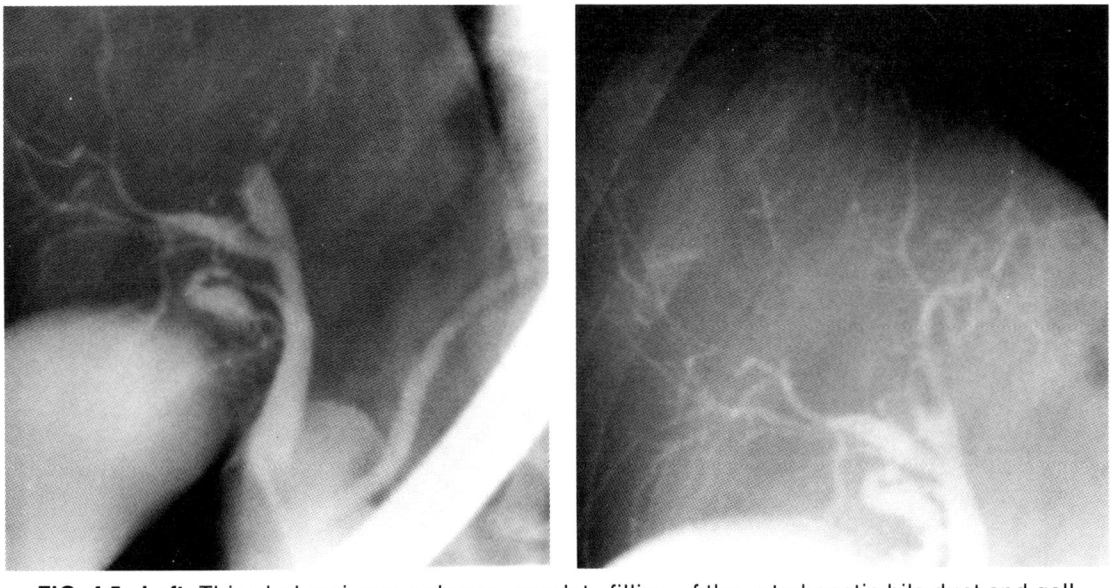

FIG. 4.5. Left: This cholangiogram shows complete filling of the extrahepatic bile duct and gallbladder and filling of the right hepatic duct. Incomplete filling of the left hepatic tree is noted. **Right:** After a catheter is passed deeply into the left hepatic duct, complete filling is accomplished. The patient has intrahepatic disease, fibrosis or cirrhosis, worse on the left, which resists retrograde filling until the catheter is inserted deeply into the duct.

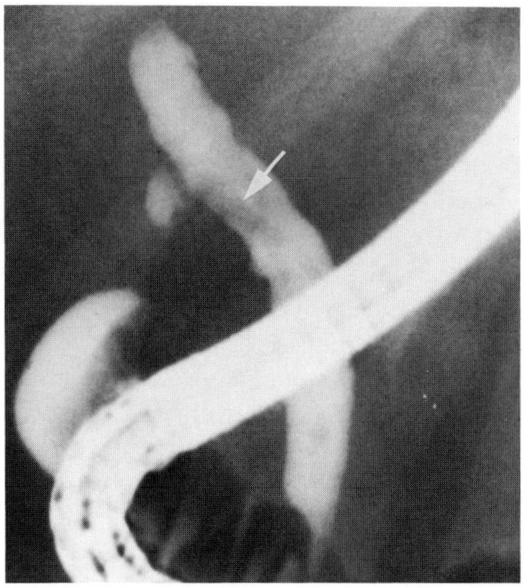

FIG. 4.6. Filling of the extrahepatic bile duct is accomplished in this study, but there is no filling of the proximal tree despite advancing the cannula deeply into the bile duct (*arrow*) and injecting contrast with pressure. The proximal bile duct tapers or narrows, suggesting a true obstruction. Entry into the proximal biliary tree can be facilitated by using a dilating catheter and guidewire, as explained in Fig. 3.15.

catheter can be advanced into the common hepatic duct, the balloon inflated, and contrast injected. With this maneuver, the biliary tree should opacify even with the presence of an obstructing stricture or an intrahepatic disease that offers high resistance, such as sclerosing cholangitis (Figs. 4.8, 4.9). If a cannula or balloon cannot be advanced deeply into the bile duct, one must continue to inject contrast with the cannula impacted in the ampulla or distal common bile duct and wait for the gallbladder to fill completely, allowing for spillover of contrast into the biliary tree. The intrahepatic ducts should then opacify if no true obstruction to retrograde flow is present. It is best to avoid overfilling the gallbladder because the patient may feel discomfort, but if the entire biliary tree is to be opacified, filling the gallbladder is necessary and should be accomplished as cautiously as possible.

On cholangiography, the intrahepatic ducts should look like branches of a tree, appearing tubular and distributed equally throughout the area of the liver (1). Morphologic changes in the intrahepatic ducts connote disease consistent with a pathologic process. These abnormalities will be discussed in Chapter 5. It is also important to observe the degree and extent of filling of the intrahepatic ducts. One should appreciate ductular structures extending to the periphery of the liver and, when this is not present, suspect an intrahepatic disease process such as primary biliary cirrhosis or other forms of cirrhosis or intrahepatic fibrosis (see Chapter 5). Although one should consider atresia of one or more intrahepatic ductular systems in the differential diagnosis of cholestasis, most of these abnormalities are encountered in childhood and are un-

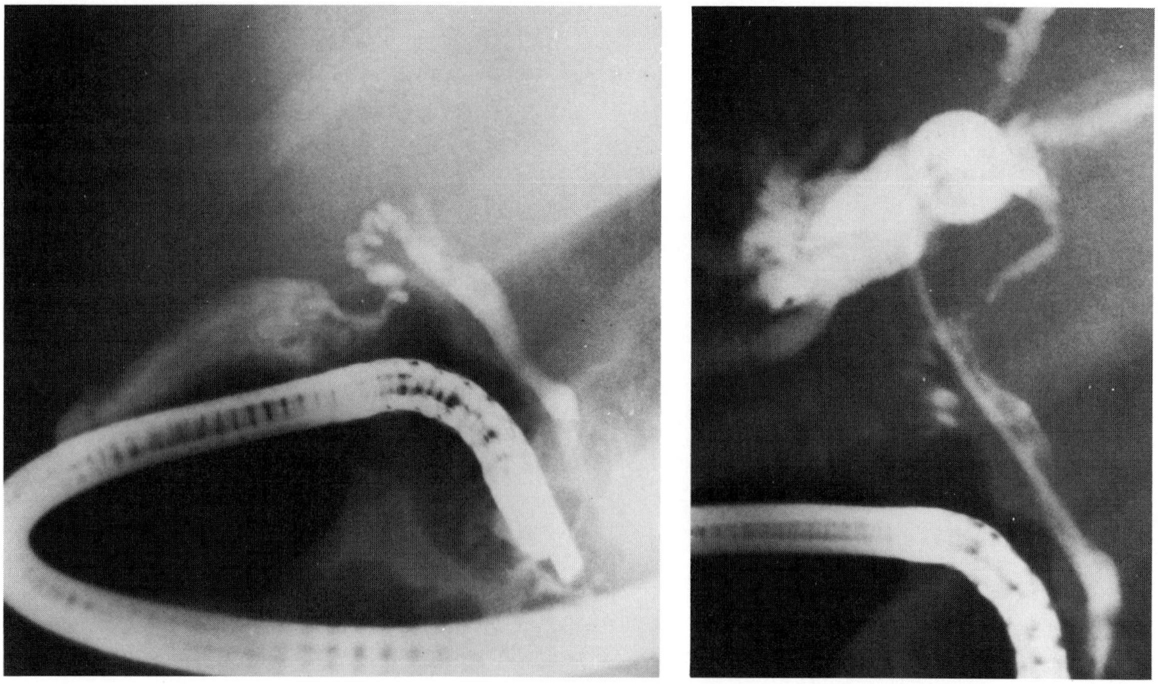

FIG. 4.7. Left: Filling of the common bile duct and gallbladder but no filling of the proximal biliary tree. **Right:** After a dilating catheter and guidewire are passed, a complete cholangiogram is obtained, demonstrating a high-grade stricture of the common hepatic duct with marked dilatation of the proximal biliary tree, suggesting a malignant obstruction.

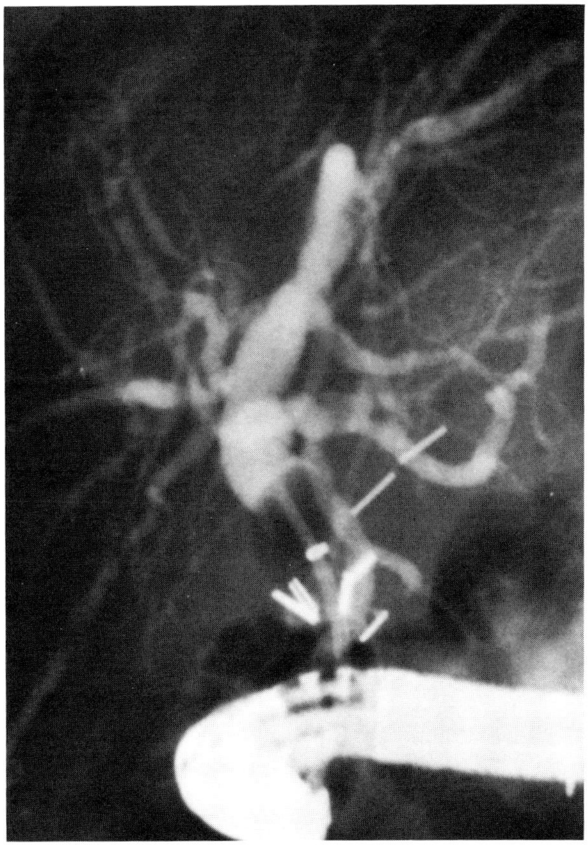

FIG. 4.8. This patient had previously undergone a choledochoduodenostomy, and because of this biliary-enteric anastamosis, contrast could not be injected into the biliary tree. A balloon was inserted and inflated and contrast injected, filling all the intrahepatic radicals.

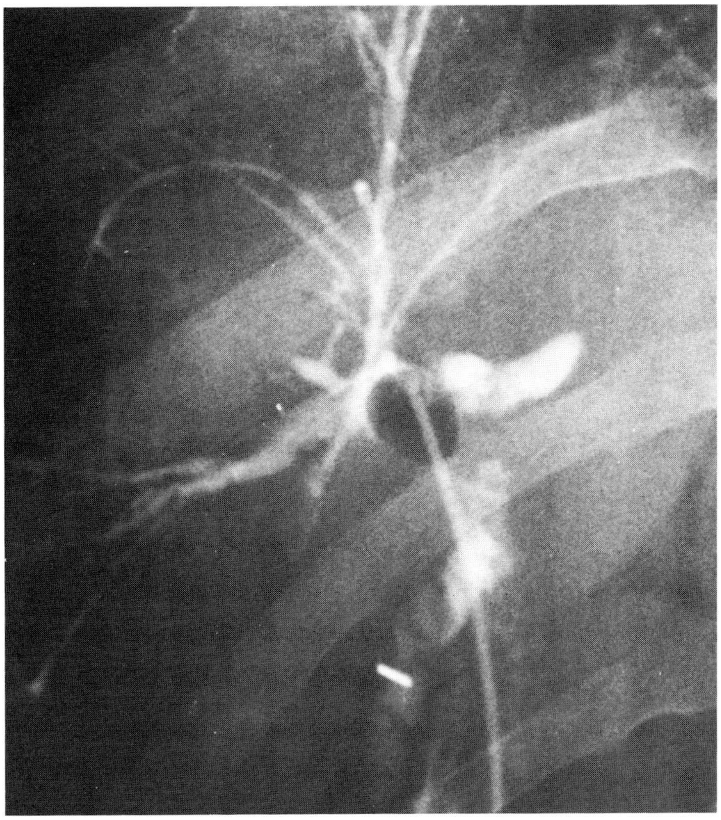

FIG. 4.9. This ERCP was performed in a patient with sclerosing cholangitis who had undergone a previous choledochojejunostomy. Complete filling of the biliary tree was accomplished after inserting a balloon catheter, inflating the balloon (large lucency at porta hepatis), and injecting contrast. Sclerosing cholangitis is evident.

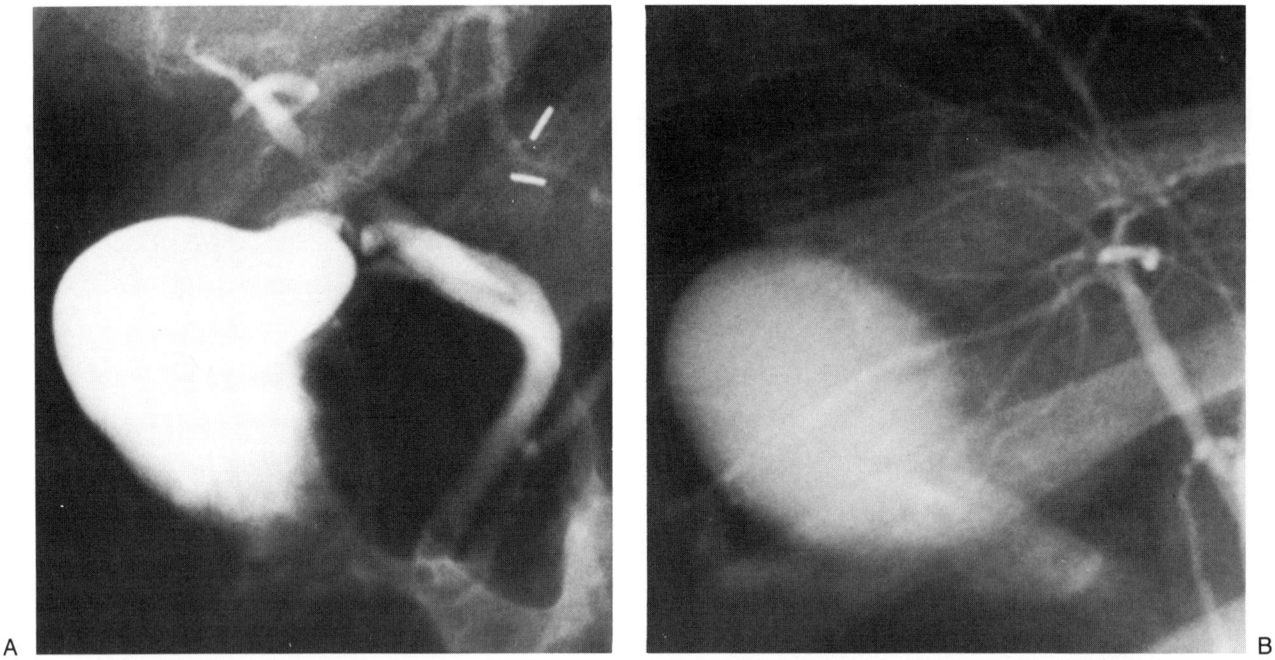

FIG. 4.10. A: This cholangiogram is complete and includes an opacified gallbladder. Dense opacification of the gallbladder may obscure small stones. **B:** This ERCP demonstrates an intrahepatic gallbladder. Note the location of the gallbladder within the parenchyma of the liver.

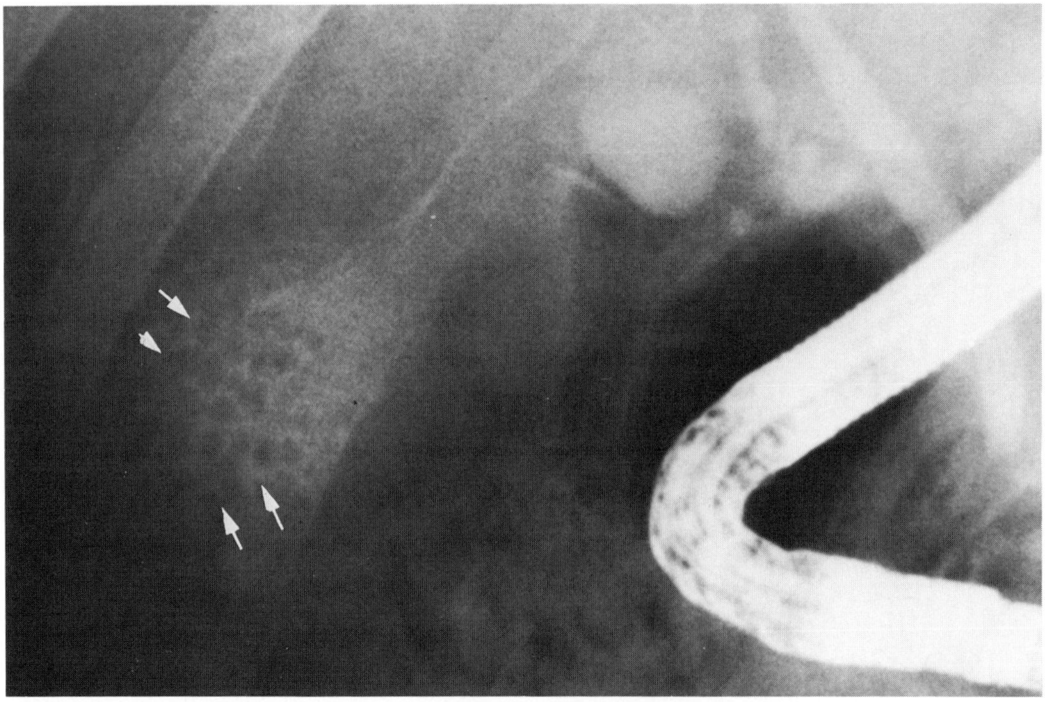

FIG. 4.11. This cholangiogram was performed using diluted, small-volume contrast injected into the gallbladder, which contains multiple small stones not previously seen on ultrasound (*arrows*).

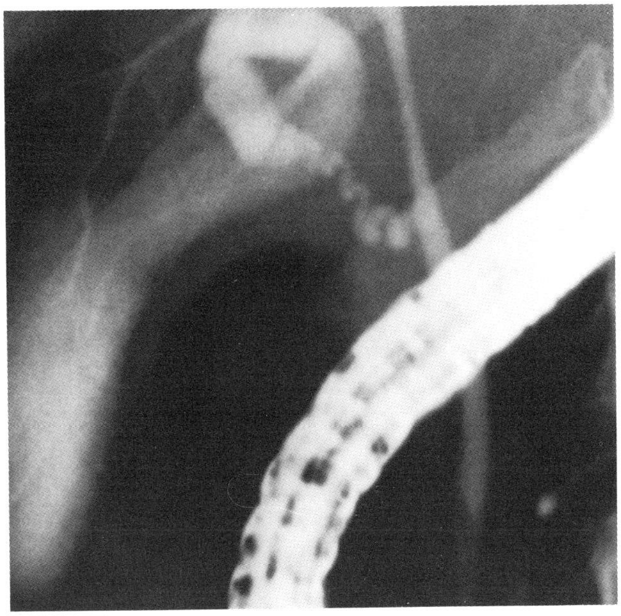

FIG. 4.12. An appropriately filled gallbladder.

common in adults (7,8). Therefore, when an adult presents with evidence of intrahepatic cholestasis or obstructive jaundice and cholangiography fails to opacify a ductular system, attempts should be made to selectively place a catheter or catheter guidewire assembly into the systems to determine a pathologic condition (for example, tumor or sclerosing cholangitis).

Variations of the normal ductular anatomy are appreciated clearly on cholangiography. These variations include cystic changes or webs, which are variations of the usual anatomy and are usually benign in nature but which may simulate an obstructive pattern. Chapters 5 and 6 describe in detail both intrahepatic and extrahepatic abnormalities encountered during cholangiography that are indicative of disease. Directed biopsies using US or CT scans are recommended to rule out the presence of a neoplasm if endoscopic brushings or biopsies are persistently negative (9–12). The ultimate determination of benignity may be laparotomy, but, to obviate unnecessary surgery for confirmation of a neoplasm or to obtain tissue, I frequently request laparoscopy before surgery in a search for evidence of malignant disease (13–15). This approach to staging is detailed in Chapter 12.

GALLBLADDER: NORMAL VARIATIONS AND DISEASE

The gallbladder is most frequently located to the right of the common bile duct in the gallbladder fossa inferior to the liver (Fig. 4.10A) (1,16,17). The exception to this location is the intrahepatic gallbladder, which is usually located within the liver, more superiorly, and in close proximity to the right hepatic duct system (Fig. 4.10B). Filling of the gallbladder should be controlled to appreciate pathologic findings: Too much contrast or contrast that is too concentrated (Fig. 4.10) will obscure findings. I routinely use 30% meglumine diatrazoate rather than 60% to obviate this problem and to provide optimal concentration. Figures 4.11 through 4.13 are examples of appropriate filling of the gallbladder, which allows for a better appreciation of filling defects as well as its mucosal appearance. Variations in the location of the gallbladder may occur as a result of congenital development and may appear as

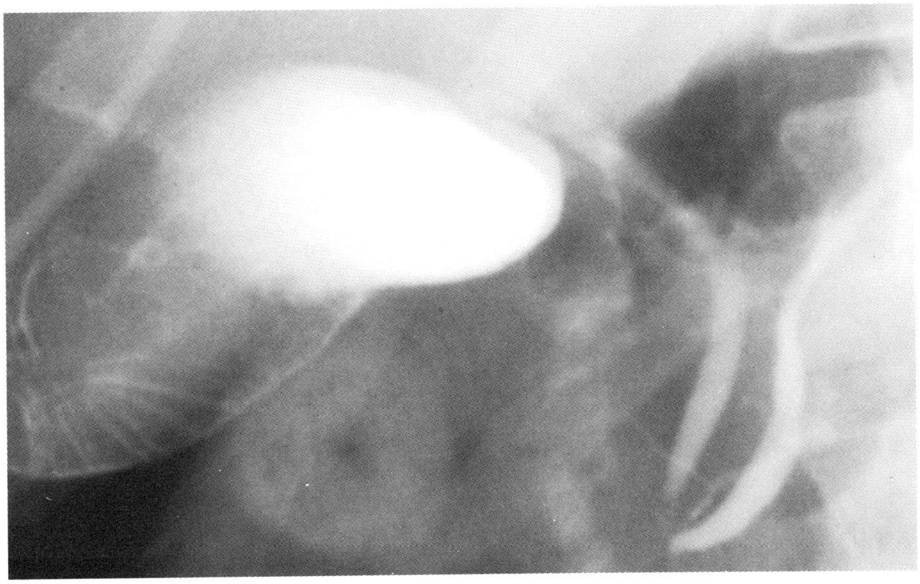

FIG. 4.13. Early filling of the gallbladder, demonstrating the mucosa of this organ.

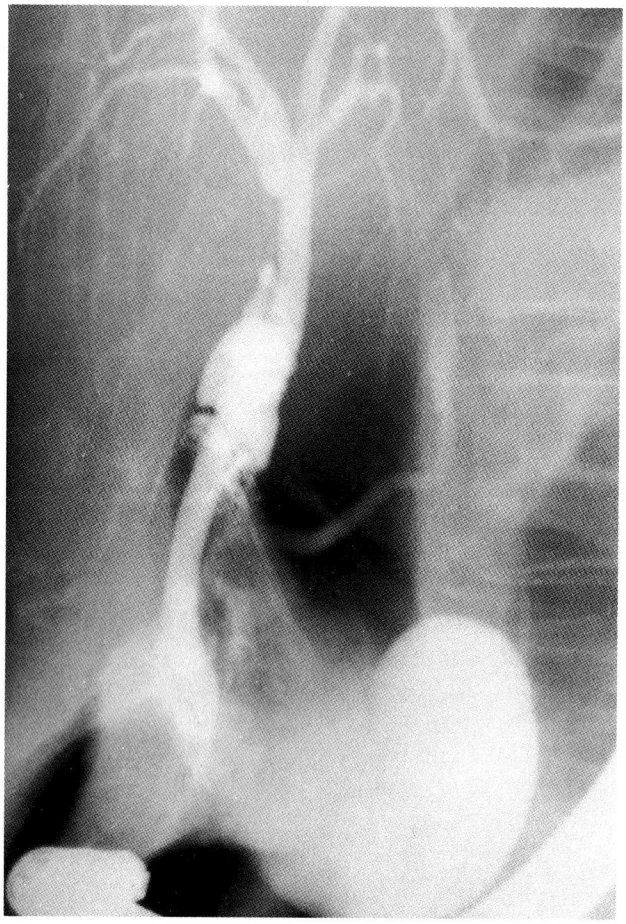

FIG. 4.14. A functional variation in which the cystic duct is wrapped around the common bile duct. The gallbladder is located medial to the bile duct, confirming partial situs inversus. A cystic duct enwrapping the bile duct may account for recurrent colicky pain. As the gallbladder contracts, the cystic duct may strangle the bile duct, producing colic.

CYSTIC DUCT: VARIATIONS AND DISEASE

The cystic duct is a tributary of the common bile duct. The takeoff of the cystic duct may vary among individuals, and the opening, or stoma, of this structure may be located anywhere from the papilla to the upper third of the common bile duct (Figs. 4.15, 4.16) (1). During retrograde cholangiography, the endoscopist can appreciate filling of the cystic duct and gallbladder and observe the retrograde filling of these structures by following the flow of contrast material during fluoroscopy. Appreciation of filling defects in either the cystic duct or gallbladder during the injection phase of the study establishes the diagnosis of cholelithiasis, which may not have been achieved by noninvasive studies such as oral cholecystogram, ultrasound, or CT scan (Fig. 4.17).

The cystic duct has many variations in its approximation to the bile duct and may, in fact, enwrap the common hepatic duct, which accounts for intermittent colicky symptoms usually occurring after eating (Fig. 4.18). During the dynamics of retrograde cholangiography, the endoscopist may appreciate these variations and enhance the study of the cystic duct by rotating the patient to provide adequate views of this structure. Four other variations of the gallbladder, including the *situs inversus* or *partial situs inversus* (Fig. 4.14) (18–20). Performing ERCP in a patient with situs inversus may present a particular challenge (21). In my limited experience with this situation, I found that placing the patient at the opposite end of the fluoroscopic table in the right lateral recumbent position with the left hip slightly elevated enabled me to intubate the patient and complete the procedure. Without prior information, a radiograph of a patient with situs inversus may be difficult to interpret. Unless the radiographs are properly oriented and labeled and an appropriate history and description are provided for the radiologist, this congenital variation is difficult to identify, especially in a patient with complete situs inversus.

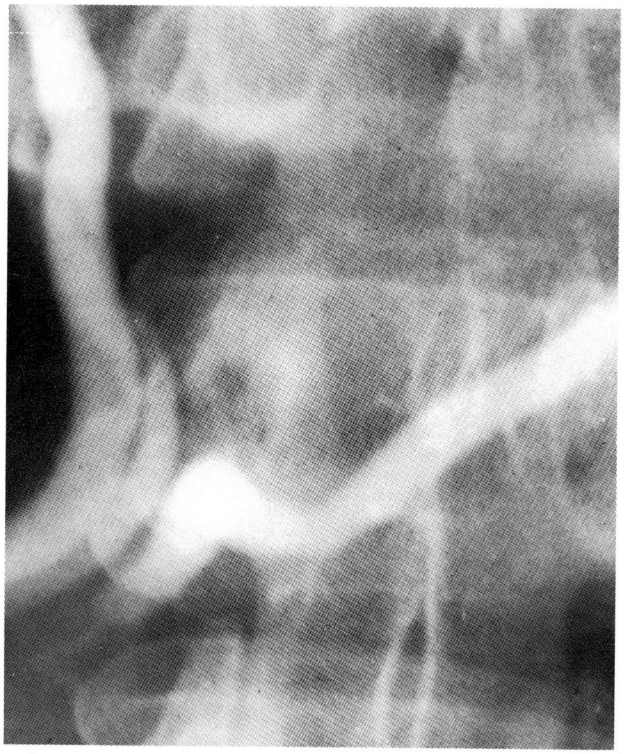

FIG. 4.15. This ERCP demonstrates 3 ductular structures arising from the ampulla. The duct to the left is the bile duct, the middle one is the cystic duct, and the duct to the right is the pancreatic duct.

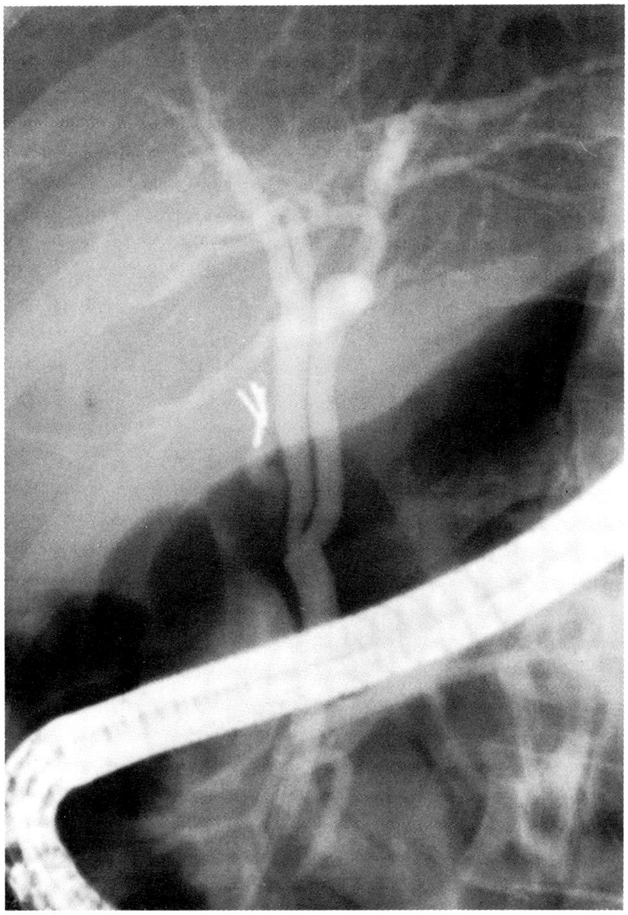

FIG. 4.16. This ERCP demonstrates an interesting variant of the bile duct. Note the short common bile duct, low bifurcation of the right and left ducts, and the cystic duct remnant arising at the bifurcation. *This variation could contribute to bile duct injury at cholecystectomy* because the right hepatic duct may be inadvertently ligated as the cystic duct. Fortunately, a misadventure did not occur in this case; the cystic duct stump was appropriately ligated, and the clips were applied in the correct position.

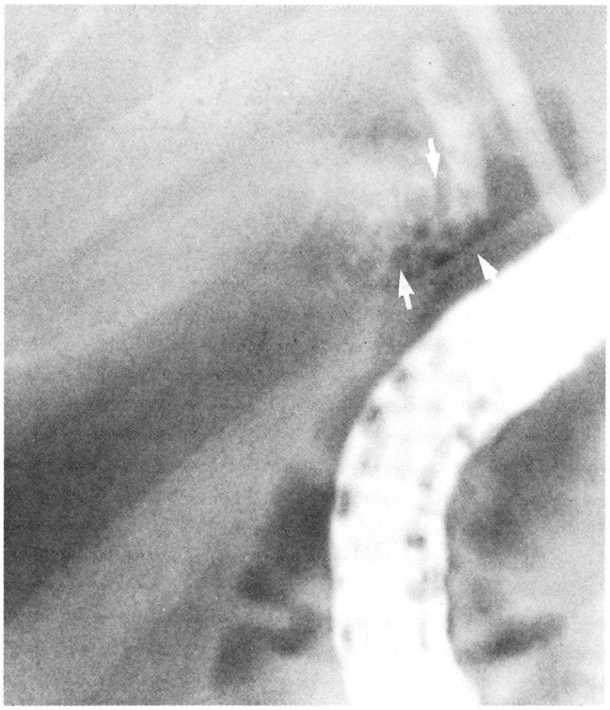

FIG. 4.17. This ERCP-cholecystogram demonstrates lucent filling defects in the cystic duct and neck of the gallbladder, which were not appreciated on other studies (*arrows*).

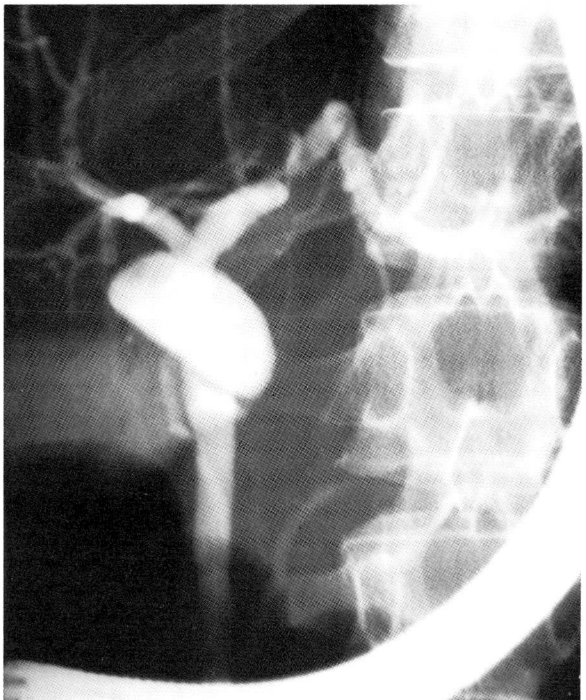

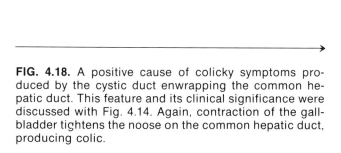

FIG. 4.18. A positive cause of colicky symptoms produced by the cystic duct enwrapping the common hepatic duct. This feature and its clinical significance were discussed with Fig. 4.14. Again, contraction of the gallbladder tightens the noose on the common hepatic duct, producing colic.

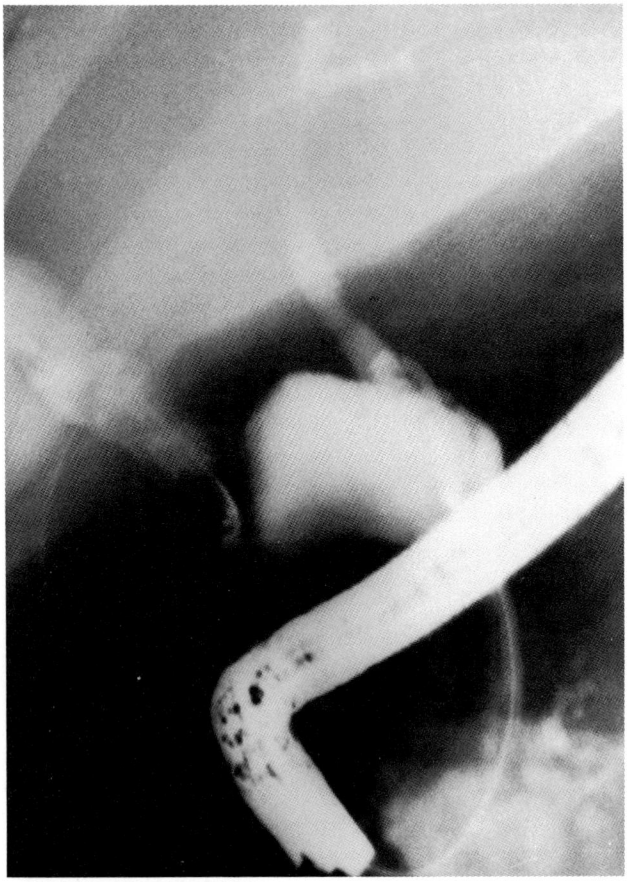

FIG. 4.19. Segmentation of the gallbladder is noted on this ERCP-cholecystogram. Note the dilated neck, narrowing of the body, and normal apex and fundus. This finding may contribute to dysfunction of the gallbladder and associated symptoms.

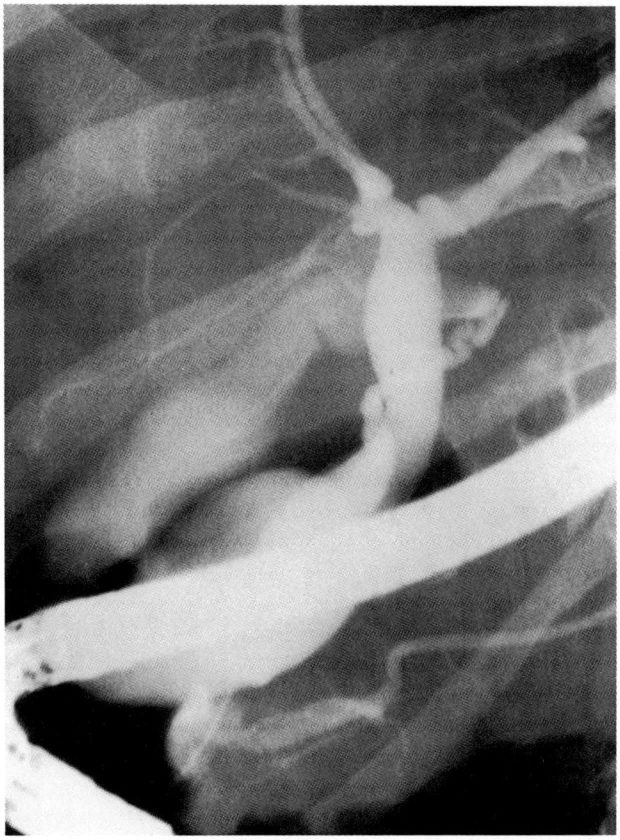

FIG. 4.20. A double gallbladder. Note the existence of two cystic ducts and two gallbladders.

phrygian cap (22) and duplication of the gallbladder (23,24), are shown in Figs. 4.19 through 4.22. These examples are unusual in their occurrence and were not anticipated because ultrasonography and CT scans were negative by interpretation. Although these illustrations demonstrate normal variants of the anatomy, these benign variations may account for alterations of the normal physiologic mechanism of gallbladder emptying, as described many years ago, and may be responsible for the presenting symptoms (25–27).

BILE DUCT AND AMPULLARY VARIATIONS

Appreciation of the papilla and ampullary region on retrograde filling is very important in understanding the physiology and function of these structures and may account for previously unexplained symptoms (28). During fluoroscopy the dynamic physiologic function of the sphincter mechanism is evident (Figs. 4.23, 4.24) (29). Also, one must pay close attention to the radiographs that demonstrate the *dividing septum,*

FIG. 4.22. Left: A large, segmented gallbladder containing multiple stones. Note the normal caliber of the bile duct and pancreas. **Right:** Repositioning the patient allows for more complete filling of the gallbladder. Note that the gallbladder is so large that it overlies the pelvic rim. These findings were not appreciated on CT scan or sonography.

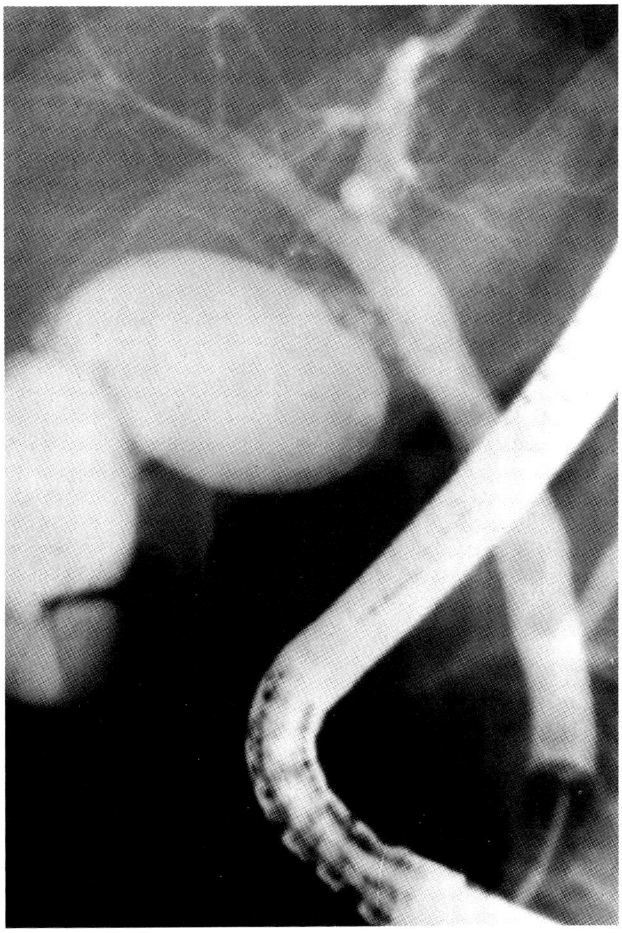

FIG. 4.21. This large, segmented gallbladder illustrates a phrygian cap. Note the occlusion balloon in the distal common bile duct, which allows for complete filling of the biliary tree and gallbladder.

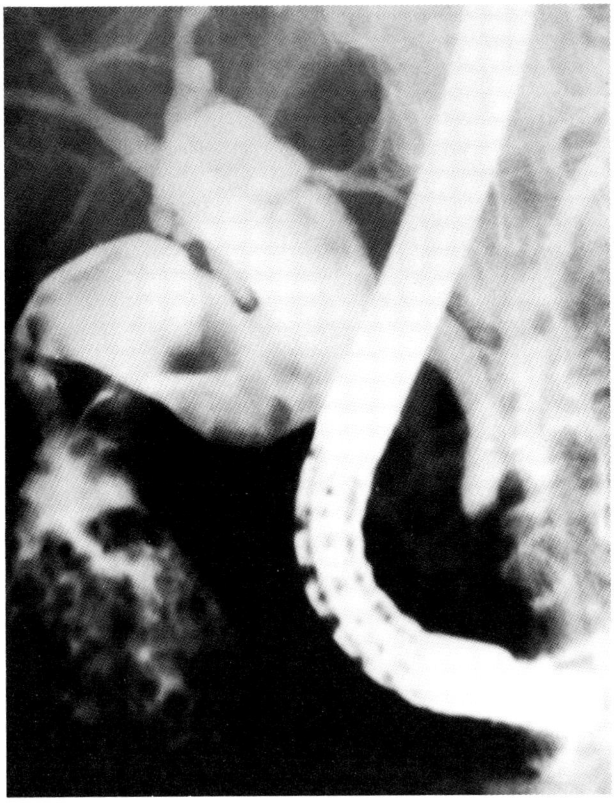

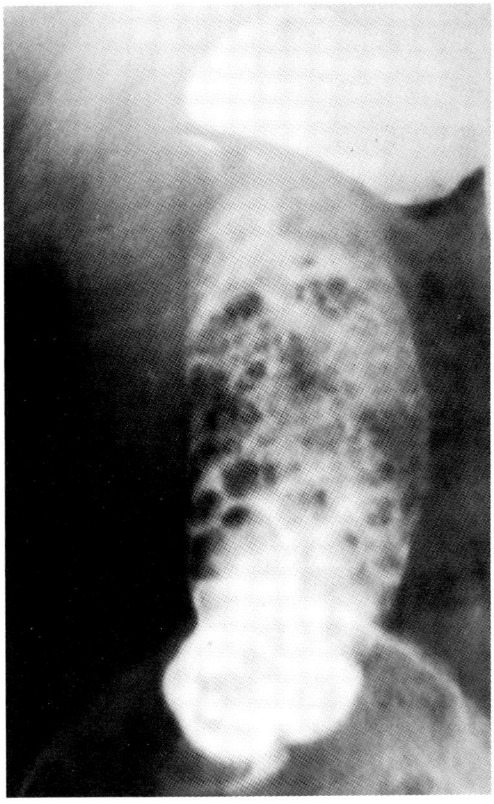

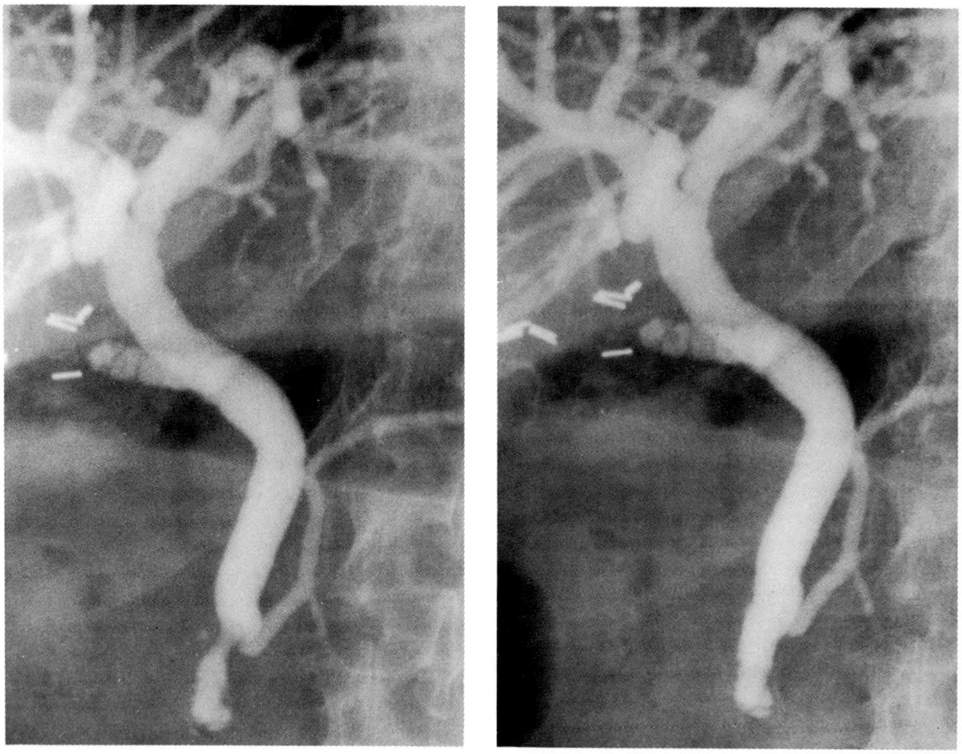

FIG. 4.23. Left: This ERCP was obtained in a patient with recurrent pain after cholecystectomy. Note the active contraction of the sphincter. No contrast is seen in the duodenum. **Right:** Despite sphincter relaxation, no contrast entered the duodenum. Further evaluation, including sphincter of Oddi manometry, was recommended in this case.

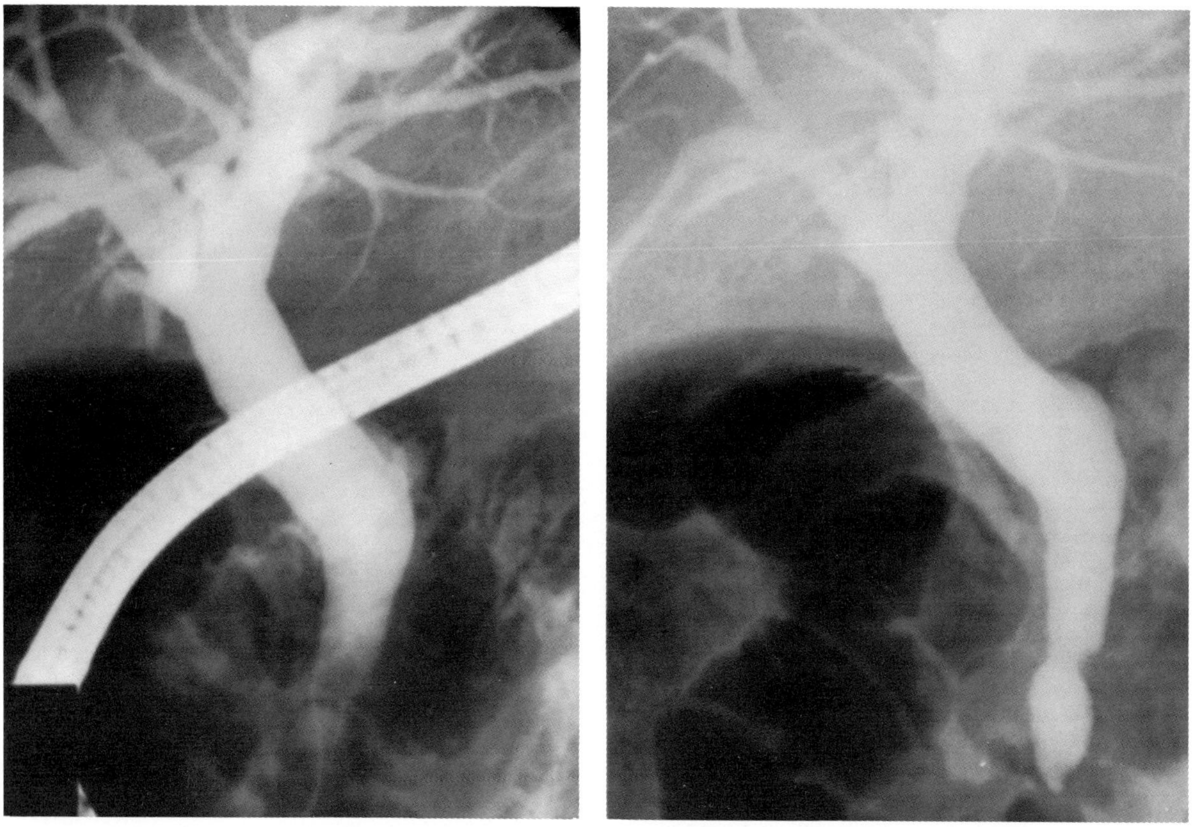

FIG. 4.24. Sphincter of Oddi spasm or dysfunction.

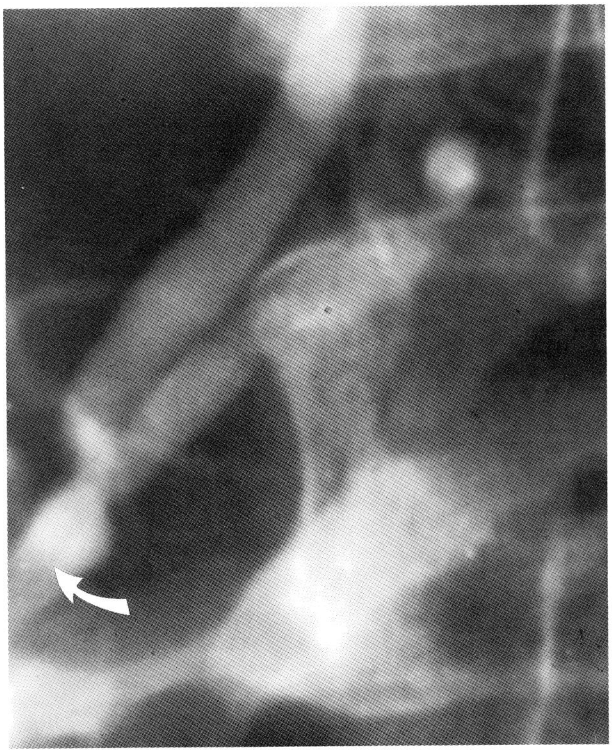

FIG. 4.25. A long common channel. Note the fine lucent line (*arrow*) in the ampulla or channel, which represents the septum.

which clearly illustrates the division of the bile duct and pancreatic duct (Fig. 4.25). Confirmation of the separation seen on radiographs provides evidence of separate openings to the duct systems (30) and accounts for the difficulty in selectively cannulating the bile duct, a potential problem in performing ERCP for the expert as well as the novice (Fig. 4.26).

Other interesting variants of the bile duct may be seen on cholangiography and should be recognized by the endoscopist. These variants may account for dysfunction of normal physiologic mechanisms and contribute to symptoms. *Webs* of the bile duct (Figs. 4.27, 4.28) may be responsible for obstructive symptoms such as cramping or colic. Treatment may include bal-

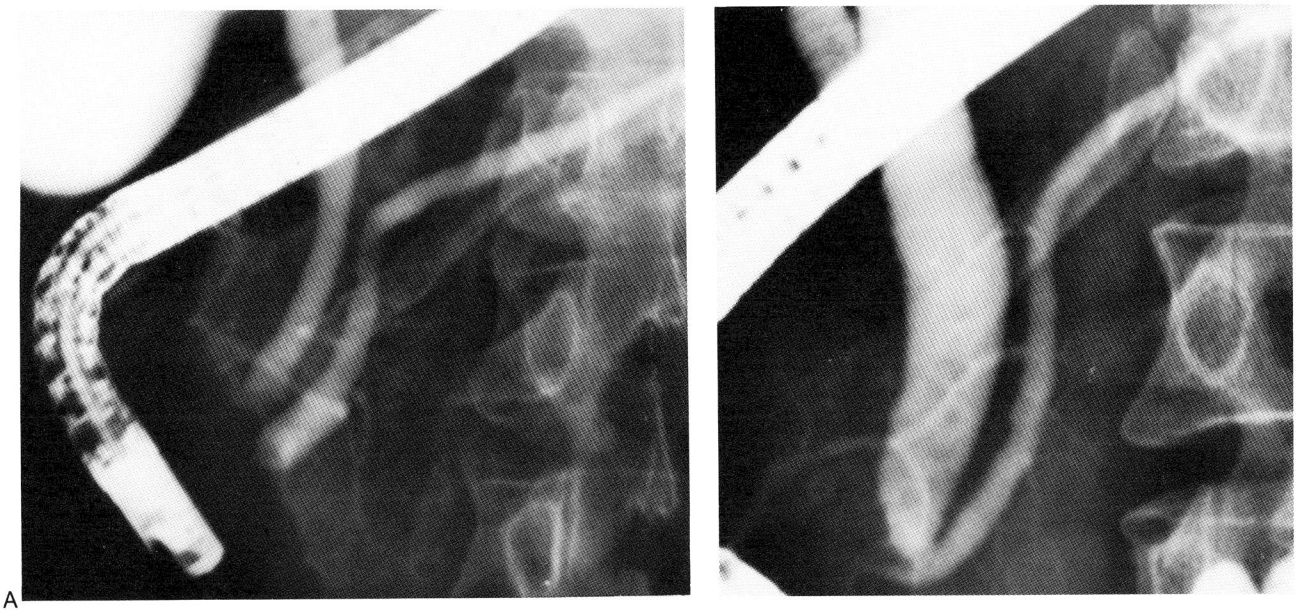

A B

FIG. 4.26. **A:** This ERCP shows separate entry of the bile duct and the pancreatic duct into the duodenum. **B:** A common channel into which both ducts enter. In this case, the bile duct enters the ampulla through the pancreatic duct. Selective entry into the bile duct may be difficult because of the acute angle of takeoff.

A 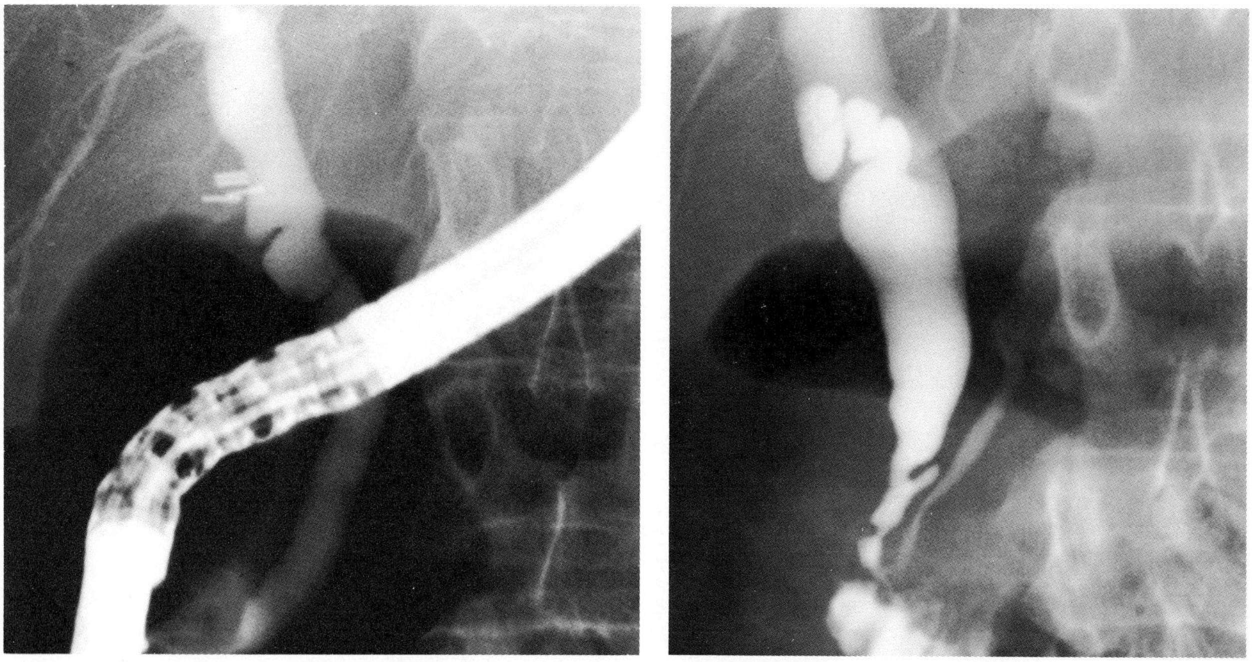 B

FIG. 4.27. A: This patient is status post cholecystectomy with 2 *webs* or *rings* noted distal to the surgical clips. **B:** A web in the distal common bile duct with a dilated proximal bile duct seen proximal to it.

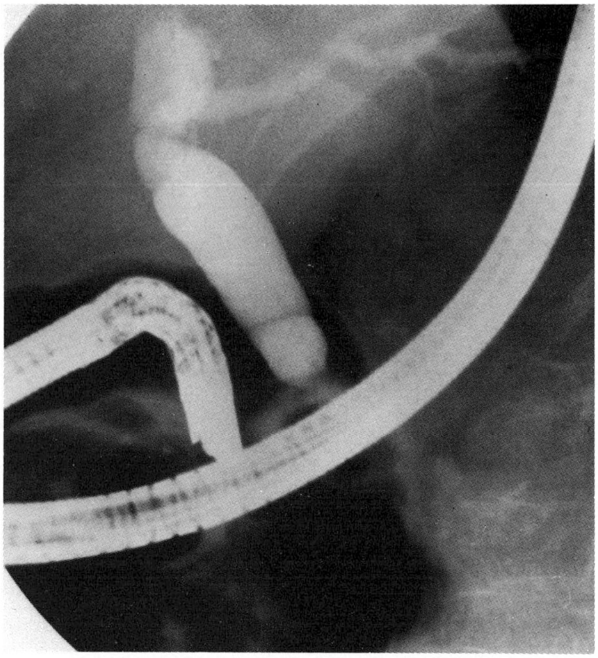

FIG. 4.28. A web in the distal portion of the dilated bile duct. It was assumed that the patient had dysfunction of the sphincter and that the web may have contributed to the symptoms. Sphincter of Oddi manometry should be performed before sphincterotomy, unless the patient has cholestatic liver tests.

loon dilatation, which is analagous to the treatment of esophageal webs, and surgical bypass. A causal relationship of symptoms should certainly be proved before undertaking aggressive treatment. *Choledochal cysts,* or true cysts of the bile duct, may account for jaundice owing to mechanical obstruction by the cyst or stones and by debris or a neoplasm (Fig. 4.29). These cysts are usually found early in life because of symptoms, and most experts advise total excision because of the high incidence of neoplasia (31–33). Figure 4.30 demonstrates an unusual finding, *duplication of the bile ducts,* (34,35), found on ERCP in a young woman who, despite a cholecystectomy, continued to experience recurrent right upper quadrant pain. Her symptoms were relieved by a sphincterotomy; only one incision was necessary for drainage of both ducts.

The question of separate openings of the pancreatic duct and bile duct has always been raised as a possible cause of difficulty in cannulating the duct of intention, usually the bile duct. The belief that a *majority* of the population has a common channel (i.e., both bile duct and pancreatic duct arising from the same orifice) rather than separate channels is a misconception. This notion was derived from anatomy and surgical textbooks and has proved to be incorrect (36). It is my opinion that the common channel exists in only 20%

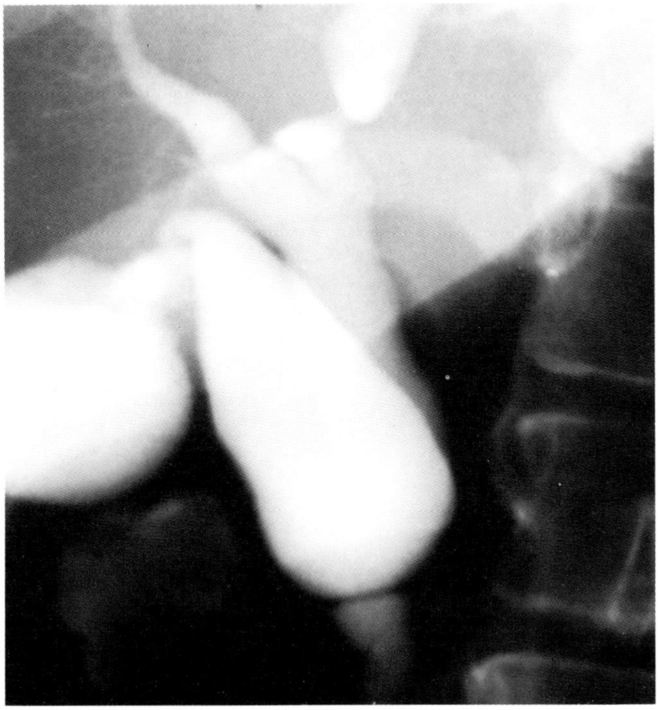

A

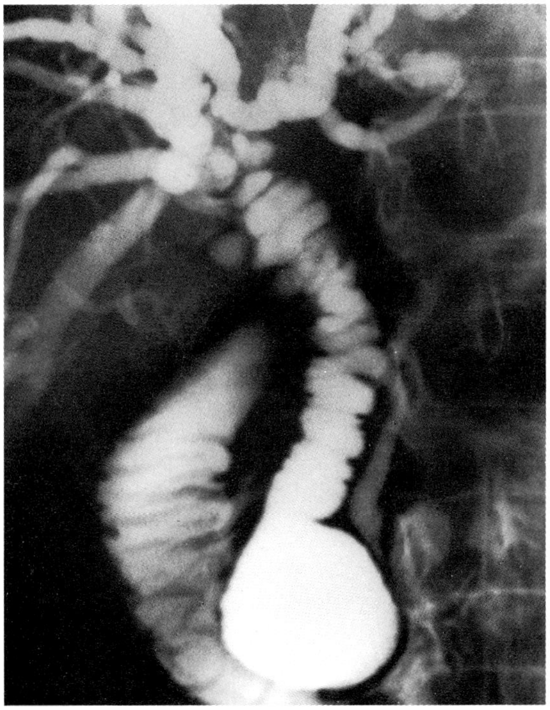

B

FIG. 4.29. **A:** This cholangiogram demonstrates a choledochal cyst arising from the mid common bile duct. Note a web in the distal duct and a dilated cystic duct. Also note intrahepatic cystic changes associated with a more diffuse involvement. **B:** A choledochocele, a cystic structure of the distal common bile duct located within the duodenum.

to 30% of the population and accounts for the difficulty that most endoscopists encounter in selectively cannulating the bile duct in these cases (Fig. 4.31). As explained in the previous chapter, selective cannulation of the pancreatic duct is usually accomplished by approaching the papilla in the middle of that structure; the bile duct arises from the uppermost margin in most patients and must be approached differently and at a more acute angle. This concept is also important in evaluating a patient with acute gallstone pancreatitis,

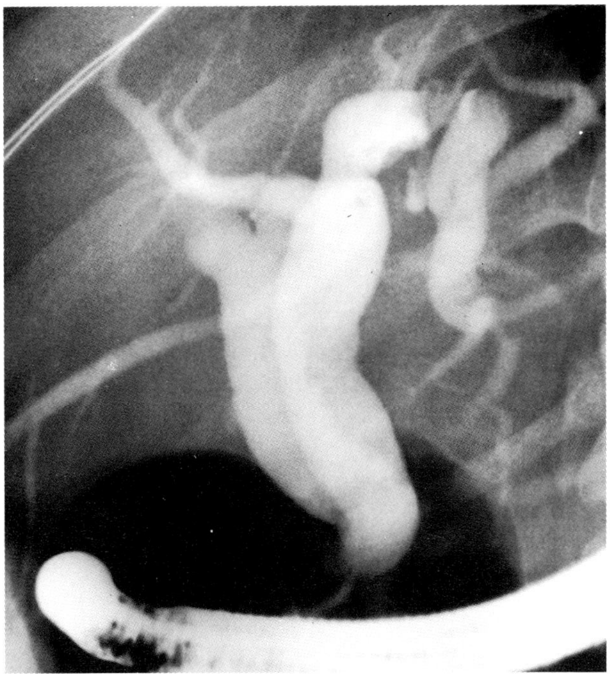

FIG. 4.30. Duplication of the bile duct. Complete filling of both ducts is noted, and dilatation to 1.5 cm is found. Although the patient underwent a cholecystectomy, the surgeon did not report this variation. A sphincterotomy was performed with relief of symptoms reported by the patient.

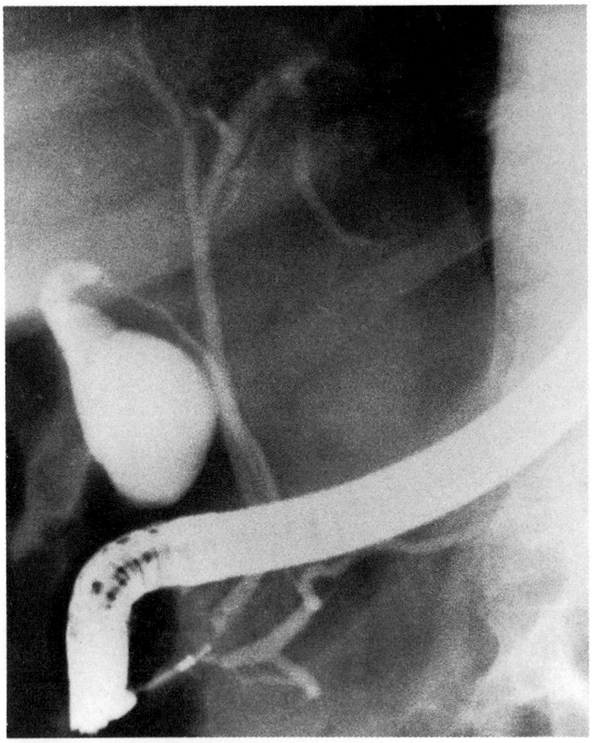

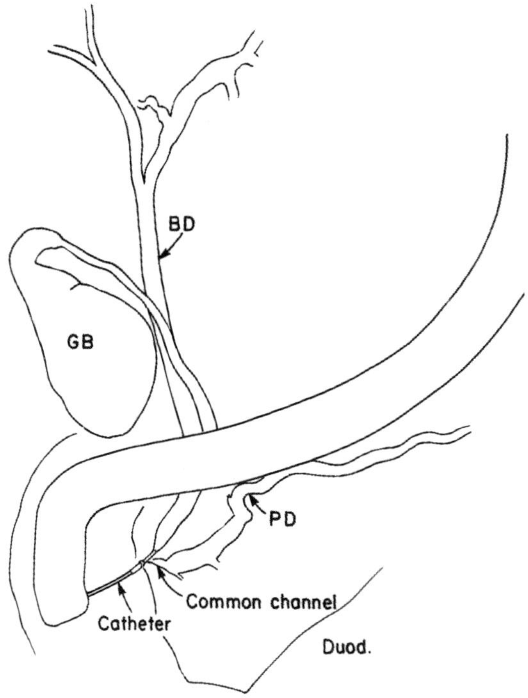

A

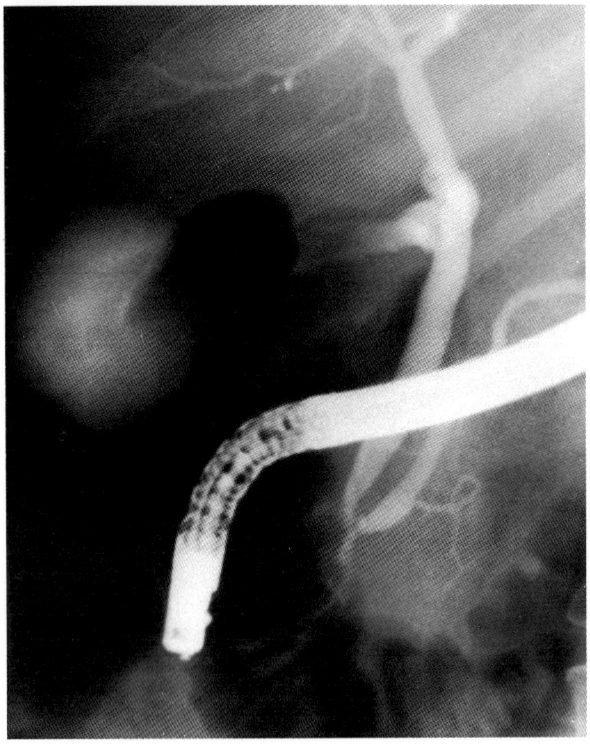

B

FIG. 4.31. A: Left: Both a cholangiogram and pancreatogram were obtained in this study, opacified after impacting the metal-tipped catheter into the ampulla. Both systems opacified with a single injection, so a common channel was confirmed. **Right:** An ERCP identifying a common channel. GB, gall bladder; BD, bile duct; PD, pancreatic duct. **B:** A common channel through which both duct systems are opacified. From reference 55, with permission.

because these patients often have a common channel into which the stone impacts, obstructing the pancreatic duct and inducing the toxic enzyme cascade (37). More people with gallstone pancreatitis have a common channel than not (Fig. 4.31). However, the percentage of subjects with a common channel is much lower than previously thought. If a common channel were as predominant as originally believed, there would be little need to describe techniques or specialized methods for selectively cannulating the bile duct. ERCP would then be considered an easier procedure to perform and complete. These issues will be addressed in more detail in Chapter 9.

NORMAL PANCREATIC SYSTEM AND VARIATIONS

Congenital pancreatic variations are discussed in detail in Chapter 9. This section describes the normal pancreatic duct system and variations, which should be appreciated because of their increasing clinical significance.

It is general knowledge that the pancreas is located posteriorly in the abdominal cavity, occupying the area medially between the second and third portions of the duodenum (the C loop) and extending laterally to the left to the spleen (38,39). The accepted normal diameter of the pancreatic duct is approximately 3 mm to 4 mm in the head, decreasing to 2 mm to 3 mm in the body and 1 mm to 2 mm in the tail (5). The *major pancreatic duct* takes off in a cephalad direction in the head of the gland; in most people, it takes a 45° to 90° turn in the neck and continues horizontally in the body and tail of the gland (Fig. 4.32). In most patients, an

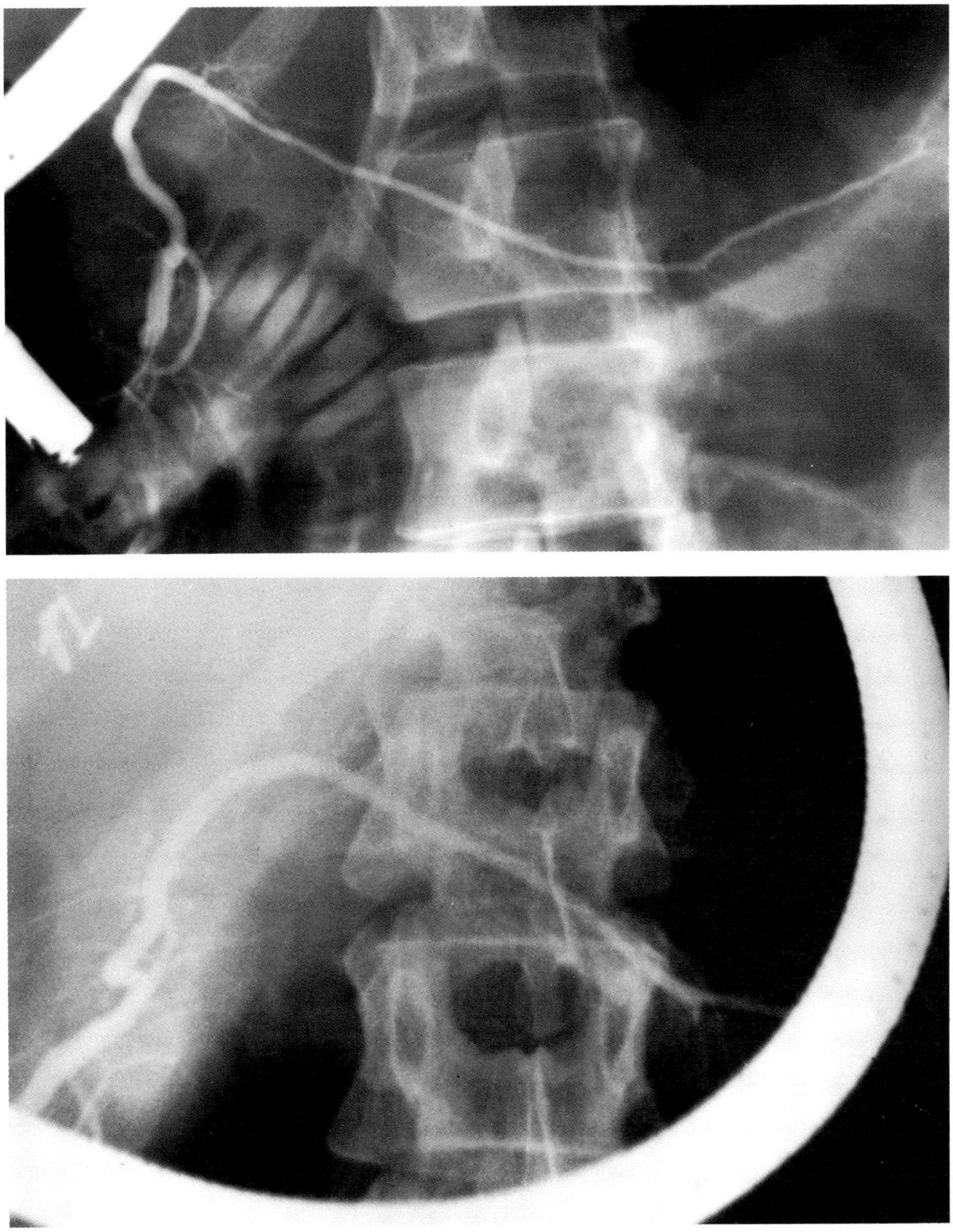

A

B

FIG. 4.32. A: A normal pancreatogram demonstrating normal contour and configuration of the duct. Filling of the duct is complete to the tail, and filling of secondary radicals is shown. The accessory duct system is also seen. **B:** A normal pancreatogram demonstrating retrograde filling of the main duct to the tail with filling of side branches throughout the length of the duct.

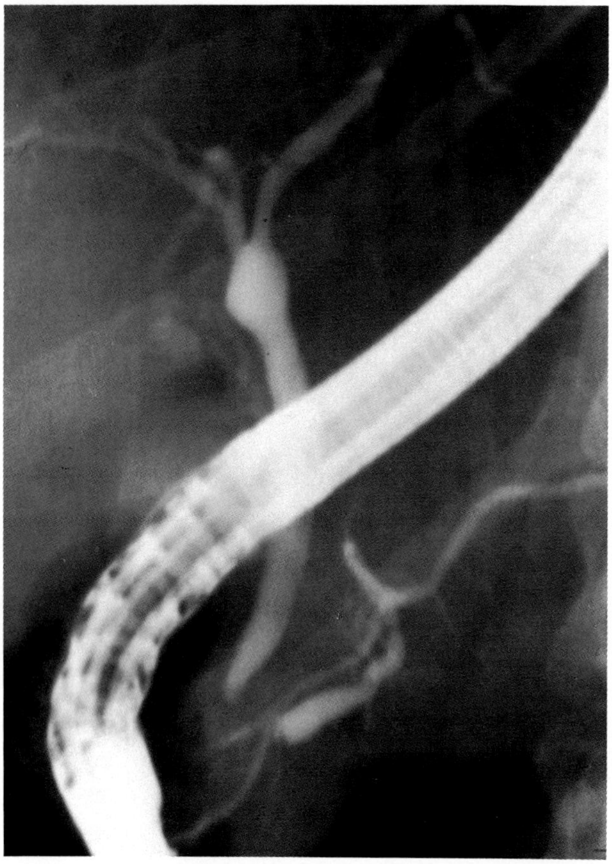

FIG. 4.33. Branching of the accessory duct. Note the parallel attitude of the accessory duct. Small uncinate branches are also present. A loop variation is apparent.

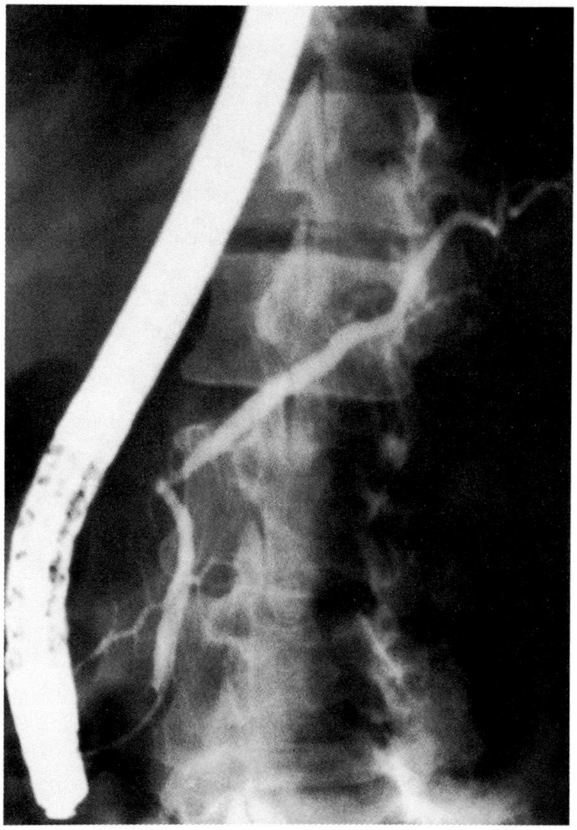

FIG. 4.34. A normal but tortuous pancreatic duct. The accessory duct is very thin in this patient. Branches of the uncinate process are also evident.

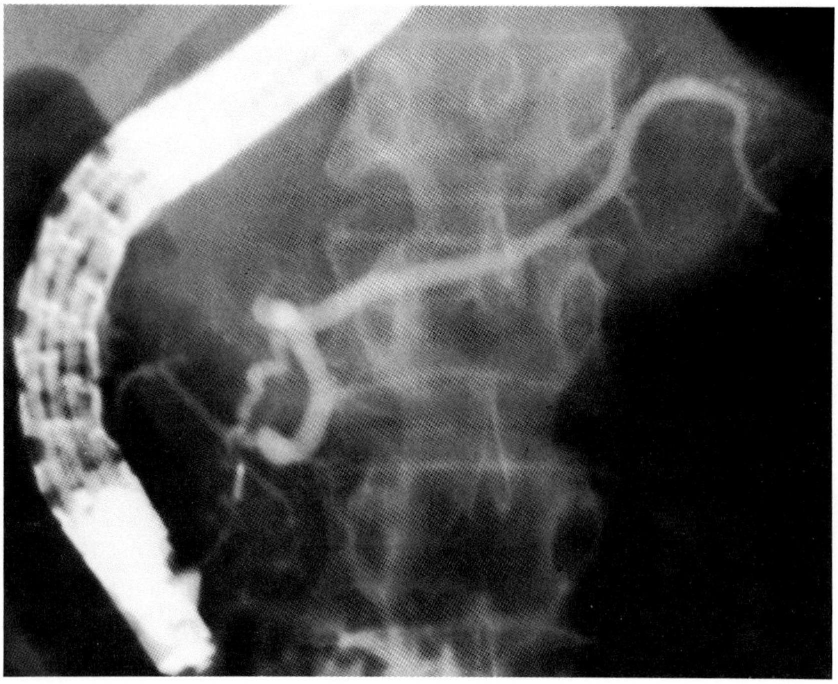

FIG. 4.35. A tortuous accessory duct and other branches in the head of the gland in this patient.

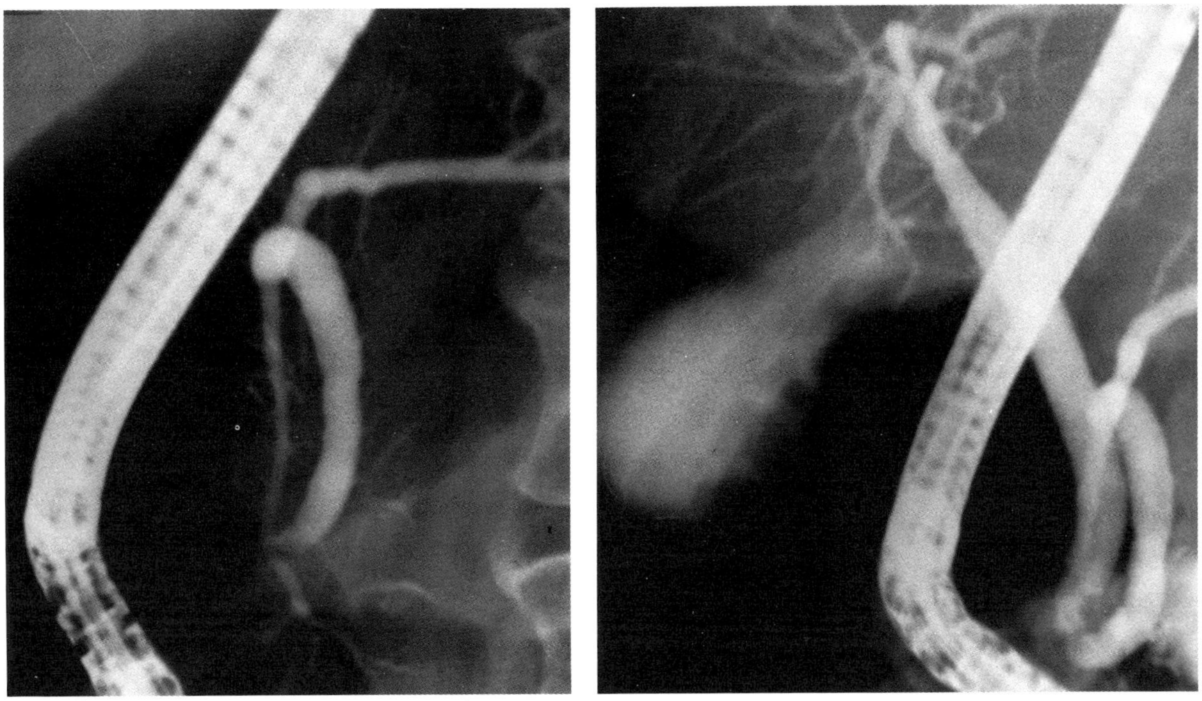

FIG. 4.36. Left: A long, vertical accessory duct arising from the major papilla. **Right:** The uncinate branches and the bile duct also arise from the major papilla, making this an unusual common channel.

accessory duct system can be identified when filling the pancreatic duct. The accessory duct is usually located superior to the major duct and slightly parallel as it separates from the major duct, entering the duodenum more perpendicularly. The accessory duct enters the second portion of the duodenum through the minor papilla, which is cephalad and lateral to the major papilla. There are many variations of the accessory duct and uncinate process, and several of these and their significance are demonstrated in Figs. 4.33 through 4.41. In most patients, the uncinate process, or ventral portion of the pancreatic duct system, is usually identified as its branches are opacified inferior to the main duct (Figs. 4.42–4.46). Identification of these structures is emphasized because opacification of these systems is important in distinguishing between benign and malignant disease.

The *side branches* of the pancreatic duct should be

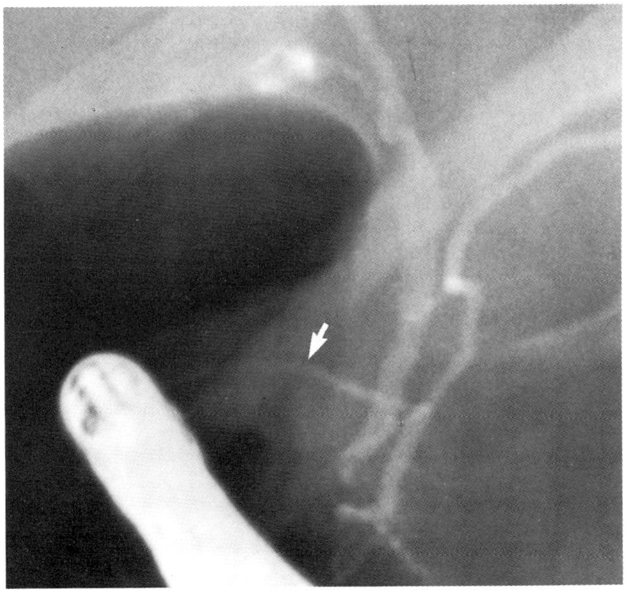

FIG. 4.37. Note the horizontal accessory duct in this patient (*arrow*) and uncinate branches.

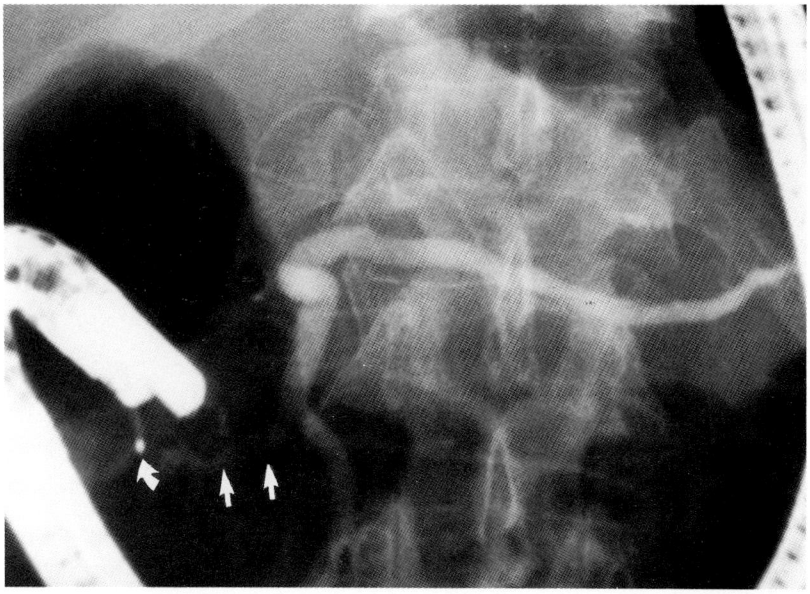

FIG. 4.38. Opacification of the entire pancreatic duct was accomplished on this examination using a needle-tip catheter inserted into the minor papilla (*curved arrow*), opacifying the accessory duct (*arrows*).

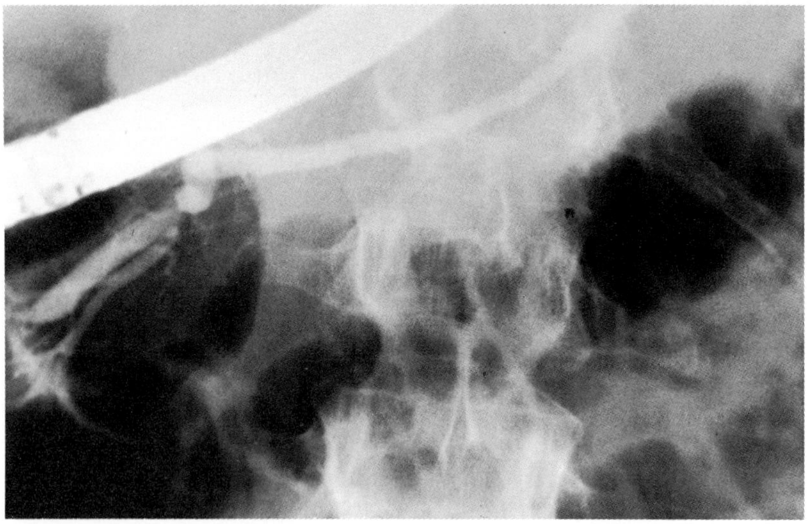

FIG. 4.39. A pancreatogram showing either an aberrant accessory duct system or a prominent uncinate branch appears inferior and parallel to the main duct.

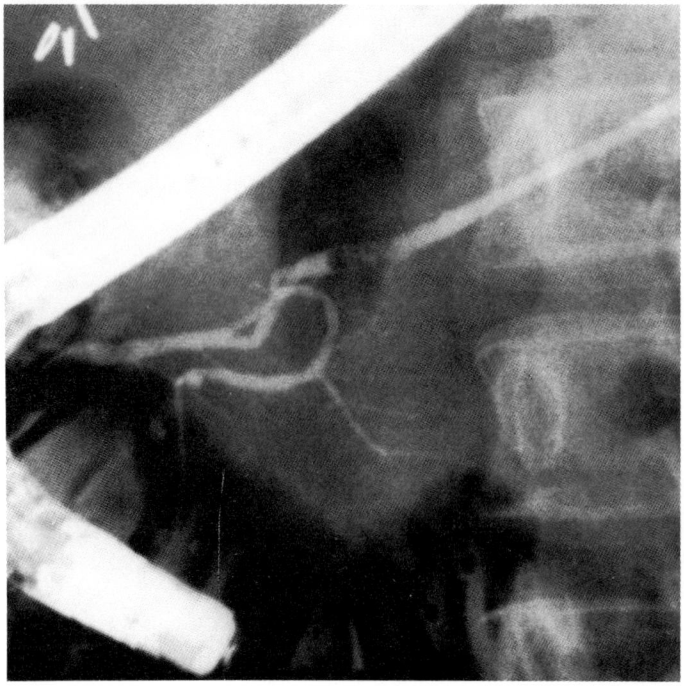

FIG. 4.40. Opacification of the pancreatic duct through an inferior branch of the uncinate process with filling of the accessory duct and dorsal pancreatic system. Air bubbles are present in the dorsal duct near the aberrant junction.

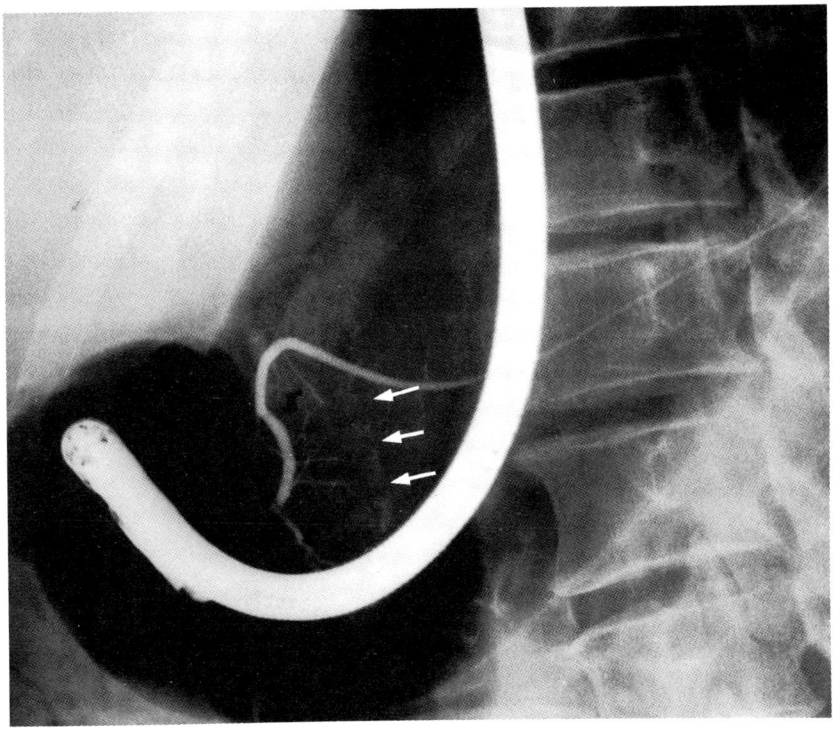

FIG. 4.41. This pancreatogram shows filling of a slender pancreatic duct with opacification of the uncinate branches and, if one looks closely, an acinargram (*arrows*). As indicated earlier, acinar filling in the head of the pancreas may represent resistance to retrograde flow compatible with an impedence related to pancreatitis or a stricture, benign or malignant.

filled or opacified completely during retrograde injection of contrast, and they should be identified on the pancreatogram (Fig. 4.32) (40–45). Appreciation of their filling during examination is possible with high-quality, high-resolution fluoroscopic equipment. Filling of the side branches is usually the most important finding in distinguishing benign from malignant disease, and one should take adequate time to identify these branches. Overfilling of these and the tertiary branches, however, may lead to acinarization and pancreatitis. The figures presented in this section reveal filling of side branches; in most examples, the fine secondary branches are seen filled completely out to the tail. Loss of these side branches may connote malig-

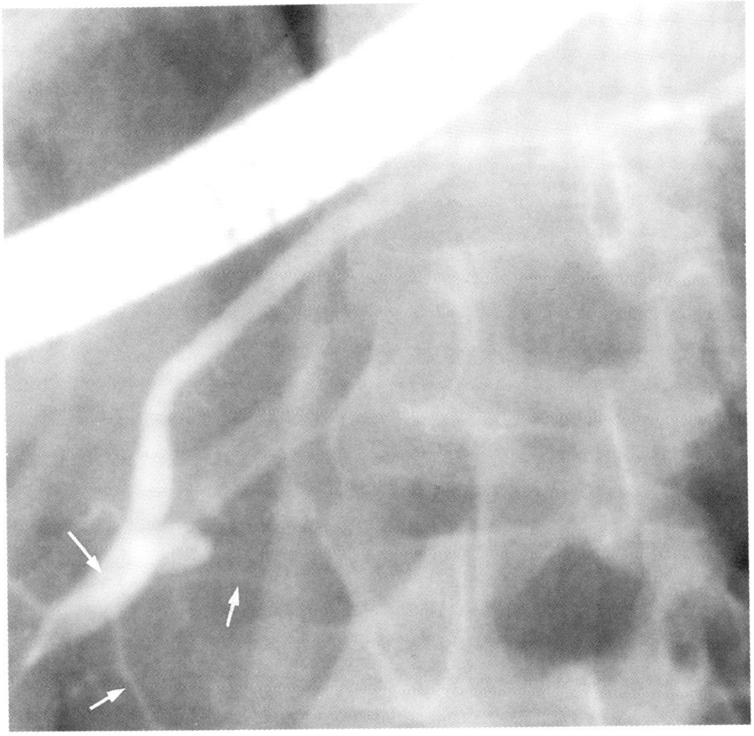

FIG. 4.42. Another example of aberrancy of the accessory duct with filling of the uncinate branches (*arrows*).

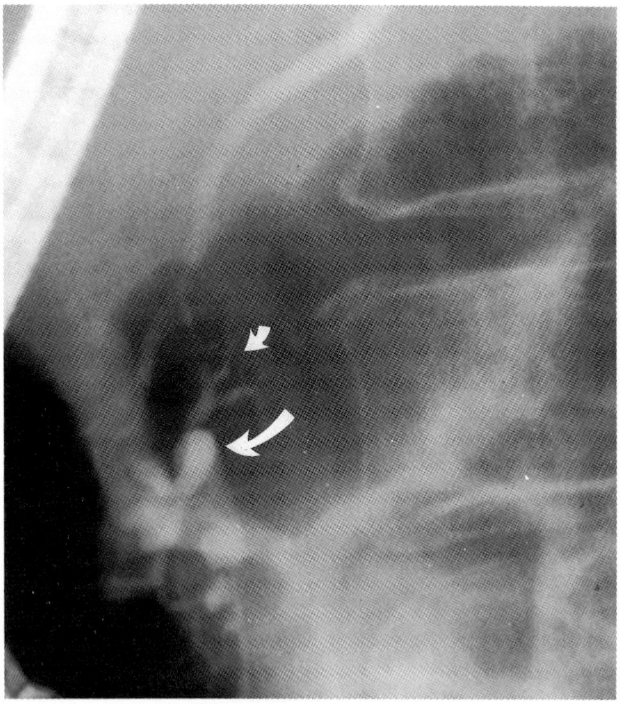

FIG. 4.43. An unusual pancreatogram demonstrating tortuosity of the duct in the head of the gland (*large arrow*) with branching in what is probably the uncinate process (*small arrow*). The presence of this configuration has affected filling of the duct in the head and, consequently, emptying of the duct, which may account for clinical symptoms and biochemical abnormalities attributed to pancreatitis.

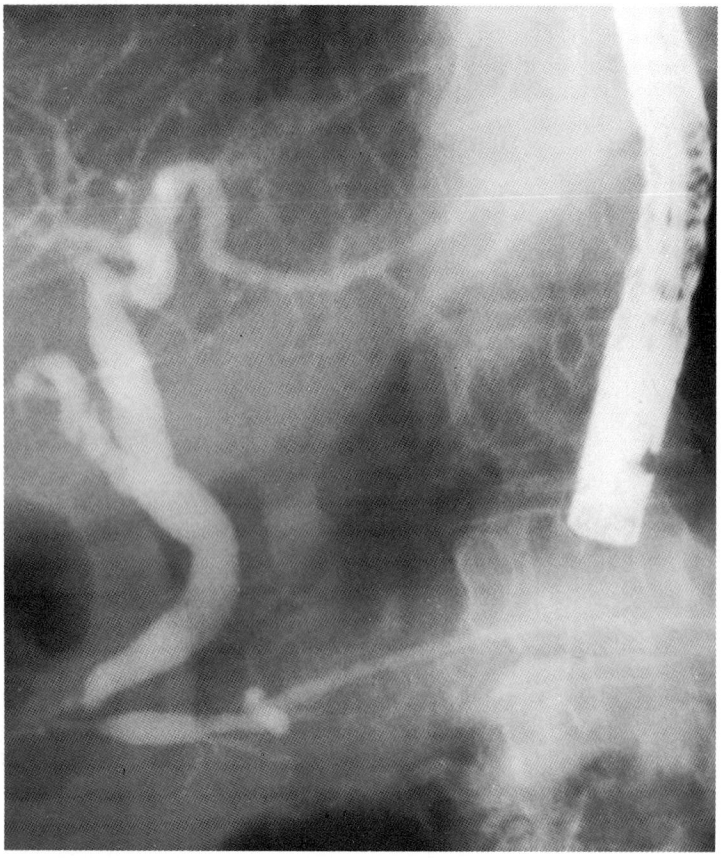

FIG. 4.44. An unusual takeoff of the pancreatic duct. This is a straight configuration of the duct interrupted by a loop. Secondary branches are normal, which rules out pancreatitis. Note the activity of the common sphincter, which is contracted in this study, delaying emptying of the bile duct and pancreatic duct.

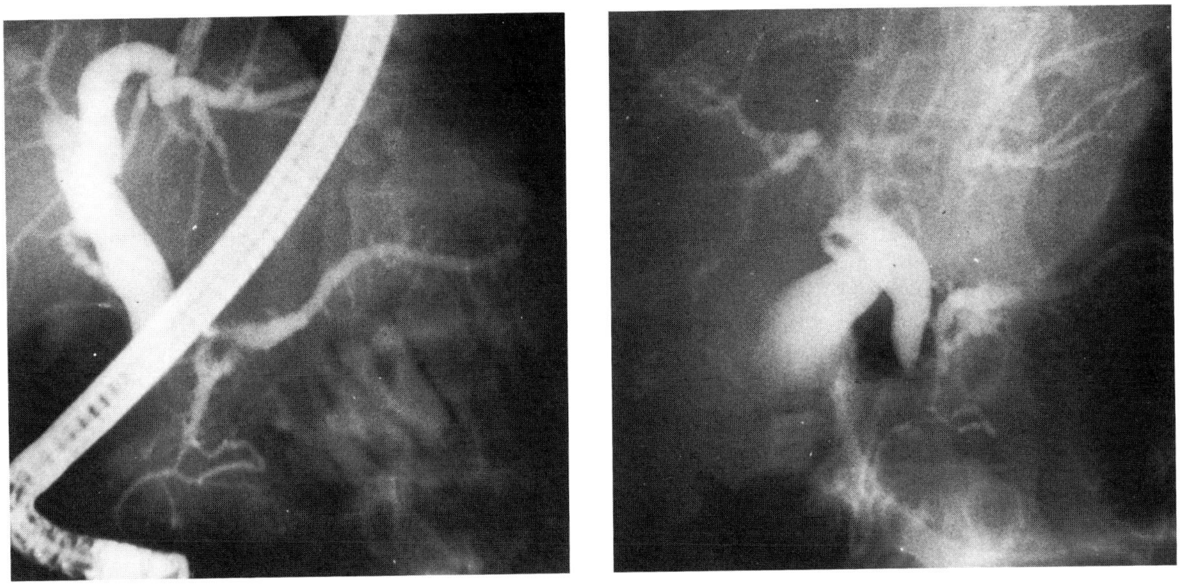

FIG. 4.45. Left: An unusual configuration of the uncinate branches. Note filling of the secondary branches. **Right:** This ERCP illustrates findings consistent with pancreatitis. Delayed emptying of the bile duct, which is dilated proximally and tapered distally, is consistent with fibrosis secondary to pancreatitis. Note the slight blunting of the secondary pancreatic branches, which is consistent with pancreatitis.

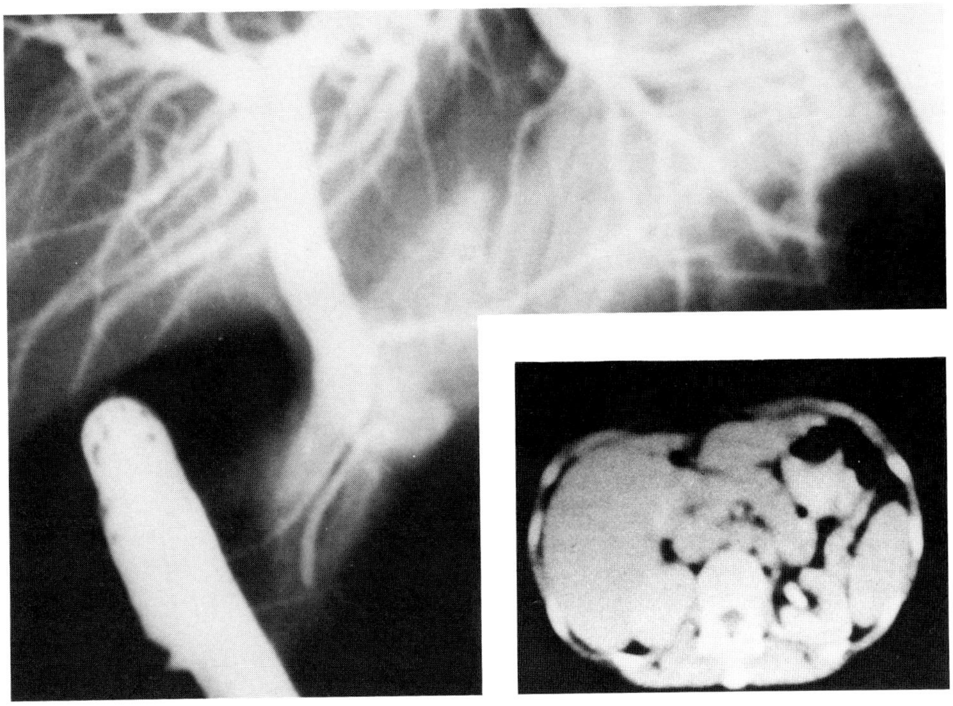

FIG. 4.46. This ERCP demonstrates a loop variation in the head of the pancreas. A CT scan of the abdomen, illustrating fullness of the head of the pancreas corresponding to a loop of the pancreatic duct.

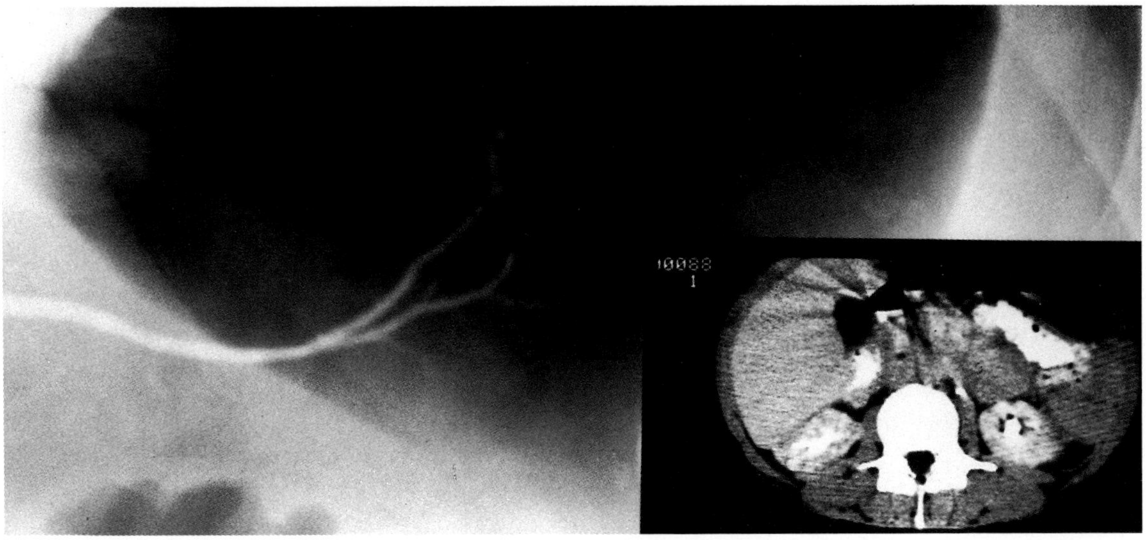

FIG. 4.47. A pancreatogram showing a bifurcation of the pancreatic duct in the tail. **Inset:** A CT scan showing enlargement of the tail of the pancreas, which was interpreted as a mass. However, this proved to be a pseudomass after obtaining the ERP, which showed the bifid tail variation.

nant disease, whereas blunting confirms inflammatory disease (Fig. 4.45).

The configuration of the pancreatic duct varies from patient to patient. In a 1983 paper, Yatto and Siegel introduced a new classification for identifying subgroups of patients with normal variations of pancreatic duct morphology seen on pancreatography (46). The significance of this paper was reflected by the earlier report that described pseudomasses of the pancreas. In that index report, *variants* of the pancreatic duct were identified at pancreatography and were consequently classified as pseudomasses or pseudotumors. The variants found at pancreatography clearly correlated to the abnormal findings on CT scans of the pancreas in which a mass had been described (47) (Figs. 4.46, 4.47). In the former report, branching of the pancreatic duct in critical locations was thought to create a pseudomass on CT scan, but the findings on pancreatography corresponded to a benign variant. Follow-up of the 24 patients reported in that paper proved the benignity of the masses seen on CT scan, thus strengthening the position of ERCP in evaluating

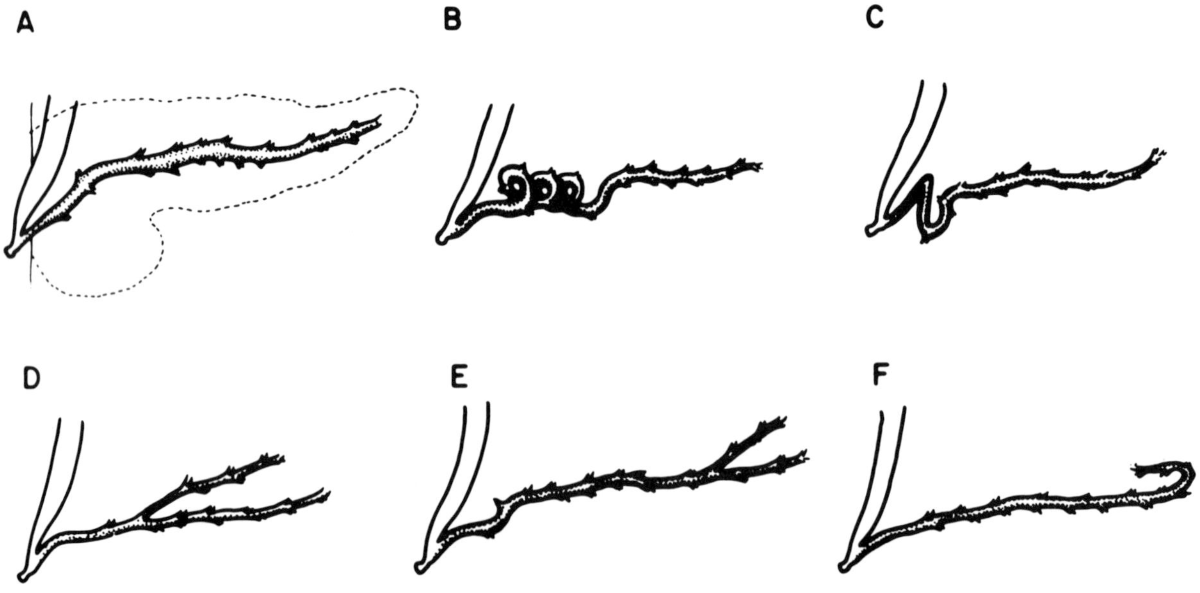

FIG. 4.48. The normal pancreatic duct and variations of the ductular system that may produce pseudomasses on CT scans. **A:** The normal configuration. **B:** The loop variation. **C:** N configuration. **D:** Bifurcations of the body. **E:** Bifurcations of the tail. **F:** Angulations of the tail. From reference 47, with permission.

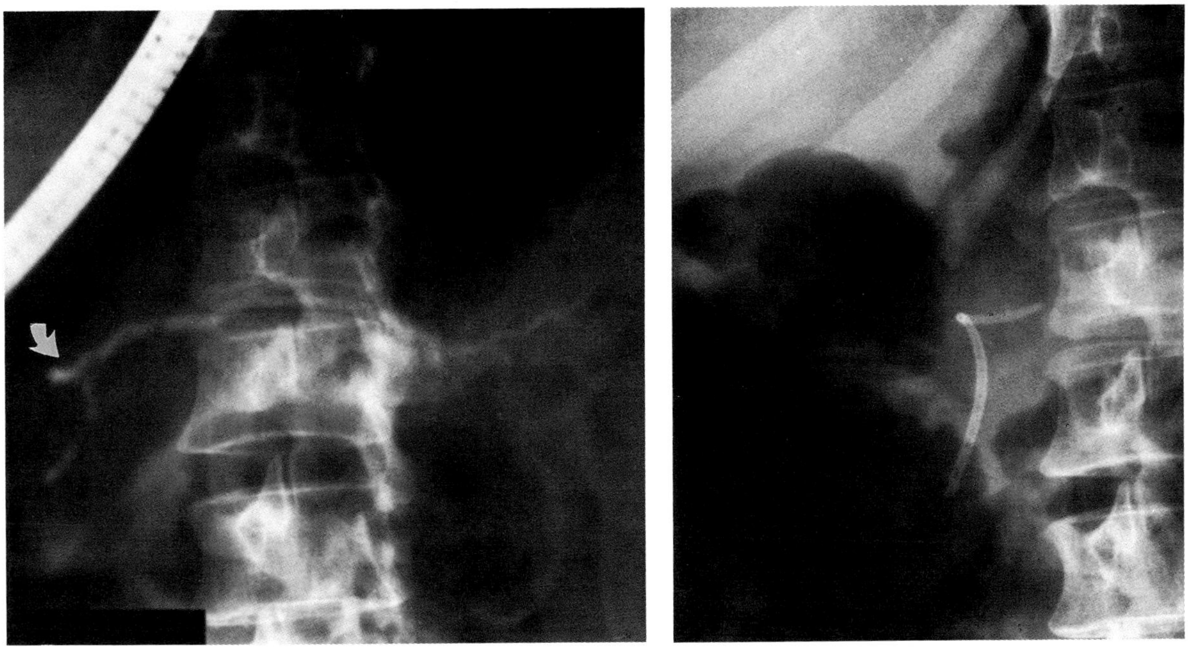

FIG. 4.49. Left: This pancreatogram shows a small loop in the head of the gland (*arrow*). **Right:** A prosthesis has been placed through the loop to provide decompression.

pancreatic disorders and especially in determining malignancy. This report attempted to correlate ERCP findings with CT findings and directed attention toward these variants for the first time. It was appropriate to introduce a new classification of pancreatic duct morphology to include these variants. Because pancreatography, unlike cholangiography, is relatively new and unfamiliar to most clinicians, a new atlas of pancreatography has ultimately been created.

This new classification of variants of the pancreas is shown in Table 4.3. Some of this material is covered in Chapter 9, so congenital variants are not described in this section. Figure 4.48 is an artist's interpretation of pancreatograms, which are variants of the normal configuration shown in Fig. 4.48A. The variants shown are common configurations found in association with pseudomasses reflected on the CT scan. If the pancreatogram correlates with the CT variation, there is no malignancy. Because the CT scan was performed to elucidate the symptoms expressed by the patient, we concluded that pancreatic duct function, usually on emptying of the stimulated secretions, was affected adversely by the variation. Most patients studied originally did well following conservative measures such as dietary restrictions and enzyme supplementation, so we recommend this type of management when the variation is first noted. Patients who manifest persistent, intractable symptoms and had loop variations were treated with prostheses with favorable results (48,49) (Figs. 4.49, 4.50).

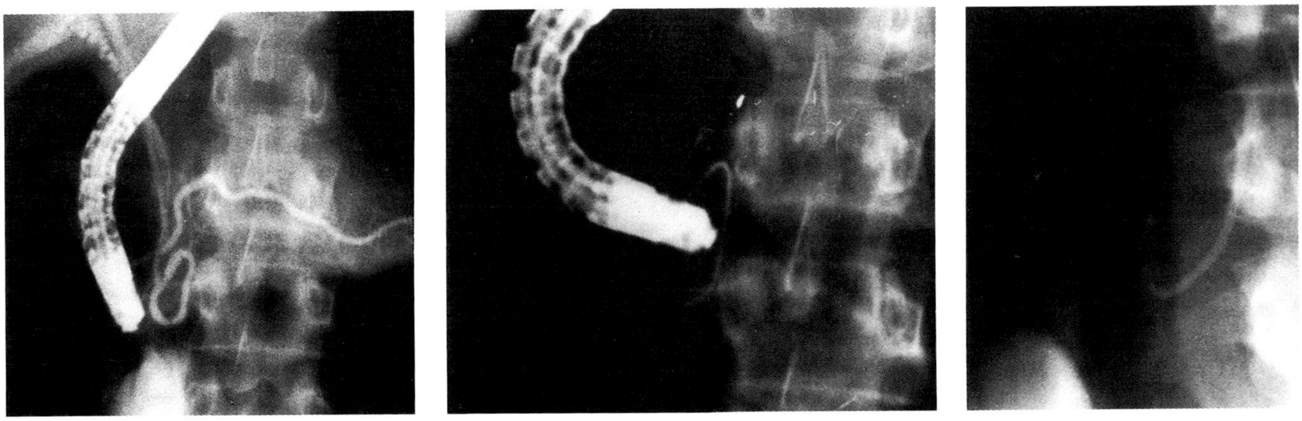

FIG. 4.50. Left: A large loop in the duct in the head of the gland. **Middle:** A guidewire is placed through and around the loop to facilitate stent placement. **Right:** The prosthesis after being placed through the loop.

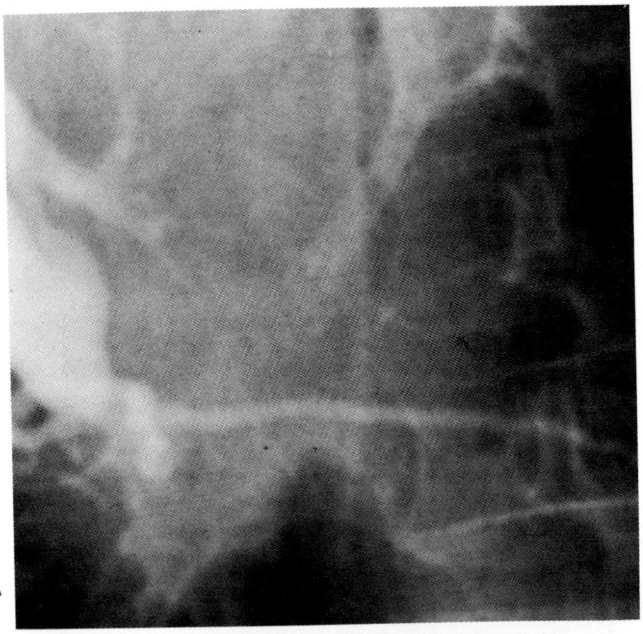

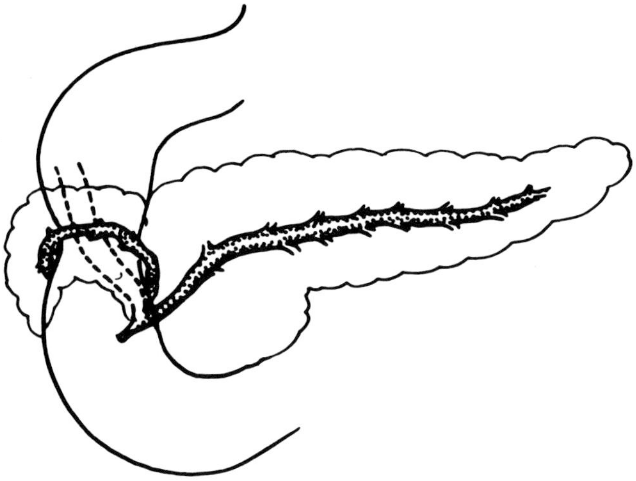

A

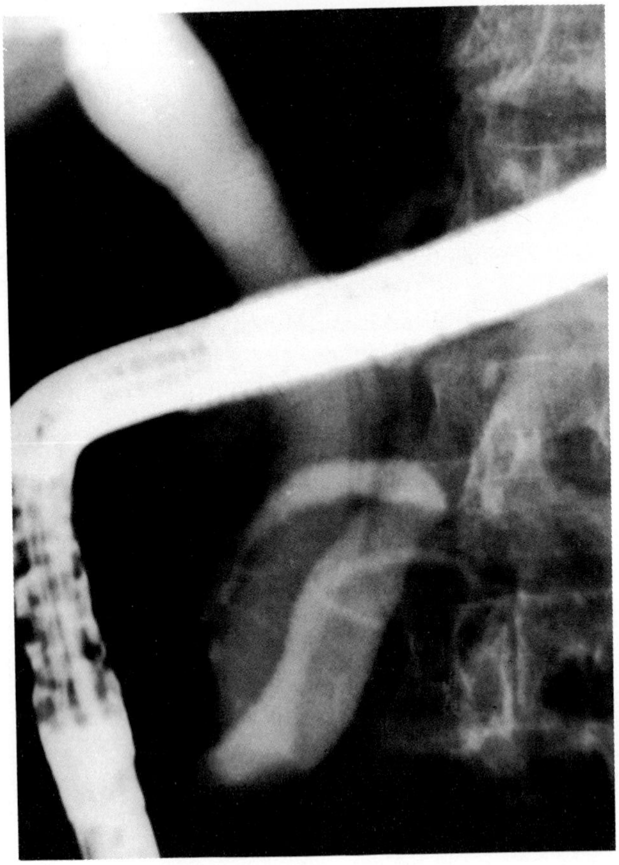

B

FIG. 4.51. A: Left: An annular pancreas completely surrounding the bile duct, producing obstruction and dilatation of the biliary tree. **Right:** Annular pancreas. Note the accessory branch and lobe enwrapping the duodenum and bile duct. **B:** An ERCP showing an annular pancreas with the main pancreatic duct directed vertically while the accessory duct completes the circle obstructing the bile duct. From reference 46, with permission.

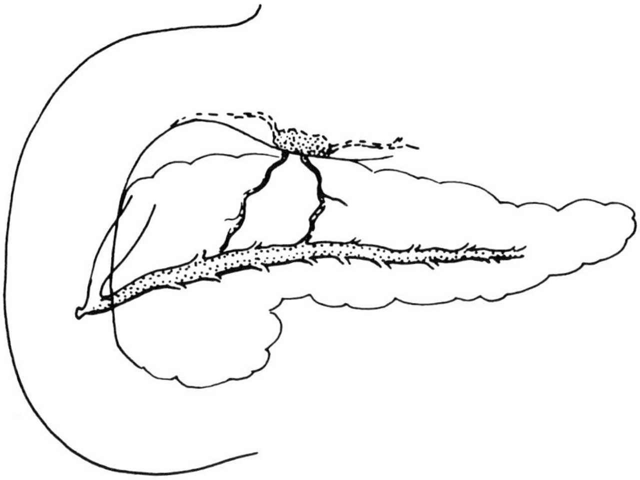

FIG. 4.52. An aberrant pancreas demonstrating the umbilicated nodule in the stomach, which may connect to the pancreatic ductal system. From reference 56, with permission.

Migration Variants

The first category of our classification is *migration variants*. This category includes both the annular pancreas and the aberrant pancreas, which are shown in Figs. 4.51 and 4.52. Both of these variants are very rare, but the annular pancreas has the potential of producing severe complications. Both the duodenum and the bile duct become entrapped by the annular growth of the pancreas, which produces intestinal obstruction, obstructive jaundice, or both. This variation may generally be managed quite satisfactorily by either primary surgical anastomosis or a bypass drainage procedure of the biliary tree and duodenum (50,51). Aberrant pancreas is more a curiosity than a problem and, when visualized and appreciated in the stomach, is identified as an umbilicated nodule usually present on the greater curvature. Very rarely is this anomaly responsible for symptoms of pancreatitis.

Fusion Variants

The next variant of pancreatography is the group classified as *fusion variants*. Included in this category are *pancreas divisum,* which is discussed in greater detail in the section on congenital variants in Chapter 9 and *functional divisum,* or an incomplete pancreas divisum. The notion that the functional divisum variant represents a fusion variant is supported by the accompanying illustration (Fig. 4.53). In the functional div-

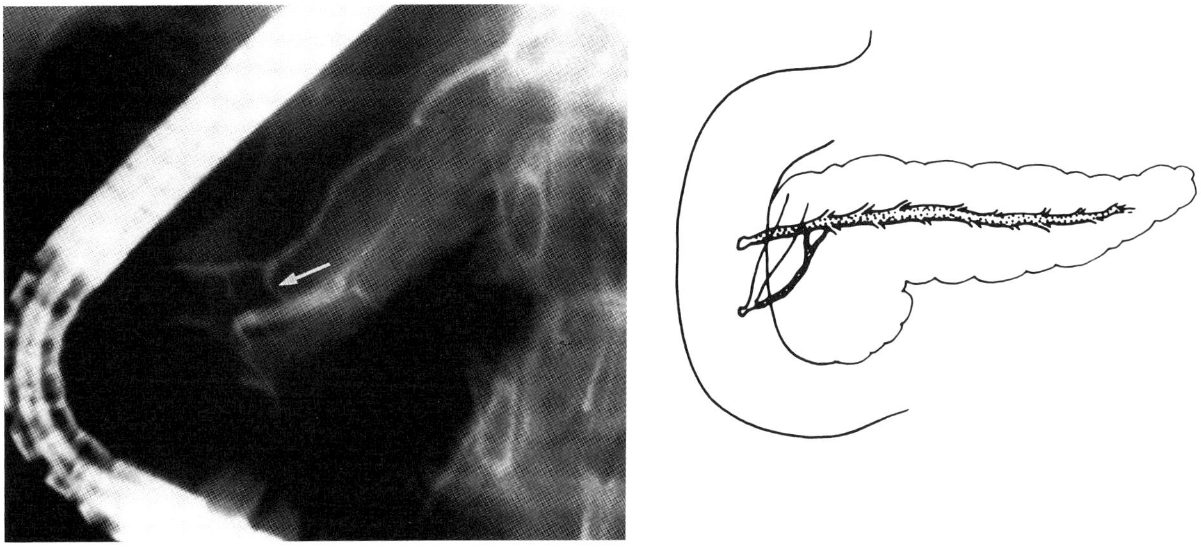

FIG. 4.53. Left: Functional pancreas divisum. Filling of the dorsal pancreatic duct is provided by a slender branch of the ventral duct that communicates with the dorsal duct (*arrow*). **Right:** A functional divisum variant with filling of the dorsal duct provided by a communicating branch of the ventral duct. From reference 46, with permission.

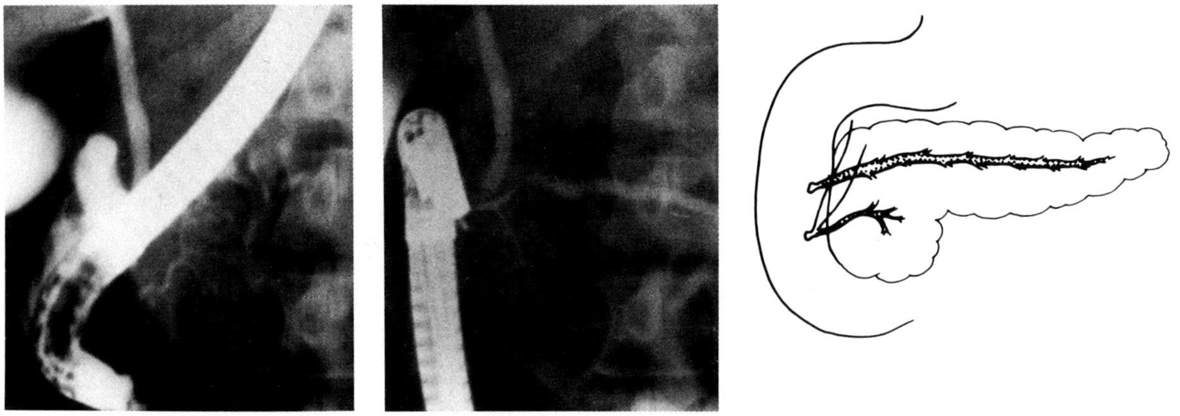

FIG. 4.54. Left: Filling of the ventral pancreatic duct with branching of that system but without filling of the dorsal duct. **Middle:** Opacification of the dorsal pancreatic duct in the same patient is obtained by cannulating the minor papilla with a needle-tipped cannula. Note the stricture of the duct in the head of the gland with a dilated duct proximal to the stricture (toward tail). **Right:** Pancreas divisum demonstrating separation of the pancreatic ducts. From reference 46, with permission.

isum example, opacification of the dorsal pancreatic duct is accomplished through the major papilla through a communicating branch of the ventral duct; in pancreas divisum, both ducts are separate and do not communicate (Fig. 4.54). The major, or ventral, duct tapers as though it terminates like the ventral rudiment of pancreas divisum (Figs. 4.55, 4.56). A closer examination of the radiographs, however, reveals opacification of the dorsal system of the pancreas connected by a narrow segment of the pancreatic duct. Because there is communication between the ventral and dorsal systems, this variation is classified as a functional divisum rather than a complete pancreas divisum. The small, thin tributary that connects the dorsal and ventral duct systems may be inadequate for increased flow volume of pancreatic juice and, at times, causes pain.

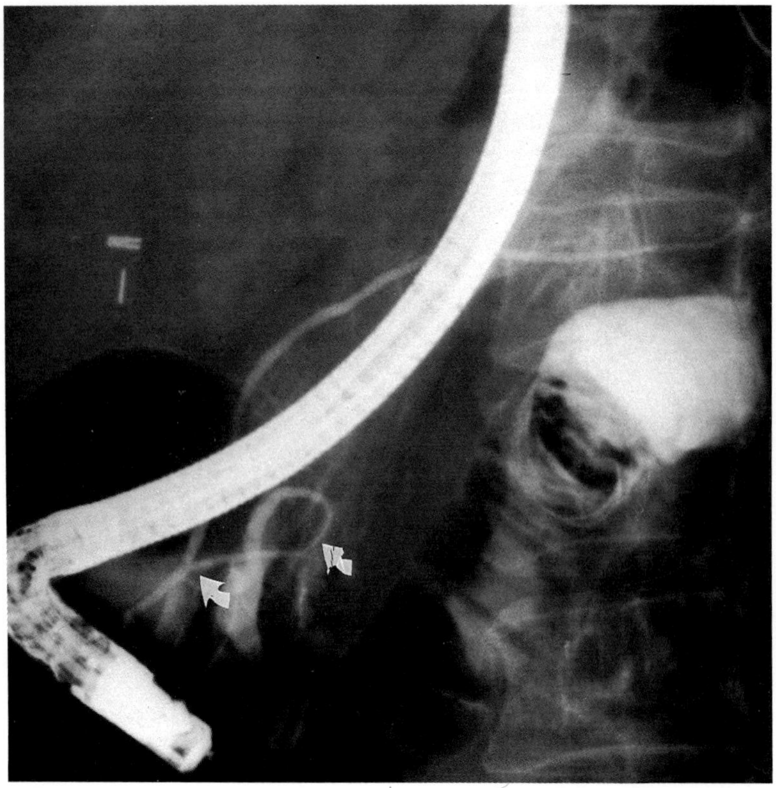

FIG. 4.55. Functional pancreas divisum with filling of the ventral duct of the pancreas. A communicating branch of this system loops inferiorly and laterally to join the dorsal or main pancreatic duct, completely opacifying the dorsal system (*arrows*).

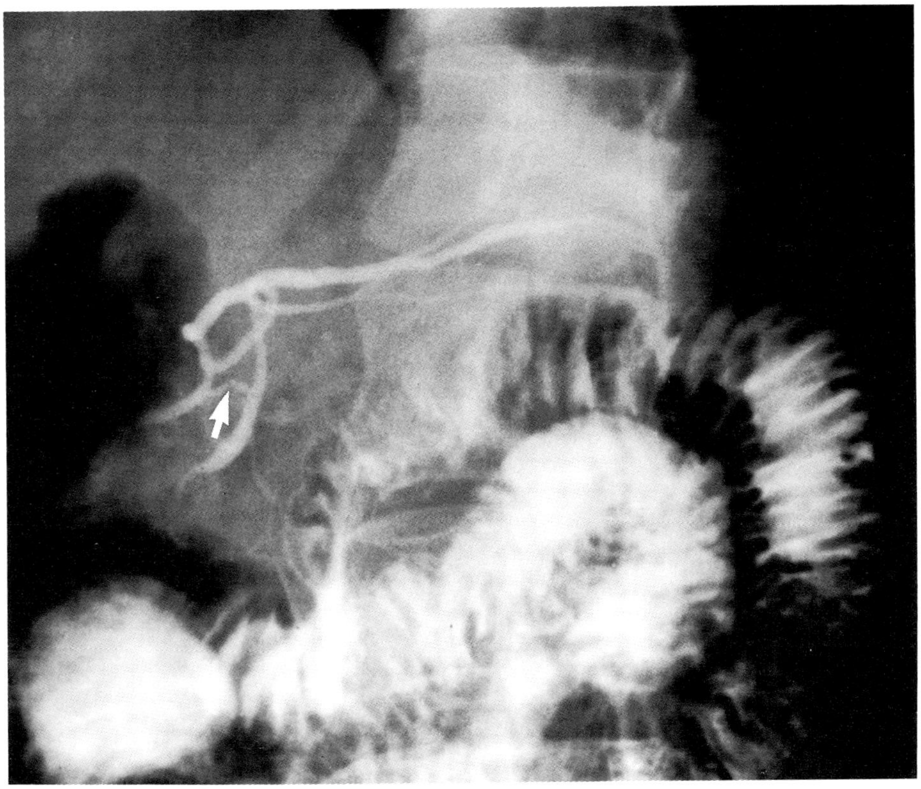

FIG. 4.56. Filling of both the ventral and the dorsal duct systems of the pancreas through the major papilla. Note a thin communicating branch between the systems, which is responsible for filling of the dorsal system (*arrow*). Another communication into the body of the dorsal duct is seen. Although this is an example of functional divisum, it could also be classified as a duplication of pancreatic ducts. From reference 46, with permission.

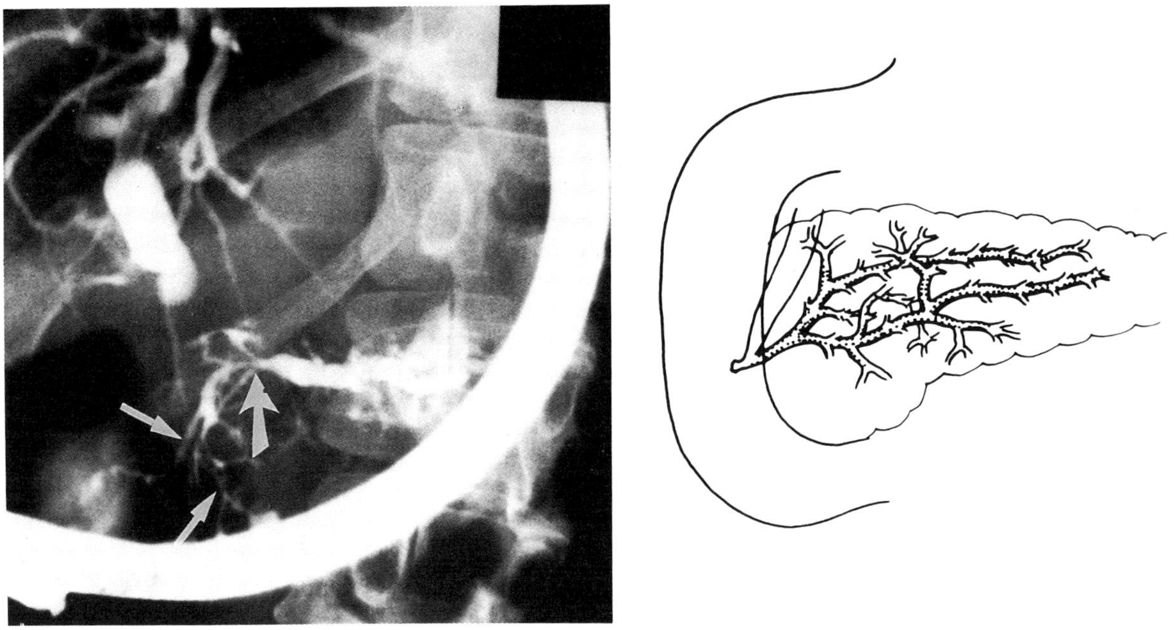

FIG. 4.57. Left: A plexus configuration of the pancreatic duct demonstrating branching of the duct in the head (*small arrows*), a stricture at the genu (*large arrow*), and dilatation of the duct proximal to the stricture (toward the tail). Blunting of the branches secondary to pancreatitis is appreciated. **Right:** A plexus configuration. From reference 46, with permission.

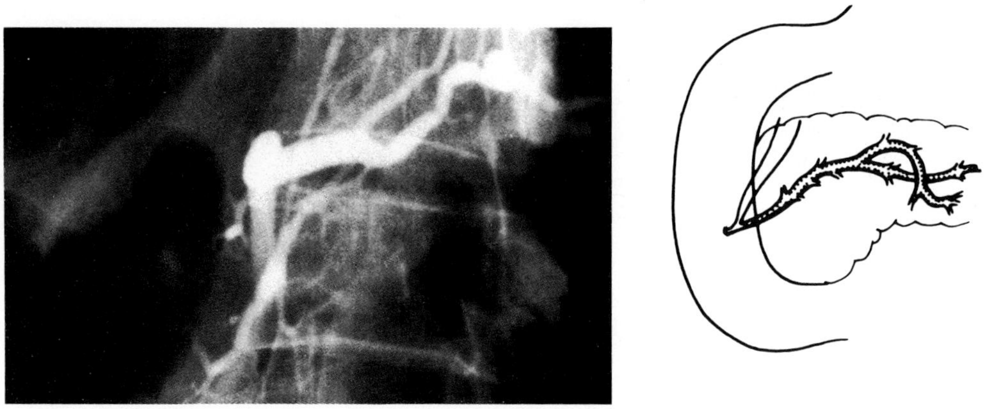

FIG. 4.58. Left: Bifurcation of the main pancreatic duct. **Right:** A bifurcation variant shown in a pancreatogram. From reference 46, with permission.

Some patients with this variation present with vague abdominal pain and may require further endoscopic manipulation or even surgery if symptoms persist.

Duplication Variants

Another group of variants, *duplication variations,* includes subcategories classified as *number variation* and *form variation*. The number variation group is further subdivided into *plexus configuration* and *bifurcations*. The plexus configuration is identified by the presence of multiple branches of the pancreatic duct located in the head of the gland (Fig. 4.57). The morphology of the ducts on pancreatography is consistent with chronic pancreatitis. The question, however, is "which appeared first, the plexus configuration variation or pancreatitis?" Although there may be disagreement over the validity of the former category, plexus configuration, most physicians and radiologists agree that the bifurcation configuration (Figs. 4.58–4.60) does exist and may be responsible for the so-called pseudotumor or pseudomass (47). Bifurcation of the pancreatic duct can occur at any location in the pancreatic duct system and, because the bifurcation is surrounded by pancreatic tissue, may appear as a mass on a CT scan. Until our first description of these variations, however, this was not appreciated, and the physician was required to prove there was no tumor. The endoscopist and radiologist participating in ERCP should be familiar with these variations to avoid making an incorrect diagnosis or false-positive conclusion.

The *form variants* are easier to appreciate and understand but were not described before our earlier pub-

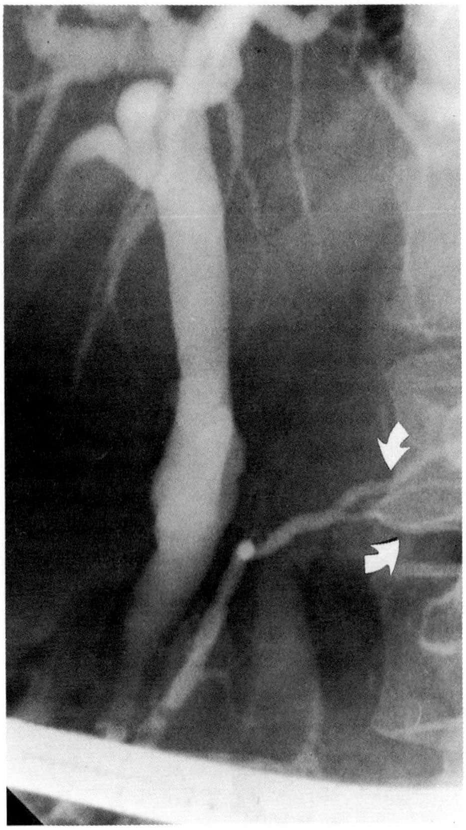

FIG. 4.59. Bifurcation of the main pancreatic duct over a vertebral body (*arrows*).

TABLE 4.3. *Variant pancreatography*

I.	Migration variants
	A. Annular pancreas
	B. Aberrant pancreas
II.	Fusion variants
	A. Pancreas divisum
	B. Functional divisum
III.	Duplication variants
	A. Number variants
	1. Plexus
	2. Bifurcations
	B. Form variants
	1. Loop
	2. Spiral
	3. N
	4. Ring

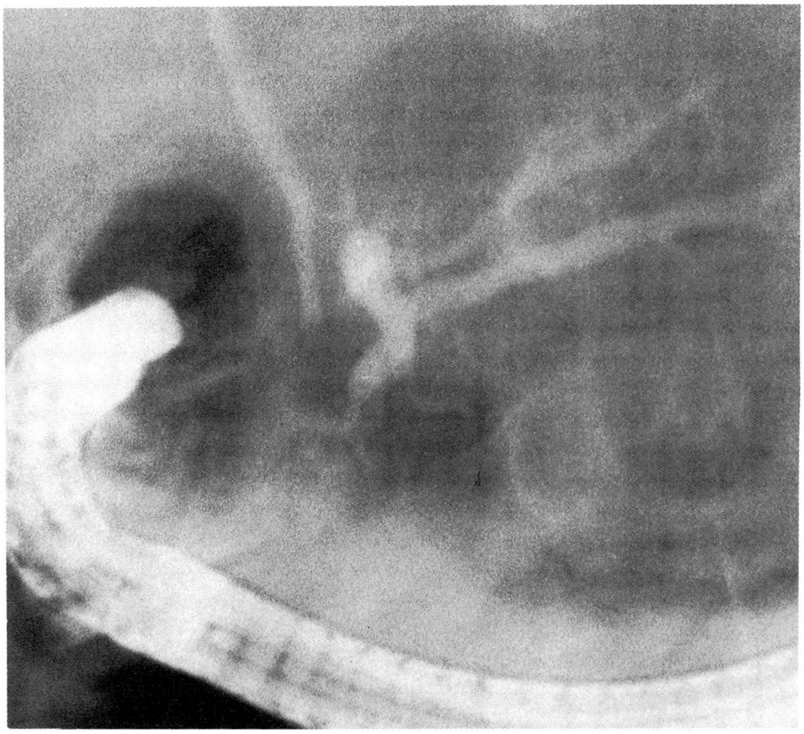

FIG. 4.60. Bifurcation of the pancreatic duct with two major ducts, or a duplication.

lication (46). Illustrations of the loop, spiral, N, and ring variations are shown and should be apparent to the reader (Figs. 4.61–4.64).

What is the significance of these variations? These variations may be responsible for the symptoms expressed by some individuals who are referred with vague discomfort in the epigastrium usually associated with meals, sometimes referred to the back, and occasionally associated with nausea, anorexia, and weight loss. It is thought that the ubiquitous symptoms associated with these variations of pancreatic duct morphology result from the impedence of the antegrade flow of pancreatic juice during peak stimulation, thus producing symptoms referable to the epigastrium. Therapeutic maneuvers in these patients will be described in Chapters 10, 12, and 13. Some of these patients, however, have benefitted either from surgical drainage without prior endoscopic decompression or from surgical drainage preceded by endoscopic decompression, which was heralded by relief of symptoms experienced prior to the therapeutic endoscopic procedure (48,49).

It is the intention of the author to familiarize readers with variations of pancreatic duct morphology because these variants may be responsible for symptoms in an otherwise healthy individual and because there are no descriptions of variant pancreatography, other than our index publication, published in the ERCP era. On another note, variations of pancreatic duct entry into the duodenum were described not only by our group

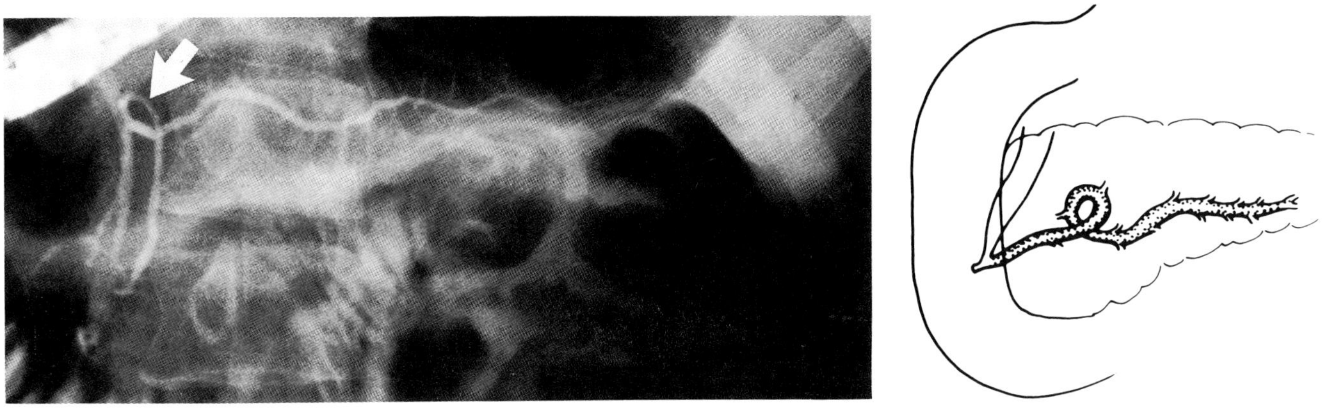

FIG. 4.61. Left: An ERP demonstrating a loop in the pancreatic duct at the genu (*arrow*). **Right:** A loop variation. From reference 46, with permission.

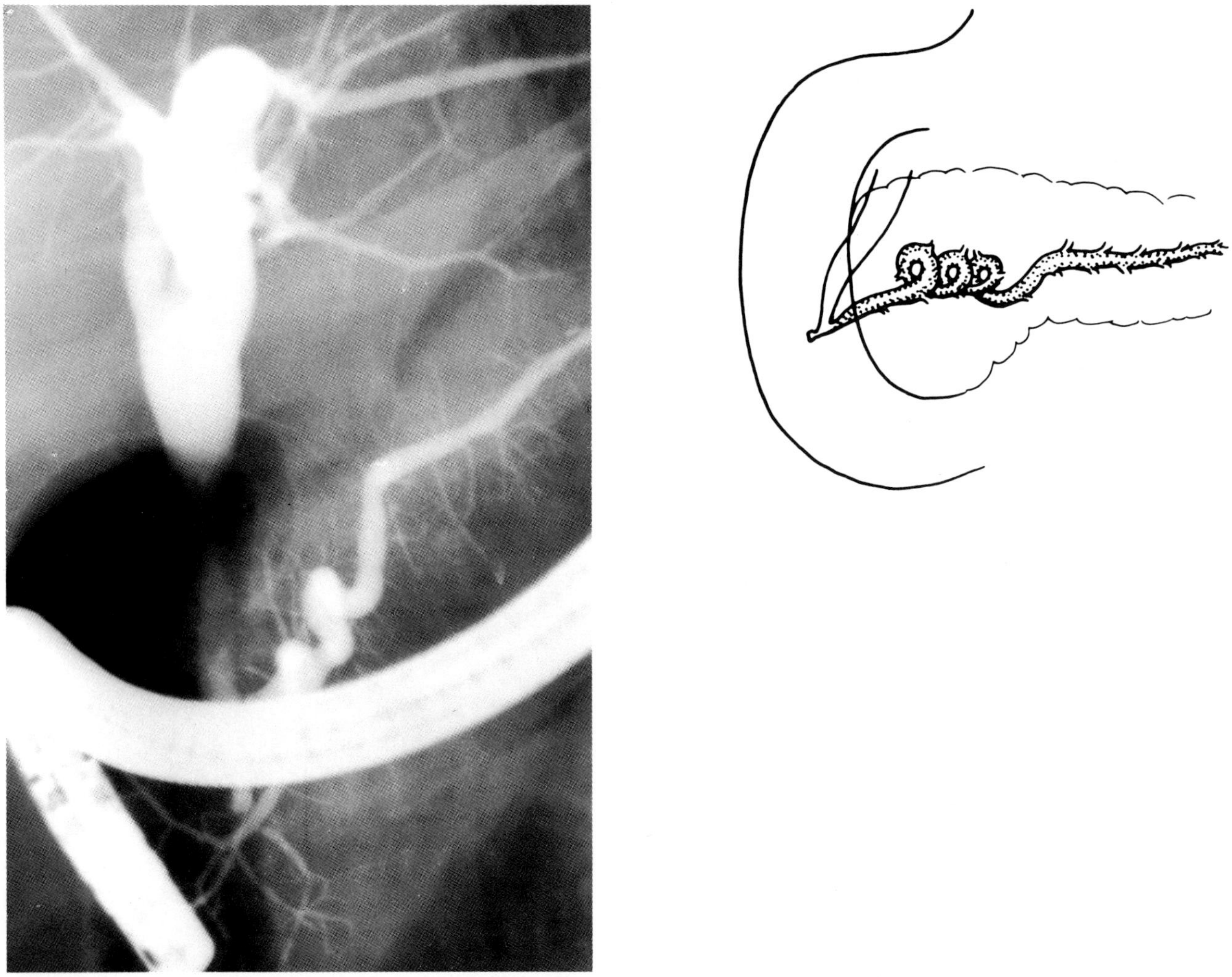

A

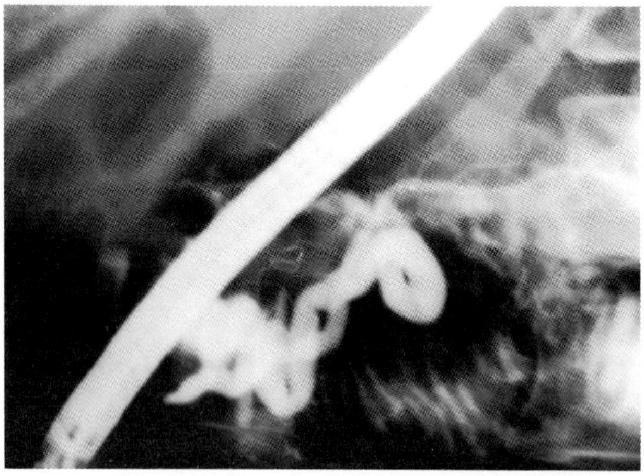

B

FIG. 4.62. A: Left: An ERCP showing spiral looping in the head-body junction of the pancreas. **Right:** A spiral variation. **B:** A pancreatogram demonstrating extreme looping of the pancreatic duct. From reference 47, with permission.

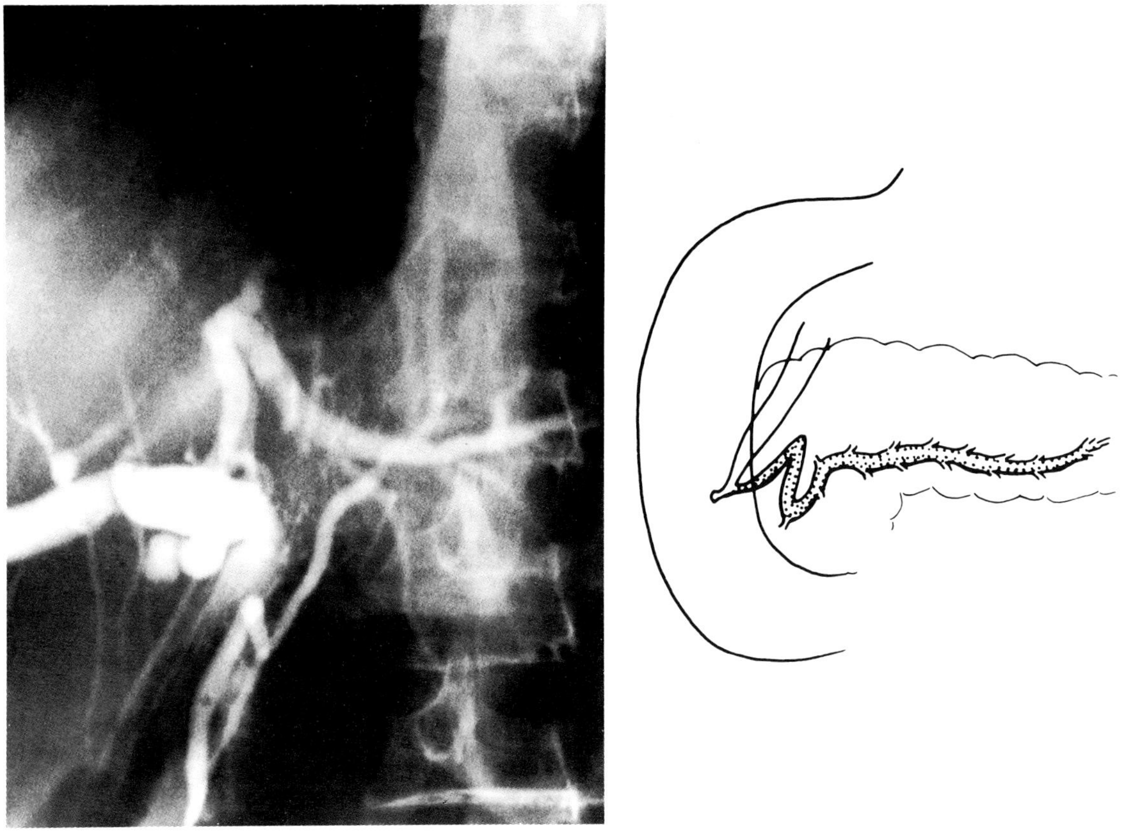

FIG. 4.63. Left: An N configuration in the head of the gland. **Right:** An N variation. From reference 47, with permission.

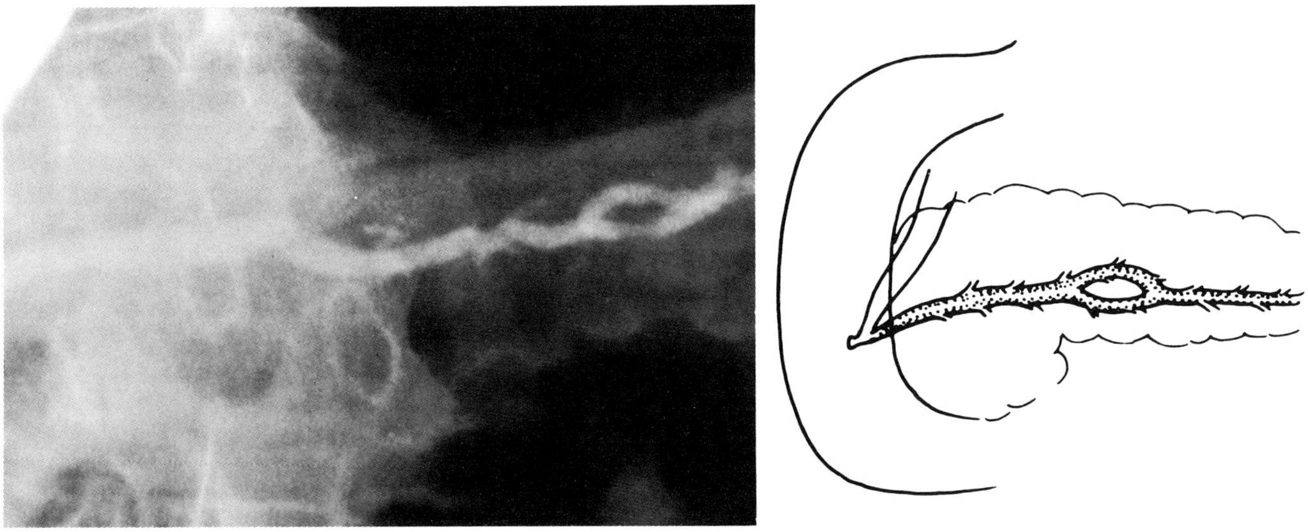

FIG. 4.64. Left: A ring variation of the pancreatic duct located in the tail of the gland. **Right:** Ring variation. From reference 46, with permission.

as an association with alcoholic pancreatitis (46) but also by Japanese and Indian workers who associated this finding with certain disease states such as gallstones and carcinoma of the gallbladder (52–55). Awareness of such variations recorded by pancreatography has become crucial in distinguishing between the normal and disease states. These illustrations are permanently recorded in our enlarging and increasingly definitive atlases of pancreatography.

REFERENCES

1. Rothman MM. Anatomy and physiology of the gallbladder and bile ducts. In: Bockus HL, ed. *Gastroenterology*. Philadelphia: WB Saunders, 1963:567–589.
2. Schwartz SI. *Principles of surgery*. New York: McGraw-Hill, 1969.
3. Glenn F. *Atlas of biliary tract surgery*. New York: MacMillan, 1963.
4. Belber JP. Endoscopic retrograde cholangiopancreatography (ERC) and the skinny needle. In: Slesinger MH, Fortron JS, eds. *Gastrointestinal diseases*. Philadelphia: WB Saunders, 1978.
5. Hamilton I, Ruddell WS, Mitchell CJ, Lintott DJ, Axon AT. Endoscopic retrograde cholangiograms of the normal and postcholecystectomy biliary tree. *Br J Surg* 1982;69:343–5.
6. Yapp RG, Siegel JH. Unexplained biliary tract dilatation in lung cancer patients. A new paraneoplastic syndrome. [Submitted for publication].
7. Thaler MM, Gellis SS. Studies in neonatal hepatitis and biliary atresia. IV diagnosis. *Am J Dis Child* 1968;116:280.
8. Hays DM. Biliary atresia: the current state of confusion. *Surg Clin N Amer* 1973;53:1257.
9. Rosenthal WS, Barone M, Siegel JH. Ultrasonic guided biopsies of the liver in suspected neoplasia. *Digestion* 1977;16:270 (abst).
10. Jennings PE, Coral A, Donald JJ, Coral A, Rode J, Lees WR. Ultrasound-guided core biopsy. *Lancet* 1989;1:1369–71.
11. Parker SH, Hopper KD, Yakes WF, Gibson MD, Ownbey JL, Carter TE. Image directed percutaneous biopsies with a biopsy gun. *Radiology* 1989;171:663–9.
12. Foutch PG, Harlan JR, Kerr D, Sanowski RA. Wire guided brush cytology: a new endoscopic method for diagnosis of bile duct cancer. *Gastrointest Endosc* 1989;35:243–7.
13. Gandolfi L, Muatori R, Solmi L, Rossi A, Leo P. Laparoscopy compared with ultrasonography in the diagnosis of hepatocellular carcinoma. *Gastrointest Endosc* 1989;35:508–11.
14. Herrera JL, Brewer TG, Peura DA. Diagnostic laparoscopy: prospective review of 100 cases. *Am J Gastroenterol* 1989;84:1051–4.
15. Watanabe M, Takatori Y, Ueki K, et al. Pancreatic biopsy under visual control in conjunction with laparoscopy for diagnosis of pancreatic cancer. *Endoscopy* 1989;21:105–7.
16. Michels NA. Blood supply and anatomy of the upper abdominal organs. Philadelphia: JB Lippincott, 1955.
17. Schwartz SI. In: Schwartz SI, ed. *Principles of surgery*. Gallbladder and extrahepatic biliary system. New York: McGraw-Hill, 1974:1221–1224.
18. Newcombe JF, Henley FA. Left sided gallbladder. A review of the literature and a report of a case associated with hepatic duct carcinoma. *Arch Surg* 1964;88:494.
19. Mayo CW, Rice RG. Cholecystitis and cholelithiasis with complete situs inversus viscerum. Report of a case. *Proc Staff Meet Mayo Clin* 1948;23:610.
20. Mayo CW, Kindrick DB. Anomalies of the gallbladder. Report of a case of left sided floating gallbladder. *Arch Surg* 1950;60:668.
21. Nordback I, Airo I. ERCP and endoscopic papillotomy in complete situs inversus. [Letter]. *Gastrointest Endosc* 1988;34:150.
22. Boyden EA. Phrygian cap in cholecystography. A congenital anomaly of the gallbladder. *Am J Roentgenal* 1935;33:589.
23. Moore TC, Hurley AG. Congenital duplication of the gallbladder. Review of the literature and report of an unusual symptomatic case. *Surgery* 1954;35:2–3.
24. Urbaim D, Jeanmart J, Janne P, et al. Double gallbladder with cholestasis: preoperative demonstration by endoscopic retrograde cholangiopancreatography. *Gastrointest Endosc* 1989;35:345–8.
25. Ivy AC, Goldman L. Physiology of biliary tract. *JAMA* 1939;113:2413.
26. Davenport HW. Physiology of the digestive tract. An introductory text. Chicago: The Yearbook Medical Publishers, 1961.
27. Edholm P. Gallbladder evacuation in the normal male induced by cholecystokinin. *Acta Radiol* 1960;53:257.
28. Boyden EA. The anatomy of the choledoduodenal junction in man. *Surg Gynecol Obstet* 1957;104:641.
29. Jacobsen B, Lanner LO, Radberg C. The dynamic variability of the choledochopancreaticoduodenal junction. A roentgen cinematographic investigation. *Acta Radiol* 1959;52:269.
30. Yatto RP, Siegel JH. The role of pancreatiobiliary duct anatomy in the etiology of alcoholic pancreatitis.
31. Alonso-Lej F, Rever WB Jr, Pessagno DJ. Congenital choledochus cyst, with a report of 2 and an analysis of 94 cases. *Int Abst Surg* 1959;108:1.
32. Longmire WP Jr, Mandiola SA, Gordon HE. Congenital cystic disease of the liver and biliary system. *Ann Surg* 1971;174:711.
33. Komi N, Takehara J, Kunitomo K. Choledochal cyst: anomalous arrangement of the pancreatiobiliary ductal system and biliary malignancy. *J Gastroenterol Hepatol* 1989;4:63–74.
34. Boyden EA. The problem of the double ductus choledochus; an interpretation of an accessory bile duct found attached to the pars superior of the duodenum. *Anat Rec* 1932;55:71.
35. Eishendrath DN. Anomalies of the bile ducts and blood vessels as the cause of accidents in biliary surgery. *JAMA* 1918;71:864.
36. Hand BH. An anatomical study of the choledoduodenal area. *Br J Surg* 1963;1:486.
37. Siegel JH, Tone P, Menikeim D. Gallstone pancreatitis: pathogenesis and clinical forms. The emerging role of endoscopic management. *Am J Gastroenterol* 1986;81:774–8.
38. Pincus IJ. Embryology, anatomy and physiology of the pancreas. In: Bockus HL, ed. *Gastroenterology*. 1965; Philadelphia: WB Saunders, 1965:877–887.
39. Kleitsch WP. Anatomy of the pancreas: a study with special reference to the duct system. *Arch Surg* 1955;71:795.
40. Siegel JH. ERCP update: diagnostic and therapeutic applications. *Gastrointest Radiol* 1978;3:311–8.
41. Siegel JH. Endoscopy and papillotomy in diseases of the biliary tract and pancreas. *J Clin Gastroenterol* 1980;2:337–47.
42. Dickinson PB, Belsito AA, Cramer GG. Diagnostic value of endoscopic cholangiopancreatography. *JAMA* 1973;225:944.
43. Vennes JA, Silvis SE. Endoscopic visualization of the bile and pancreatic ducts. *Gastrointest Endosc* 1972;18:149.
44. Kasugai T, Kuno V, Kobayashi S, et al. Endoscopic pancreatocholangiography I. The normal endoscopic pancreatocholangiogram. *Gastroenterology* 1972;63:217.
45. Kasugai T, Kuno N, Kizu M, et al. Endoscopic pancreaticocholangiography. II. The pathological endoscopic pancreatocholangiogram. *Gastroenterol* 1972;63:227.
46. Yatto RP, Siegel JH. Variant pancreatography. *Am J Gastroenterol* 1983;78:115–8.
47. Siegel JH, Yatto RP. Anamolous pancreatic ducts causing pseudomass of the pancreas. *J Clin Gastroenterol* 1983;5:33–6.
48. Siegel JH. Evaluation and treatment of acquired and congenital pancreatic disorders: endoscopic dilatation and insertion of endoprostheses. *Am J Gastroenterol* 1983;78:696 (abst).
49. Cooperman AM, O'Shea JS, Hammerman H, Siegel JH. Pancreatic variants, symptoms and surgery: an ongoing saga. *Gastroenterology* 1987;92:1354 (abst).
50. Yogi Y, Shibue T, Hashimoto S. Annular pancreas detected in adults, diagnosed by endoscopic retrograde cholangiopancreatography: report of four cases. *Gastroenterol Jpn* 1987;22:92–9.

51. Dowsett JF, Rode J, Russell RC. Annular pancreas: a clinical, endoscopic, and immunohistochemical study. *Gut* 1989;30:130–5.
52. Kato O, Hattori K, Suzuki T, Tachino F, Yuasa T. Clinical significance of anomalous pancreaticobiliary union. *Gastrointest Endosc* 1983;29:94–8.
53. Kinoshita H, Nagata E, Hirohashi K, Sakai K, Yasutsugu Y. Carcinoma of the gallbladder with an anomalous connection between the choledochus and the pancreatic duct. *Cancer* 1984;54:762–9.
54. Mirsa SP, Divivedi M. Pancreaticobiliary ductal union. *Gut* 1989;31:1144–9.
55. Yatto RP, Siegel JH. The role of pancreatiobiliary duct anatomy in the etiology of alcoholic pancreatitis. *J Clin Gastroenterol* 1984;6:419–23.

CHAPTER 5

Intrahepatic Cholestasis

An essential component of the performance of ERCP is the ability to interpret both the fluoroscopic images and the radiographs obtained during ERCP. Some endoscopists work in conjunction with a radiologist and therefore rely on the interpretation of the accompanying specialist, and they are not compelled to interpret the films or diagnosis. This, I believe, is a shortcoming because the endoscopist should be completely familiar with not only the endoscopic techniques but the radiographic techniques and the findings. Often the endoscopist must make a decision for therapy based on the findings at ERCP and should be capable of providing therapy simultaneously. Delaying therapy for an official interpretation of the films may lead to other complications and perhaps a lost opportunity to assist in the care of the patient.

After excluding hepatocellular causes of cholestasis and jaundice by history or appropriate laboratory studies, one would recommend cholangiography to define the anatomy of the biliary tree. Adhering to the algorithm in Table 2.2, an endoscopist should perform an ERCP or percutaneous cholangiogram after a screening ultrasound, which is employed to determine whether dilated or nondilated bile ducts are associated with the presenting symptoms and findings. Utilization of ERCP in patients with intrahepatic disease is attributed largely to the experience of the endoscopist. In an earlier work, Sherlock and associates determined that ERCP is a more exact procedure in patients with nondilated ducts, whereas percutaneous cholangiography (PTC) has a higher success rate in patients with a dilated intrahepatic tree (1). This study was performed early in the development of ERCP skills, and the results reflect the authors' inexperience. This statement is certainly no longer true. Experienced endoscopists should successfully opacify the biliary tree, dilated or not, in more than 95% of attempts and the duct of intention (providing or confirming the diagnosis) in at least 94% of attempts (2) (Table 2.2).

Cholangiography, which provides morphology and definition of the bile ducts, is very exact and, thus, confirmatory in suspected disease (3). Occasionally, patients with *acute hepatitis* or *chronic hepatitis,* whose clinical states vary from the usual, require cholangiography to delineate the cause of cholestatic jaundice, but ERCP, although it is more sensitive, may not be necessary in such situations if one conducts a complete assessment of laboratory studies, physical findings, and scanning imaging (4–10). ERCP is certainly complementary to appropriate serologic studies and

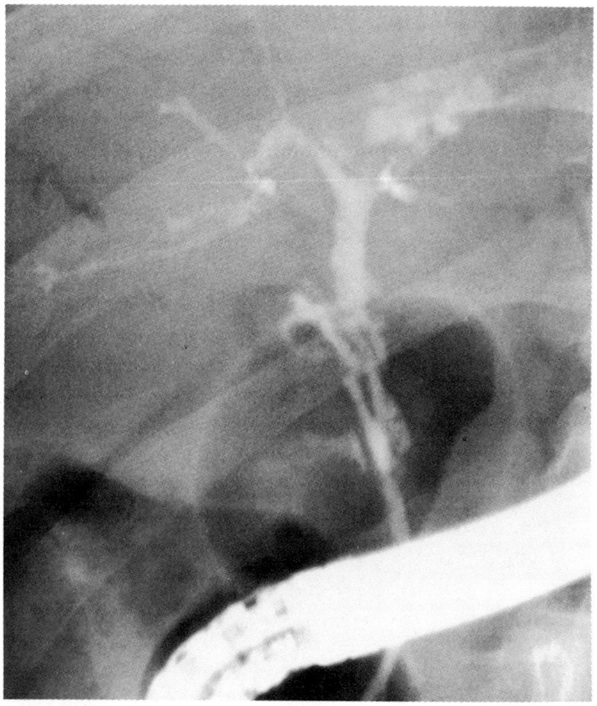

FIG. 5.1. A classic cholangiogram of sclerosing cholangitis showing a paucity of intrahepatic ducts with areas of beading with strictures and dilatation. Evidence of extrahepatic disease is also apparent.

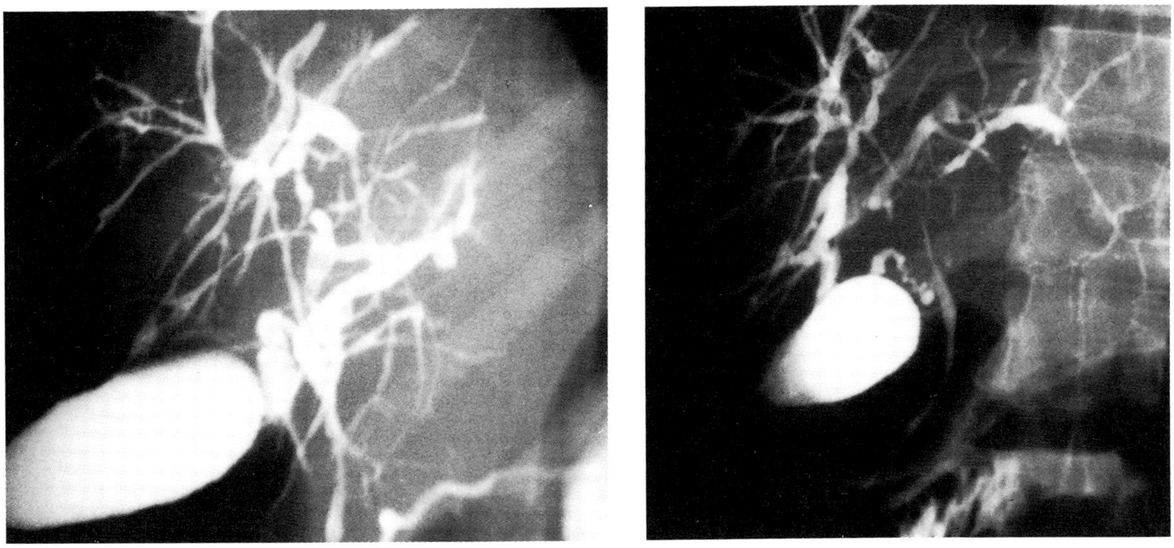

FIG. 5.2. Left: Another classic example of intrahepatic and extrahepatic sclerosing cholangitis with beading, strictures, and dilatation. **Right:** Profound evidence of sclerosing cholangitis. Specific changes affecting both the intra- and extrahepatic ducts are noted and present a stringlike appearance.

liver biopsy, but specific findings on cholangiography are confirmatory for *primary sclerosing cholangitis* and *primary biliary cirrhosis,* especially when other modalities are not diagnostic or equivocal (Figs. 5.1–5.8) (11–22). In diseases affecting the hepatic parenchyma, random percutaneous biopsies may be nondiagnostic, inconsistent with, or nonspecific for disease, whereas cholangiography usually corroborates the diagnosis (23). Certainly the question of coexisting malignancy—for example, *cholangiocarcinoma*—in

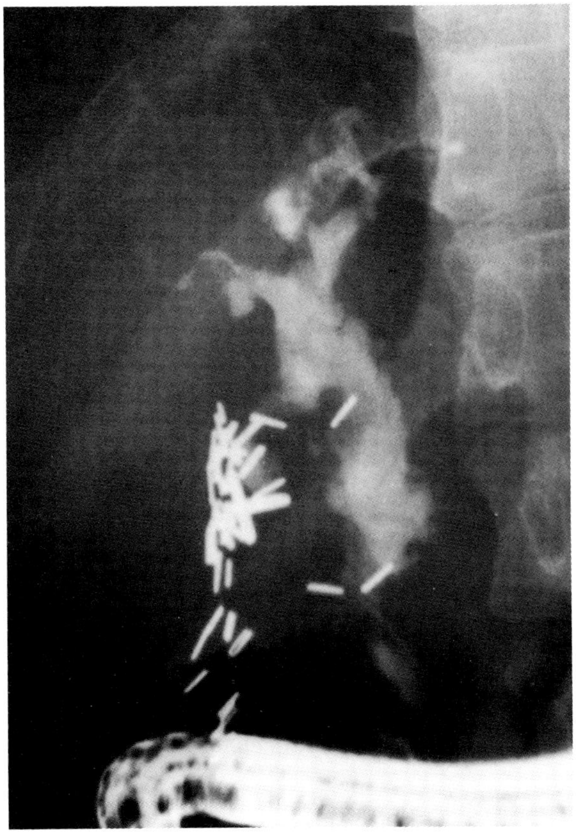

FIG. 5.3. Severe changes of both extrahepatic and intrahepatic disease consistent with sclerosing cholangitis. The patient had undergone previous cholecystectomy. Note the dilated bile ducts and diffuse irregularities of both the extra- and intrahepatic systems.

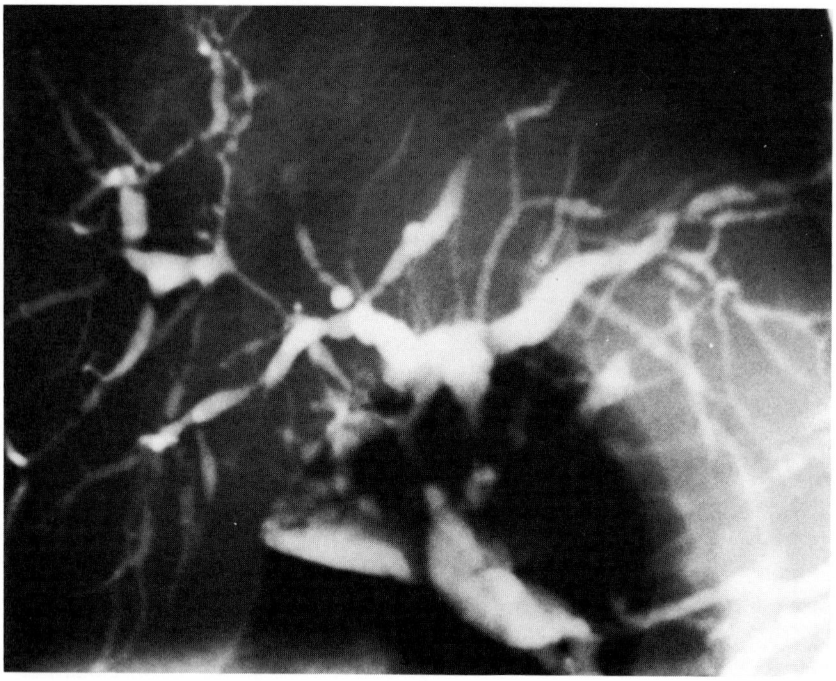

FIG. 5.4. Diffuse intra- and extrahepatic changes of sclerosing cholangitis.

patients with sclerosing cholangitis is troublesome. Adequate brushings or tissue should be obtained from the affected ducts for histologic and cytologic evaluation prior to other therapeutic maneuvers, chemotherapy, or radiotherapy (24–25).

Cirrhosis of any cause presents a characteristic radiograph, in many cases, and the cholangiogram is helpful in formulating a differential diagnosis (Figs. 5.9–5.17). Cholestasis associated with *chronic hepatitis,* cirrhosis, and coexisting portal hypertension often requires ERCP for definition because performance of a liver biopsy in individuals with coagulopathy is contraindicated (Fig. 5.18). Few noninvasive tests confirm or support *hepatocellular carcinoma,* but in most cases, the cholangiogram is specific (Figs. 5.19, 5.20) (26). *Metastatic disease* to the liver, (intrahepatic without evidence of extrahepatic obstruction),

Text continues on page 69.

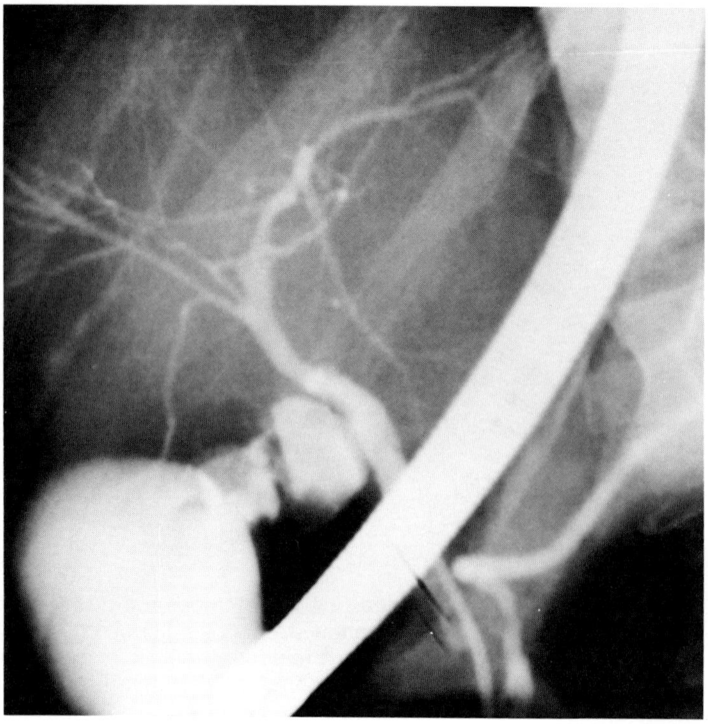

FIG. 5.5. A cholangiogram obtained in a study carried out on a middle-aged woman who presented with abnormal immunologic studies, including an elevated IgM; an elevated alkaline phosphatase; and gamma glutamyl transpepsidase. Findings of thin, tapered intrahepatic ducts consistent primary biliary cirrhosis are noted.

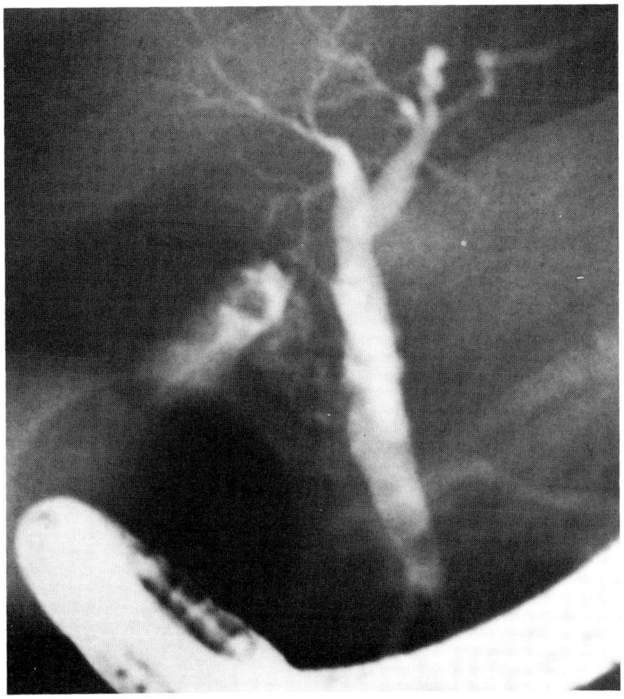

FIG. 5.6. A cholangiogram obtained in a patient with negative mitochondrial antibodies but with cholestatic parameters and pruritis. Note the thin, tapered intrahepatic ducts consistent with primary biliary cirrhosis. In this example, the ducts do not demonstrate arborization and do not extend to the periphery of the liver.

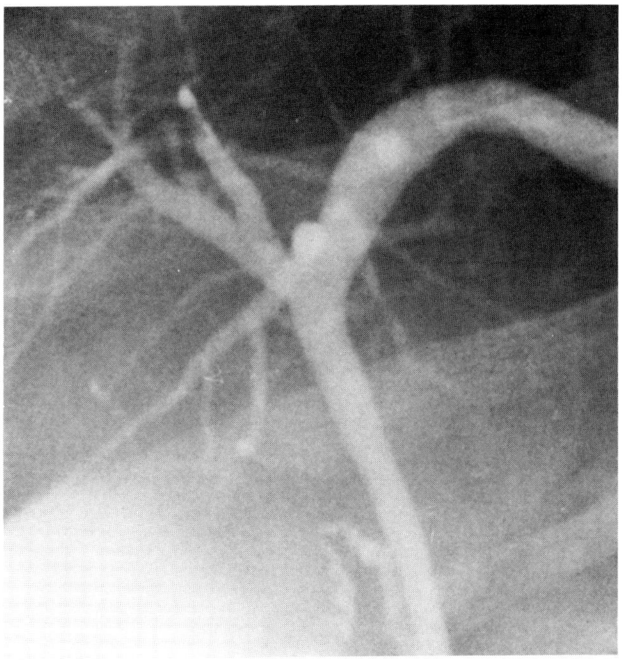

FIG. 5.8. A cholangiogram consistent with primary biliary cirrhosis. Note the paucity of intrahepatic ducts and failure of the ducts to extend to the periphery of the liver. Also note the dilated left hepatic duct, which is probably a congenital variant in this patient.

A

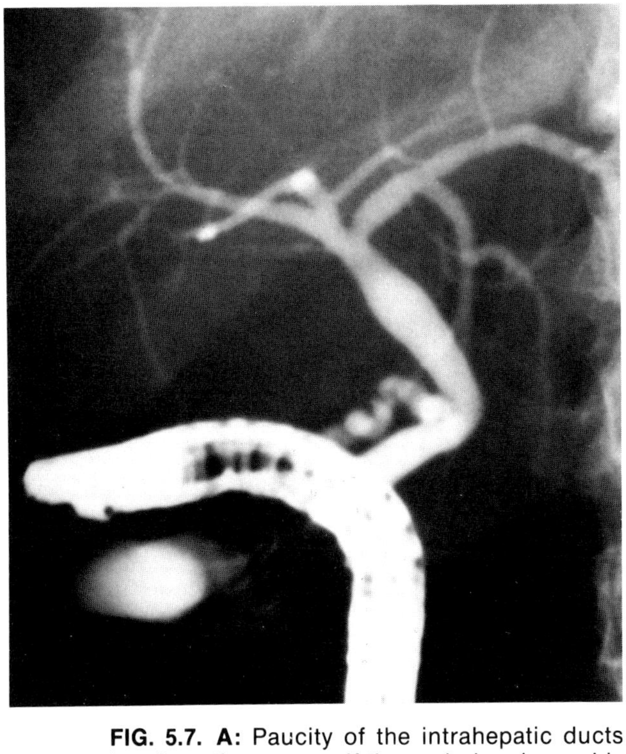

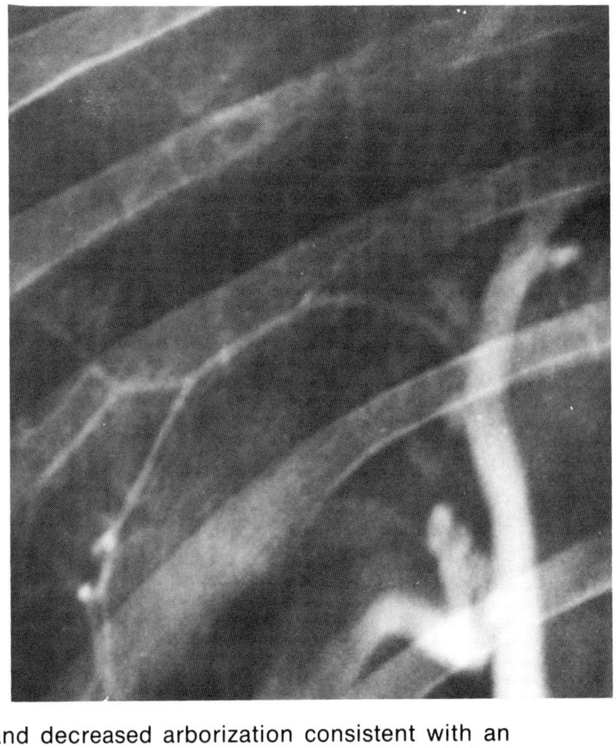

B

FIG. 5.7. A: Paucity of the intrahepatic ducts and decreased arborization consistent with an intrahepatic process. If these cholangiographic findings are correlated with the patient's clinical history and appropriate serologic studies, primary biliary cirrhosis would be included in differential diagnosis. **B:** A cholangiogram compatible with primary biliary cirrhosis. Note the incomplete filling of the intrahepatic ducts and rigidity of these ducts.

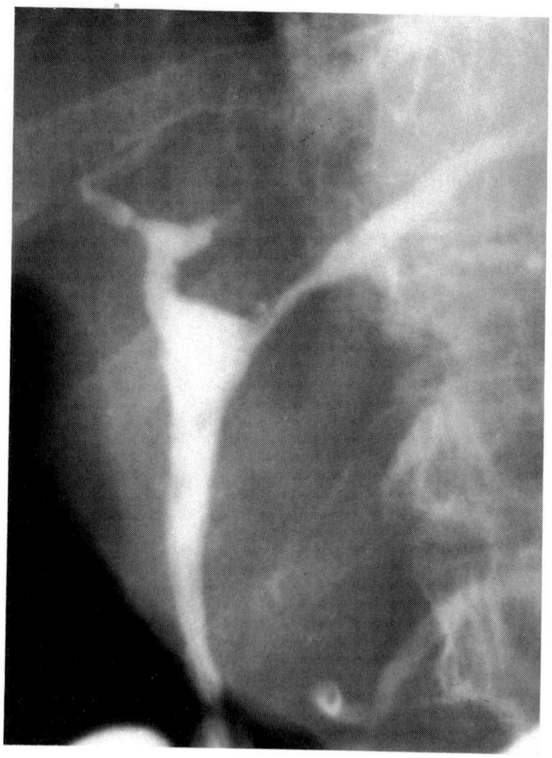

FIG. 5.9. Incomplete filling of the intrahepatic ducts, probably owing to a cirrhotic nodule. The patient had a prior history of hepatitis in the past. Postnecrotic nodules in the liver account for displacement of the major ducts and prevent filling of other ducts.

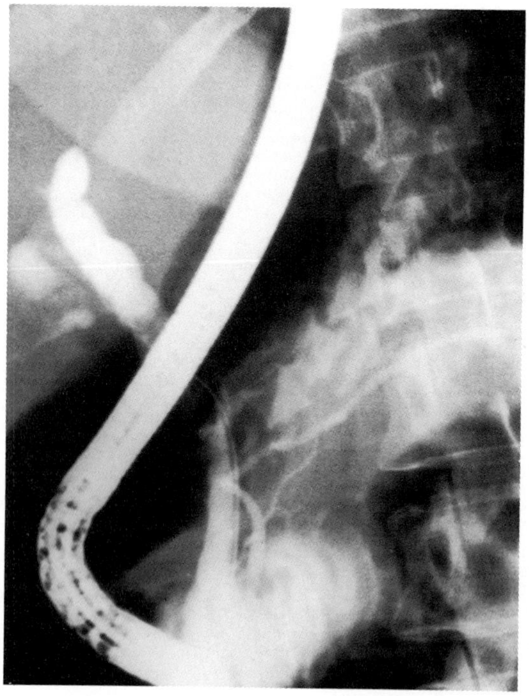

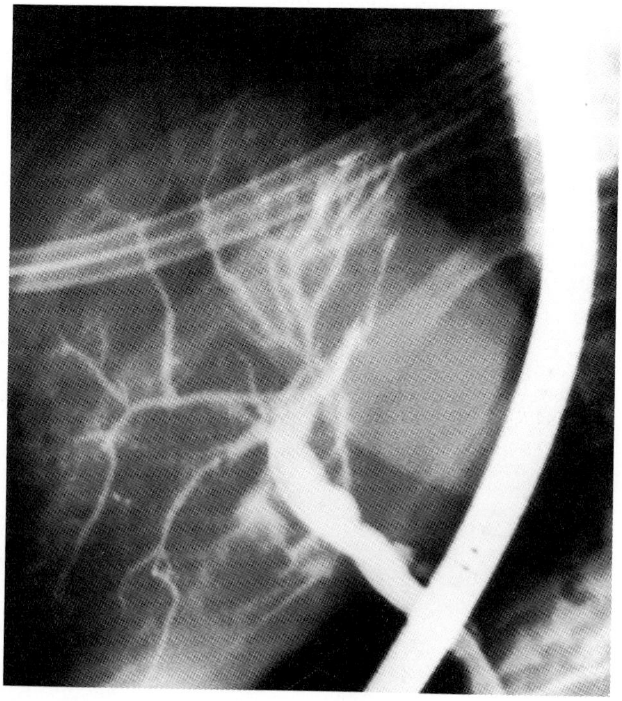

FIG. 5.10. Left: Deep cannulation of the bile duct was accomplished in this study. The bile duct is dilated, and little or no filling of the intrahepatic ducts is noted on this cholangiogram. **Right:** A cholangiogram obtained after deep cannulation of the bile duct using a catheter and guidewire. Compression of the porta hepatis by a cirrhotic nodule prevented retrograde filling until the catheter was passed through the obstruction. The intrahepatic ducts are rigid and sparce in the compressed left lobe. Note the filling of liver sinusoids and parenchyma consistent with regenerative nodules. Similar cholangiographic findings have been seen in patients with chronic active hepatitis.

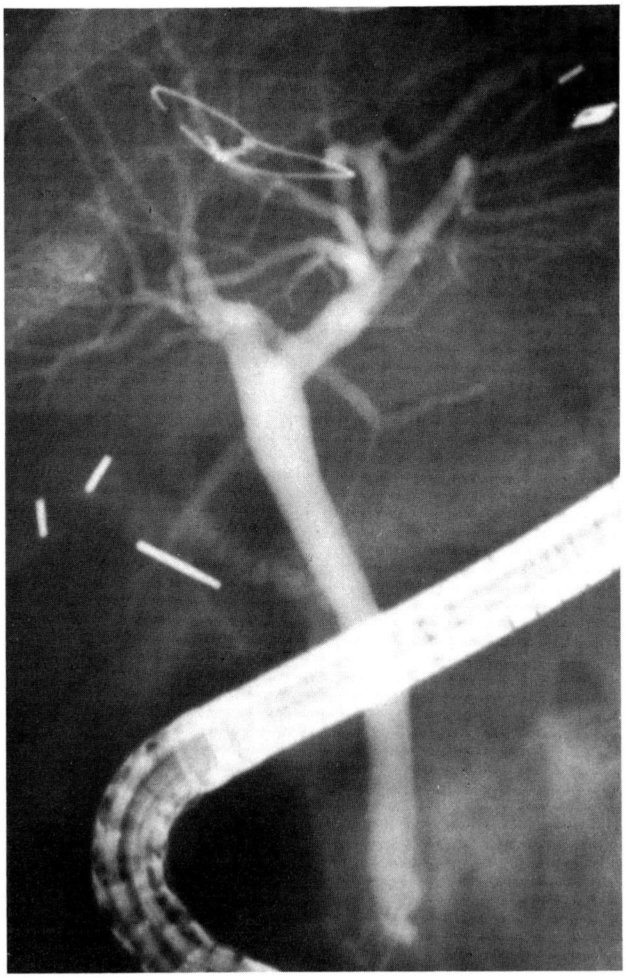

FIG. 5.11. Changes of intrahepatic ducts in a patient with cardiac cirrhosis (note metal sutures in sternum). Attenuation of intrahepatic ducts and, particularly, an abnormal area are evident in the right lobe of the parenchyma, which resulted from erratic regeneration of the ducts.

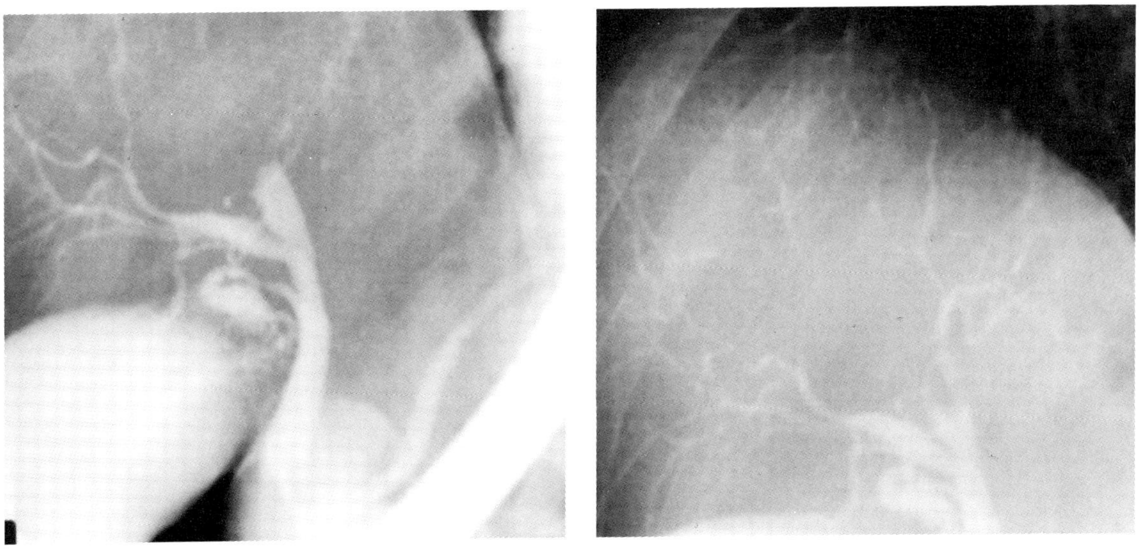

FIG. 5.12. Left: Incomplete filling of left lobe of the liver. The ducts of the right lobe are thin, tapered, and attenuated secondary to fibrotic changes. **Right:** The left hepatic duct system is opacified after selective cannulation of the bile duct; again, note sparce distribution of intrahepatic ducts that are attenuated. The midportion of the liver is not opacified despite deep cannulation because of fibrosis. The middle lobe ducts are completely stenotic.

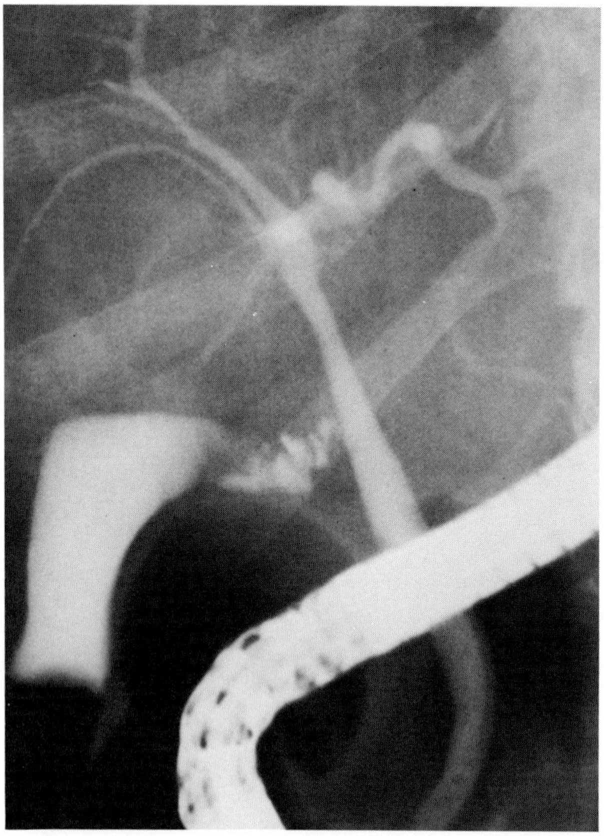

FIG. 5.13. A cholangiogram suggesting that the stretched, attenuated ducts of the right lobe of the liver are secondary to a cirrhotic nodule. Note the blunting of the apex of the gallbladder, which is lying on distended bowel. Appreciation of such normal variations of the anatomy avoid misdiagnoses. On fluoroscopy, during the dynamic portion of the examination, the apex of the gallbladder was normal on expiration and flattened on inspiration.

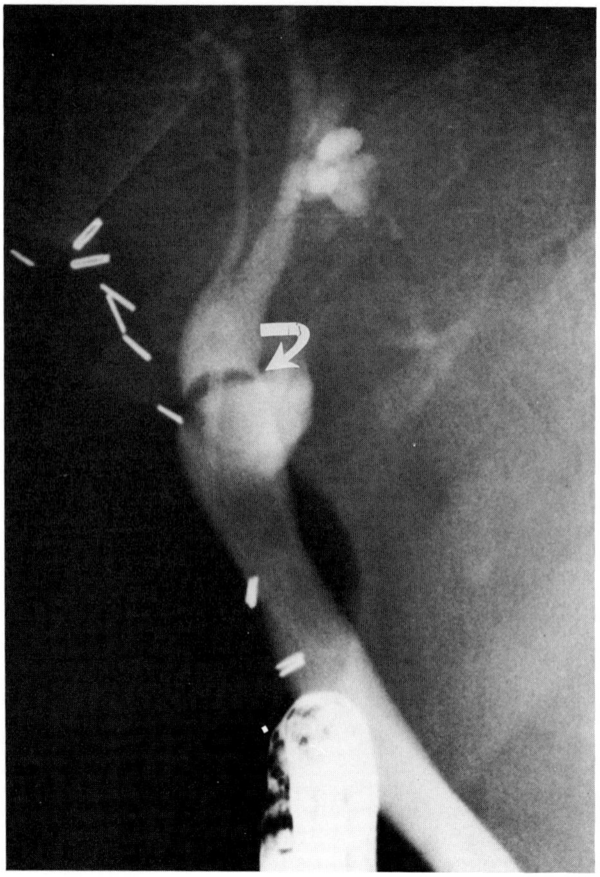

FIG. 5.14. A distended common bile duct resulting from injection of contrast. Poor filling of the intrahepatic ducts is a direct result of cirrhosis. Even after placement of a balloon into the porta hepatis (proximal lucency) (*arrow*), the right duct system filled poorly. The left system demonstrated more filling but comparable findings. The intrahepatic ducts are tapered and attenuated by fibrosis, with no filling of the periphery of the liver.

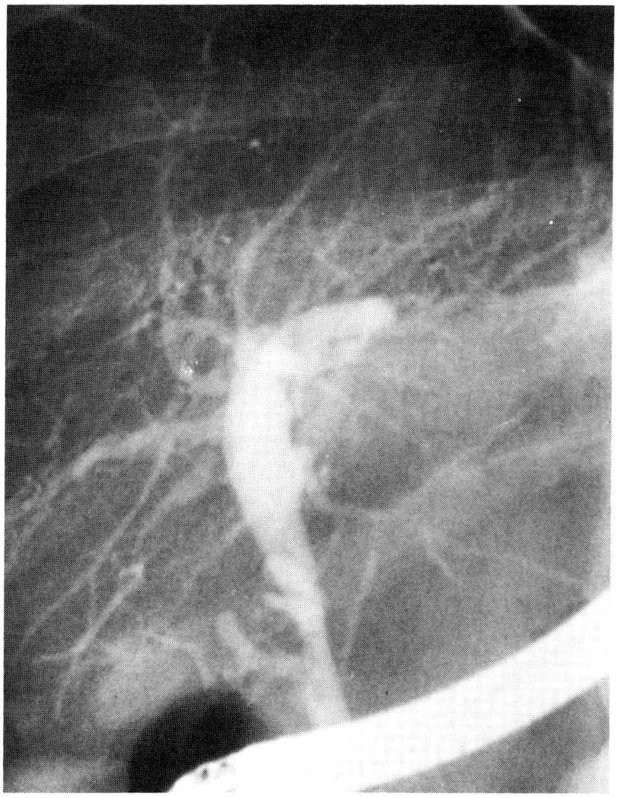

FIG. 5.15. Filling of most of the intrahepatic tree is appreciated on this study, but attenuation of the ducts is present, confirming a diffuse process consistent with chronic active hepatitis or cirrhosis.

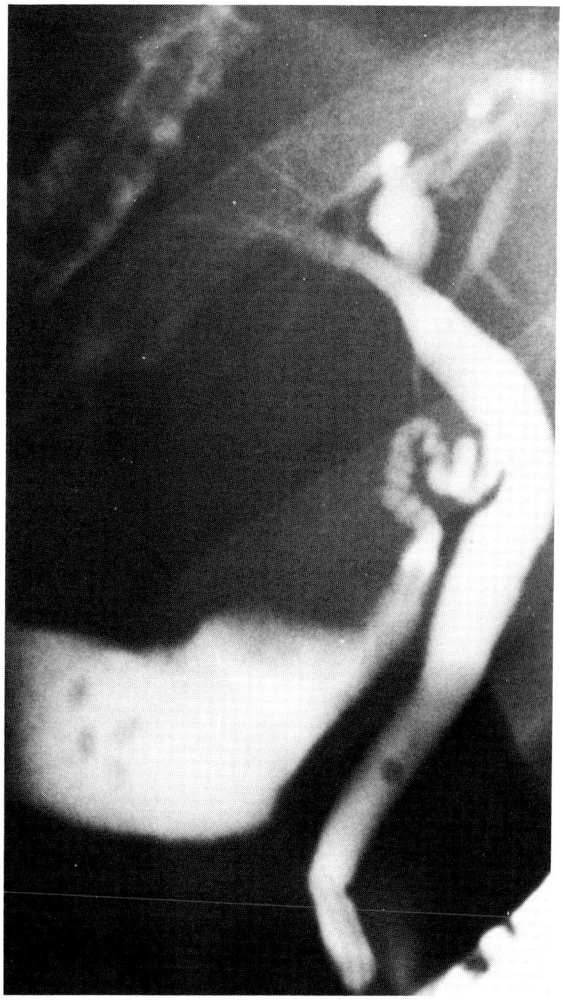

FIG. 5.16. Evidence of cholelithiasis is seen on this ERCP study. An air bubble artifact is present in the distal common bile duct. Poor filling of the intrahepatic tree is noted and is worse on the right. These findings are compatible with fibrosis, and, because of the presence of gallstones, biliary cirrhosis may be responsible for the attenuated ducts.

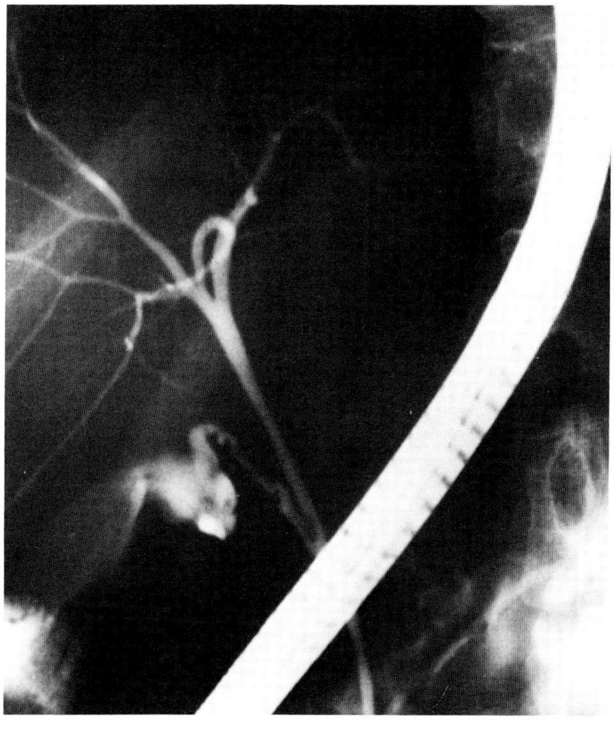

FIG. 5.17. Thin, tapered bile ducts with areas of separation characteristic of fatty infiltration, another intrahepatic cause of cholestasis.

A
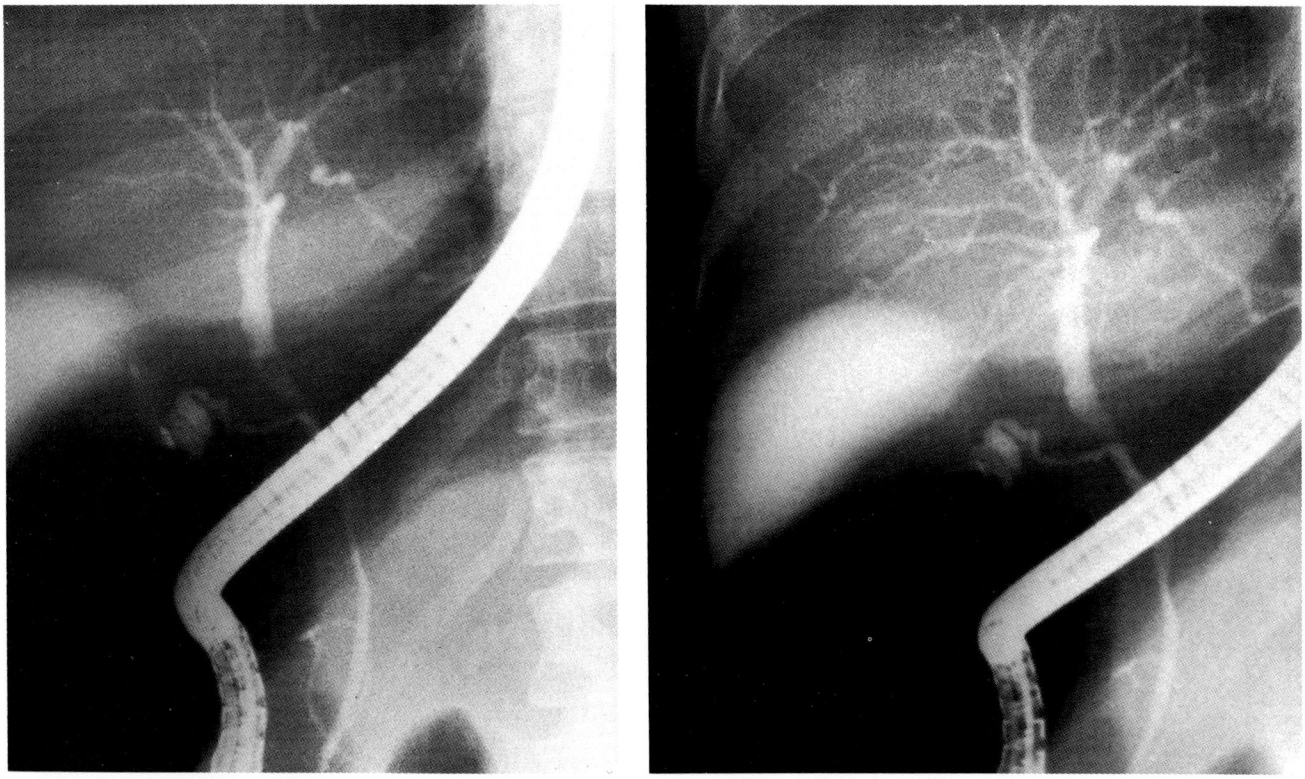

FIG. 5.18. A: This ERCP shows incomplete filling of the biliary tree secondary to chronic hepatitis and active cirrhosis. Portal hypertension was evident clinically. **B:** After deep cannulation of the bile duct, complete filling of the biliary tree is noted. Attenuation of the ducts is confirmatory for intrahepatic disease. Again note the displaced gallbladder secondary to a distended bowel.

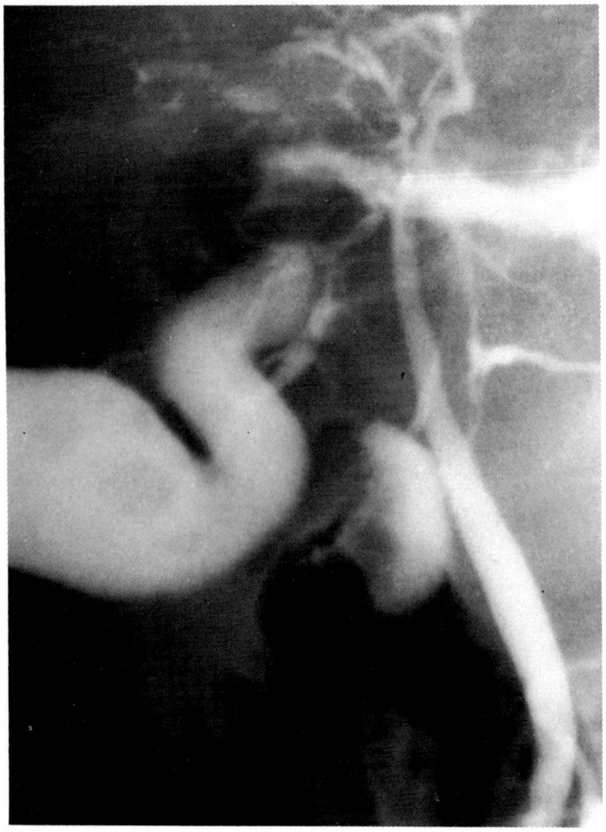

FIG. 5.19. Attenuation of the intrahepatic biliary tree. Pruning and disruption of the ducts secondary to hepatocellular carcinoma and incidental gallstones are evident.

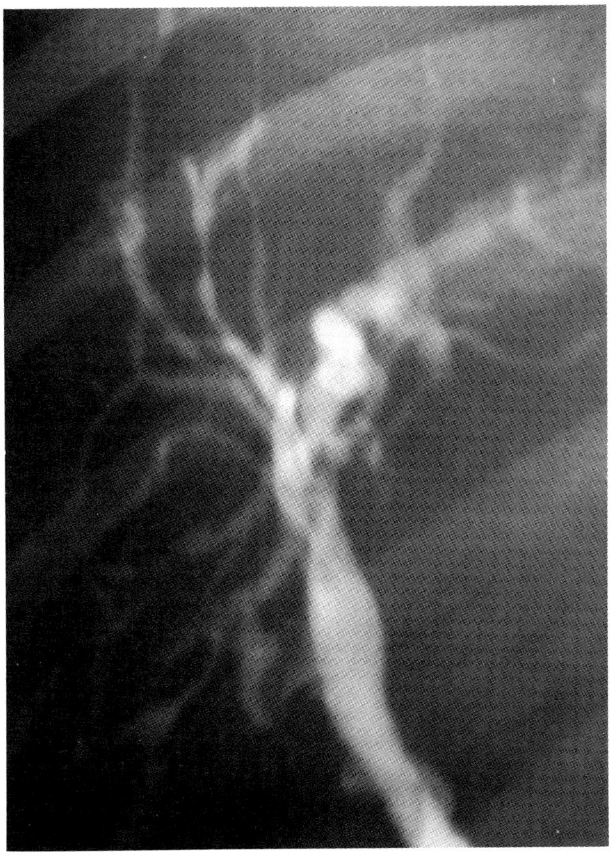

FIG. 5.20. Diffuse changes of the intrahepatic biliary tree secondary to hepatocellular carcinoma. Note attenuation, pruning, and displacement of the ducts, which are diffuse and present throughout the liver.

Text continued from page 62.
another cause for cholestatic jaundice, may present with nondilated biliary radicals, but its appearance is usually varied (Figs. 5.21–5.24) (27–29). One can appreciate encasement of the biliary radicals, which I believe are analagous to the more specific confirmatory findings reported on angiography, especially because the biliary radicals and vascular structures are parallel in the triads. In addition, cholangiography graphically illustrates displacement of liver radicals resulting from metastatic nodules. In order to provide appropriate therapy, it is imperative to differentiate the etiology of cholestasis and to determine whether it is due to metastatic disease or intrahepatic disease resulting from a toxic drug reaction (hypersensitivity) or chemotherapy (30–44). Figure 5.25 illustrates diffuse, intrahepatic changes following long-term arterial perfusion of the liver with 5-FUDR. These changes, which are temporal, are reversible in some cases and can simulate the cholangiographic changes seen with sclerosing cholangitis; often, after discontinuing the medication, the biliary morphology returns to the preperfusion status.

Diffuse changes of the entire biliary tree (45–49) and liver (50–54) have been demonstrated by ERCP in patients with AIDS-related infections such as *cytomeg-*
Text continues on page 73.

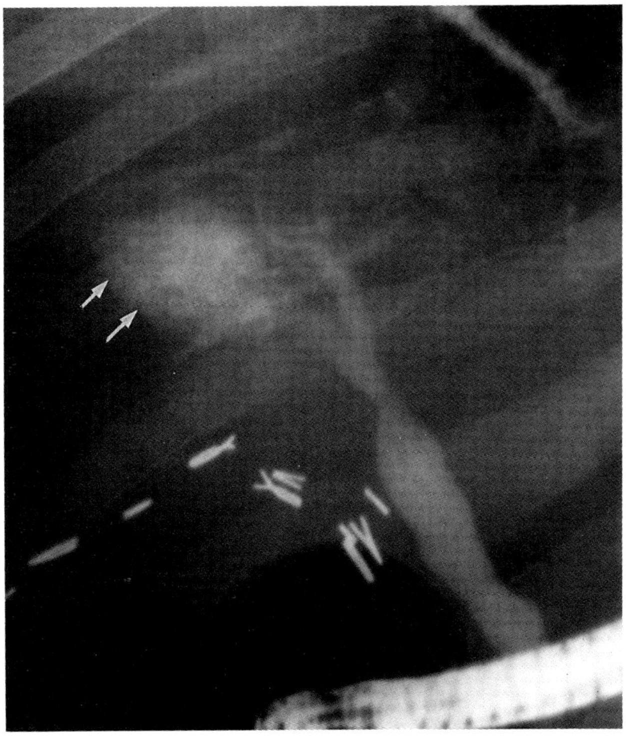

FIG. 5.21. This ERCP shows displaced, attenuated biliary radicals with minimal filling of the intrahepatic ducts. The collection of contrast in the right lobe (*arrows*) may be secondary to filling of necrotic space.

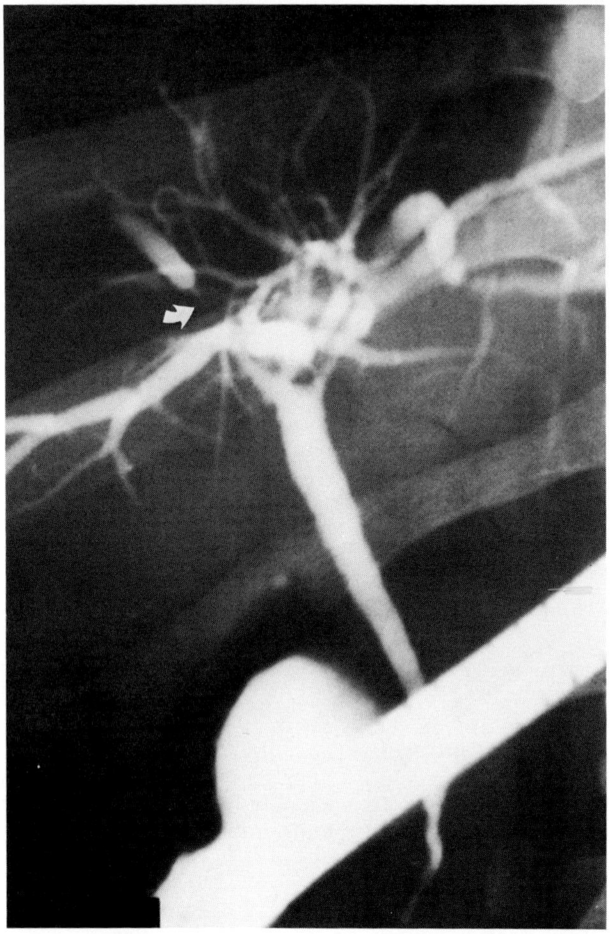

A

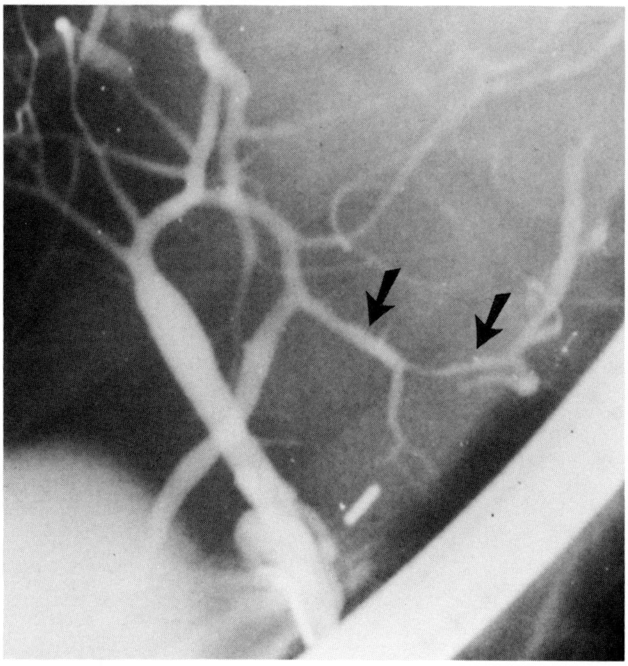

B

FIG. 5.22. **A:** Evidence of metastatic disease to the liver, more evident in the right lobe, is noted on this ERCP. Attenuation, stretching, and displacement of the ducts are present. Encasement of one duct is highlighted by an arrow. **B:** Another example of metastatic disease. Attenuation and displacement of the ducts is evident especially in the left lobe (*arrows*).

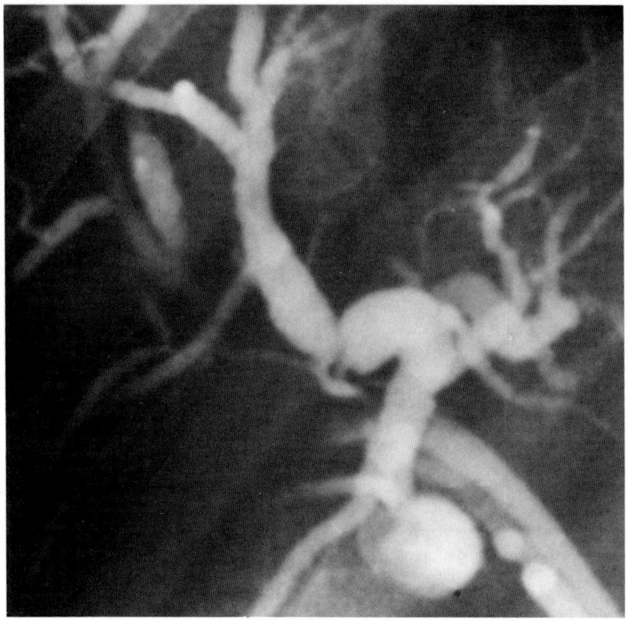

FIG. 5.23. Evidence of metastatic disease to the liver. Note encasement of the branches of the right lobe, which is associated with tapering and pruning.

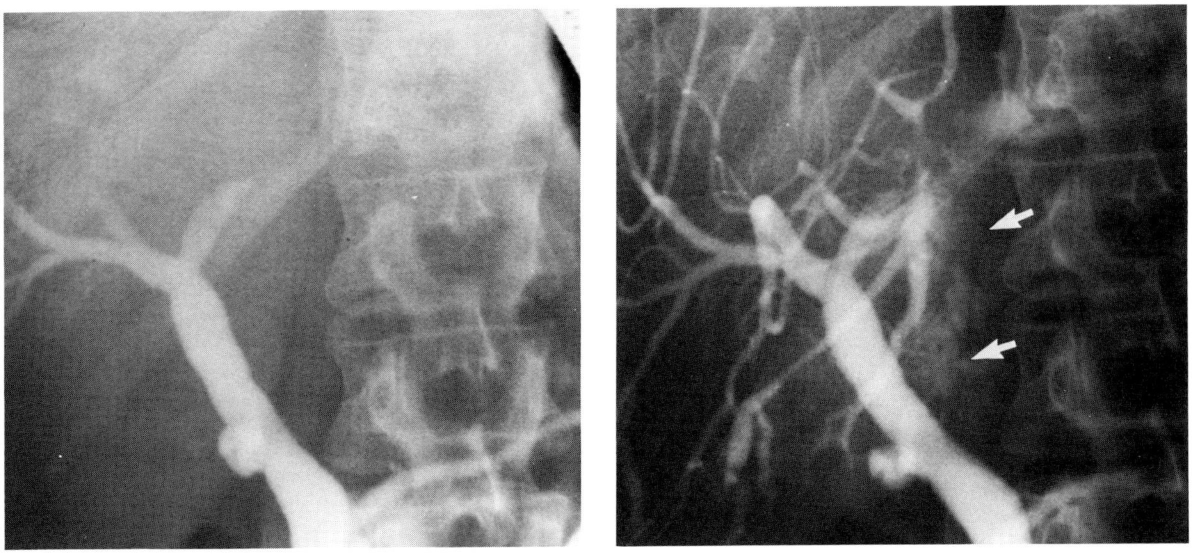

FIG. 5.24. Left: A cholangiogram in a patient with metastatic carcinoma to the liver. Incomplete filling of the biliary tree is seen on initial injection of contrast. **Right:** Diffuse intrahepatic changes in the liver after deep insertion of the cannula, filling all radicals. Radicals of the right lobe are attenuated and displaced, whereas the left lobe fills incompletely. Encasement and pruning of these radicals are noted. Parenchymal filling (*arrows*) indicates necrotic changes.

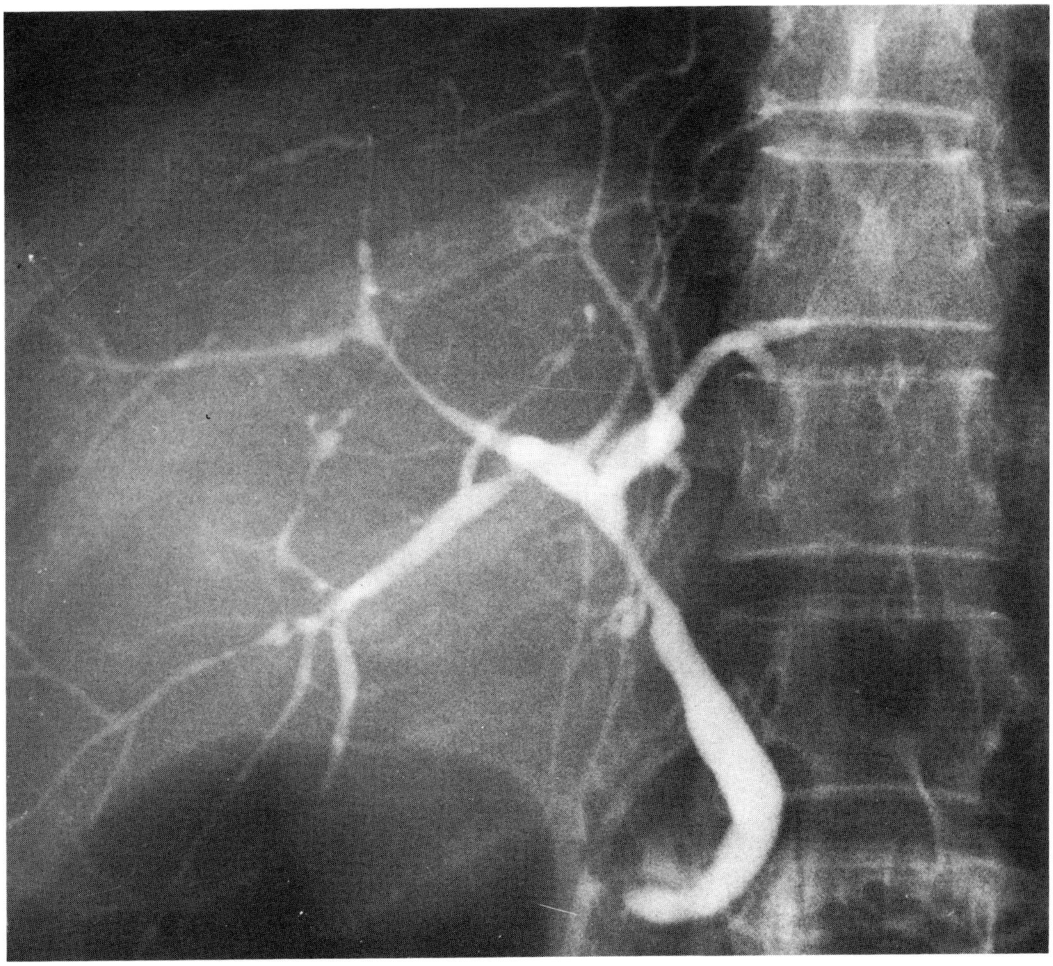

FIG. 5.25. ERCP of a patient with metastatic colon cancer to the liver treated with intraarterial perfusion 5-FUDR. A diffuse intrahepatic process developed, simulating sclerosing cholangitis. After the drug was discontinued, the liver morphology returned to normal on cholangiography. The infusion pump catheter is seen at the junction of the mid- and lower portions of the common bile duct. From reference 44, with permission.

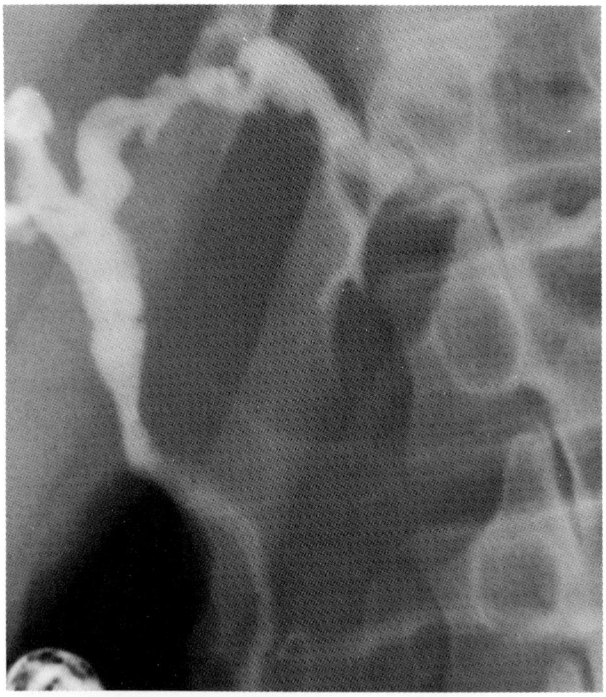

A

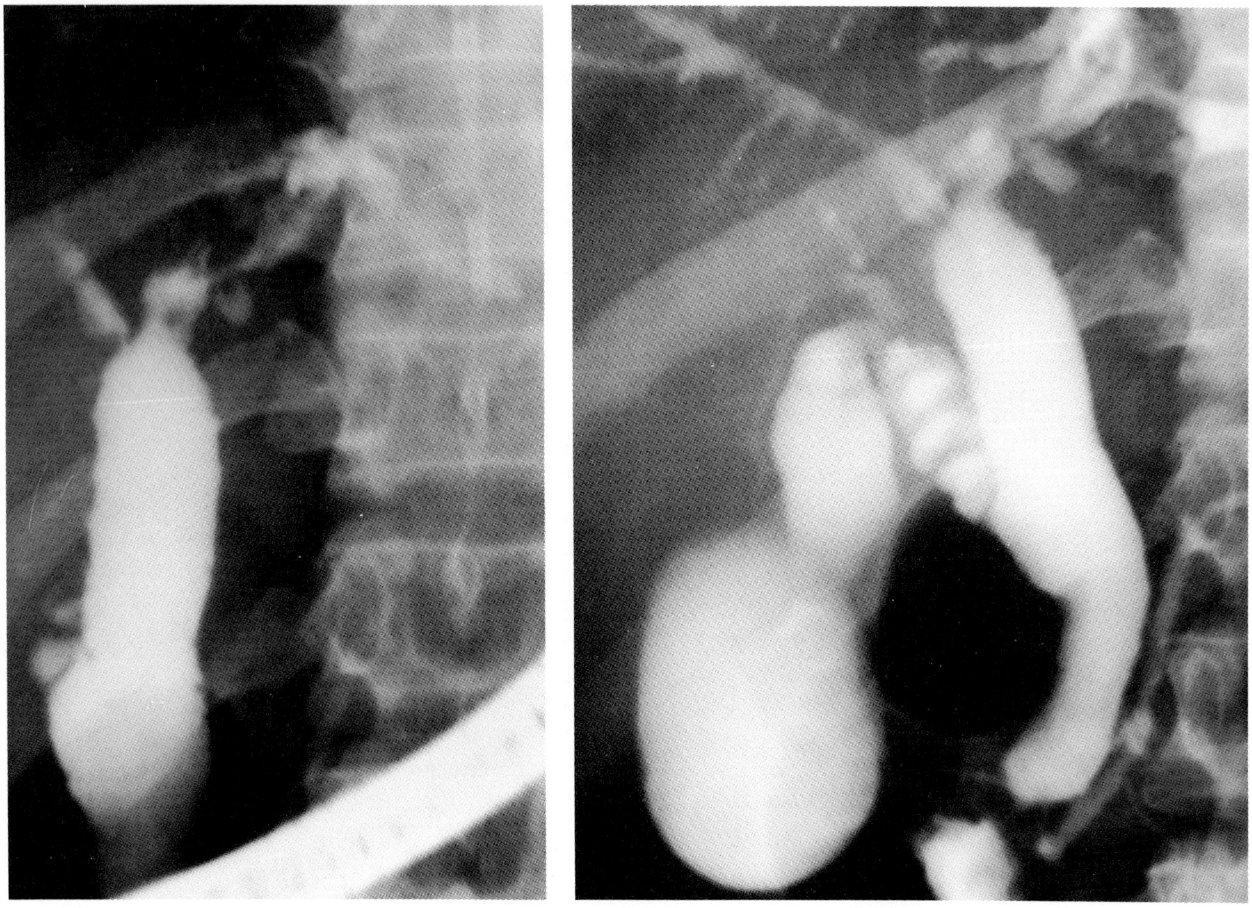

B

FIG. 5.26. A: Diffuse intrahepatic changes seen on cholangiography obtained in a former I.V. drug abuse patient who presented with a positive HIV test and biochemical evidence of cholestasis. Cytomegalovirus infection of the biliary tree has been shown to produce these changes. **B: Left:** A dilated bile duct with serrations. Strictures and irregularity of the intrahepatic ducts are seen, consistent with inflammatory disease found in a patient with AIDS. **Right:** More filling of the intrahepatic ducts and gallbladder after a catheter is placed more deeply into the duct. Note evidence of papillary stenosis.

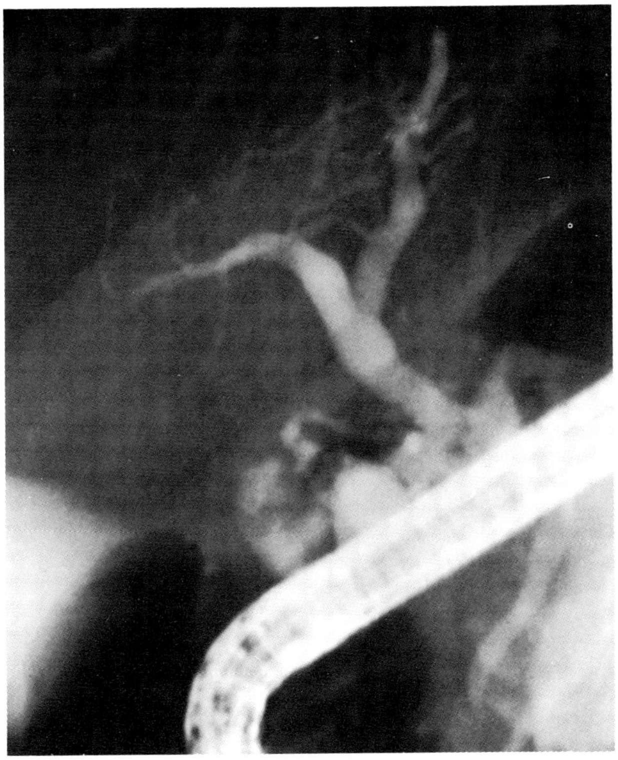

FIG. 5.27. Incomplete filling of the intrahepatic ducts in a patient with AIDS. Attenuation of the smaller radicals is noted. These findings are compatible with a diffuse, intrahepatic process such as chronic active hepatitis. Luetic hepatitis was confirmed on biopsy.

Text continued from page 69.
alovirus disease, herpes virus, and *cryptosporidia*. In my experience, ERCP has been confirmatory in AIDS-related cholecystitis, cholangitis (Fig. 5.26), and papillary stenosis, and sphincterotomy and/or placement of prostheses have mollified this syndrome, improving the cholestatic picture. One patient with AIDS was found on cholangiography to have severe intrahepatic changes consistent with hepatocellular disease (Fig. 5.27), and the differential diagnosis included prescription drug–induced cholestasis (he had been on numerous medications) versus intercurrent disease. Luetic hepatitis was found on liver biopsy (55).

Cystic diseases of the liver, which include congenital disease and hydatid disease, may be responsible for cholestasis, cholangitis, or other symptoms such as abdominal pain and fullness secondary to the mass effect of the cysts. Fig. 5.28 is a cholangiogram obtained in a patient with Caroli's disease who presented with recurrent sepsis attributed to multiple intrahepatic cysts. In this example, the cysts, which communicate with the bile duct as shown in the cholangiogram, became infected. One must also be aware that neoplastic changes can occur in these cysts, and these patients should be followed closely to detect degenerative changes that may be associated with neoplasia. The increasing utilization of ERCP in confirming the diagnosis of cystic diseases of the liver and bile ducts and in providing therapeutic decompression, in some cases, is gaining wide acceptance (56–63).

A striking example of a solitary, communicating liver cyst is shown in Figure 5.29. The patient, a young woman, presented with an elevated alkaline phosphatase and right upper quadrant discomfort. All tests for parasites were negative, and no abnormal immunologic studies were found. A CT scan revealed the presence of a cystic mass in the right lobe of the liver, and the ERCP demonstrated the large, communicating cyst.

Figure 5.30 shows a remarkable example of cystic disease of the liver. This patient had increasing abdominal discomfort and girth. The CT scan shows nearly total occupation of the liver with cysts, and the ERCP demonstrated displacement and attentuation of the intrahepatic ducts without communication with the cysts.

The utility of ERCP in the diagnosis and management of intrahepatic disease is therefore well appreciated, and our increasing reliance on its performance is based on its specificity (see Table 2.1).

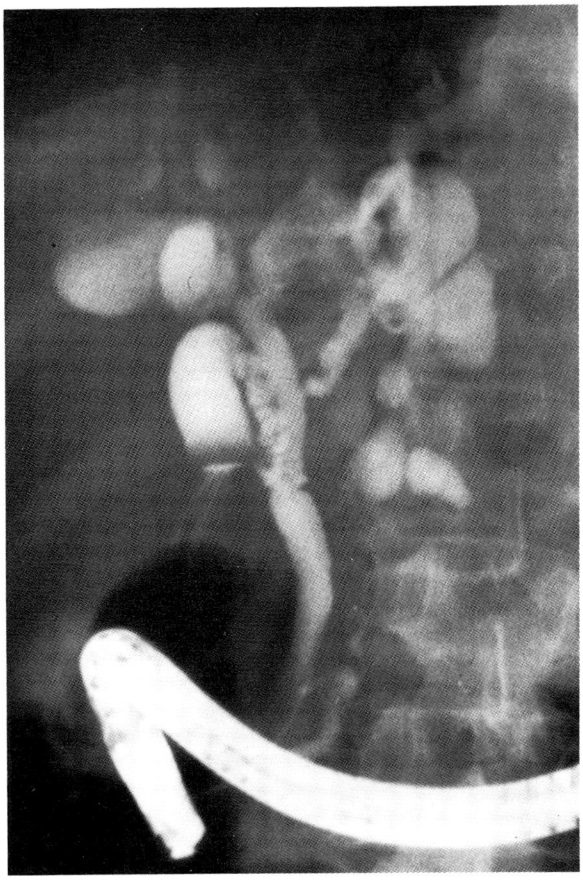

FIG. 5.28. A cholangiogram demonstrating communicating intrahepatic cysts consistent with Caroli's disease. The patient presented with sepsis secondary to infection of the cysts.

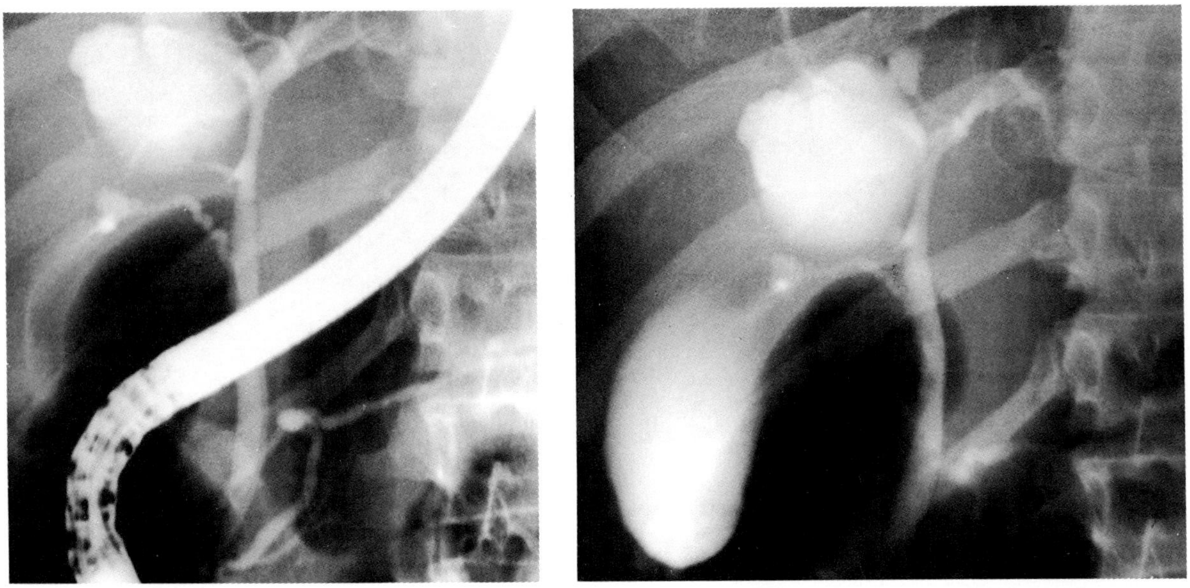

FIG. 5.29. A communicating solitary liver cyst in a patient in whom a CT scan demonstrated a cystic mass.

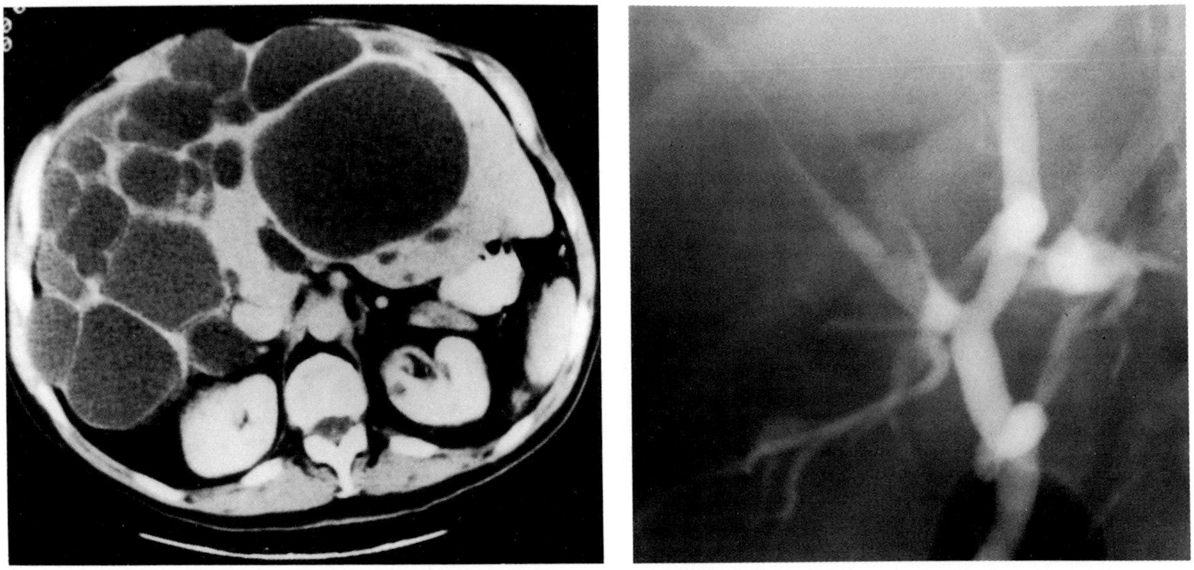

FIG. 5.30. Left: A CT scan showing multiple intrahepatic cysts occupying most of the liver. **Right:** The cholangiogram in this case demonstrates pruning and attenuation of the intrahepatic ducts without evidence of communication. These changes are secondary to compression of the ducts by the intrahepatic cysts.

REFERENCES

1. Elias E, Hamlyn AN, Jain S, et al. A randomized trial of percutaneous transhepatic cholangiography with the Chiba needle versus endoscopic retrograde cholangiography for bile duct visualization in jaundice. *Gastroenterology* 1976;71:439.
2. Siegel JH. Endoscopic approach to management of hepaticopancreatico-biliary disorders. In: Bengmark S, ed. *Progress in surgery of the liver, pancreas and biliary system*. Dordreeht, The Netherlands: Martinus Nijhoff, 1988:57–94.
3. Ayoole EA, Vennes JA, Silvis SE, et al. Endoscopic retrograde intrahepatic cholangiography in liver diseases. *Gastrointest Endosc* 1976;22:156.
4. O'Connor KW, Snodgrass PJ, Swonder JE, Mahoney S, et al. A blinded prospective study comparing four current noninvasive approaches in the differential diagnosis of medical versus surgical jaundice.
5. Gupta S, Owshalimpur D, Cohen G, Margules R, Herrera N. Scintigraphic detection of segmental bile duct obstruction. *J Nucl Med* 1982;23:89–91.
6. Takeda I, Nakano S, Watahiki H. Diagnostic ability of hepatobiliary scintigraphy. *Gastroenterol Jpn* 1982;17:201–6.
7. Borsch G, Wegener M, Wedmann B, Kissler M, Glocke M. Clinical evaluation, ultrasound, cholescintigraphy, and endoscopic retrograde cholangiography in cholestasis. A prospective comparative clinical study. *J Clin Gastroenterol* 1988;10:185–90.
8. Salem S, Vas W. Ultrasonography in evaluation of the jaundiced patient. *J Can Assoc Radiol* 1981;32:30–4.
9. Huang MJ, Kiaw YF, Wu CS. Comparison of intravenous radionuclide c cholescintigraphy and endoscopic retrograde cholangiography in the diagnosis of intrahepatic gallstones. *Br J Radiol* 1981;54:302–6.
10. Ginestal-Cruz A, Pinto-Correia J, Camilo E, Grima N, et al. Combined approach to the differential diagnosis of cholestastic percutaneous transhepatic cholangiography, ultrasonography, and liver biopsy. *Gastrointest Radiol* 1981;6:177–83.
11. Summerfield JA, Elias E, Hungerford MB, et al. The biliary system in primary biliary cirrhosis: a study by endoscopic retrograde cholangiopancreatography. *Gastroenterology* 1976; 70:240.
12. Legg DA, Carlson HC, Dickson ER, et al. Cholangiographic findings in cholangiolitic hepatitis. Syndrome of primary biliary cirrhosis. *Am J Roent* 1971;113:16.
13. Siegel JH. Endoscopic management of benign biliary strictures, biliary tract fistulae and sclerosing cholangitis. In: Jacobson IM, ed. *ERCP. Diagnostic and therapeutic applications*. New York: Elsevier Scientific Publications, 1989.
14. Legge DA, Carlson HC, Ludwig J. Cholangiographic findings in diseases of the liver: a post mortem study. *Am J Roent* 1971;113:34.
15. Elias E, Summerfield JA, Dick K, et al. Endoscopic retrograde cholangiopancreatography in the diagnosis of jaundice associated with ulcerative colitis. *Gastroenterology* 1974;67:907.
16. Sivak MV Jr, Farmer RG, Lalli AF. Sclerosing cholangitis: its increasing frequency of recognition and associated with inflammatory bowel disease. *J Clin Gastroenterol* 1981;3:261–6.
17. Wiesner RH, La Russo NF. Clinicopathologic features of the syndrome of primary sclerosing cholangitis. *Gastroenterology* 1980;79:200–6.
18. Chapman RWG, Orborgh BAM, Rhodes JM, et al. Primary sclerosing cholangitis: a review of its clinical features, cholangiography and hepatic histology. *Gut* 1980;21:870–7.
19. MacCarty RL, LaRusso NF, Wiesner RH, et al. Primary sclerosing cholangitis: findings on cholangiography and pancreatography. *Radiology* 1983;149:39–44.
20. Ludwig J, MacCarty RL, LaRusso NF, Krom RA, Wiesner RH. Intrahepatic cholangiectases and large-duct obliteration in primary sclerosing cholangitis. *Hepatology* 1986;6:560–8.
21. Theilmann L, Stiehl A. Detection of large intrahepatic cholangiectases in patients with primary sclerosing cholangitis by endoscopic retrograde cholangiography. *Endoscopy* 1990;22:49–50.
22. Panes J, Borda JM, Bruguera M, Cortes M, Rodes J. Localized sclerosing cholangitis? *Endoscopy* 1985;17:121–2.
23. Hamilton I, Lintott DJ, Ruddell WS, Axon AT. The endoscopic retrograde cholangiogram and pancreatogram in chronic liver disease. *Clin Radiol* 1983;34:417–22.
24. Wee A, Ludwig J, Coffey RJ, et al. Hepatobiliary carcinoma associated with primary sclerosing cholangitis and chronic ulcerative colitis. *Hum Pathol* 1985;46:719–726.
25. MacCarty RL, LaRusso NF, May GR, et al. Cholangiocarcinoma complicating primary sclerosing cholangitis: cholangiography features. *Radiology* 1985;156:43–46.
26. Lee NW, Wong KP, Siu KF, Wong J. Cholangiography in hepatocellular carcinoma with obstructive jaundice. *Clin Radiol* 1984;35:119–23.
27. Severini A, Ellomi M, Cozzi G, Pizzetti P, Spinella P. Lymphomatous involvement of intrahepatic and extrahepatic biliary ducts. PTC and ERCP findings. *Acta Radiol Diagn* 1981;22:159–63.
28. Hoerder U, Heyder N, Riemann JF. Endoscopic-radiological findings in metastatic obstructive jaundice. *Endoscopy* 1983;15:12–5.
29. Vilgrain V, Erlinger S, Belghiti J, Degott C, et al. Cholangiographic appearance simulating sclerosing cholangitis in metastatic adenocarcinoma of the liver. *Gastroenterology* 1990;99:850–3.
30. Plaa GL, Priestly BG. Intrahepatic cholestasis induced by drugs and chemicals. *Pharmacol Rev* 1977;28:207–60.
31. Zimmerman HJ. *Hepatotoxicity*. New York: Appleton-Century-Crofts, 1978.
32. Van Thiel DH, de Bell R, Mellow M, Widerlite L, Phillips E. Tolazamidehepatotoxicity.*Gastroenterology*1974;67:506–10.
33. Lolndice TA, Lang JA. Tolazamide-induced hepatic dysfunction. *Am J Gastroenterol* 1978;69:31–3.
34. Raichel J, Goldberg SB, Ellenberg M, Schaffner F. Intrahepatic cholestasis following administration of cholorpropamide: report of a case with EM observations. *Am J Med* 1960;28:654–60.
35. Nakao NL, Gelb AM, Stenger RJ, Siegel JH. A case of chronic liver disease due to tolazamide. *Gastroenterology* 1985;89:192–195.
36. Balch CM, Urist MM, McGregor ML. Continuous regional chemotherapy for metastatic colorectal cancer using a totally implantable infusion pump.
37. Humberman MS. Comparison of systemic chemotherapy with hepatic arterial infusion in metastatic colorectal carcinoma. *Semin Oncol* 1983;10:238–48.
38. Niederhuber JE, Ensminger W, Gyves J, et al. Regional chemotherapy of colorectal cancer metastatic to the liver. *Cancer* 1984;53:1335–43.
39. Weiss GR, Garnik MB, Osteen RT, et al. Long-term hepatic arterial infusion of 5-fluorodeoxidine for liver metastasis using an implantable infusion pump. *J Clin Oncol* 1983;1:337–44.
40. Kemeny N, Daly I, Oderman P, et al. Hepatic artery pump infusion: toxicity and results in patients with metastatic colorectal carcinoma. *J Clin Oncol* 1984;2:595–600.
41. Hohn D, Melnick J, Stagg R, et al. Biliary sclerosis in patients receiving hepatic arterial infusions of floxuridine. *J Clin Oncol* 1985;156:335–7.
42. Botet JF, Watson RC, Kemeny N, et al. Cholangitis complicating intraarterial chemotherapy in liver metastasis. *Radiology* 1985;156:335–7.
43. Pien EH, Zeman RK, Benjamin SB, et al. Iatrogenic sclerosing cholangitis following hepatic arterial chemotherapy infusion. *Radiology* 1985;156:329–30.
44. Siegel JH, Ramsey WH. Endoscopic biliary stent placement for bile duct stricture after hepatic artery infusion of 5-FUDR. *J Clin Gastroenterol* 1986;8:673–676.
45. Viteri AL, Green JF. Bile duct abnormalities in the acquired immune deficiency syndrome. *Gastroenterology* 1987;92:2014–8.
46. Margulis SJ, Honig CL, Soave R, Govoni AF, Mouradian JA, Jacobson IM. Biliary tract obstruction in the acquired immunodeficiency syndrome. *Ann Intern Med* 1986;105:207–10.

47. Schneiderman DJ, Cello JP, Laing FC. Papillary stenosis and sclerosing cholangitis in the acquired immunodeficiency syndrome. *Ann Intern Med* 1987;106:546–9.
48. Dolmatch BL, Laing FC, Federle MP, Jeffrey RB, Cello JP. AIDS-related cholangitis: radiographic findings in nine patients. *Radiology* 1987;163:313–6.
49. Cello JP. Acquired immunodeficiency syndrome cholangiopathy: spectrum of disease. *Am J Med* 1988;86:539–46.
50. Lebovics E, Thung SN, Schaffner F, et al. The liver in the acquired immunodeficiency syndrome: a clinical and histologic study. *Hepatology* 1985;5:293–8.
51. Glasgow BJ, Anders K, Layfield LJ, et al. Clinical and pathologic findings of the liver in the acquired immune deficiency syndrome. *Am J Clin Pathol* 1985;83:582–8.
52. Nakanuma Y, Liew CT, Peters RL, et al. Pathologic features of the liver in acquired immune deficiency syndrome (AIDS). *Liver* 1986;6:158–166.
53. Schneiderman DJ, Arenson DM, Cello JP, Margaretten W, Weber TE. Hepatic disease in patients with the acquired immune deficiency syndrome (AIDS). *Hepatology* 1987;7:925–30.
54. Jacobson MA, Cello JP, Sande MA. Cholestasis and disseminated cytomegalovirus disease in patients with the acquired immunodeficiency syndrome. *Am J Med* 1988;84:218–24.
55. Musher DM, Hamill RJ, Baughn RE. Effect of human immunodeficiency virus (HIV) infection in the course of syphil and on the response to treatment. *Ann Intern Med* 1990;113:872–881.
56. Wildhirt E, Ormann W. Congenital cyst dilatation of the intrahepatic bile ducts (Caroli syndrome). *Dtsch Med Wochenschr* 1987;112:1038–42.
57. Missavage AE, Sugawa C. Caroli's disease: role of endoscopic retrograde cholangiopancreatography. *Am J Gastroenterol* 1983;78:815–7.
58. Trink W, Sassaris M, Hunter FM. Endoscopic papillotomy in Caroli's disease: twenty-year followup of a previously reported case. *Endoscopy* 1985;17:81–3.
59. Lapointe R, Gamache A, Pare P. Bile duct cyst with cystlithiasis: a case report. *Can J Surg* 1984;27:271–3.
60. Rattner DW, Schapiro RH, Warshaw AL. Abnormalities of the pancreatic and biliary ducts in adult patients with choledochal cysts. *Arch Surg* 1983;118:1068–73.
61. Kyle S, Stubbs RS, Stewart RJ. Choledochal cyst: case reports and current concepts. *Aust N Z J Surg* 1988;58:895–8.
62. Vignote ML, Mino G, de la Mata M, de Dios JF, Gomez F. Endoscopic sphincterotomy in hepatic hydatid disease open to the biliary tree. *Br J Surg* 1990;77:30–1.
63. Bahar RH, Al-Mohannadi S, Wafai I, Al-Suhaili AR, Abdel-Dayem HM. Acute intrahepatic biliary obstruction caused by hydatid cysts. Correlation between various imaging techniques. *Clin Nucl Med* 1988;13:334–6.

CHAPTER 6

Extrahepatic Cholestasis: Obstructive Jaundice

The algorithm referred to in Chapter 2, Table 2.2, is most helpful in the evaluation and management of patients presenting with jaundice and cholestasis. In the present climate of cost containment, early utilization of specific tests, examinations, and procedures is paramount to providing a diagnosis and implementation of therapy. In an earlier report, my colleagues and I advocated the early utilization of ERCP and outlined its utility in the management of obstructive jaundice (1,2) (Table 6.1). In these index reports, we suggested that patients be evaluated initially in an outpatient or office environment where a careful history, a physical examination, and baseline laboratory studies may be obtained on initial presentation. Ultrasonography or CT scans can be subsequently obtained as preadmission studies. If possible, the admission to a hospital should be arranged only after obtaining these necessary preliminary studies, and an ERCP should be scheduled for the day of admission. If the ERCP examination is incomplete, a PTC may be scheduled and available on day two of the hospital admission. If ERCP or PTC fail to provide a diagnosis or to establish decompression of an obstructed biliary tree, or if surgery is the preferred treatment, the surgery should be planned and scheduled for day three of the hospital stay. Utilizing this efficient schema for diagnostic and therapeutic evaluation and intervention is critical to the efficient delivery of health care and can save valuable health dollars.

TABLE 6.1. *Extrahepatic obstruction (cholestasis and jaundice)*

Primary neoplasm
Cholangiocarcinoma
Carcinoid tumor
Others
Metastatic disease
Stone disease
Chronic cholecystitis, Mirizzi's syndrome
Inflammatory diseases of pancreas
Neoplastic diseases of pancreas
Cystic disease
Choledochocele
Choledochal cyst
Injury to bile duct
Iatrogenic
Inflammatory
Dysfunction sphincter of Oddi (papillary stenosis)
Paraneoplastic

In this chapter, cholangiograms that demonstrate both usual and unusual causes of extrahepatic cholestasis or obstructive jaundice will be illustrated. More illustrations of obstructive lesions will be presented in Chapters 10 through 13. Lesions or strictures of the common hepatic duct and bifurcation, the proximal extrahepatic ducts, will be the first described in this section, and lesions affecting the more distal bile duct will follow. Much has been written regarding the classification and treatment of tumors of the bifurcation of the biliary tree (3–9), and an enlarged bibliography is included in Chapter 12. Table 6.2 is the accepted classification that attempts to clarify the extent of involvement of tumor growth, either primary or secondary, into the bifurcation, encroaching upon the right and left hepatic ducts. This description identifies segmental obstruction resulting from tumor encroachment at the bifurcation. Several illustrations are presented to confirm these points (Figs. 6.1–6.7). Both benign and neoplastic diseases of the common hepatic duct can produce intrahepatic dilatation. The accompanying

TABLE 6.2. *Bifurcation tumors*

Type 1	A lesion encroaching upon the common hepatic duct with no extension into bifurcation
Type 2	A lesion of the hepatic duct encroaching upon the bifurcation producing obstruction to both major ducts
Type 3	Diffuse lesion of the hepatic ducts involving major ducts, extending into the liver and encroaching upon subsegments and lobules of the liver

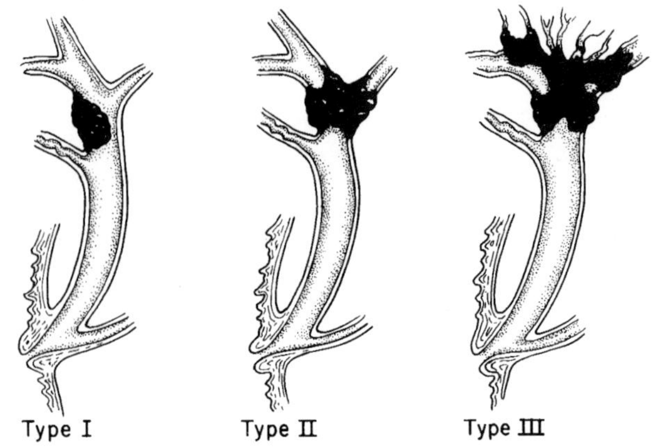

FIG. 6.1. Bifurcation tumors.

illustrations are presented to emphasize this effect. Mirizzi's syndrome, a benign obstructive phenomenon associated with chronic cholecystitis, cholelithiasis, and lymphadenopathy, produces compression of the common hepatic duct and, usually, cholestasis and jaundice (10–15). This entity is safely demonstrated and confirmed by ERCP (Figs. 6.8, 6.9) or PTC. Although noninvasive methods of diagnosis and confirmation have been reported (10,14,15), cholangiography is more definitive in any obstructive disorder (16–19). The status of the patient will determine whether the obstruction caused by the inflammatory mass in Mirizzi's syndrome is best treated surgically. Endoscopic decompression, however, certainly remains an option if the patient is at risk for surgery. Other benign causes of obstruction of the bile duct include iatrogenic or acquired strictures resulting from surgical trauma

Text continues on page 82.

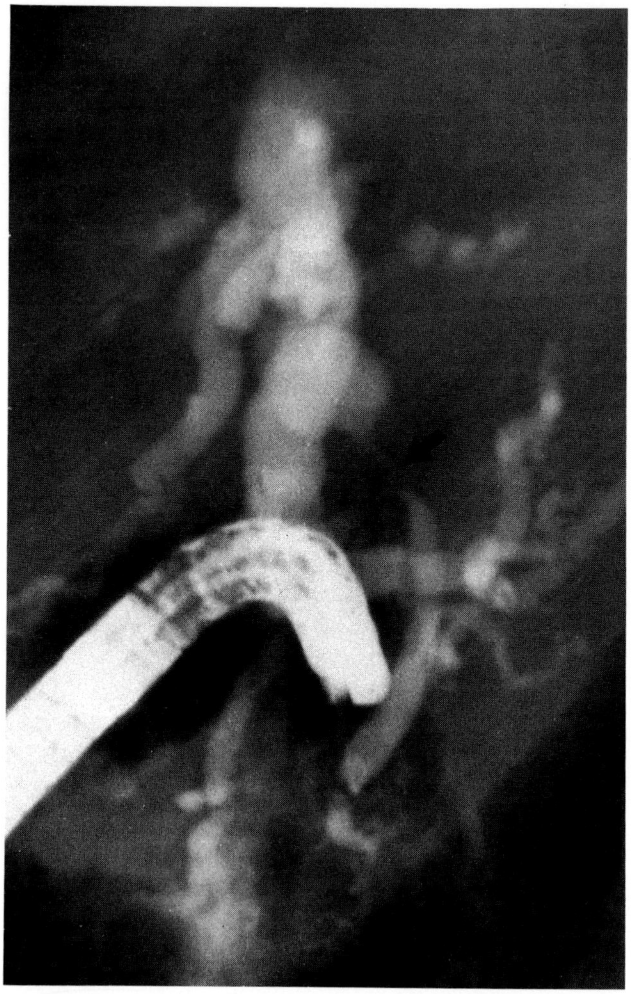

FIG. 6.3. A high-grade obstruction of the common hepatic duct (*arrow*). Opacification of the proximal biliary tree shows no encroachment of tumor onto bifurcation. This is another example of a Type 1 lesion.

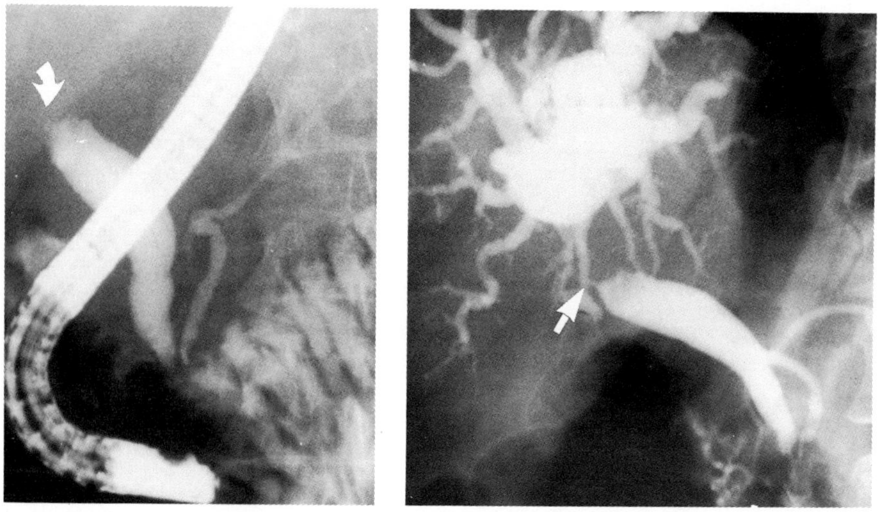

FIG. 6.2. Left: ERCP showing obstruction of the common hepatic duct (*arrow*). **Right:** After insertion of a catheter and guidewire through the obstruction, a high-grade stricture is noted in the common hepatic duct (*arrow*) with dilatation of both the right and left ducts. This is a Type 1 lesion.

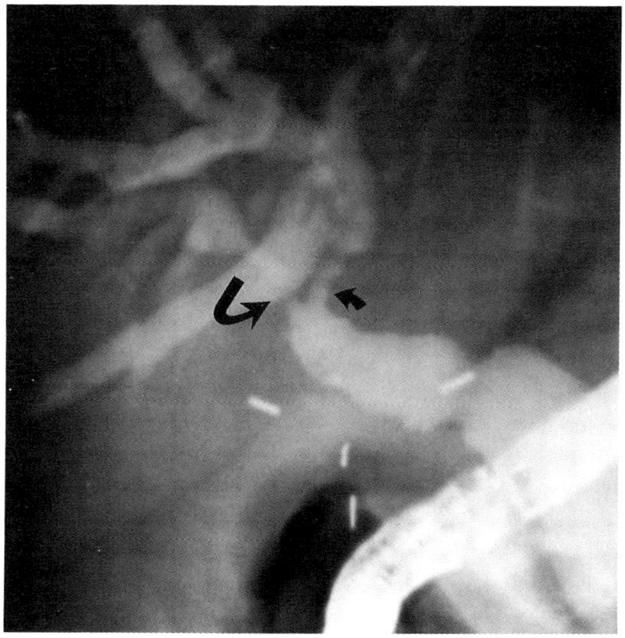

FIG. 6.4. A stricture at the bifurcation with bilateral involvement (*arrows*). Although the tumor extends into the bifurcation, no other structures are encroached upon. This is an example of a Type 2 lesion.

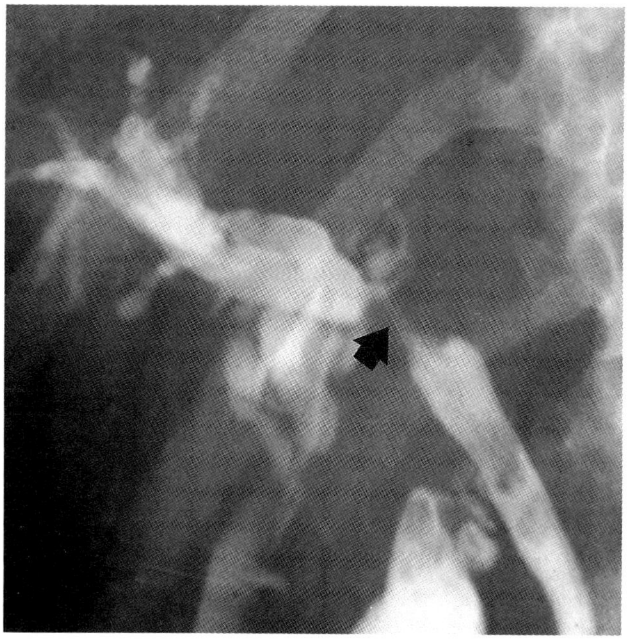

FIG. 6.6. A high-grade obstruction at the bifurcation with dilatation of the right hepatic system (*arrow*). The left system was not opacified. This is another example of a Type 3 lesion.

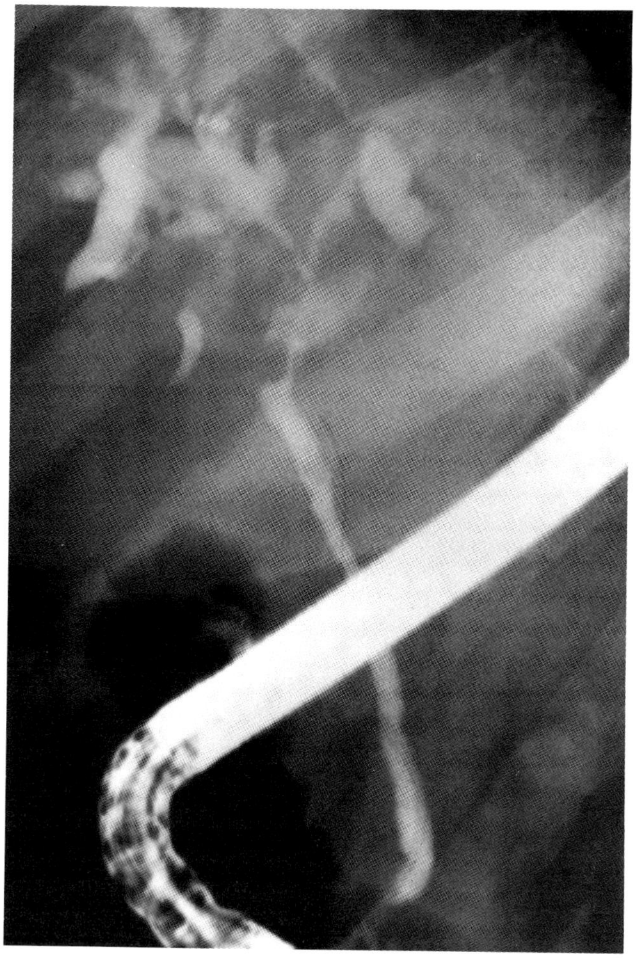

FIG. 6.5. Diffuse involvement of the bile ducts at the bifurcation and a high-grade stricture of the left hepatic system extending into the liver parenchyma. The right hepatic duct is not opacified. This is an example of a Type 3 lesion.

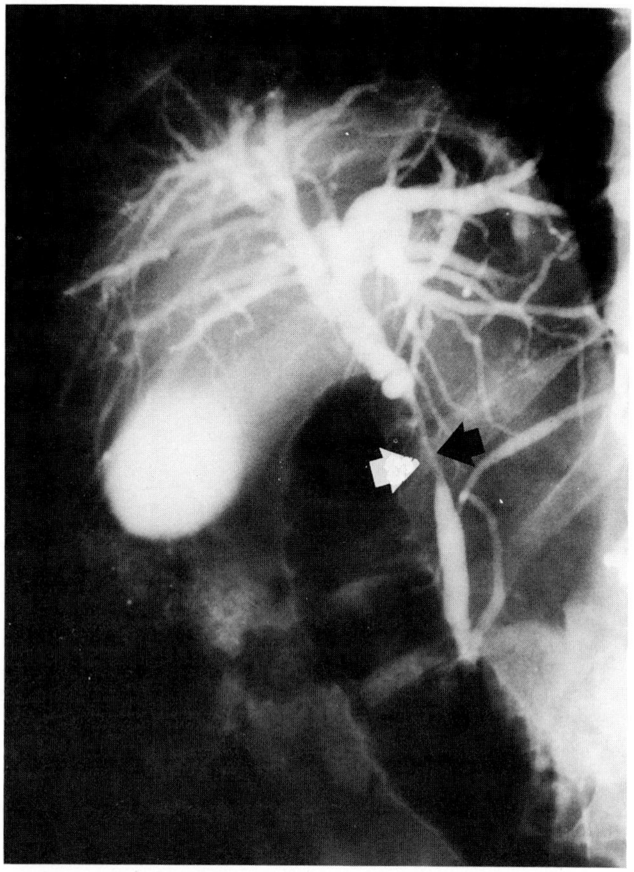

FIG. 6.7. A stricture of the bile duct distal to the cystic duct (*arrows*). No abnormality of the pancreatic duct is seen. This finding is consistent with a cholangiocarcinoma.

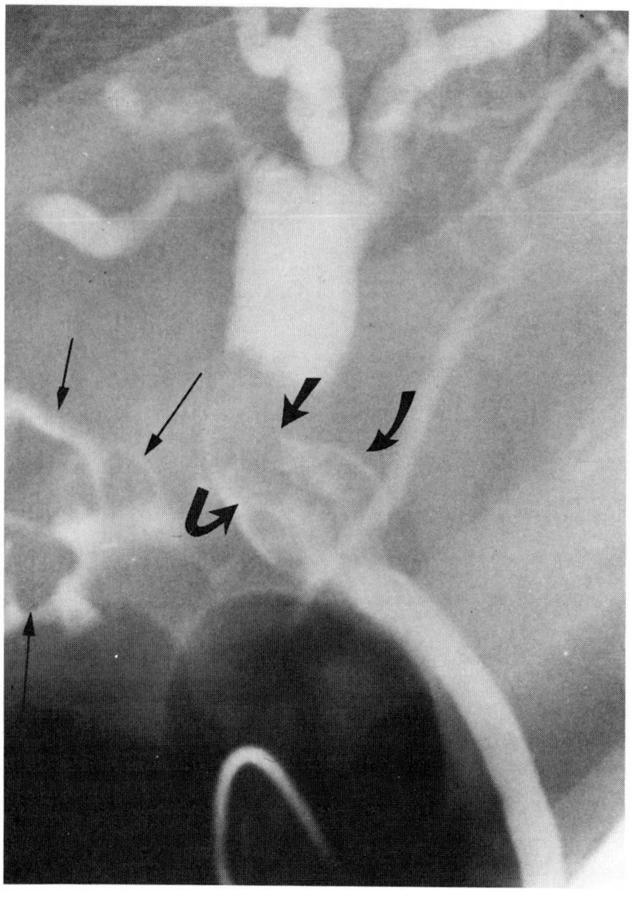

FIG. 6.8. A cholangiogram of a patient with Mirizzi's syndrome. Note the lucent stones in the gallbladder (*small arrows*) and encroachment of the bile duct and the common hepatic duct containing stones that produce high-grade obstruction (*large arrows*).

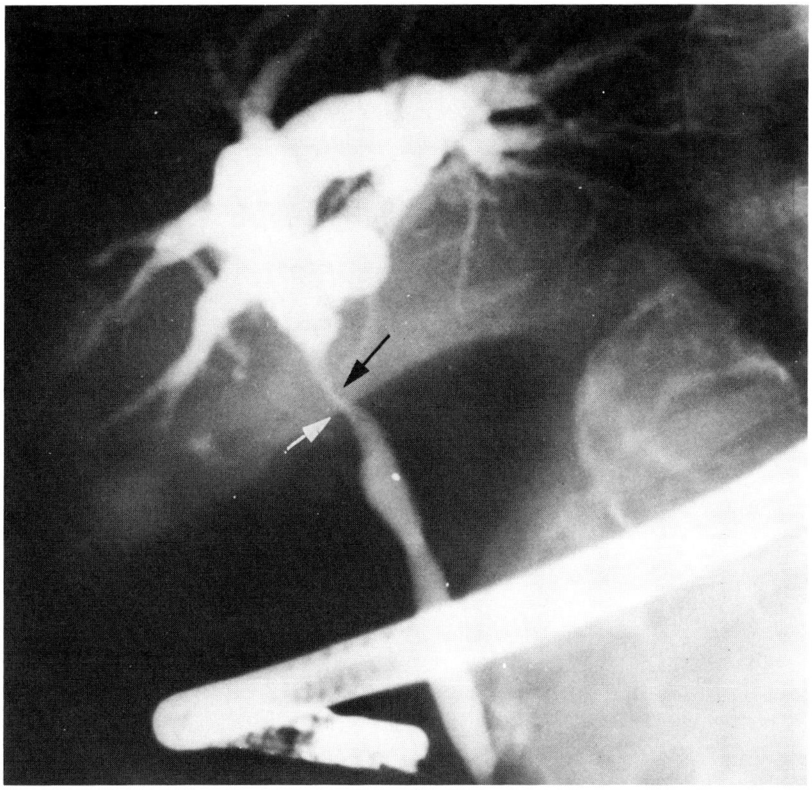

A

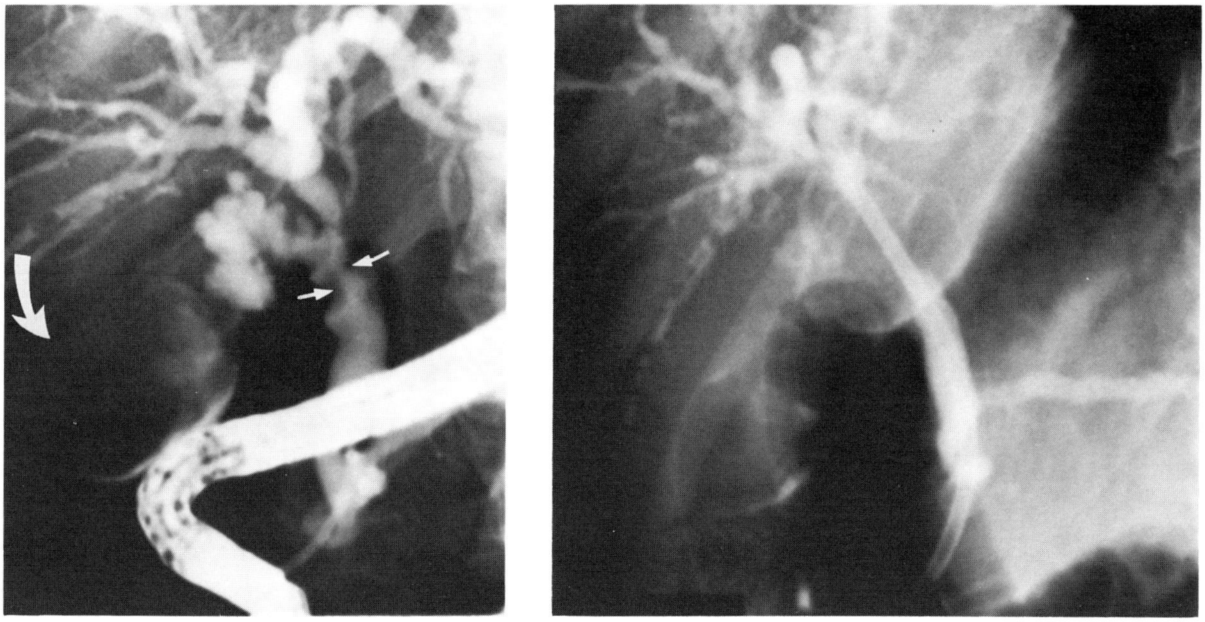

B

FIG. 6.9. A: Strictures of the common hepatic duct with nodular indentations of duct secondary to lymphadenopathy (*arrows*). Note the small amount of contrast in the cystic duct and gallbladder. These findings are compatible with Mirizzi's syndrome. **B: Left:** Irregularity of the common hepatic duct. Note the indentations (*arrows*), which are due to lymphadenopathy. The gallbladder contains large, lucent stones (*curved arrows*). **Right:** A large-caliber prosthesis has been placed for decompression.

Text continued from page 78.
to the duct, including ligation of the duct (Fig. 6.10), and chronic inflammatory changes secondary to stone disease. Iatrogenic strictures are discussed in Chapters 12 and 13.

Among other malignant causes of biliary obstruction, carcinoma of the gallbladder producing obstruction of the common hepatic duct is somewhat similar in appearance to cholangiocarcinoma, but the distinction may be made only at surgery (6,20–23). Abnormal

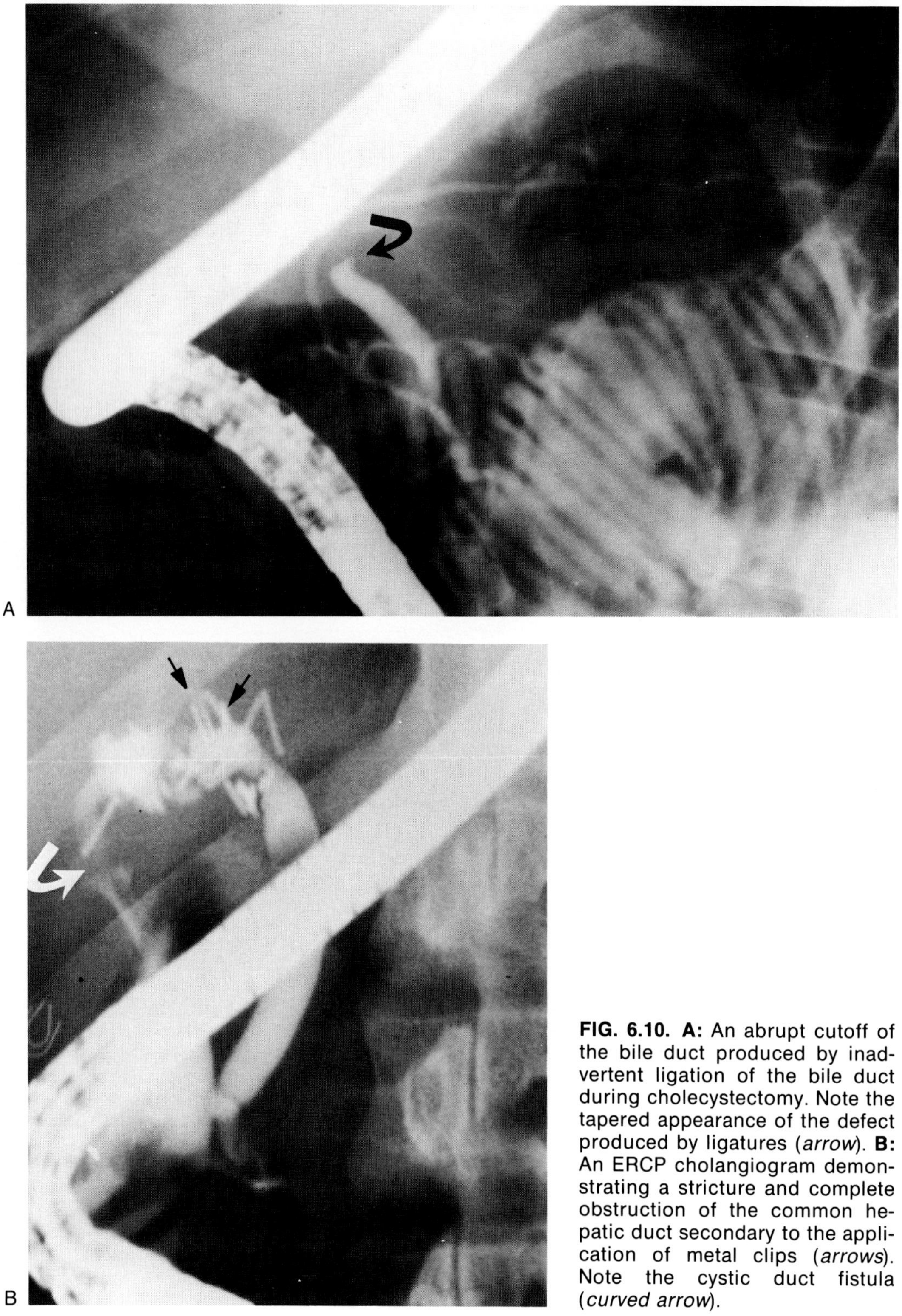

FIG. 6.10. A: An abrupt cutoff of the bile duct produced by inadvertent ligation of the bile duct during cholecystectomy. Note the tapered appearance of the defect produced by ligatures (*arrow*). **B:** An ERCP cholangiogram demonstrating a stricture and complete obstruction of the common hepatic duct secondary to the application of metal clips (*arrows*). Note the cystic duct fistula (*curved arrow*).

findings of the gallbladder are often identified by ERCP (Figs. 6.11, 6.12), which may elucidate the etiology; also, at times, the gallbladder may fail to opacify. Invasion of the right lobe of the liver is not uncommon with gallbladder cancer because of the close proximity of the two organs.

Both common hepatic and common bile duct strictures are best evaluated by cholangiography (19). Although PTC can easily demonstrate the level of obstruction, more information—ostensibly mucosal abnormalities, infiltrative processes, and compression abnormalities—is obtained with ERCP. The additional information obtained through ERCP includes material obtained by utilization of biopsy forceps or cytology

A

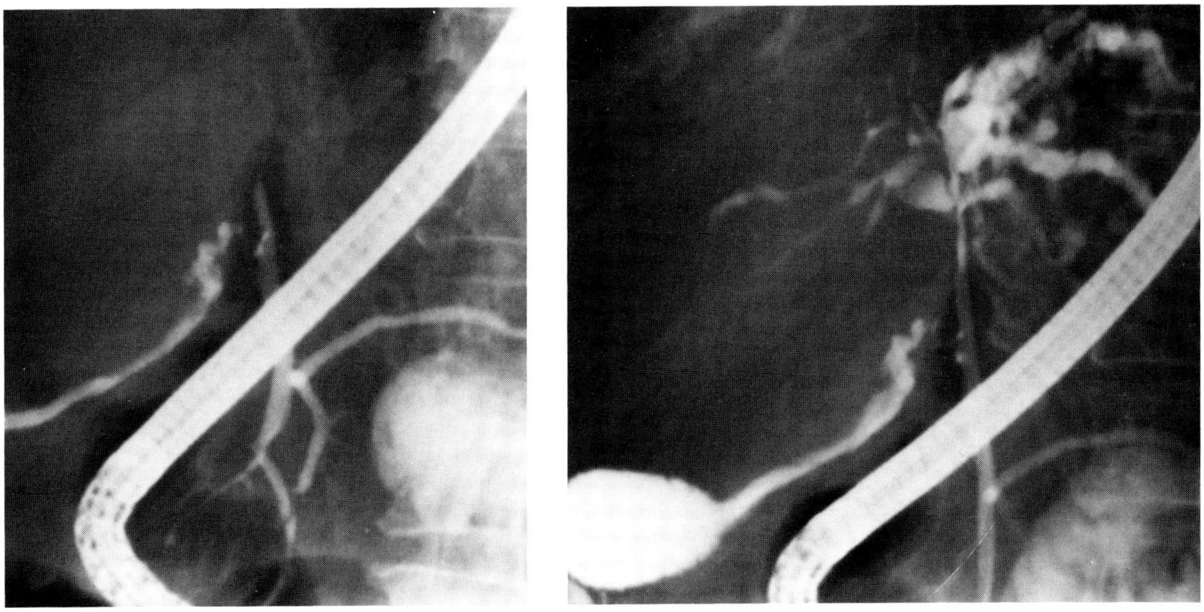

B

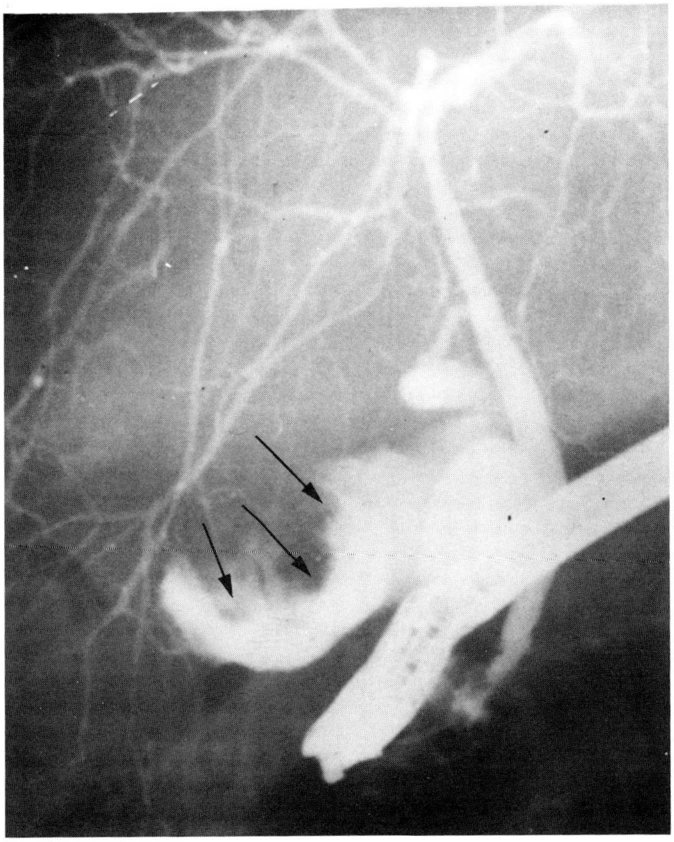

FIG. 6.11. A: Left: Obstruction of the common hepatic duct caused by a neoplastic process arising from the gallbladder. Note the thin, straight cystic duct upon which indentations are present and consistent with lymph nodes or a tumor mass. **Right:** After traversing the stricture, a dilated left system is apparent. Metastatic disease of the right lobe of the liver is confirmed by the typical appearance of the intrahepatic ducts. These changes consist of attenuation, encasement, and displacement. **B:** A radiograph showing a defect in the gallbladder (*arrows*), which represents a carcinoma of that organ.

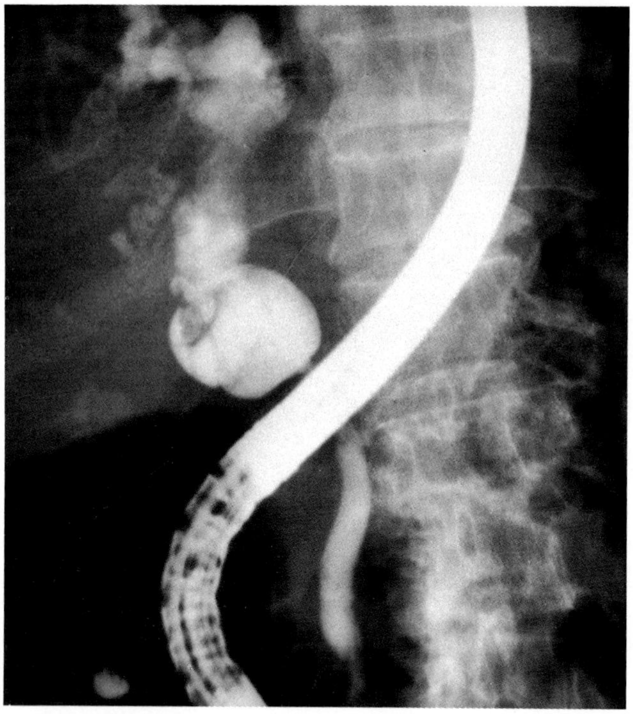

FIG. 6.12. A stricture of the common hepatic duct just proximal to the cystic duct and gallbladder mass secondary to carcinoma of the gallbladder.

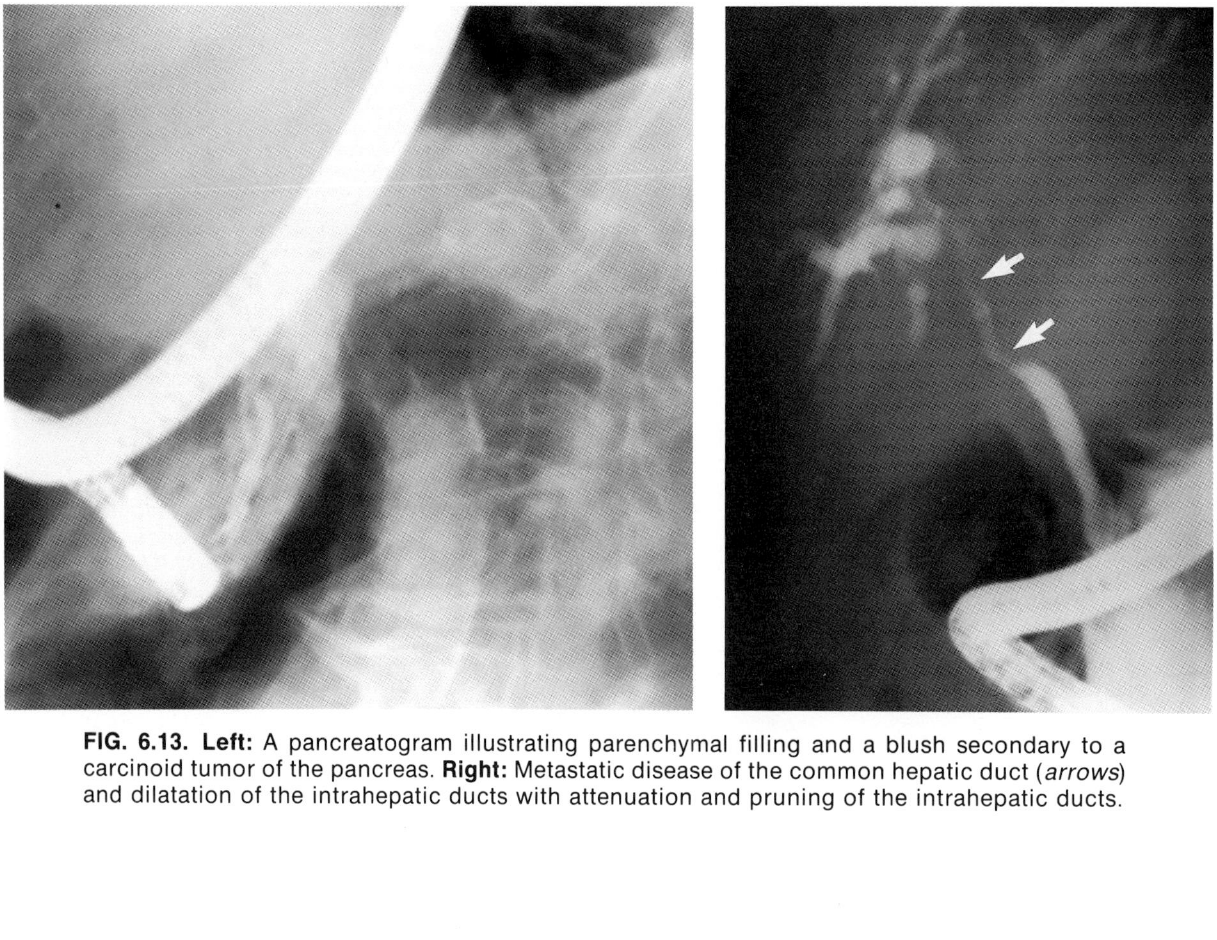

FIG. 6.13. Left: A pancreatogram illustrating parenchymal filling and a blush secondary to a carcinoid tumor of the pancreas. **Right:** Metastatic disease of the common hepatic duct (*arrows*) and dilatation of the intrahepatic ducts with attenuation and pruning of the intrahepatic ducts.

brushes (Figs. 6.13–6.16) for confirmation of the diagnosis. Biopsy and cytology can be obtained with PTC, but the morbidity associated with it is usually greater than that with ERCP (24). Chapter 14 discusses the utility of per oral choledochoscopy, which, as a direct method, provides visualization of the bile duct using a mother/daughter endoscope system. If possible, assessment of bile duct strictures is best made under direct visualization, and biopsies obtained in this manner have a higher yield than those obtained indirectly, although several recent reports emphasize the utility of brush cytology and indirectly obtained biopsies (25). Newer cytology brushes, especially those advanced over a guidewire, offer a higher yield than standard ones.

Text continues on page 89.

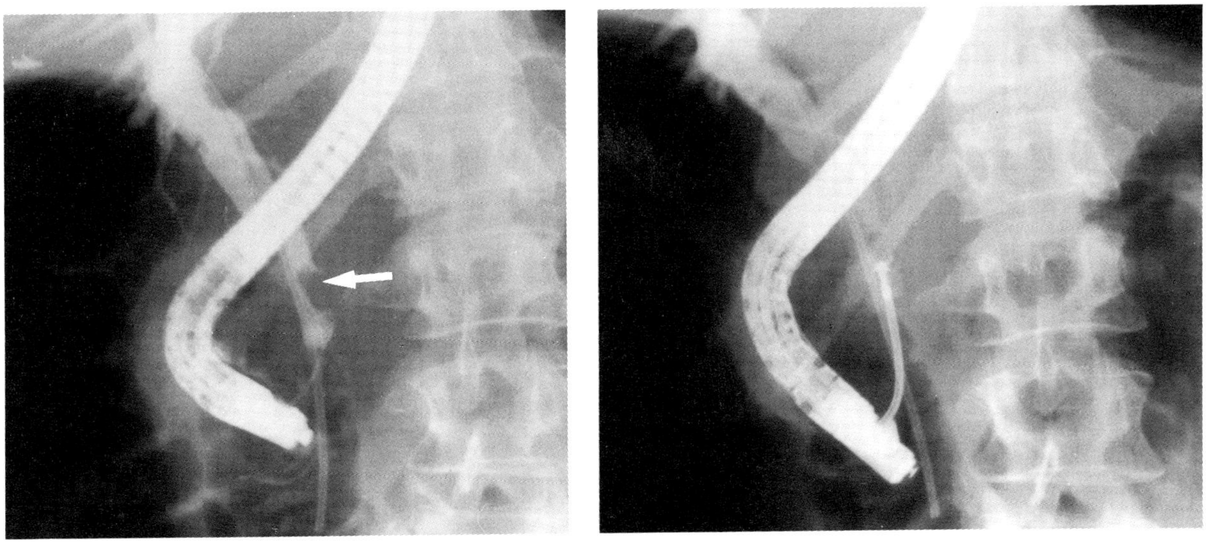

A

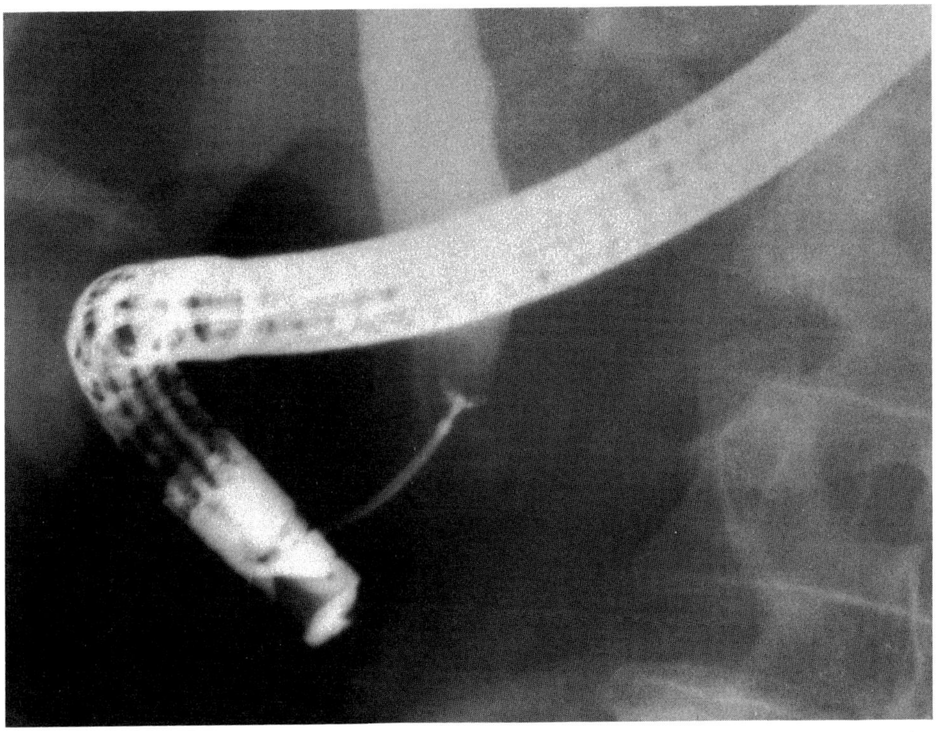

B

FIG. 6.14. A: Left: An ERCP illustrating a persistent filling defect in the distal common bile duct (*arrow*). Note the stent in place to provide decompression. **Right:** After a sphincterotomy is performed, the biopsy forcep is inserted into the bile duct up to the mass, and biopsies are obtained. **B:** The open biopsy forcep is placed into the distal common bile duct to obtain tissue from the distal obstructing lesion.

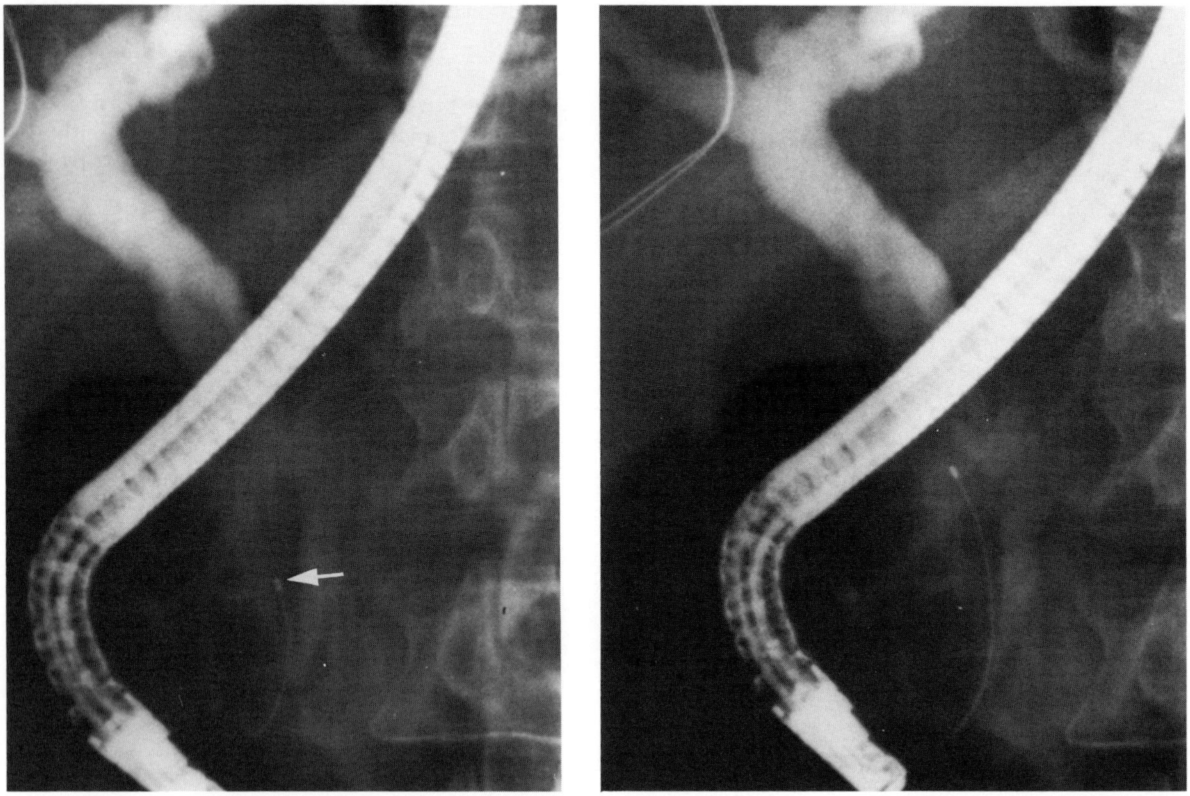

FIG. 6.15. Left: The opaque distal tip of a cytology brush is placed into the distal common bile duct to obtain specimen (*arrow*). **Right:** The brush has been extended out of the sheath to brush the lesion for cytology specimen.

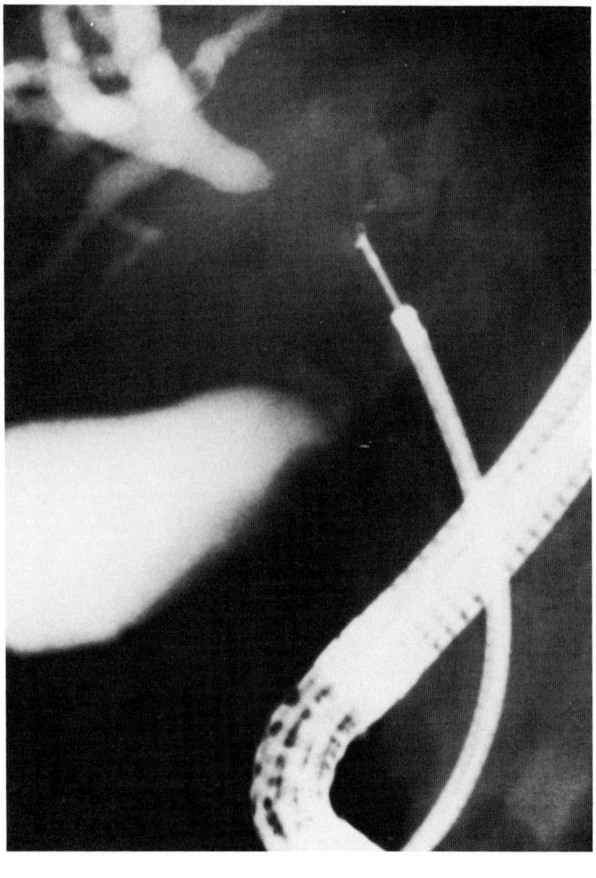

FIG. 6.16. A mother-daughter endoscope system is being used to obtain tissue from a direct biopsy of a lesion in the common hepatic duct. Note that the biopsy forcep is being extended from the daughter endoscope.

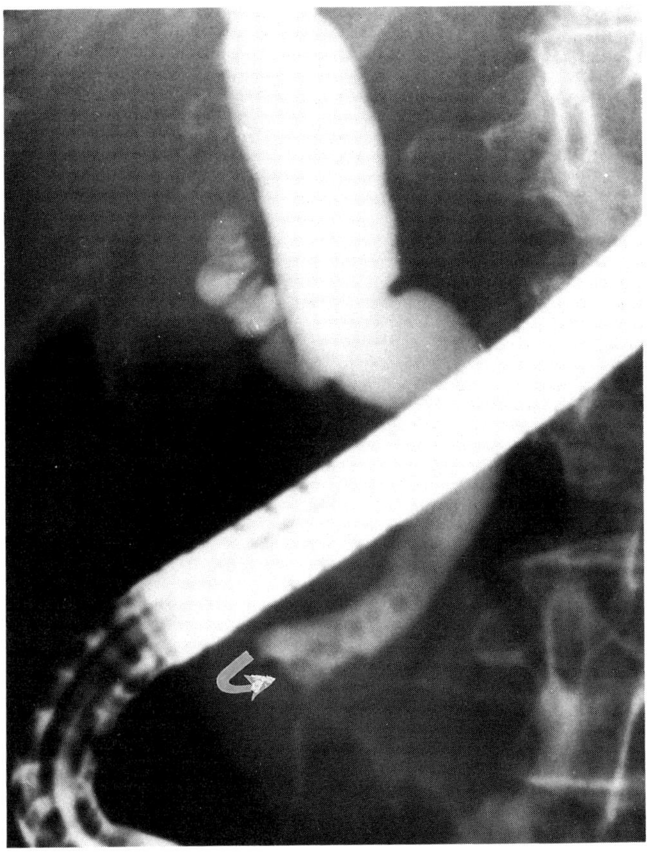

A

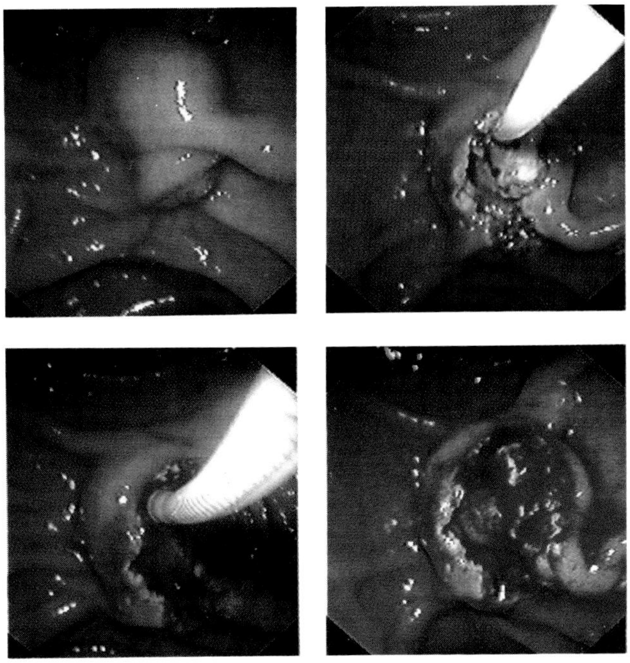

B

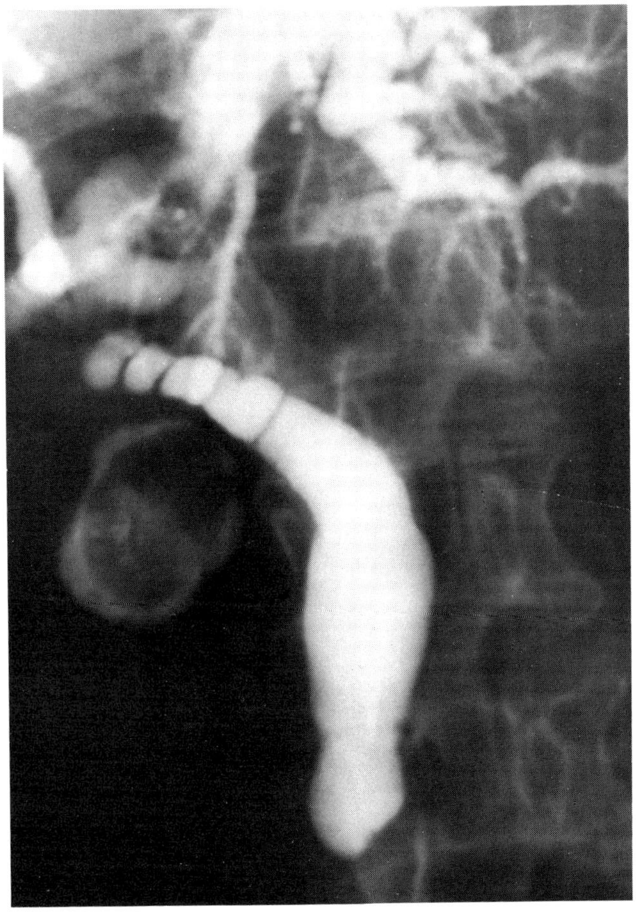

C

FIG. 6.17. A: A cholangiogram obtained in a patient presenting with a cholestatic picture. Note the irregularity of the distal common bile duct (*arrow*) consistent with a periampullary tumor. **B:** A series of videoendoscopic pictures taken during ERCP. **Top left:** Prominent ampulla. **Top right:** Sphincterotomy in progress. **Bottom left:** Sphincterotomy completed, biopsy being obtained. **Bottom right:** Tumor noted in ampulla after completion of sphincterotomy. **C:** A dilated biliary tree secondary to an ampullary tumor that has produced a deformity of the distal duct. Note the large gallstone in the gallbladder.

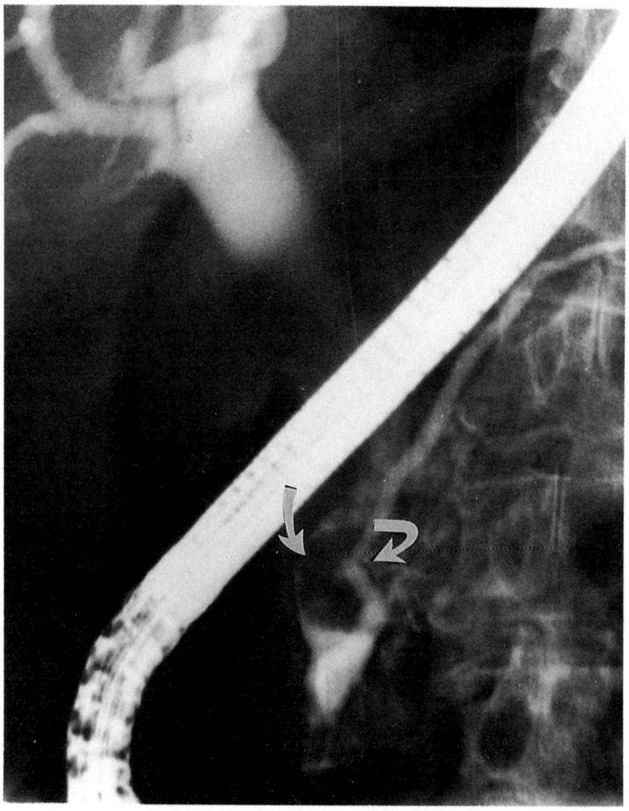

FIG. 6.18. A persistent filling defect in the distal common bile duct (*arrows*). The defect was thought to be a stone but, after a sphincterotomy, proved to be a mass, a periampullary neoplasm.

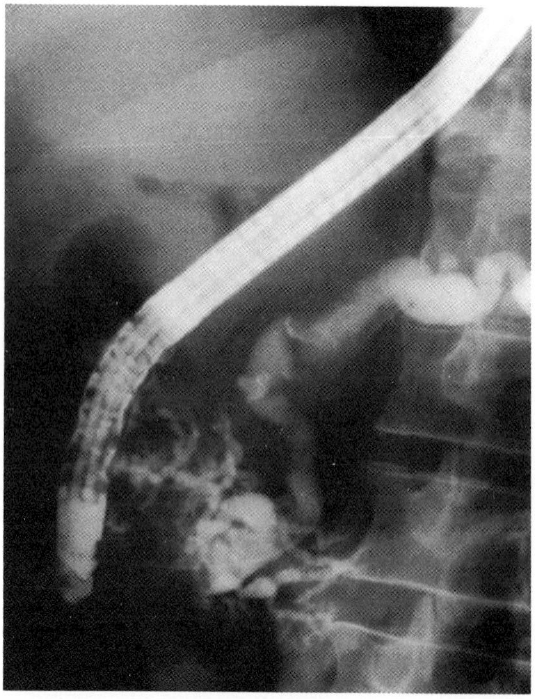

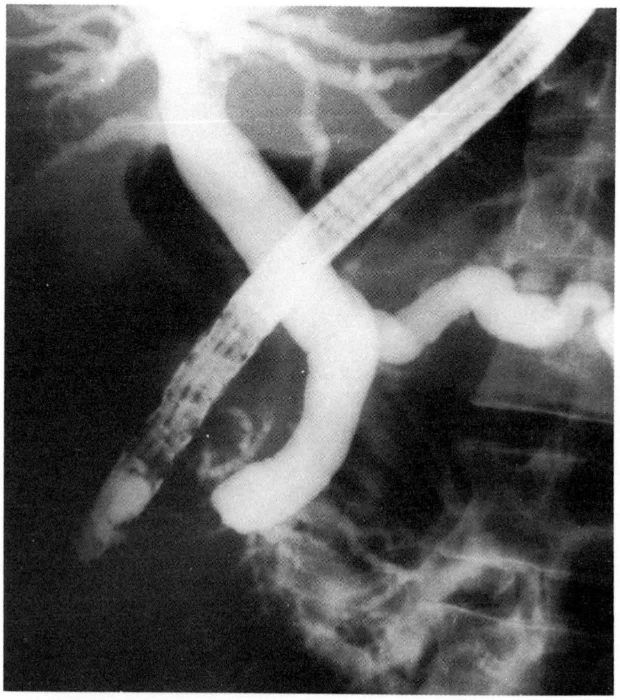

FIG. 6.19. Left: Dilatation of the pancreatic duct with dilated secondary radicals in the head of the pancreas. **Right:** Irregularity of the distal common bile duct secondary to a periampullary-ampullary neoplasm after sphincterotomy.

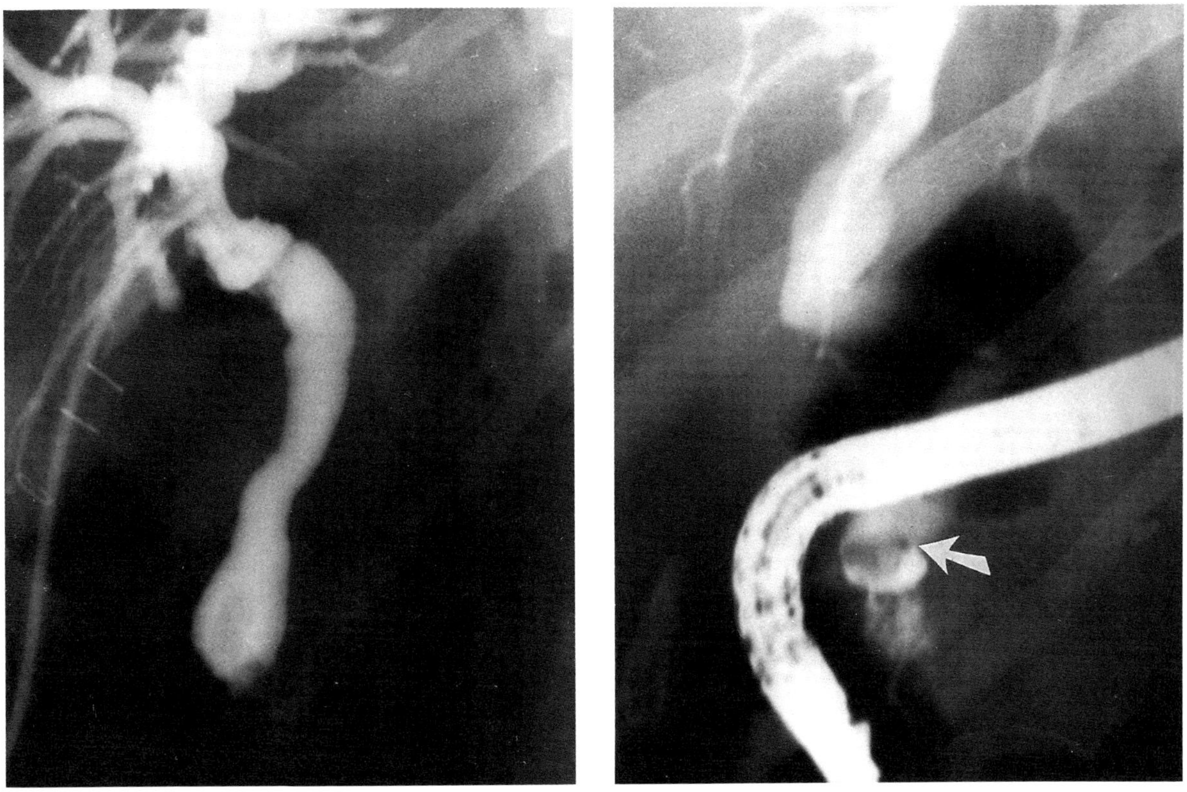

FIG. 6.20. Left: Another example of a periampullary tumor in a cholangiogram obtained via a T-tube. Irregularity of the dilated distal duct is evident. **Right:** The ERCP has highlighted the mass in the distal common bile duct (*arrow*).

Text continued from page 85.

Dilatation of the entire biliary tree emanating from the papilla of Vater can be attributed to primary neoplasm of the ampulla of vater or periampullary tumors (26–28) (Figs. 6.17–6.21); pancreatic neoplasm (Figs. 6.22, 6.23); pancreatitis (Figs. 6.24–6.27); choledochal cysts (Fig. 6.28); paraneoplastic syndrome, a syndrome presumably secondary to "humors" secreted by a primary tumor (29) (Figs. 6.29, 6.30); metastatic diseases; benign fibrosis (Figs. 6.31, 6.32); and stone disease (Figs. 6.33–6.36).

Dilatation of the biliary tree is occasionally not attributable to a definable disease or obstructive process. On three occasions, I found a normal papilla and ampulla that were cannulated without difficulty. The bil-

Text continues on page 94.

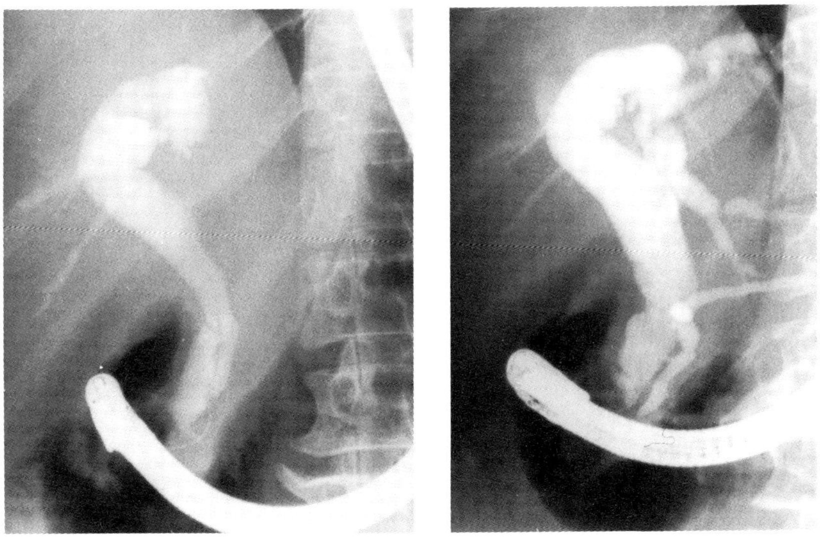

FIG. 6.21. Left: A dilated bile duct with irregularity of the distal duct. **Right:** After filling of a normal pancreatic duct, the diagnosis of a periampullary tumor is more evident.

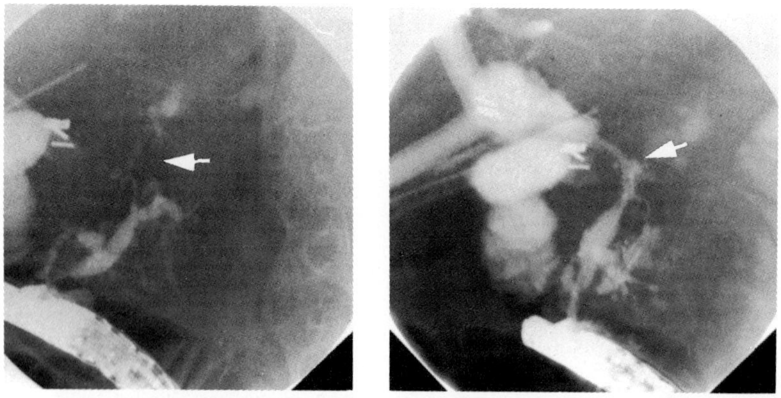

FIG. 6.22. Left: A stricture of the pancreatic duct (*arrow*) in the head of the gland. Little filling is seen proximal to the stricture. The patient has had a subtotal gastrectomy. **Right:** A corresponding stricture of the distal bile duct produced by a neoplasm of the pancreas. Despite the presence of a T-tube, the common bile duct is dilated.

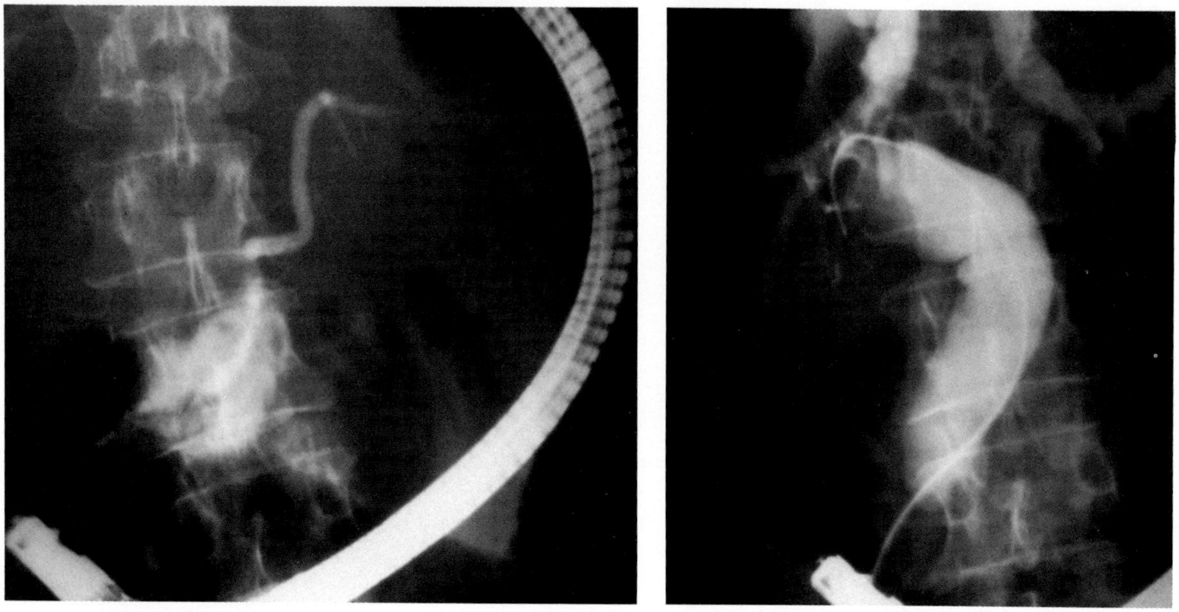

FIG. 6.23. Left: Filling of the pancreatic duct in a patient who has undergone a previous Bilroth II gastrectomy. Note the extravasation of contrast or tumor blush in the head of the gland. **Right:** A dilated bile duct. The stricture of the distal bile duct was traversed by a guidewire and catheter, which facilitated opacification of the duct. These findings are compatible with a neoplasia.

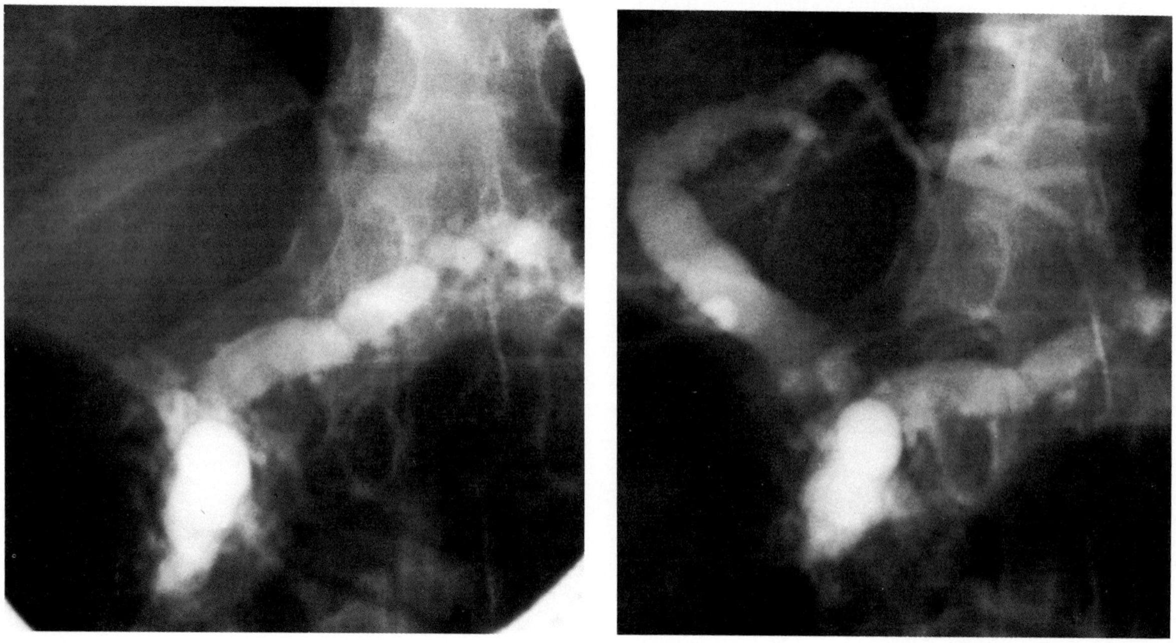

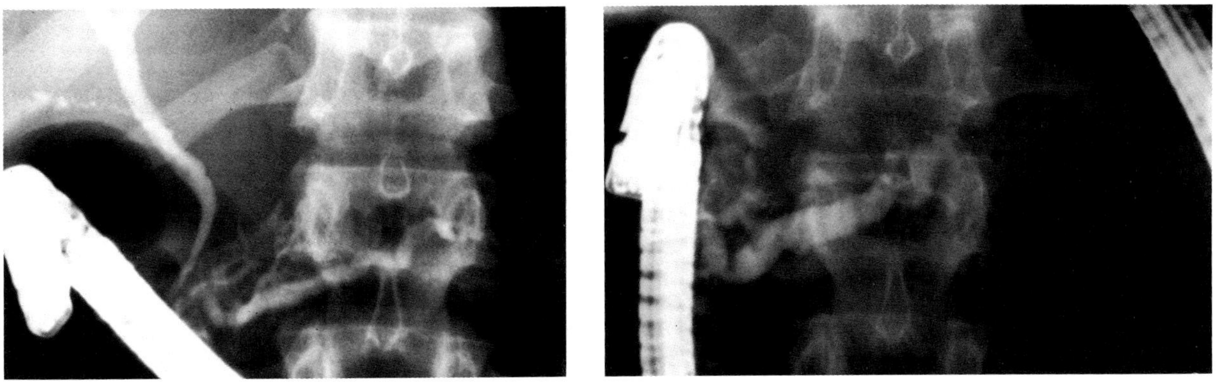

FIG. 6.25. Left: A long, smooth, tapered distal common bile duct, which is consistent with fibrosis secondary to chronic pancreatitis. **Right:** Complete filling of the pancreatic duct demonstrating dilatation and tortuosity of the duct consistent with chronic pancreatitis.

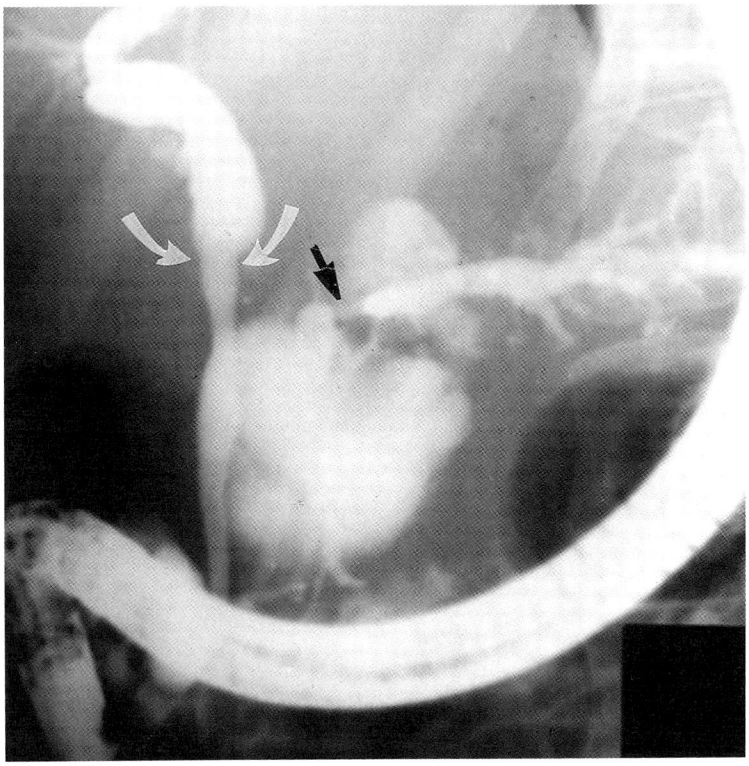

FIG. 6.26. Changes in both duct systems. Cystic changes of the pancreatic duct are present with a large communicating cyst in the head of the gland, a proximal stricture (*black arrow*), and another communicating cyst proximal to the stricture. Note the long, narrow segment of the lower bile duct, which is compressed by the fibrotic changes in the head of the gland. The bile duct proximal to the head of the pancreas (*curved arrows*) is dilated.

FIG. 6.24. Left: An ERCP showing a markedly dilated pancreatic duct that is tortuous in configuration. Note the dilated, blunted secondary radicals of the pancreatic duct. **Right:** A cholangiogram demonstrating a dilated bile duct emanating from the ampullary region and corresponding to a neoplasm of the pancreas. These findings are often seen in benign disease, making radiographic diagnosis difficult. Correlation with the clinical history, endoscopic ultrasonography, and CT scans and histologic confirmation are necessary to confirm the diagnosis.

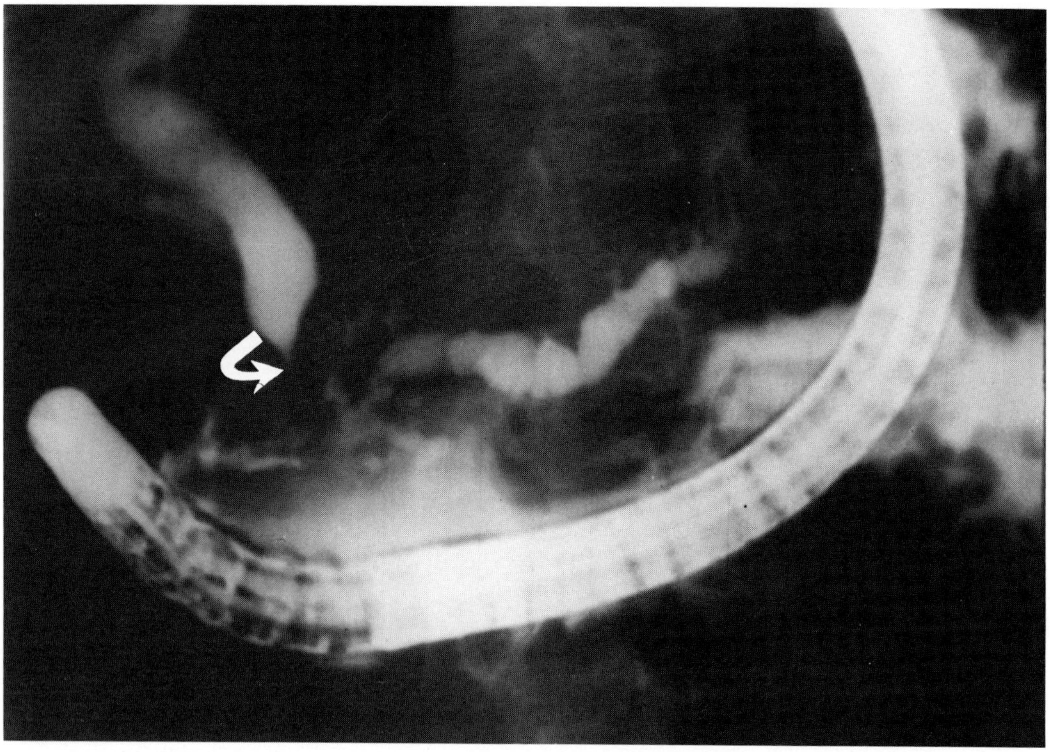

FIG. 6.27. An ERCP obtained in a patient who had undergone a Bilroth I resection and who presented with a history of recurrent pancreatitis. A smooth stricture of the distal common duct (*arrow*) is evident along with stricturing of the pancreatic duct in the head. The main pancreatic duct is dilated and tortuous, consistent with chronic pancreatitis.

A

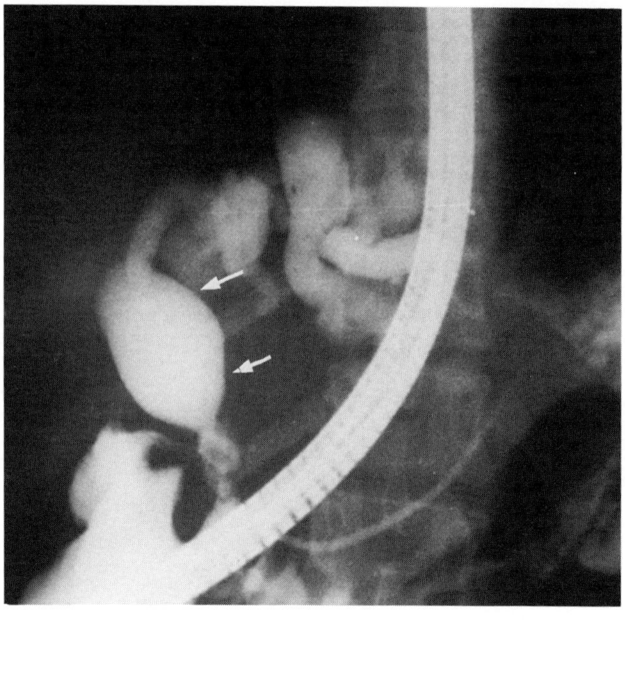

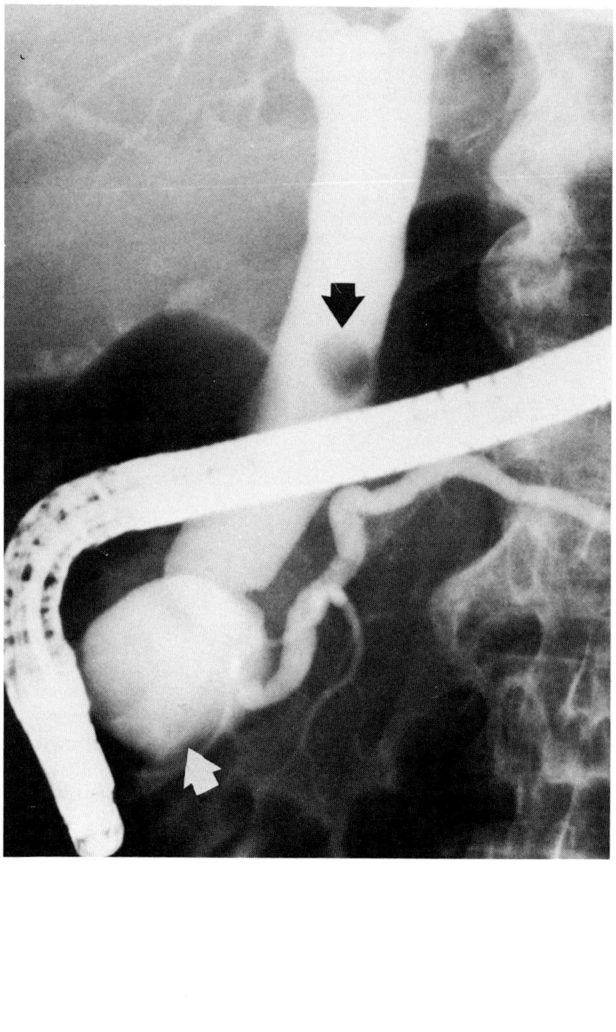

B

FIG. 6.28. A: A choledochal cyst (*arrows*) producing proximal dilatation of the biliary tree. **B:** A choledochocele in the distal bile duct (*white arrow*) producing dilatation to that system. An incidental stone is apparent in the bile duct (*black arrow*). The pancreatic duct is seen draining into the cyst, but it is not dilated.

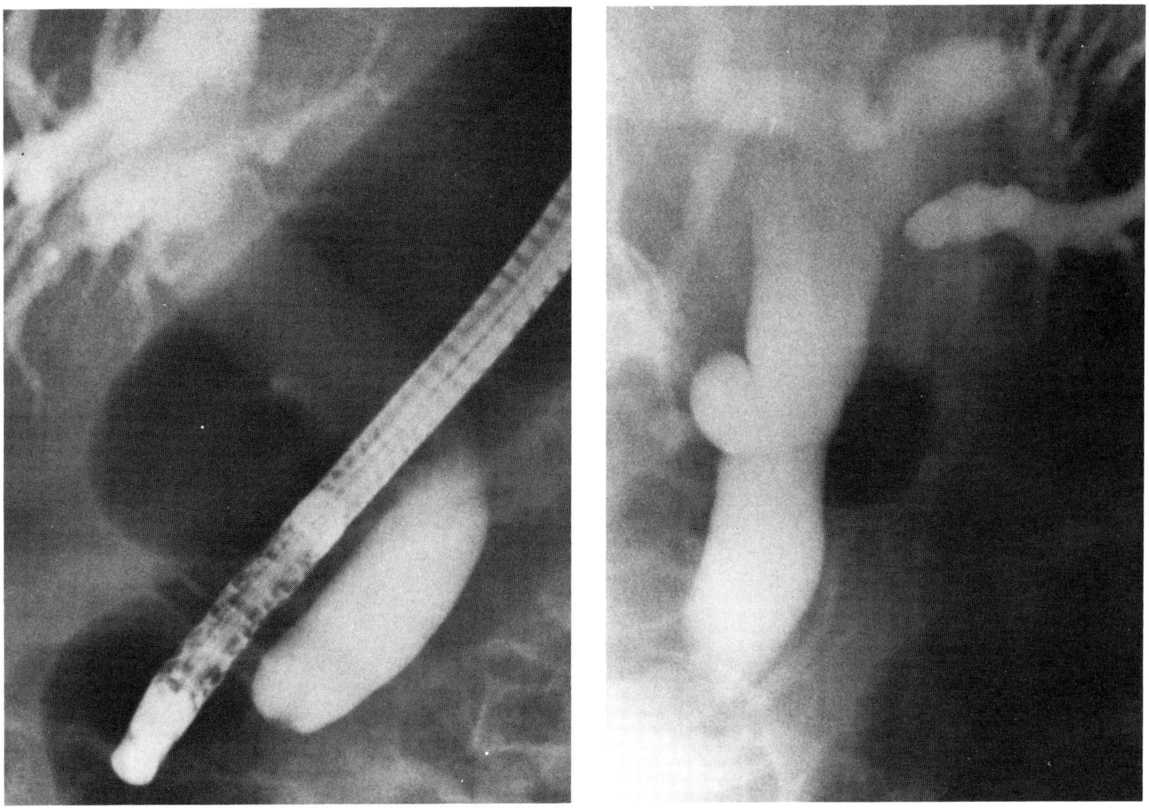

FIG. 6.29. Left: A dilated bile duct. The dilatation emanates from the ampulla. No stones or other filling defects or strictures are present. The patient had a history of carcinoma of the lung. **Right:** Delayed emptying of the bile duct without evidence of obvious obstruction.

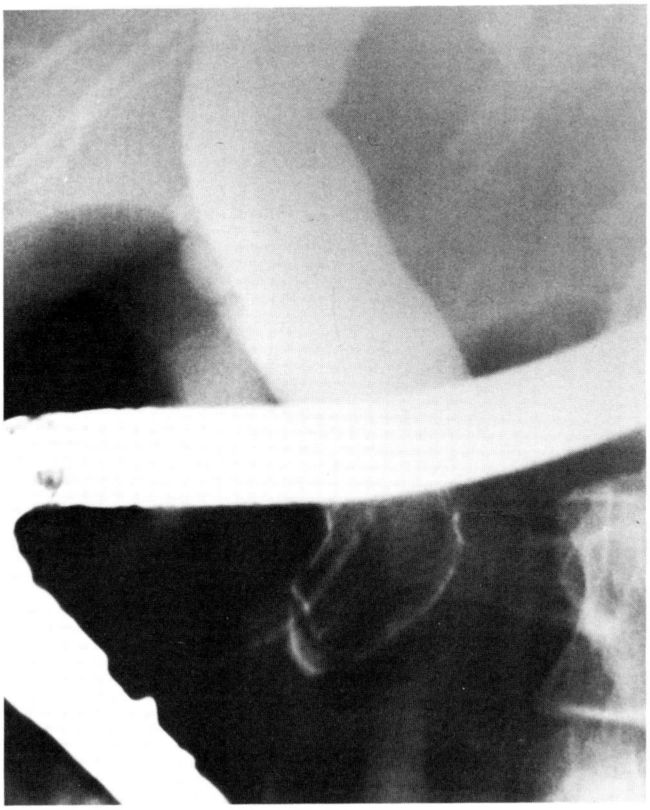

FIG. 6.30. An ERCP demonstrating a markedly dilated bile duct found in a patient with discogenic disease. Air is noted in the distal common bile duct after sphincterotomy. No obvious filling defect or stricture was present, and brush cytology was negative.

Text continued from page 89.
iary tree, however, was dilated markedly to the ampullary region, but no obstructing lesion or stricture was evident (Figs. 6.29–6.32). All patients did have an underlying neoplastic process, carcinoma of the lung, which probably produced a humor resulting in dilatation of the biliary tree. This syndrome has therefore been designated "paraneoplastic" (29). A fourth patient with this syndrome was found to have lumbar disc disease, but an occult neoplasm is suspected. This latter patient's biliary dilatation may have occurred as a result of impingement on vital structures, including sympathetic and parasympathetic nerves (myenteric plexus) denervating the periampullary region and accounting for the dilatation (30,31). Cholestasis was present in all patients, but they were not jaundiced. Because of cholestatic chemistries, a CT scan was performed, which demonstrated a dilated biliary tree. The ERCP was then requested.

Benign stenosis of the distal bile duct may be sub-

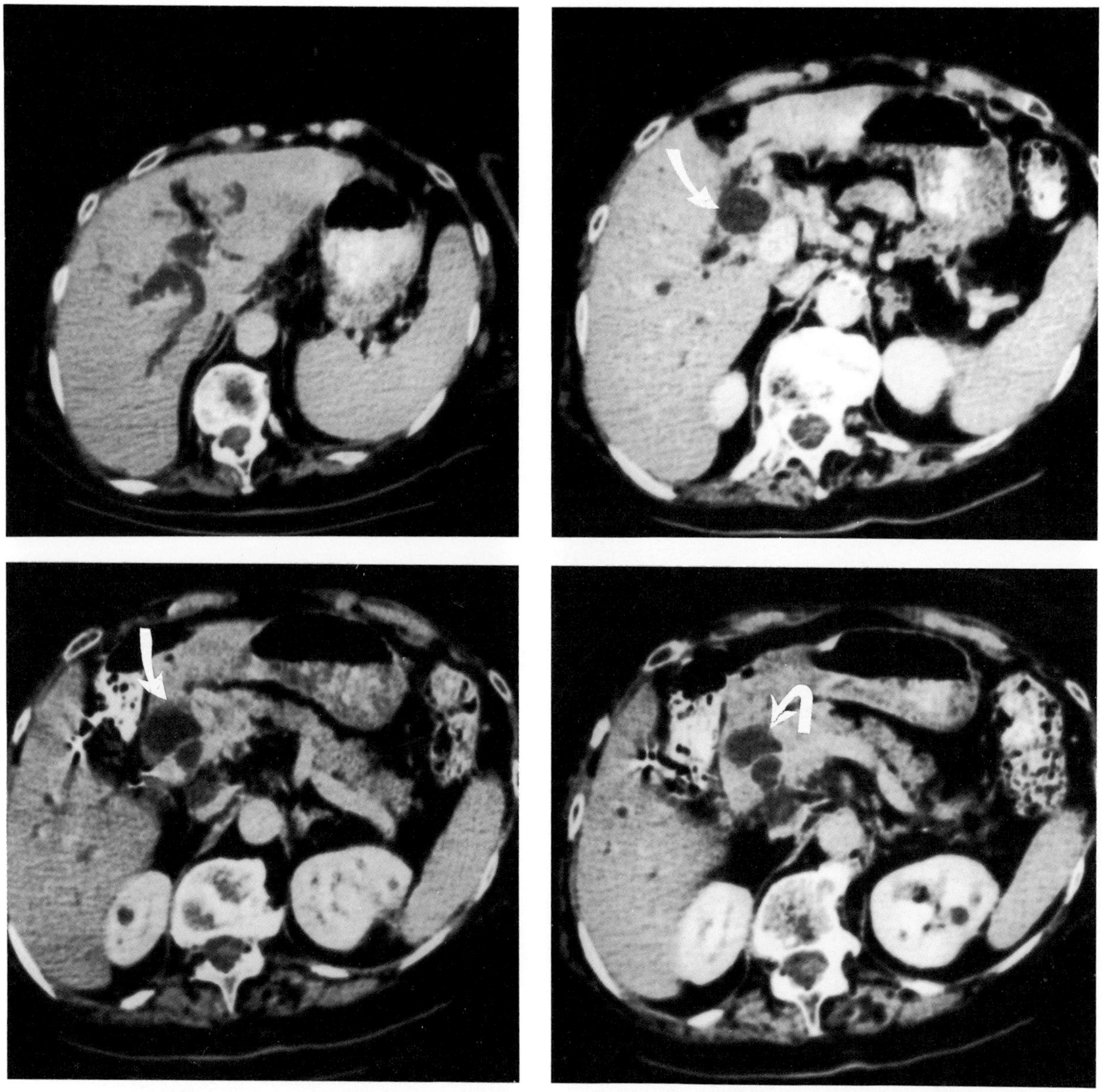

FIG. 6.31. A four-part CT scan. **Upper left:** Dilated intrahepatic ducts. **Upper right:** A dilated bile duct (*arrow*). **Lower left:** A dilated distal bile duct (*arrow*). **Lower right:** The dilated bile duct seen at the level of the head of the pancreas. No masses are evident, yet the findings are compatible with obstruction. No obstructive lesion is demonstrated, so this case can be classified as paraneoplastic.

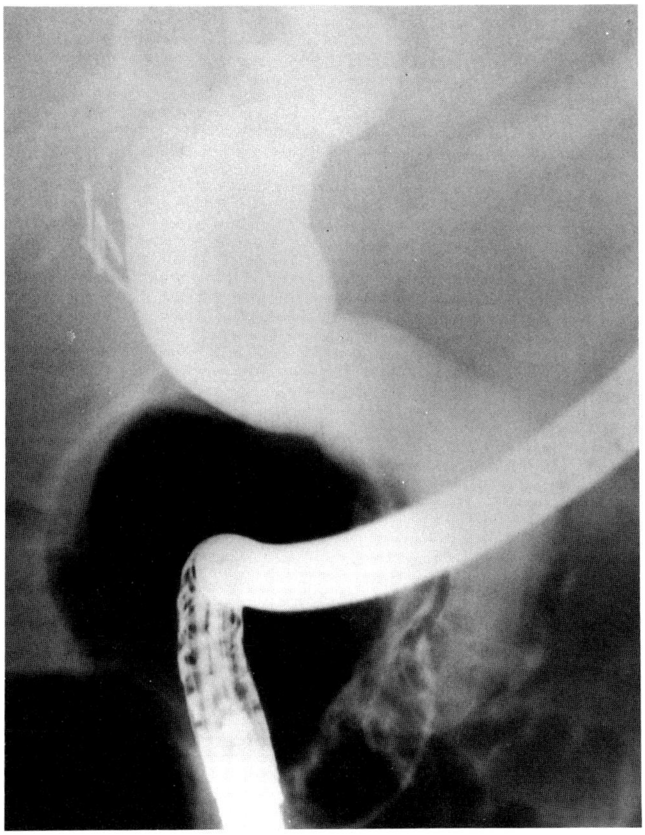

FIG. 6.32. An opacified dilated bile duct. Dilatation of the duct is seen down to the ampullary region.

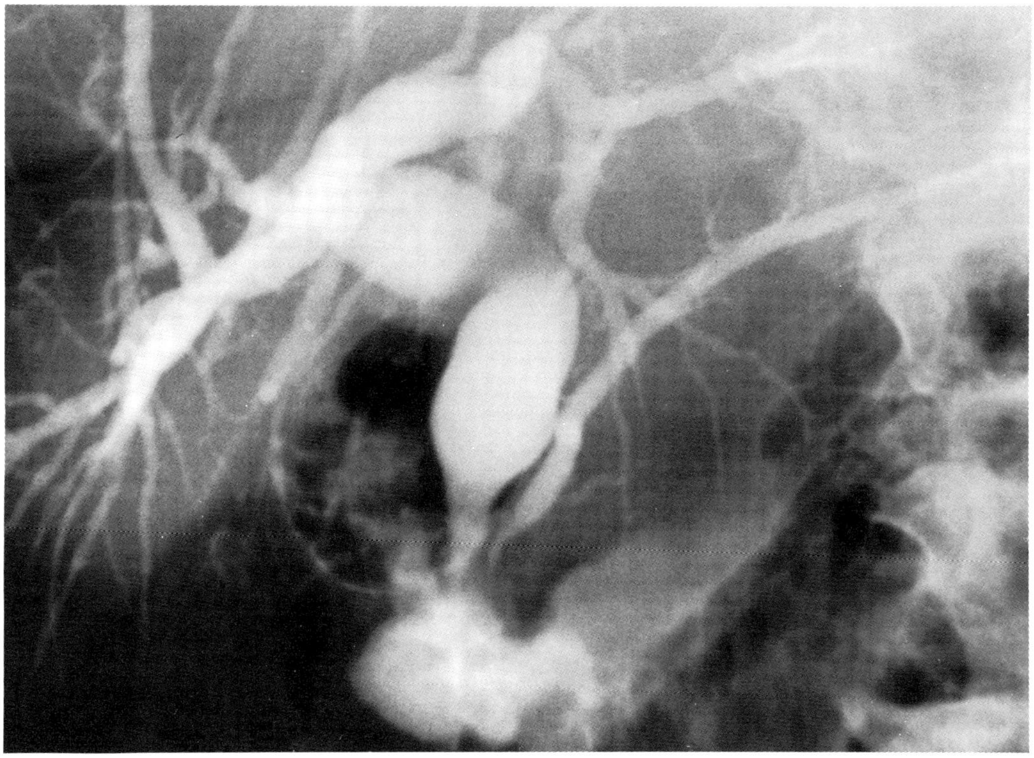

FIG. 6.33. A dilated common bile duct (CBD), a tapered distal duct, and delayed emptying consistent with papillary stenosis.

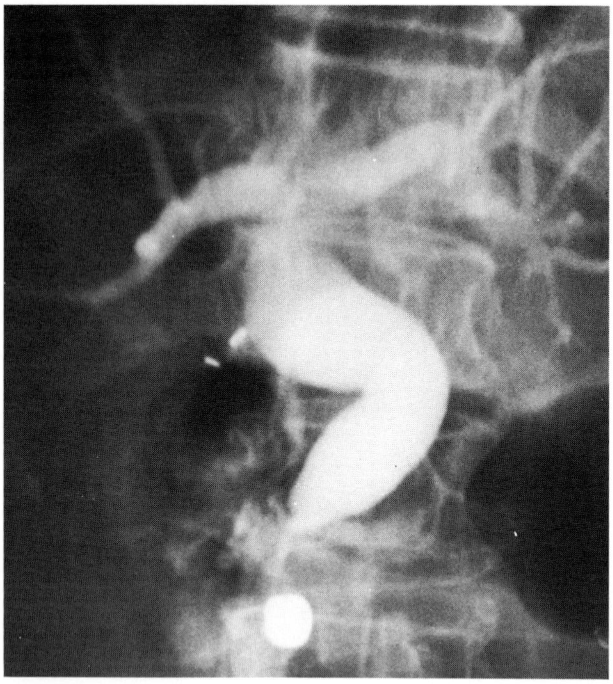

FIG. 6.34. A markedly dilated bile duct, tapered distal end, and delayed emptying consistent with papillary stenosis.

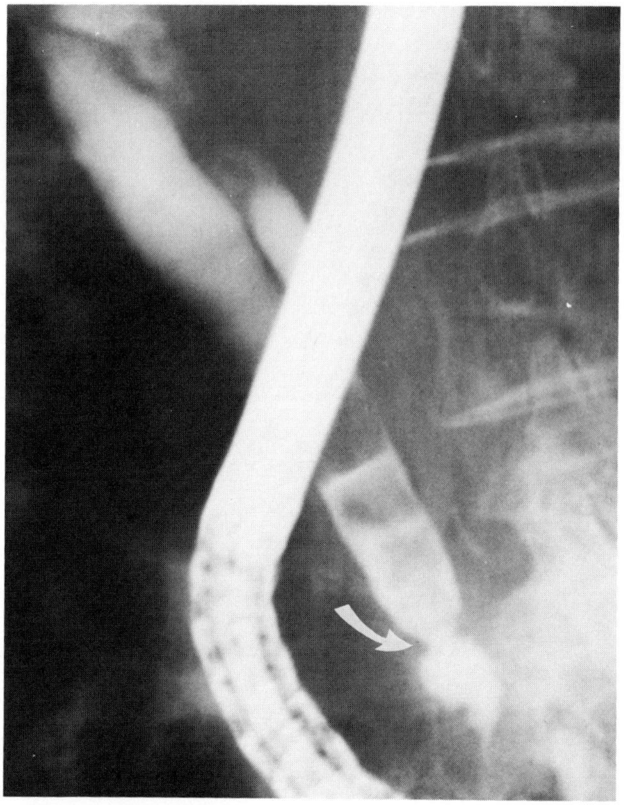

FIG. 6.36. A slightly dilated bile duct filled with several large stones. Note the activity of the sphincter of Oddi (*arrow*).

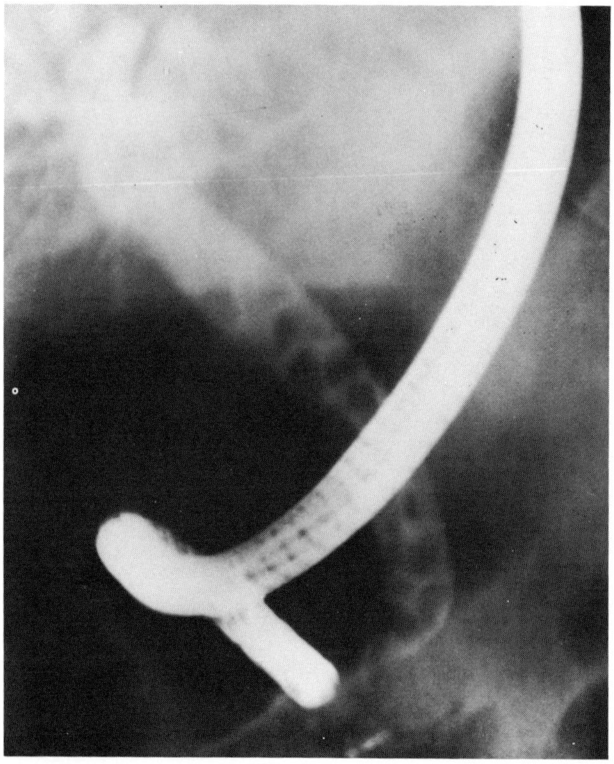

FIG. 6.35. Multiple stones in the common bile duct found in a patient presenting with jaundice and cholangitis.

sequent to long-standing inflammatory disease, usually secondary to sludge or stone passage. Examples of benign stenosis are shown in Figs. 6.33 and 6.34. Patients with this entity usually present with acute or chronic pain, evidence of cholestasis, dysfunction of the sphincter of Oddi, and delayed emptying on timed density radiographs. Attempts to classify this entity have been the subject of many papers, but it remains difficult to define unless the patient presents with cholestatic disease and a dilated bile duct (32) (Table 6.3). To date, the most reliable test to confirm dysfunction is sphincter of Oddi manometrics. This subject is covered in greater detail in Chapters 8 and 10.

Stone disease, another cause of extrahepatic jaundice, presents in many ways, varying from asympto-

TABLE 6.3. *Papillary stenosis*

Criteria for diagnosis
Clinical
Biochemical
Radiographic
Timed density studies
Sphincter of Oddi manometry; pharmacologic augmentation

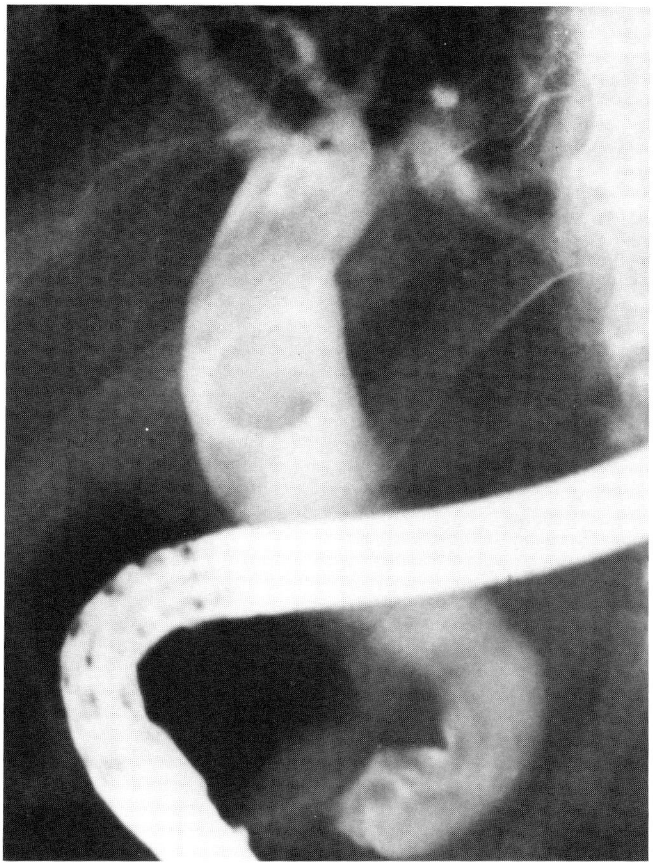

FIG. 6.37. A dilated bile duct. There are several stones floating in the common hepatic duct, which were displaced by the cannula and contrast.

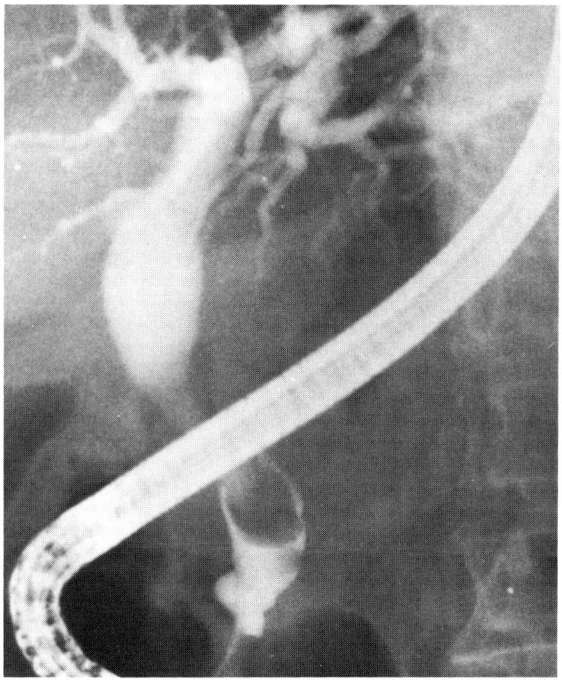

FIG. 6.38. A large common bile duct stone in the distal duct. The catheter dislodged the stone so that contrast material could be injected. The mid common bile duct is incompletely filled on this radiograph. There is no stricture present.

matic disease to life-threatening cholangitis. Figures 6.35 through 6.38 are illustrative examples of common bile duct stones. The approach to the management of stone disease is presented in Chapters 10 and 11.

Of course, with the advent of interventional techniques, both endoscopic and radiographic decompression of an obstructed biliary tree has been accomplished successfully using both therapeutic disciplines. Treatment modalities and techniques utilizing ERCP, sphincterotomy, hydrostatic dilatation and decompression procedures such as stents will be discussed in detail in chapters 10, 12, and 13.

REFERENCES

1. Siegel JH, Yatto RP. Approach to cholestasis—an update. *Arch Int Med* 1982;142:1877–9.
2. Siegel JH, Schapiro M, Hughes RW Jr. Endoscopy, obstructive jaundice, and DRG's: the buck stops in the hospital bank account. *Am J Gastroenterol* 1986;82:1783–4.
3. Dillon E, Peel AL, Parkin GJ. The diagnosis of primary bile duct carcinoma (cholangiocarcinoma) in the jaundiced patient. *Clin Radiol* 1981;32:311–7.
4. Rohrmann CA Jr, Ansel HJ, Ayoole EA, Silvis SE, Vennes JA. Endoscopic retrograde intrahepatic cholangiogram: radiographic findings in intrahepatic disease. *Am J Roentgenol* 1977;128:45–52.

5. Okuda K, Kubo Y, Okazaki N. Clinical aspects of intrahepatic bile duct carcinoma including hilar carcinoma; a study of 57 autopsy proven cases. *Cancer* 1977;39:232–46.
6. Huibregtse K. *Endoscopic biliary and pancreatic drainage*. Stuttgart, Germany: George Thieme Verlag, 1988.
7. Huibregtse K, Cheng J. Management of malignant biliary strictures. In: Barkin J, O'Phelan CA, eds. *Advanced therapeutic endoscopy*. New York: Raven Press, 1990.
8. DeViere J, Baize M, De Toenf J, Cremer M. Long term followup of patients with hilar malignant stricture treated by endoscopic internal biliary drainage. *Gastrointest Endosc* 1988;34:95–101.
9. Siegel JH. Endoscopic approach to management of hepatico-pancreatico-biliary disorders. In: Bengmark S, ed. *Progress in surgery of the liver, pancreas and biliary system*. Dordrecht, The Netherlands: Martinus Nijhoff, 1988.
10. Ravo B, Epstein H, LaMendola S, Ger R. The Mirizzi syndrome: preoperative diagnosis by sonography and transhepatic cholangiography. *Am J Gastroenterol* 1986;81:688–90.
11. Mirizzi PL. Syndrome del conducto hepatico. *J Int Chir* 1948;8:731–7.
12. Koehler RE, Melson GL, Lee JKT, et al. Common hepatic duct obstruction by cystic duct stone. Mirizzi syndrome. *Am J Roentgenol* 1979;132:1007–9.
13. Starling JR, Matallan RH. Benign mechanical obstruction of the common hepatic duct (Mirizzi syndrome). *Surgery* 1980;88:737–40.
14. Balthazar EJ. The Mirizzi syndrome: inflammatory stricture of the common hepatic duct. *Am J Gastroenterol* 1975;64:144–8.
15. Joseph S, Carvajal S, Odwin C. Sonographic diagnosis of Mirizzi's syndrome. *JCU* 1985;13:199–201.
16. Richter JM, Silverstein MD, Shapiro R. Suspected obstructive jaundice: a decision analysis of diagnostic strategies. *Ann Intern Med* 1983;99:46–51.
17. Baron RL, Stanley RJ, Lee JK, Koehler RE, Levitt RG. Computed tomographic features of biliary obstruction. *AJR* 1983; 140:1173–8.
18. Bondestam S, Taavitsainen M, Jappinen S, Korhola O. Ultrasound examination and cholescintigraphy in cholestasis. *Acta Radiol* 1981;22:421–6.
19. Borsch G, Wegener M, Wedmann B, Kissler M, Glocke M. Clinical evaluation, ultrasound, cholescintigraphy, and endoscopic retrograde cholangiography in cholestasis. A prospective comparative clinical study. *J Clin Gastroenterol* 1988;10:185–90.
20. Musher DR, Madayag MA, Tobias H. Carcinoma of the gallbladder: a diagnosis aided by endoscopic retrograde and percutaneous hepatic cholangiography. *Am J Gastroenterol* 1976;66:79–83.
21. Walker JM, Kanzer BF. Carcinoma of the cystic duct mimicking the Mirizzi syndrome. *Am J Gastroenterol* 1982;73:936–8.
22. Piehler J, Cinchlow R. Primary carcinoma of the gallbladder. *Surg Gynecol Obstet* 1978;147:929–42.
23. Kelly T, Chamberlain T. Carcinoma of the gallbladder. *Am J Surg* 1982;143:737–47.
24. Kreek MJ, Balint JA. "Skinny needle" cholangiography—results of a pilot study of a voluntary prospective method for gathering risk data on new procedures. *Gastroenterology* 1980; 78:598.
25. Foutch PG, Harlan JR, Kerr D, Sanowski RA. Wire-guided brush cytology: a new endoscopic method for diagnosis of bile duct cancer. *Gastrointest Endosc* 1989;35:243–7.
26. Makipur H, Cooperman A, Danzi JT, Farmer RG. Carcinoma of the ampulla of Vater: a review of 38 cases with emphasis on treatment and prognostic factors. *Ann Surg* 1976;183:341–4.
27. Knox RA, Kingston RD. Carcinoma of the ampulla of Vater. *Br J Surg* 1986;73:72–3.
28. Cooperman AM. Periampullary cancer. *Semin Liver Dis* 1983;3:181–92.
29. Yapp RG, Siegel JH. Unexplained biliary tract dilatation in lung cancer patients: a new paraneoplastic syndrome. [Submitted for publication].
30. Ahmed MN, Carpenter S. Anatomic neuropathy and carcinoma of the lung. *Can Med Assoc J* 1975;113:410–2.
31. Ogilvie H. Large intestine colic due to sympathetic deprivation. *Br Med J* 1948;2:671–3.
32. Geenen JE, Hogan WJ, Dodds WJ, Toouli J, Venu RP. The efficacy of endoscopic sphincterotomy after cholecystectomy in patients with sphincter of Oddi dysfunction. *N Engl J Med* 1989;320:82–7.

CHAPTER 7

Periampullary Findings: Atlas of Duodenoscopy

Access to the papilla of Vater is possible after entering the duodenum and positioning the duodenoscope in an enface position. The major advantage of ERCP over percutaneous cholangiography is the fact that the mucosa of the upper gastrointestinal (GI) tract is available for examination and may provide essential information specific to the disease spectrum and symptom complexes, especially inflammatory and neoplastic diseases of the papilla. The newer, wide-angle duodenscope is capable of examining the distal esophagus when properly flexed in a position permitting visualization of the lumen (Fig. 7.1). Naturally, the stomach can be carefully examined before entering the duodenum. It is advisable to examine the entire stomach and the gastroesophageal junction, which may yield significant pathology. Examination of the gastroesophageal junction is made easier using the side-viewing endoscope because of the ease of retroflexion and visualization of this juncture as a natural function of this endoscope (Fig. 7.2) (see Chapter 2).

The stomach should be regarded not as a conduit through which the endoscope passes to reach the ampulla but as a significant organ (Figs. 7.2–7.5). Evaluation of its physiologic function can be determined by carrying out a proper examination. During the dynamic portion of the examination, observation of peristaltic activity is critical to determining function of the stomach and enables the endoscopist to rule out infiltrative disease. Extrinsic compression of the posterior wall of the stomach yields vital information consistent with pancreatic disease, both benign and malignant. Pancreatic pseudocysts may compress the posterior wall of the stomach, restricting the gastric lumen and affecting its distensibility. Assessment of the function of the gastric antrum as to pliability and rigidity is also important in the total evaluation of the stomach for both inflammatory and malignant disease. Rigidity of the gastric antrum is significant and should be ascertained during the examination.

The pylorus is identified and traversed in a manner previously described. The duodenal bulb is often seen briefly in transit, unless the endoscopist pauses to view its walls adequately. Once again, disease states can be confirmed with a proper examination (Figs. 7.6–7.9). When approaching the ampullary region, the endoscopist should always carry out a careful examination of the periampullary structures; in my opinion, this is best performed using the duodenoscope (Figs. 7.10–7.13).

A series of endoscopic views of normal and abnormal papillae is presented in Figs. 7.14 through 7.35, with commentary regarding each in the accompanying legends.

The presence of *periampullary diverticula* may pose a problem in identifying the papilla and properly orienting this structure for cannulation. Several endoscopic views of diverticula are presented in Figs. 7.36 through 7.44. For purposes of teaching and orientation, the papilla is identified, and its position on the wall of the stoma of the diverticulum is identified and classified. A papilla located within a diverticulum is in the most difficult location for identification and cannulation, especially when it lies on the inferior wall of the diverticulum. Assessing the papilla in this situation can be challenging at times, and most of the accepted rules for cannulation, such as straightening the endoscope with the patient in a prone position, are forgotten because the main objects are to identify the papilla and to provide a cholangiopancreatogram. If there are more than one diverticula, straightening the endoscope to 60 cm to 65 cm allows identification of the diverticulum in which the papilla is located. The longitudinal fold will be seen leading toward the diverticulum, con-

Text continues on page 109.

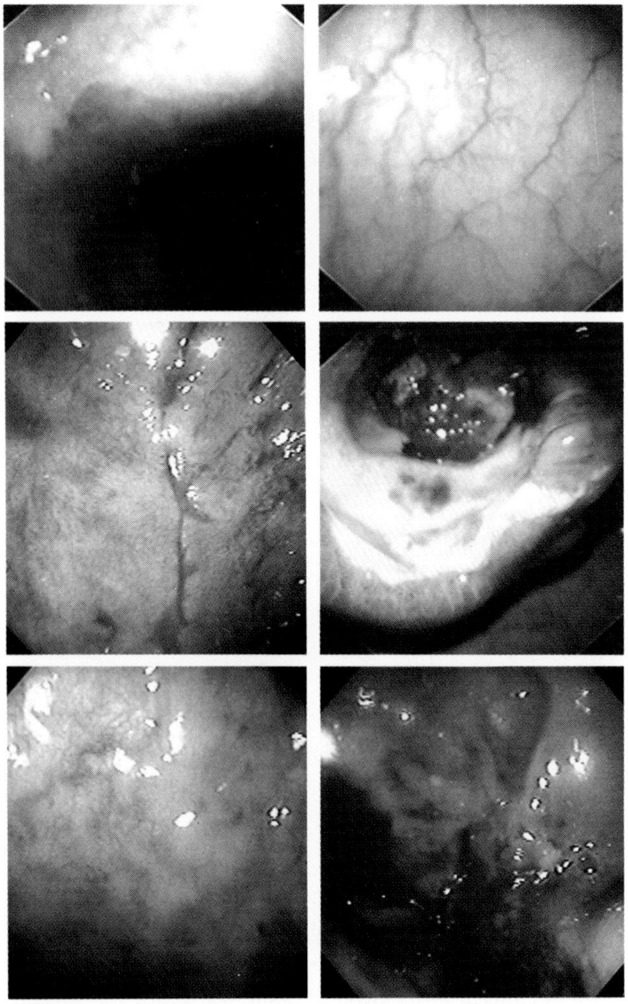

FIG. 7.1. Top left: The junctional mucosa of the gastroesophageal junction (the "Z" line) seen with a duodenoscope. **Top right:** A videoendoscopic view of the distal esophagus showing normal color of the mucosa and vascular pattern. **Middle left:** The esophagogastric junction, revealing evidence of esophagitis. **Middle right:** A lesion of the gastroesophageal junction (squamous cell carcinoma) seen on retroflexion of the videoduodenoscope. **Bottom left:** Esophageal varices on a videoendoscopic picture obtained in a patient with sclerosing cholangitis. **Bottom right:** Bleeding esophageal varices.

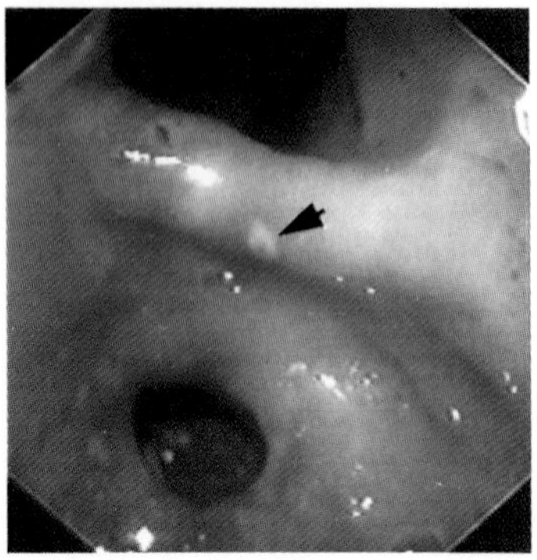

FIG. 7.2. A videoduodenoscopic image of the gastric antrum demonstrating a small ulcer on the angularis (*arrow*). Note the retroflexed view toward the fundus.

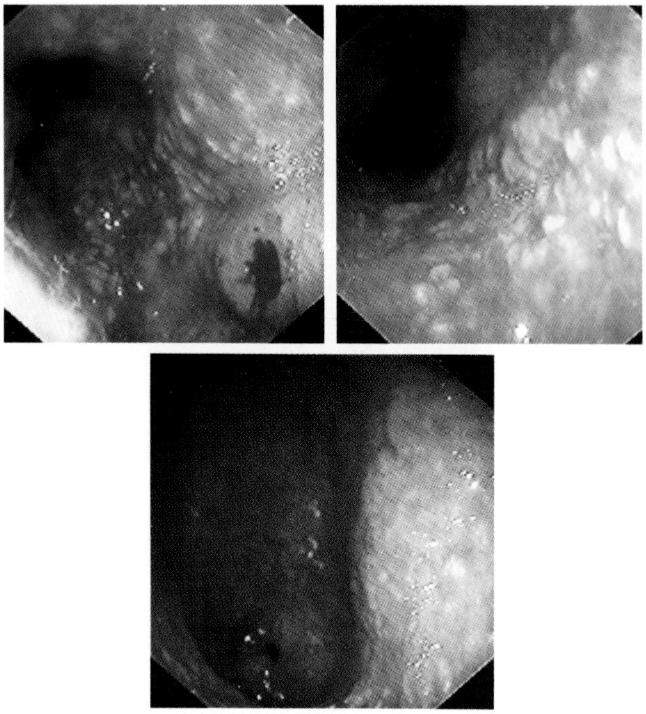

FIG. 7.3. Top left: A videoduodenoscopic picture of the stomach showing evidence of severe gastritis with obvious friability. **Top right:** A close-up view of inflammatory nodules of the stomach. **Bottom:** A view of the gastric antrum and pylorus.

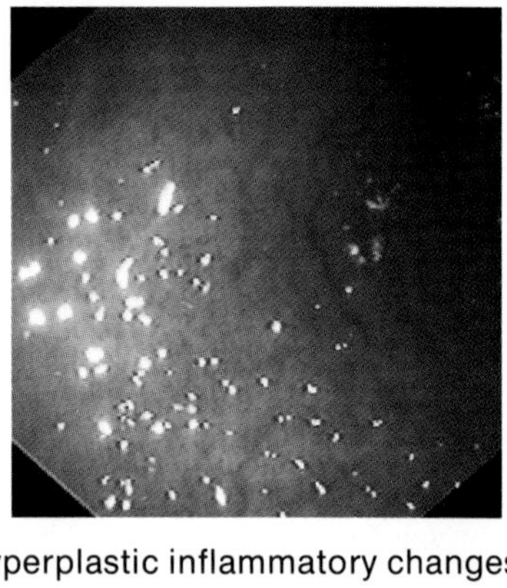

FIG. 7.4. Hyperplastic inflammatory changes of gastritis.

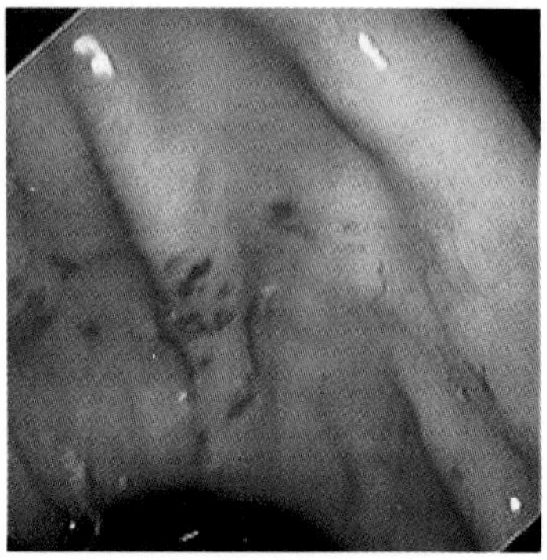

FIG. 7.5. A videoduodenoscopic image of erosive gastritis of the lesser curvature of the stomach.

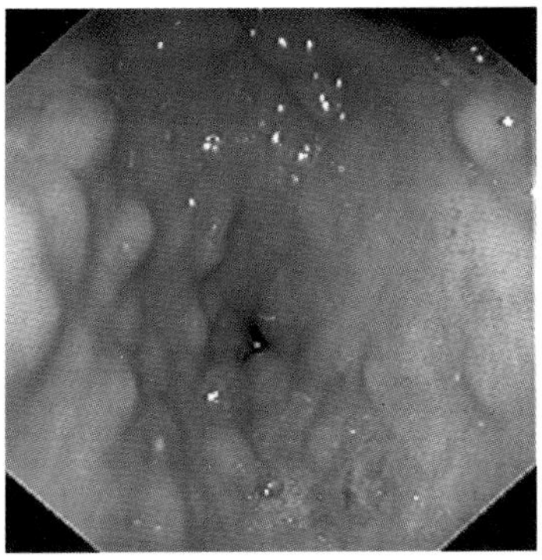

FIG. 7.6. A videoduodensocopic image of hypertrophic Brunner's glands seen in the duodenal bulb.

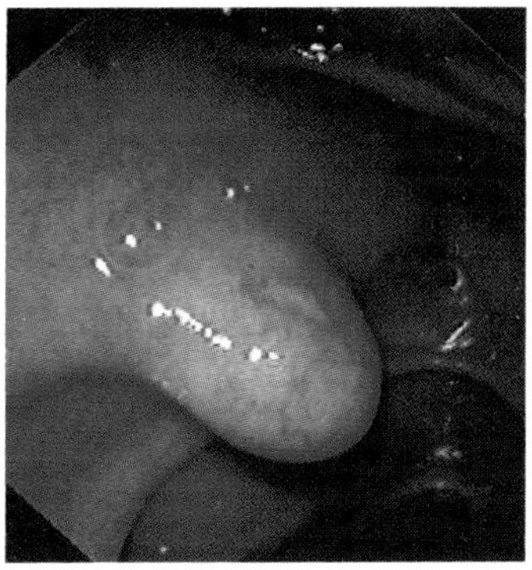

FIG. 7.7. An inflammatory, erosive nodule identified at the junction of the first and second portions of the duodenum.

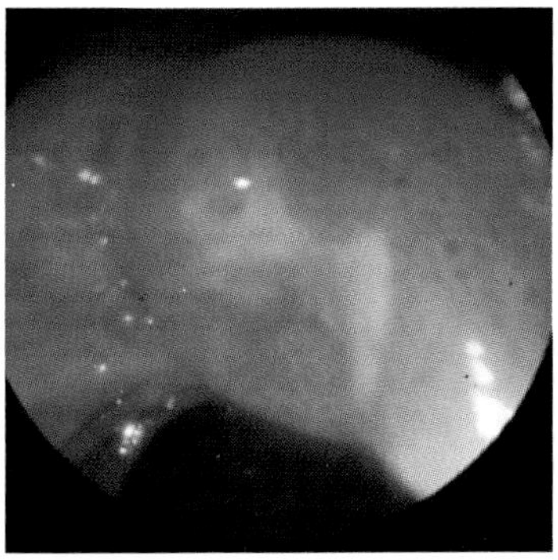

FIG. 7.8. For contrast, this fiberoptic image demonstrates an ulceration of the duodenum at the junction of the first and second portions of the duodenum.

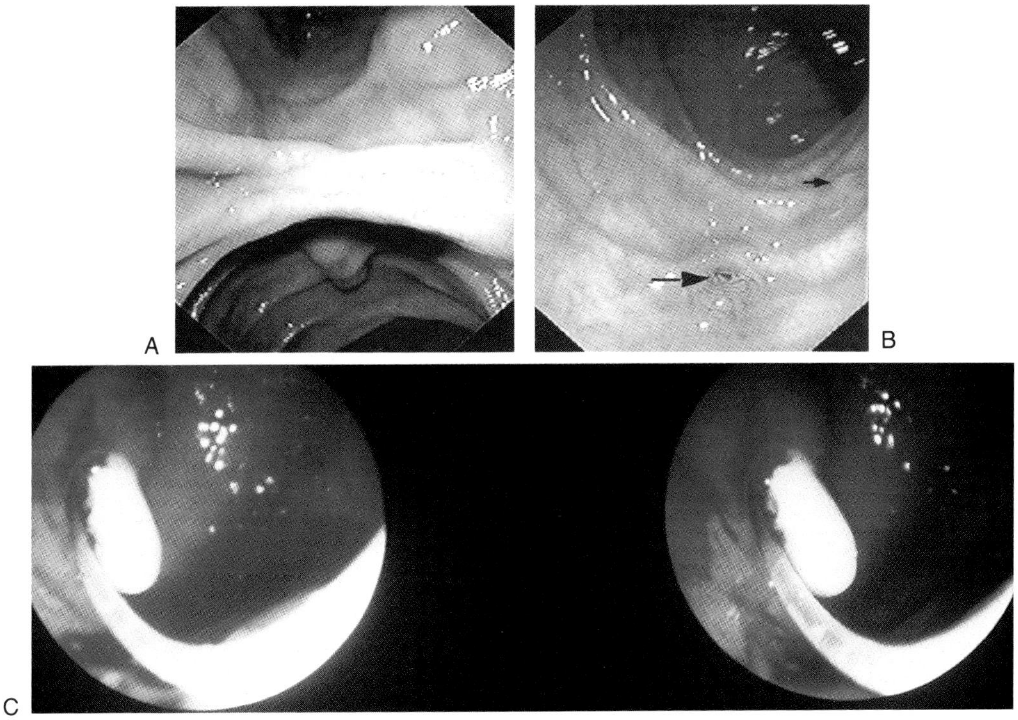

FIG. 7.9. A: After the endoscopist has entered the proximal duodenum, the minor papilla is seen at 1:00. The major papilla is evident in the distance. B: An endoscopic view of a less-obvious papilla in the second portion of the duodenum. The eroded center probably resulted from passage of a stone or sludge (*lower arrow*). The minor papilla is situated at 3:00 (*upper arrow*). C: An unusual fiberoptic view of an abdominal drain in the duodenum that had perforated the duodenal wall. A cannula is used to enter the cavity into which the drain was placed to inject contrast for identification of the fistulous tract.

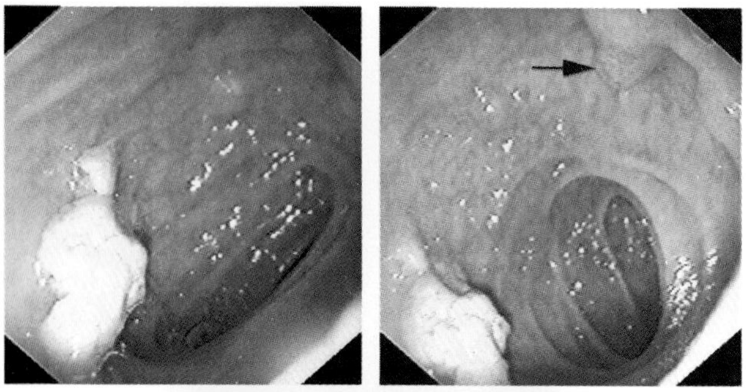

A

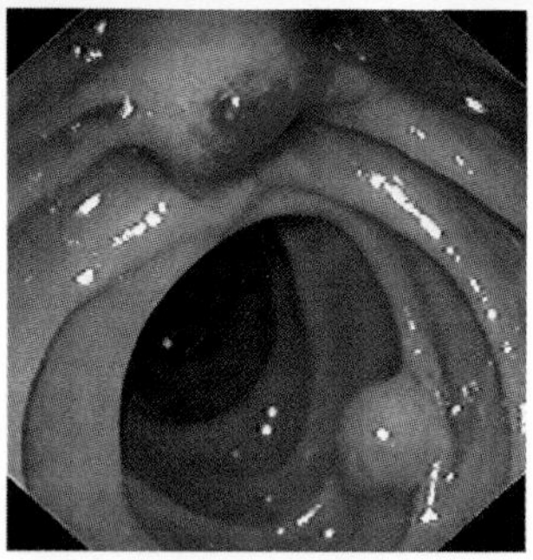

B

FIG. 7.10. A: Left: A videoendoscopic view of the second portion of the duodenum obtained using a forward-viewing instrument. The mass on the medial wall is an adenocarcinoma, but, because of improper orientation using a forward-viewing endoscope, it was confused for a large papilla. **Right:** After repositioning of the forward-viewing endoscope, the papilla can be seen at 1:00 (*arrow*). This orientation would be more accurate and usual using a duodenoscope. **B:** A duodenoscopic picture showing the major papilla in the upper portion of the picture (11:00), slightly irritated after cannulation. The cystic structure in the lower portion of the picture at 5:00 represents an aberrant minor papilla.

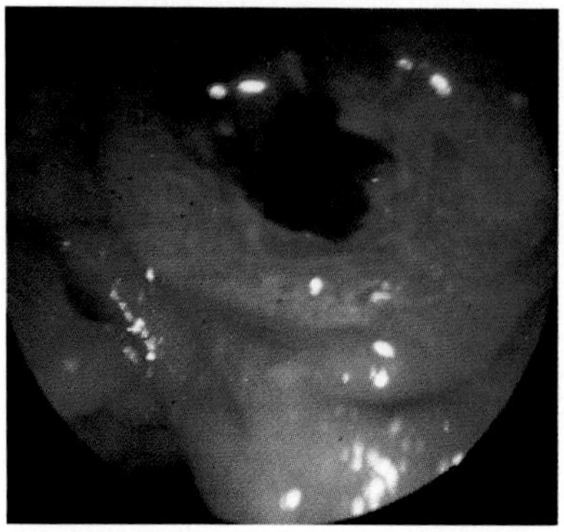

FIG. 7.11. A fiberoptic picture of an eroded papilla after passage of a stone.

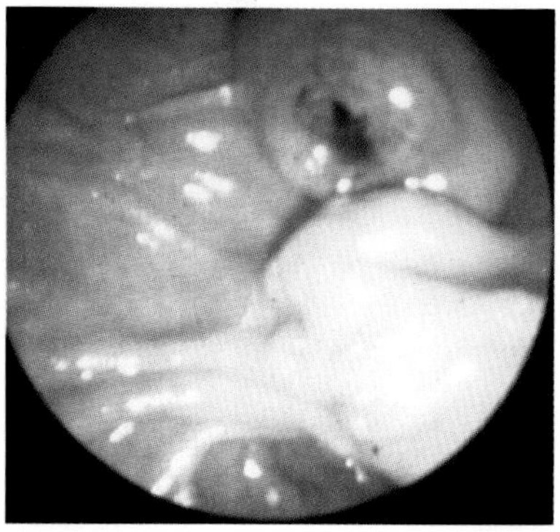

FIG. 7.12. Another example of an eroded papilla after stone passage.

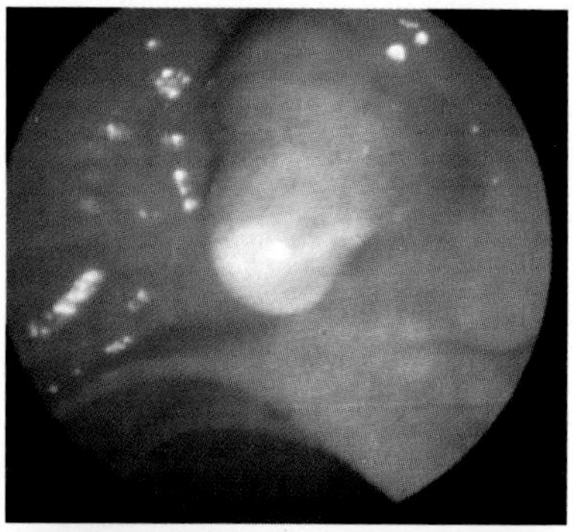

A

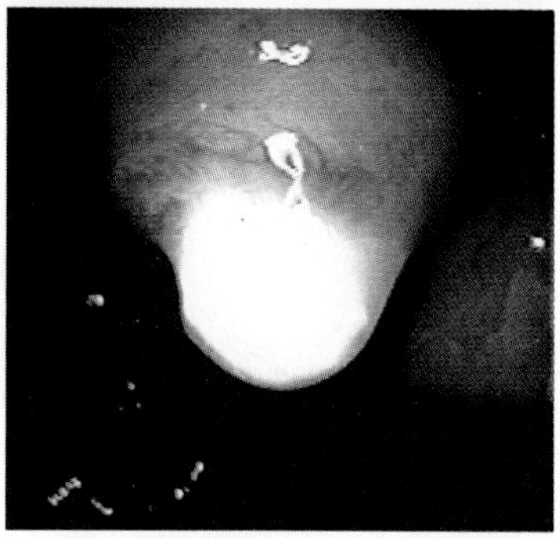

B

FIG. 7.13. A: A prominent and distended papilla with purulent material exuding from its opening. This finding is classical for suppurative cholangitis. **B:** A prominent papilla containing a white defect that proved to be a pancreatic stone that obstructed the duct and was responsible for pancreatitis. After the stone was dislodged and a sphincterotomy was performed, the pancreatitis resolved.

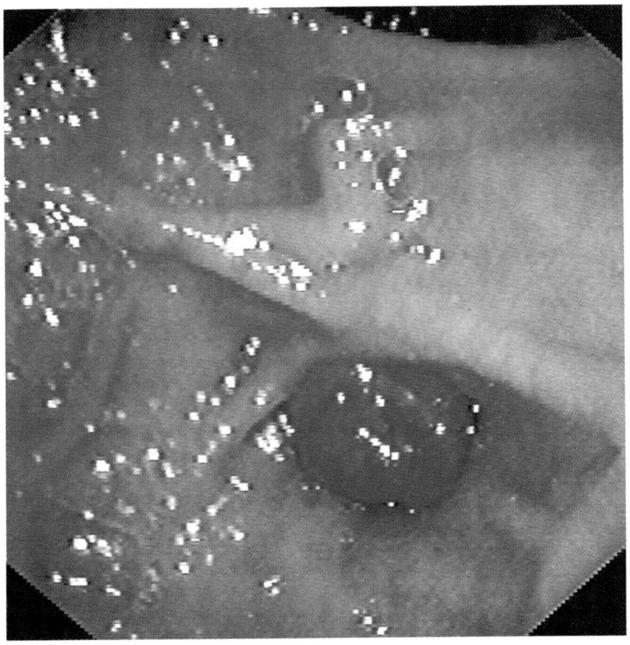

FIG. 7.14. An example of acute papillitis, which is identified by the beefy red inflammatory changes of the papilla.

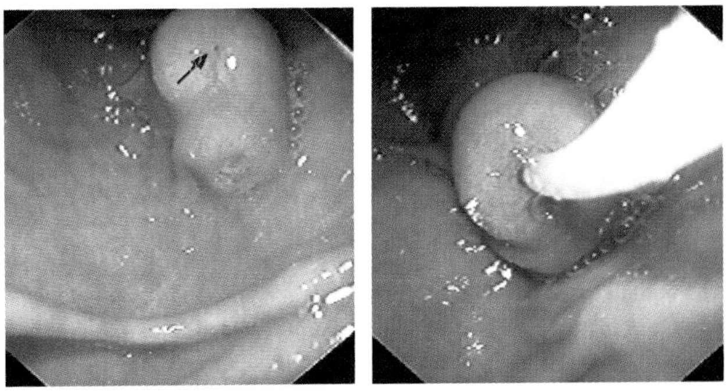

FIG. 7.15. **Left:** A prominent ampulla containing a bulge, which is located cephalad and is due to an impacted stone. The small dot in the middle of the bulge (*arrow*) is the opening to a fistula, which developed from stone erosion. The papilla is inferior to the prominent ampulla. **Right:** A cannula has been placed into the fistulous opening to obtain a cholangiogram.

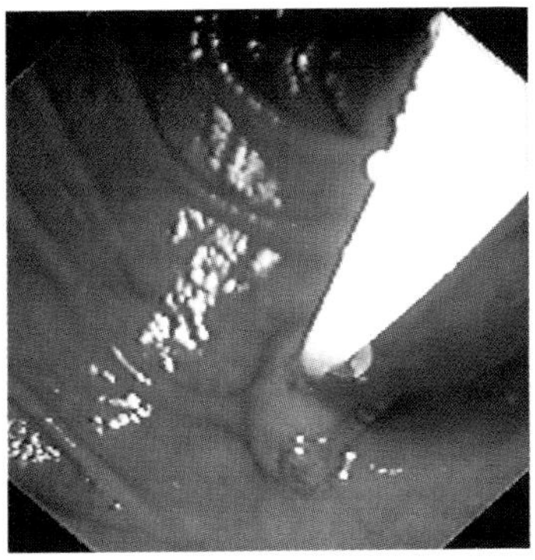

FIG. 7.16. A cannula is placed into a fistulous opening on the ampulla. In addition to stone passage, these fistulas may result from surgical exploration when a probe or dilator is passed into the bile duct, perforating that portion of the ampulla which is least resistant to pressure. This area lacks the usual sphincter fibers and can be penetrated by a stone or probe.

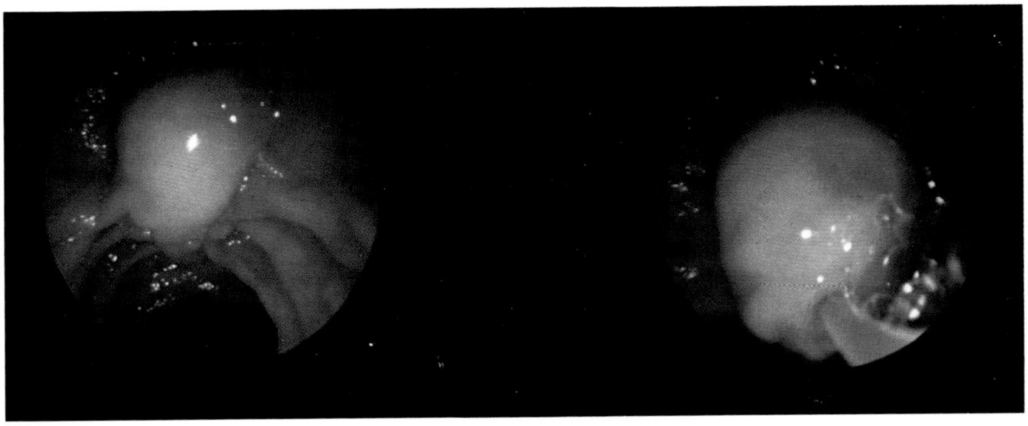

FIG. 7.17. **Left:** A very prominent ampulla and a fistulous opening at the most cephalad portion. The red mucosa represents bile duct mucosa. **Right:** A cannula is placed into the papillary orifice to obtain a cholangiogram. Often, contrast will be seen flowing out of the fistulous tract unless the cannula is inserted deeply beyond the fistulous opening.

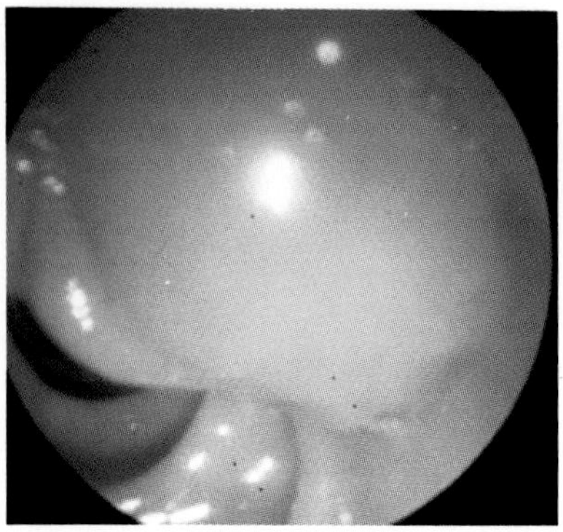

FIG. 7.18. An endoscopic picture of a choledochocele. The choledochocele is a congenital variant and a type of choledochal cyst occurring at the junction of the bile duct and duodenal wall.

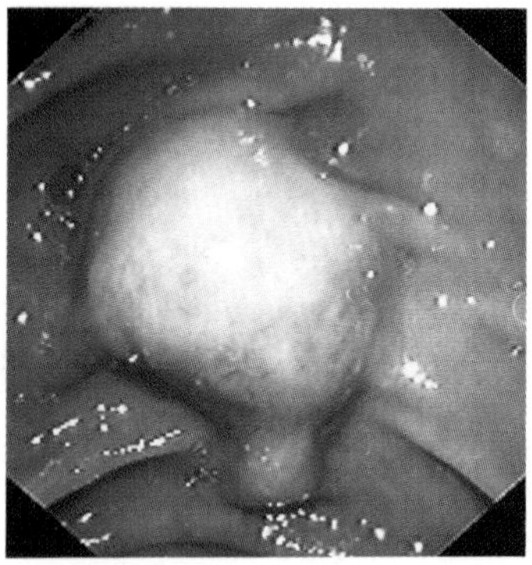

FIG. 7.19. An endoscopic image of a prominent cystlike ampulla. Impacted stones account for the cystic changes.

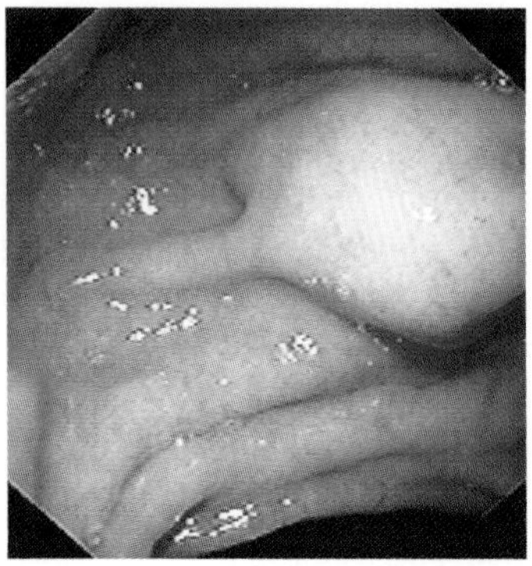

FIG. 7.20. An endoscopic image of a prominent cystlike ampulla. Impacted stones account for the cystic changes.

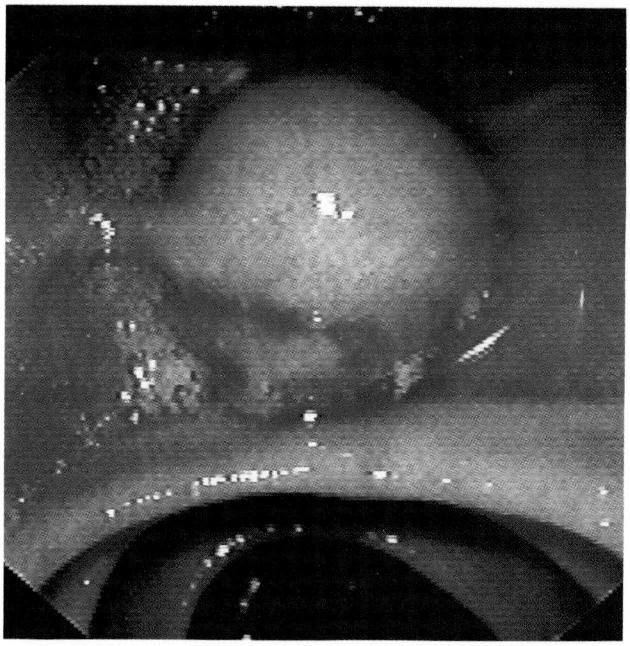

FIG. 7.21. An endoscopic image of a prominent cystlike ampulla. Impacted stones account for the cystic changes.

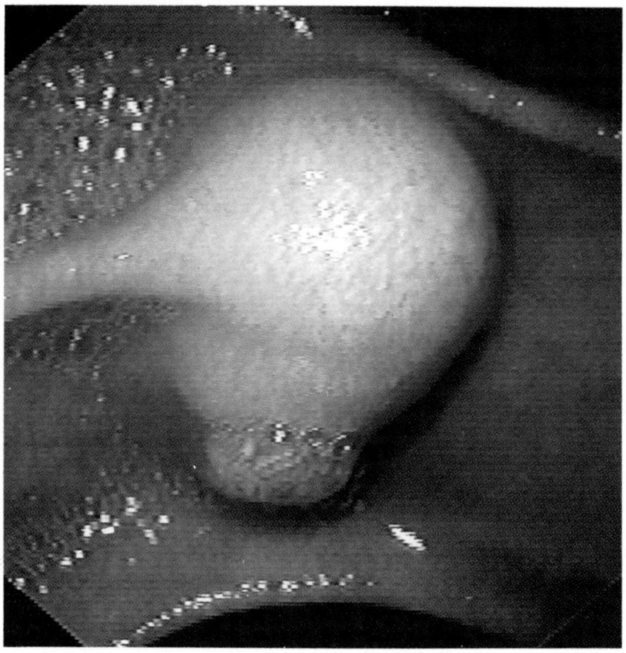

FIG. 7.22. An endoscopic image of a prominent cystlike ampulla. Impacted stones account for the cystic changes.

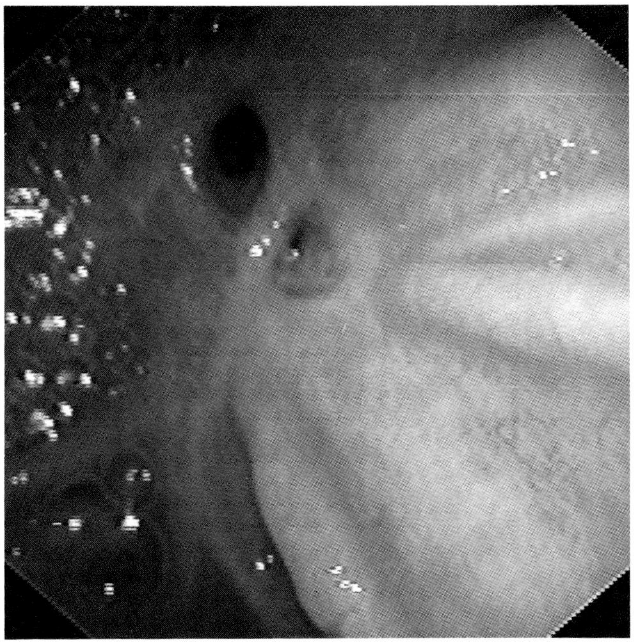

FIG. 7.23. The ampullary region in a patient who has undergone a surgical sphincteroplasty of both the bile duct and the pancreatic duct. Patent stomata are noted.

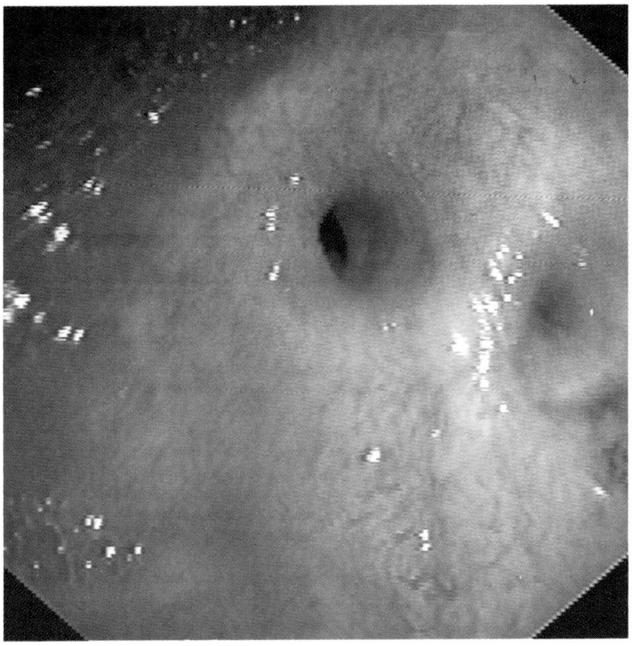

FIG. 7.24. An endoscopic picture taken in a patient who had undergone a surgical sphincterotomy of both the bile duct and the pancreatic duct. In this case, the bile duct stoma was quite adequate, but the pancreatic stoma was stenosed.

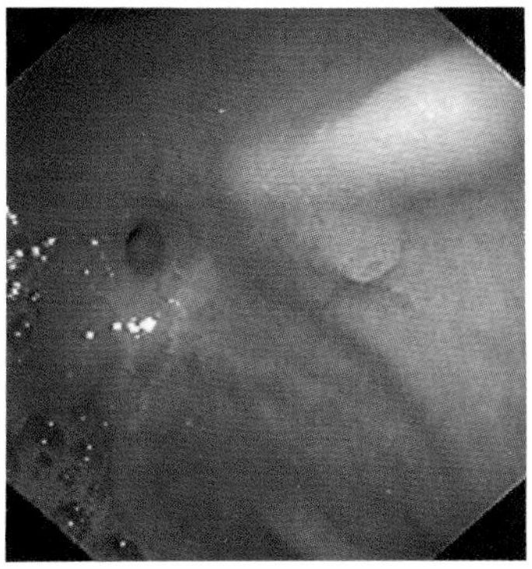

FIG. 7.25. An ampullary region after endoscopic sphincterotomy of the bile duct. The stoma is patent and adequate. The minor papilla is right of the sphincterotomy, just beneath the fold.

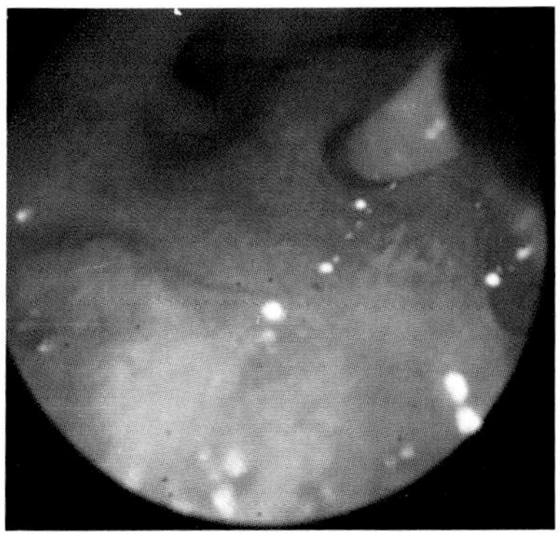

FIG. 7.26. An ampullary region after endoscopic sphincterotomy. A cannula is placed into the pancreatic orifice. After an endoscopic or surgical sphincterotomy of the bile duct, the pancreatic orifice is usually located inferior to the bile duct stoma, is usually flat and not prominent, and requires gentle palpation with the cannula. In the case of stenosis of the pancreatic orifice, a needle-tip catheter or a guidewire is used to cannulate the pancreatic duct selectively.

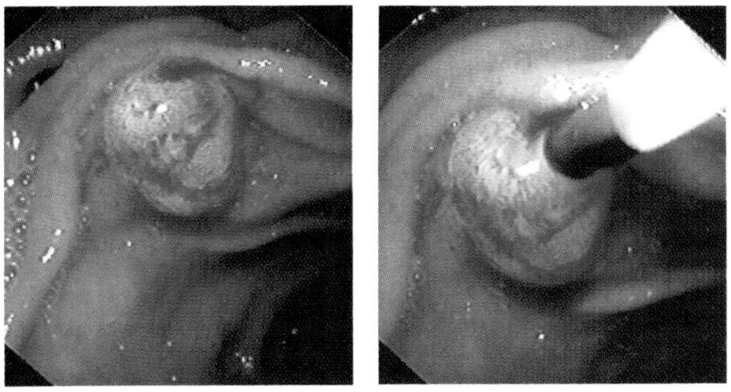

FIG. 7.27. Left: A prominent papilla. **Right:** When the cannula is inserted, the opening is obvious.

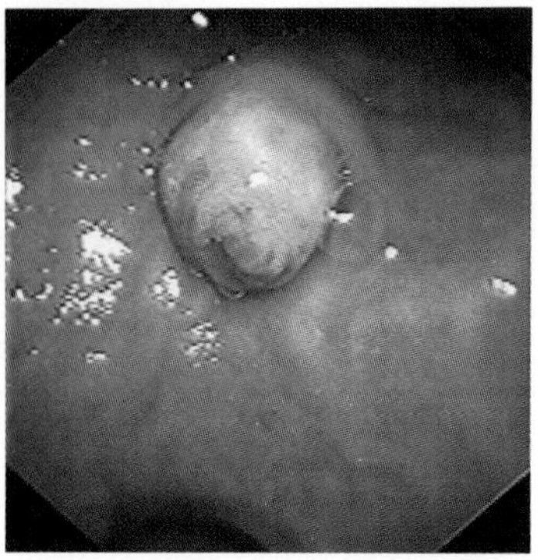

FIG. 7.28. A prominent papilla with an open orifice.

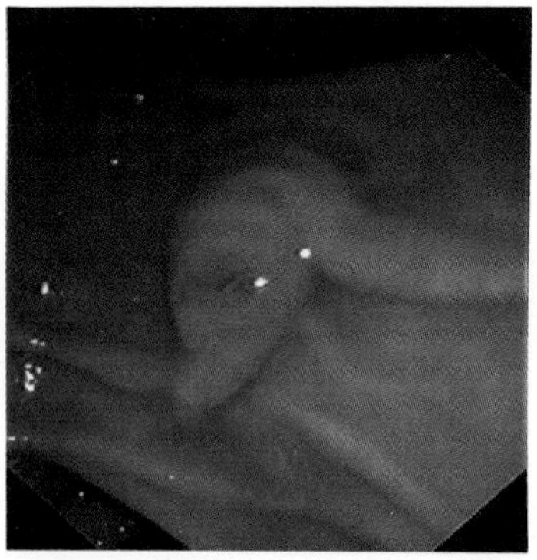

FIG. 7.29. Another example of a prominent papilla with an open orifice.

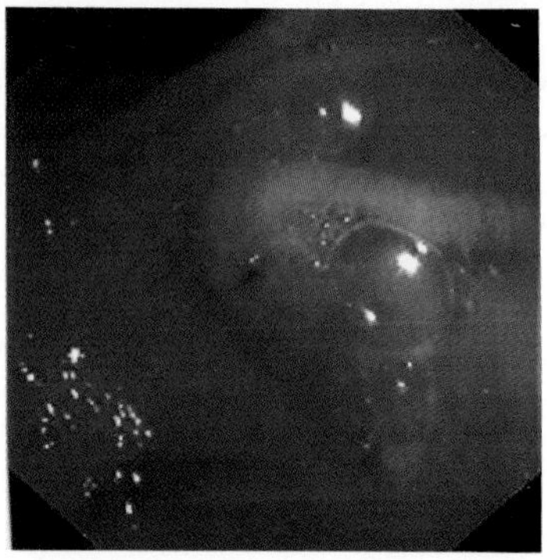

FIG. 7.30. Open orifice on a prominent papilla.

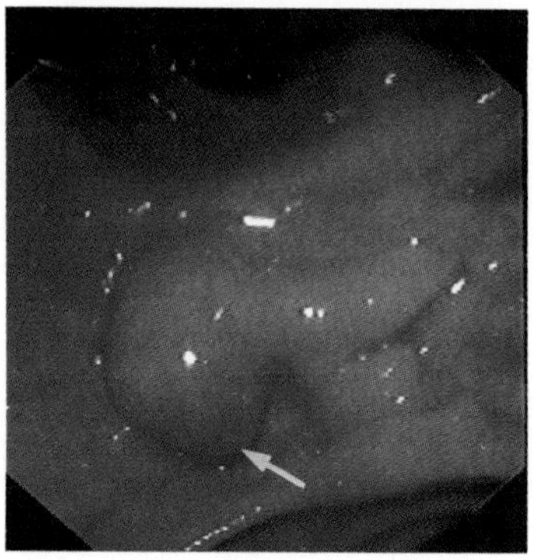

FIG. 7.31. An eccentric papilla with the opening inferior to the bulge (*arrow*).

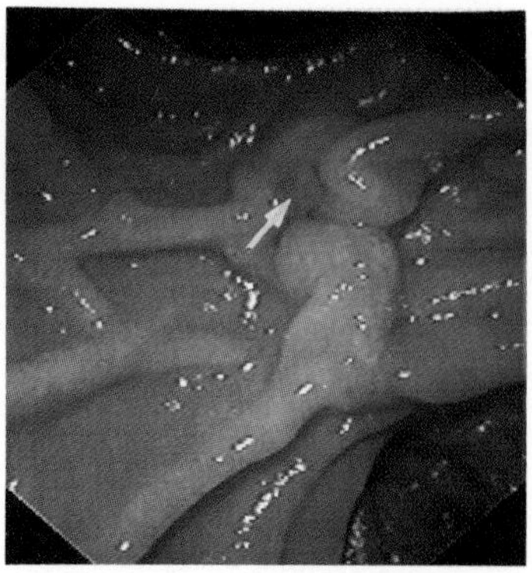

FIG. 7.32. A papilla surrounded by mucosal folds. A careful search and gentle palpation exposes the opening in the middle of the folds (*arrow*).

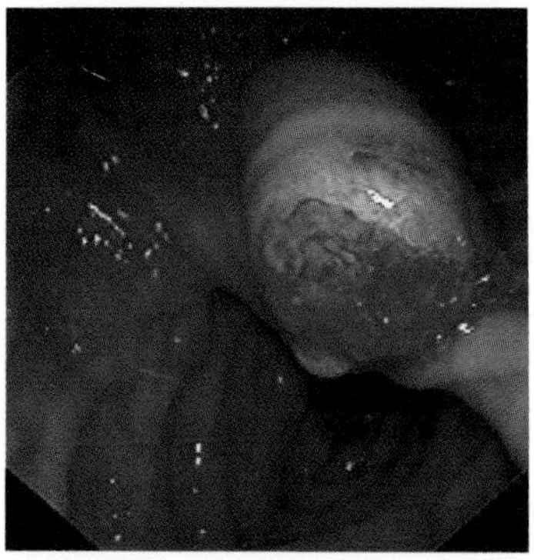

FIG. 7.33. A very prominent, elongated papilla that is enlarged because of an intraampullary adenomacarcinoma.

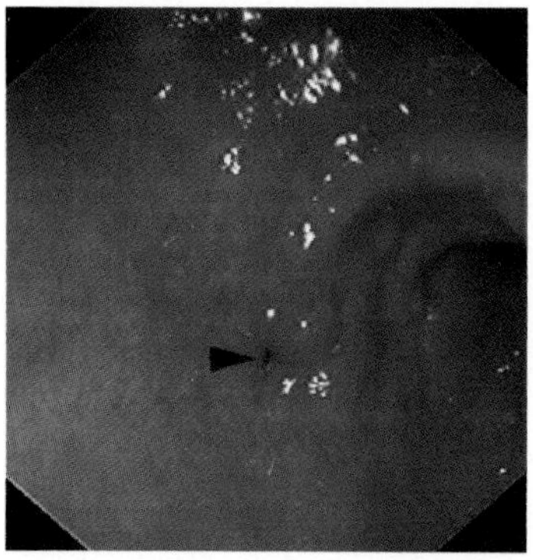

FIG. 7.34. A tiny opening of a stenosed choledochoduodenostomy at the junction of the first and second portions of the duodenum (*arrow*). The patient presented with a "sump syndrome," which resulted from the stenosed enterostomy, preventing egress of bile and refluxed gastrointestinal contents.

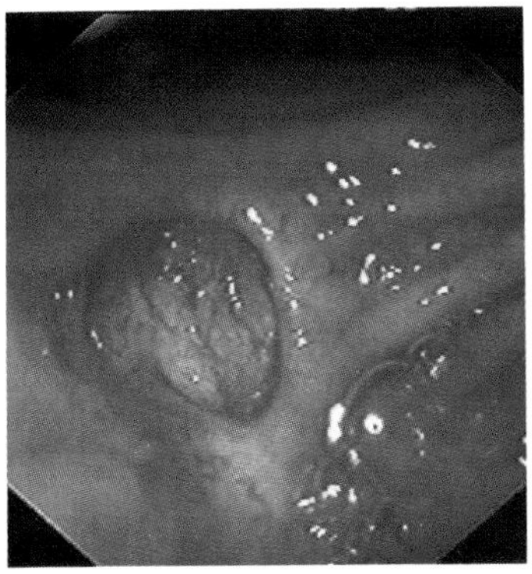

FIG. 7.35. A wide-open choledochoduodenostomy, which appears like a diverticulum. Despite its adequate opening, a sump syndrome developed but was relieved after a retained stone was removed following a sphincterotomy.

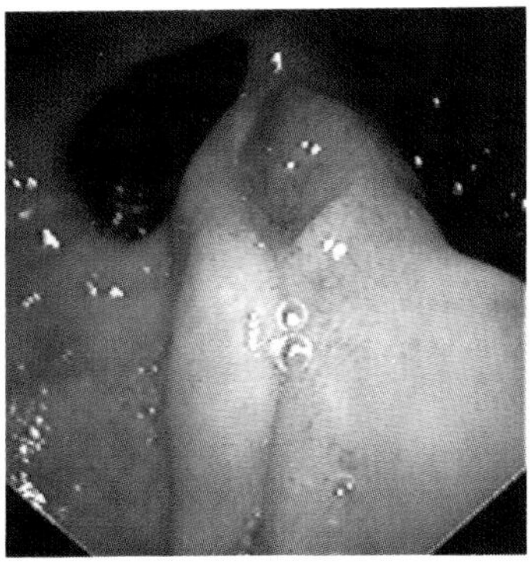

FIG. 7.36. An example of periampullary diverticulum with the papilla in the center of a "pantaloon" diverticulum.

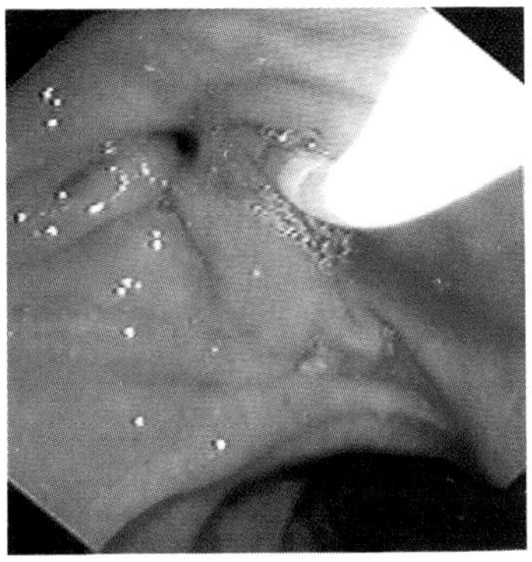

FIG. 7.37. Periampullary diverticulum with the papilla located on the lateral wall.

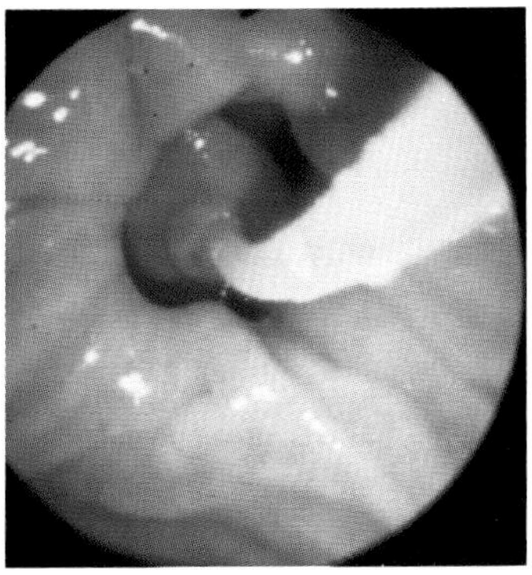

FIG. 7.38. An example of the papilla located deep in the diverticulum, with the cannula shown in the papilla.

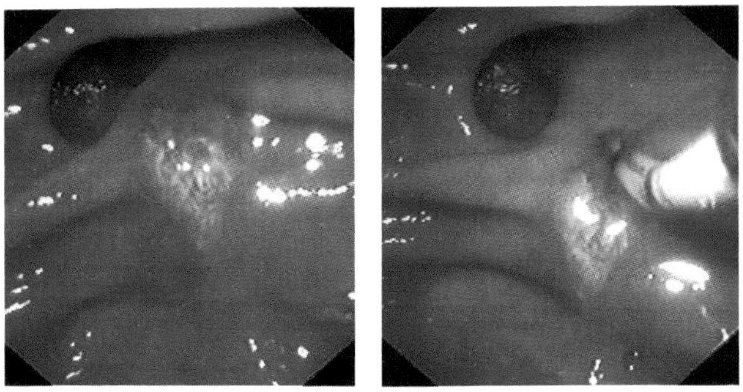

FIG. 7.39. Left: The papilla is located on the inferiolateral wall of this diverticulum. **Right:** The cannula is deeply inserted into the papilla.

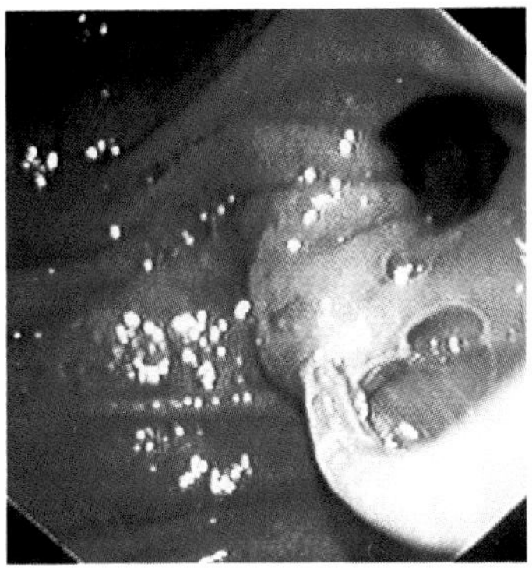

FIG. 7.40. The cannula is being inserted into the papilla, which is located on the medial wall.

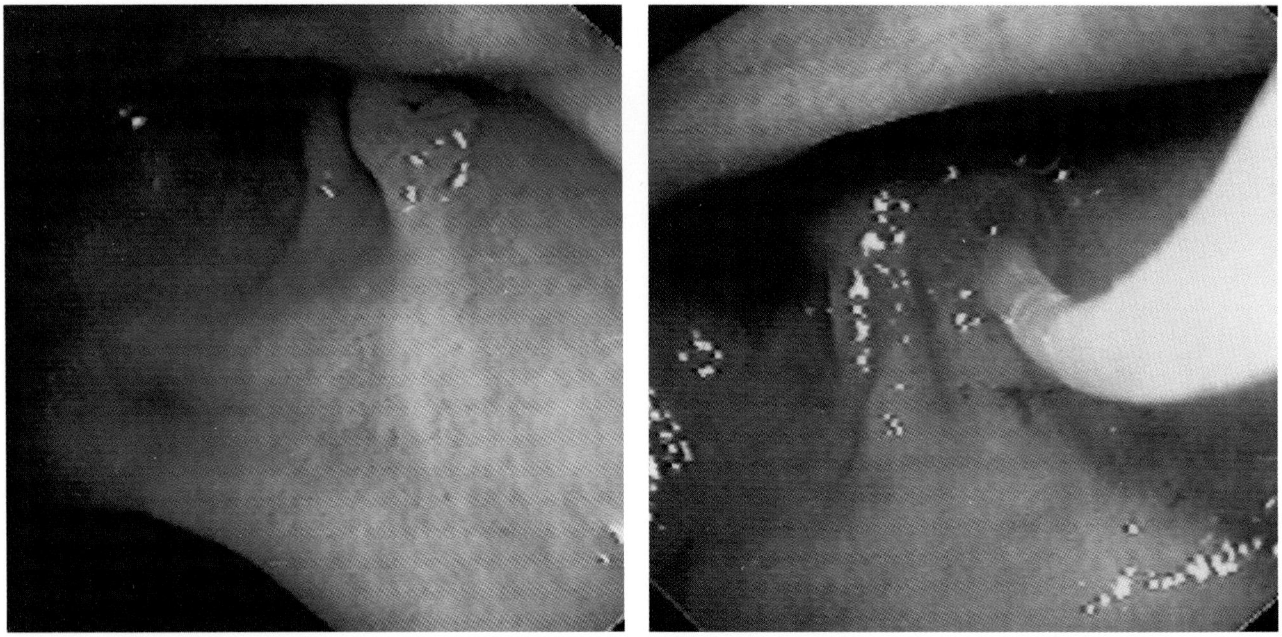

A B

FIG. 7.41. A: A concealed papilla, which is inferior to a fold and lateral to the diverticulum. **B:** The cannula has been inserted into the papilla.

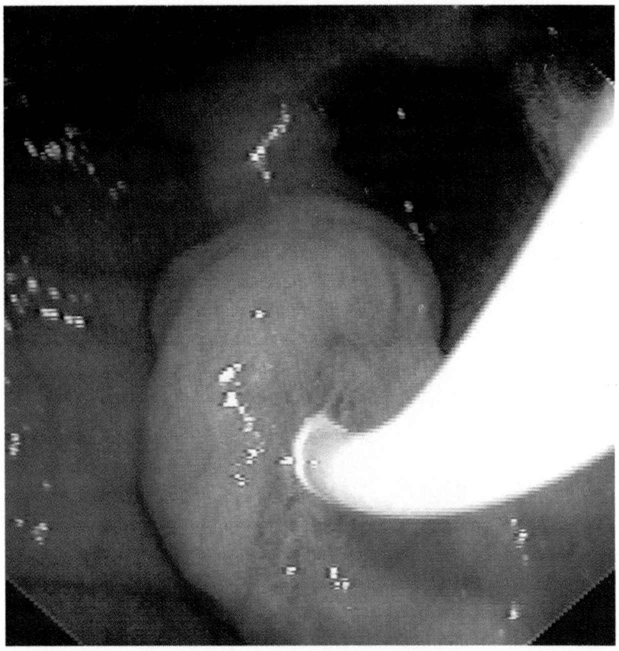

FIG. 7.42. The cannula has been deeply inserted into the papilla located on the inferior medial wall of a large diverticulum. Because of an impacted stone, a submucosal injection occurred, which is represented by the blue color of the swollen tissue.

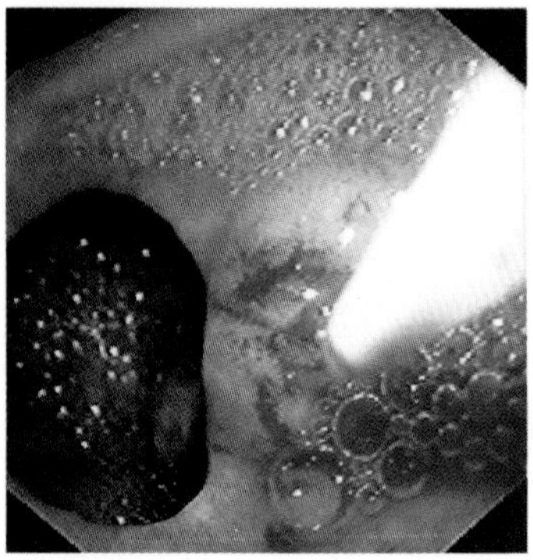

FIG. 7.43. A periampullary diverticulum with its papillary orifice within the diverticulum, which is inaccessible to cannulation. A needle knife is poised in preparation to perform a fistulotomy.

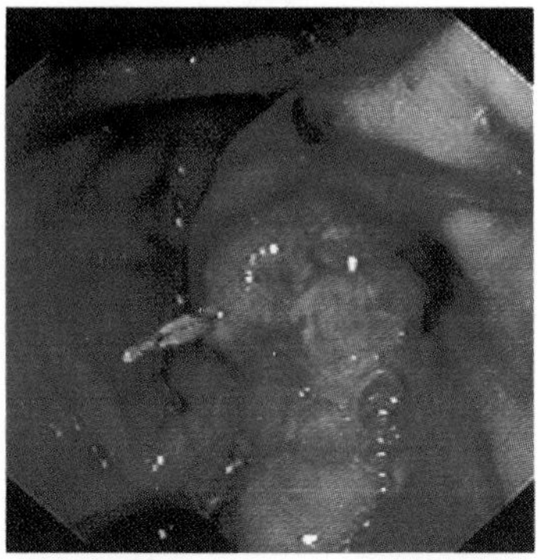

FIG. 7.44. A periampullary diverticulum. The papilla is located on the medial wall. This patient had previously undergone a surgical sphincteroplasty: Note the granulation tissue and suture material near the sphincterotomy.

Text continued from page 99.

firming that the papilla is located within that diverticulum. Also, the minor papilla, which is almost never located in a diverticulum, can be used to identify the major papilla, which will be located in the visualized diverticulum distal to the minor papilla. Performing sphincterotomy in patients with periampullary diverticula is discussed in Chapter 10. Dysfunction of the sphincter of Oddi can result from the anatomic changes or alterations associated with a periampullary diverticulum. The presence of a foreign body, such as a bezoar, may interfere with the physiologic emptying of the bile duct and pancreatic duct and may be responsible for both biliary colic and pancreatitis. If the papilla is lying in the inferior position, abutting the diverticulum wall, dysfunction of the papilla is likely. One can demonstrate this phenomenon by carefully examining the papilla and studying its movement during peristaltic activity. Peristaltic activity may compress the diverticulum and, ultimately, the papilla, producing physiologic dysfunction. A sphincterotomy can be performed in this situation, especially if the bile duct is dilated and if the patient has presented with abnormal liver function studies.

Periampullary lesions such as tubular or villous adenomata or other polypoid lesions can be responsible for recurrent biliary tract or pancreatic duct disorders. Figure 7.45 shows a pedunculated polyp whose stalk was large enough to produce gastric outlet obstruction as the polyp prolapsed into the stomach. At other times, the stalk produced intermittent obstruction to the pancreatic duct responsible for pancreatitis.

It is important for the endoscopist to demonstrate that both the bile and pancreatic ducts are not contained in the polyp stalk before considering transection. These vital structures are often contained in the stalk, and a serious misadventure would occur following a polypectomy, performed either surgically or endoscopically. Therefore, I recommend that, *before performing a polypectomy on a polyp located in the periampullary region, the endoscopist attempt an ERCP to identify the ductular structures*. Once the lo-

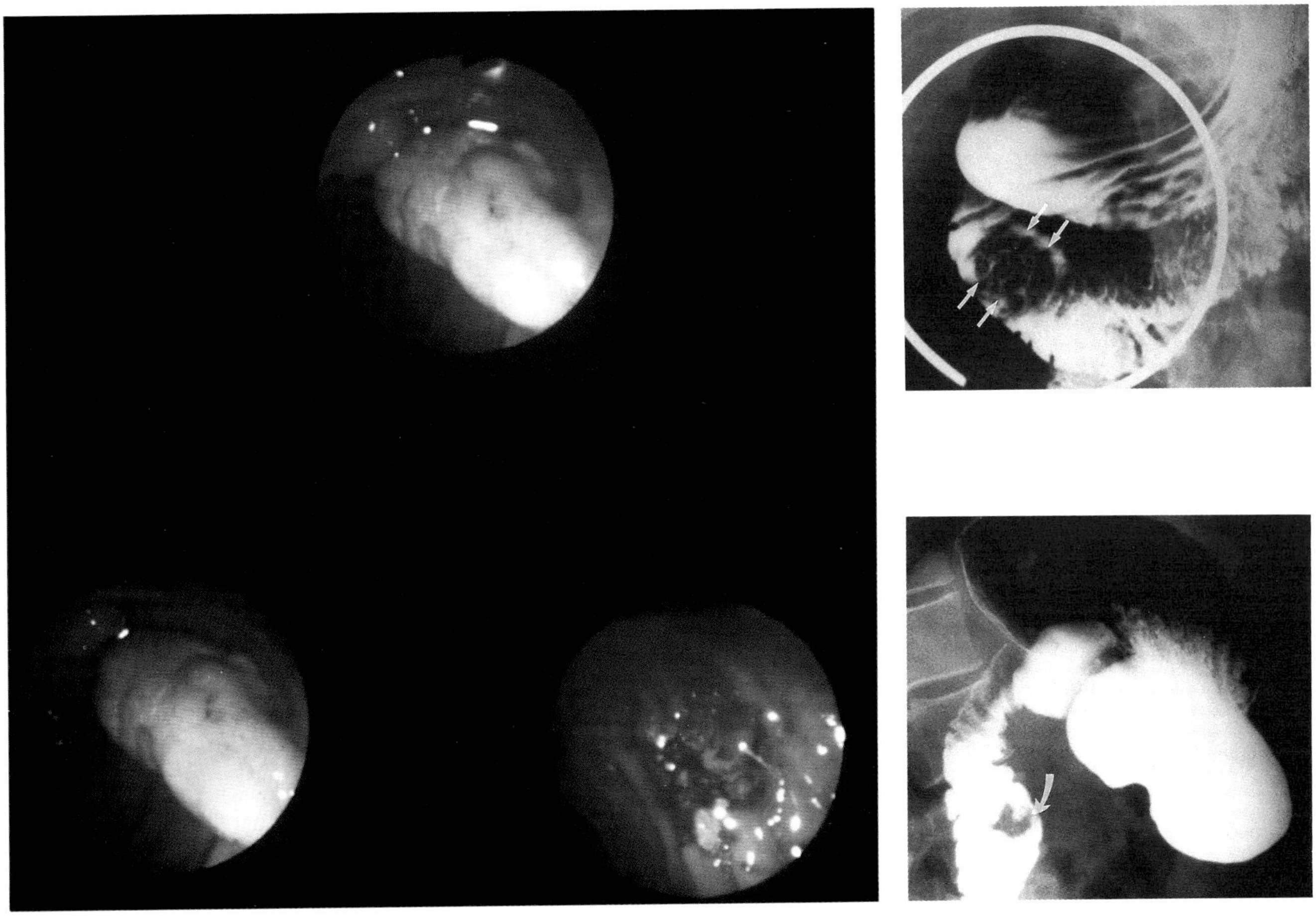

A B

FIG. 7.45. A: Two views of a large polyp. The third picture was taken after polypectomy. **B: Top:** Compression is applied to the abdominal wall to delineate the dimensions of the polyp (*arrows*). **Bottom:** A radiograph of a GI series demonstrating a large filling defect in the second portion of the duodenum (*arrow*).

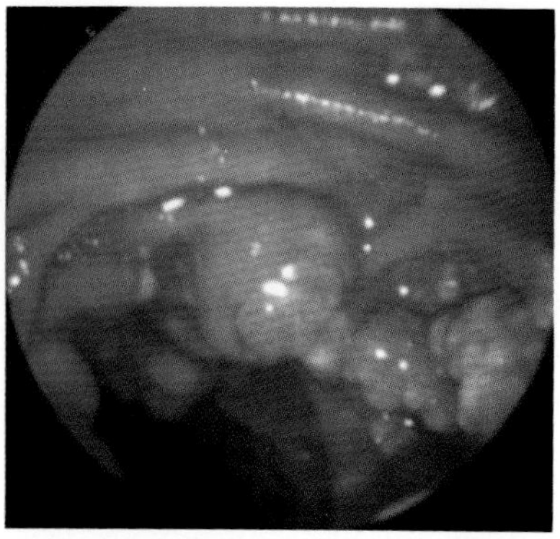

FIG. 7.46. An extensive lesion of the duodenum on a fiberoptic photograph. The lesion proved to be a carcinoma of the duodenum.

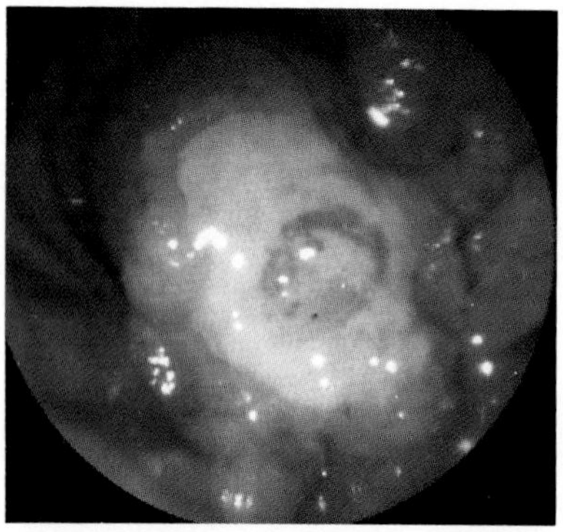

FIG. 7.47. A fiberoptic endoscopic picture of an ampullary carcinoma.

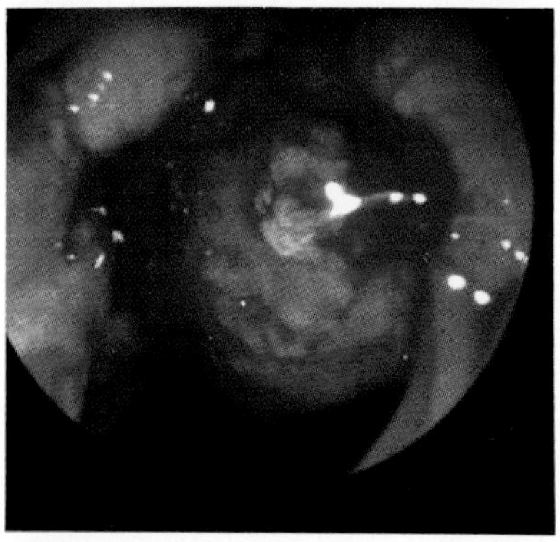

FIG. 7.48. Another ampullary carcinoma.

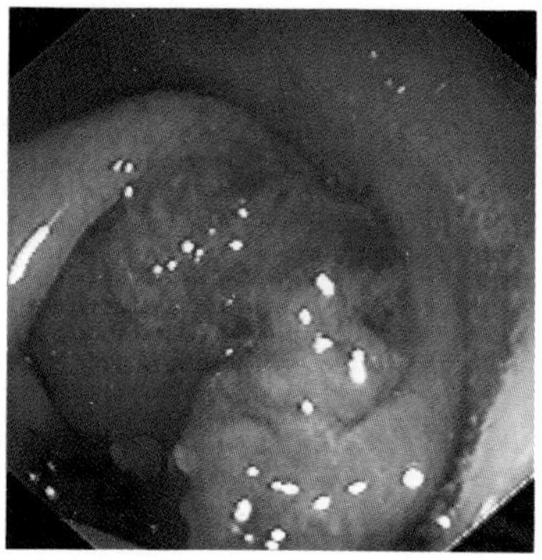

FIG. 7.49. A videoduodenoscopic picture of a duodenal carcinoma.

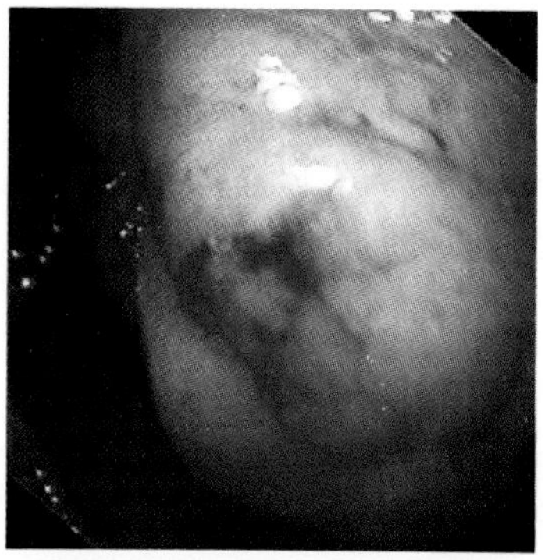

FIG. 7.50. A videoduodenoscopic picture of an ampullary carcinoma.

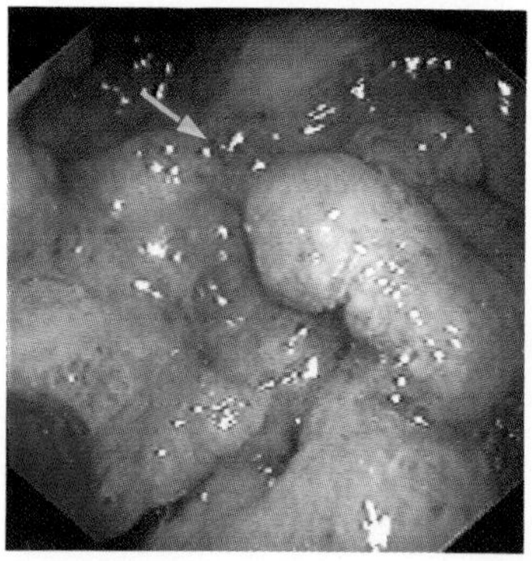

FIG. 7.51. An extensive ampullary carcinoma. The opening of the papilla is seen at 11:00 (*arrow*).

cation of the vital structures is confirmed, a polypectomy can be performed, as demonstrated in the lower half of Fig. 7.45A.

Ampullary carcinoma often produces obstruction to the bile duct and, occasionally, the pancreatic duct. Patients with an ampullary tumor usually present with evidence of cholestatic jaundice and occasionally pancreatitis. If surgery is not being considered for a patient with an ampullary carcinoma, decompression of one of both systems should be attempted. This is illustrated in Chapter 12. The photographs in this series demonstrate the varied endoscopic appearances of ampullary carcinomas (Figs. 7.46–7.53). Figure 7.54 is the endoscopic appearance of an invasive pancreatic carcinoma. Often an ulcerating mass of the duodenum is found associated with an invasive pancreatic tumor. Its presence increases the difficulty in maneuvering the duodenoscope and requires skill and extra patience to provide both a diagnostic study and decompression. Careful examination of any duodenal lesion is paramount to management. Multiple biopsies should be obtained to confirm the diagnosis because definitive sur-

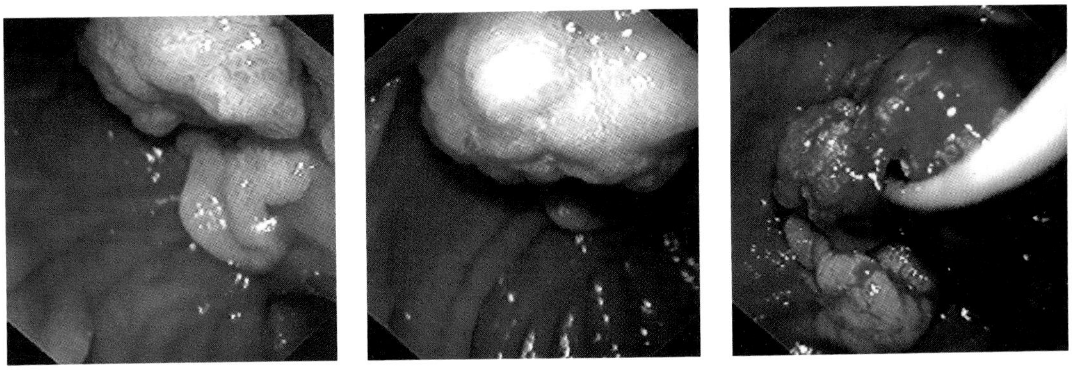

FIG. 7.52. Left, middle: A large mass extending down the descending duodenum. The opening is found between a large, bulky area and the descending duodenum. A sphincterotome was used to create an opening into the duct. **Right:** A catheter entering the opening into the bile duct.

gery or radiotherapy can offer cure or prolonged palliation. Of course, the best method for identifying an ampullary lesion is endoscopic, and I strongly advocate using the cannulating endoscope for this purpose because the lesion is visualized enface and visualized directly.

In my experience, carcinoid tumors have produced obstruction to the biliary tree (Fig. 7.55), and, in one patient, a carcinoid lesion of the ampulla became metastatic to the liver.

An endoscopic examination of a patient with jaundice may provide additional information regarding the underlying disease (for example, demonstrating esophageal varices as a consequence of portal hypertension and identifying erosions or ulcers that substantiate the cause of gastrointestinal bleeding). This contribution and observation will be most important in the patient's management and care. For the evaluation of patients with jaundice, however, I advise that the endoscopist *use the side-viewing endoscope for examination of the duodenum and ampullary region,* because the forward-viewing endoscope does not provide an adequate view of the second portion of the duodenum. Also, most of the time, the ampullary region is seen tangentially and rarely enface, causing an incomplete examination and failure to view the papilla. If the endoscopist feels more comfortable using the forward-viewing instrument to examine the esophagus and stomach adequately, he or she can complete that examination with the forward-viewing endoscope and then can pass the side-viewing instrument for examination of the papilla and subsequent cannulation. It has been my experience that, when using the forward-viewing endoscope, orientation of the structures in the duodenum is inaccurate, accounting for inappropriate diagnoses. For example, a lesion thought to be ampullary when seen with the forward-viewing endoscope was actually a lesion located on the lateral wall when visualized with the side-viewing instrument (Fig. 7.10).

If a patient is jaundiced, the endoscopic examination should be performed with two objectives in mind: to establish a diagnosis and to provide therapy. These objectives *cannot* be fulfilled using a forward-viewing instrument. Also, an *ERCP should not be attempted or performed in a patient presenting with cholestasis or a suspicion of obstruction of either duct system unless the endoscopist is capable of performing a ther-*

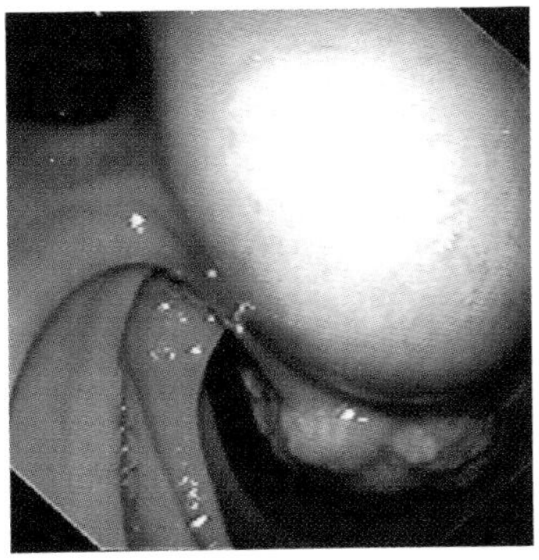

FIG. 7.53. An ampullary carcinoma in the distal bile duct producing cystic dilatation of the bile duct proximal to the obstruction. This dilated segment was entered using a needle knife (see Chapter 10).

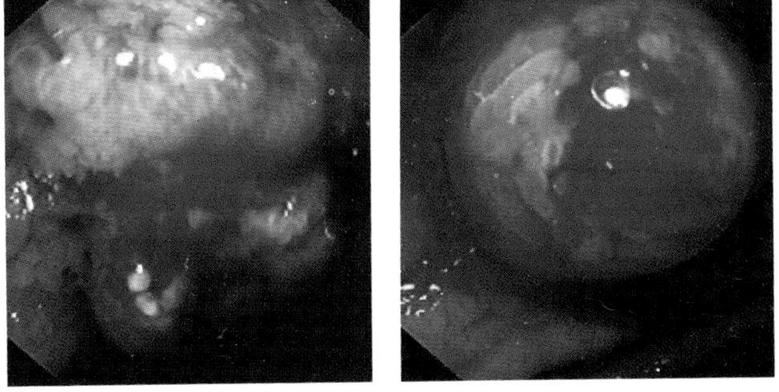

FIG. 7.54. Left: A carcinoma of the pancreas invading the duodenal lumen. **Right:** The distended papilla was found proximal to the mass.

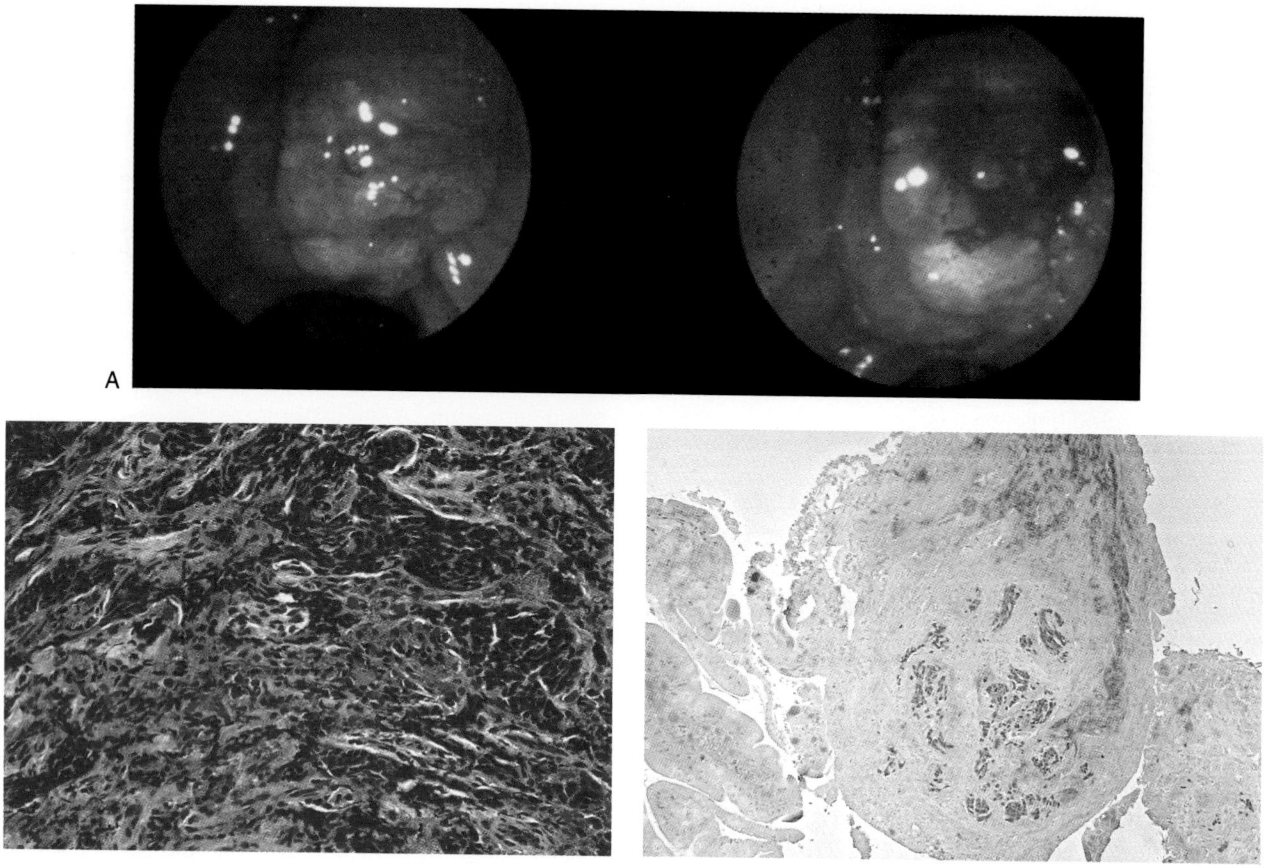

A

B

C

FIG. 7.55. A: Left: The endoscopic appearance of an ampullary mass. **Right:** The same mass after a biopsy was taken. **B:** An H & E stain of the tissue obtained from the lesion. Note the darker stained areas. **C:** A silver stain of the tissue confirming a carcinoid tumor of the ampulla.

apeutic drainage procedure. Therefore, an inexperienced endoscopist or one who does not perform sphincterotomy or insertion of prostheses should not attempt an ERCP for practice or experience unless he or she can provide decompression via a therapeutic procedure. Alternatively, a surgeon or radiologist should be available to provide immediate decompression after an ERCP demonstrates evidence of obstruction. Even an experienced endoscopist fails to provide decompression occasionally, but the experienced endoscopist at least attempts the procedure with a specific goal. I advise others, and use it as my personal policy, to have a good working relationship with a skilled radiologist who can assist with either primary decompression or a rendezvous procedure. Nurturing a supportive, mutual relationship with a surgeon is paramount to establishing a pancreaticobiliary referral center. If the endoscopist does have personal experience with percutaneous procedures and is unable to provide endoscopic decompression, the patient can be turned on the table into the appropriate position and a PTC with catheter insertion performed. Therefore, the therapeutic endoscopist can provide an array of services, obviating the need for unnecessary surgical procedures performed because of persistent failures caused by inexperience.

CHAPTER 8

Advantages and Limitations of Endoscopic Manometry of the Sphincter of Oddi

J. Delmont and A. G. Harris

For the past 15 years, gastroenterologists have been able to record sphincter of Oddi (SO) pressure quite easily during routine endoscopy: A basal pressure at the duodenocholedochopancreatic junction is found, always higher than that measured in the lumen of the ducts above and in the duodenum below. Superimposed phasic activity, unrelated to duodenal motility, can be easily detected by using perfused catheters. This represents the definition of a sphincter.

HISTORICAL REVIEW

The paper published by Ruggero Oddi (1) in an Italian journal was written in French, the prevailing scientific language at that time (1887). In spite of its mediocre quality, it created a certain interest, and this is probably why this sphincter still bears Oddi's name. The concept of a sphincter in this area was not new, because Glisson (2) described it succinctly but accurately as early as 1681. Claude Bernard, in his splendid *Mémoire sur le Pancréas* (3), which was recently translated into English by the Royal Physiological Society (4), perfectly described the pancreatic ducts and their junction with the bile duct in humans and various animals. He referred to a "contractile aperture." Fine anatomic dissection allowed Hendrickson (5) and subsequently Boyden (6) to progress further, but, as Claude Bernard wrote, one should not expect too much from anatomic dissection when attempting to understand physiology. In 1977 Floquet et al. (7) and in 1982 Velasco Suarez (8) reported that although the SO is not anatomically distinguishable from the smooth muscle fibers of the duodenum, it is a functional entity similar to the lower sphincter of the esophagus. This deserves to be strongly stressed.

Ruggero Oddi's personal contribution is important in reference to the physiology of the SO. One year after his anatomy paper, he published a remarkable article on the physiology and pathophysiology of SO pressure (9). Using a column of mercury, he indicated that the stimulation or section of the vagus nerves does not modify it. Unfortunately, this second paper was written in Italian and went unnoticed. Nevertheless, it justifies retaining his name for the sphincter.

Subsequently, surgeons studied extensively the physiology of the SO in humans by *indirect* measurements of pressure or flow in the bile duct, either during surgery or postoperatively through a T-tube. These studies were initiated by Bergh (10) as early as 1940. However, strict conditions must be respected (11). These studies culminated with the combination of pre- and postoperative electromyography (12,13).

The emergence of ERCP in 1969 allowed direct access to the SO. In 1974, Vondrasek et al. (14) recorded the first pressure measurements using indwelling microsensors. The following year Nebel (15) was the first to record pressures from the SO using perfused catheters. This is the most widespread technique employed today because, as shown by the Milwaukee school, it provides additional information. Indeed, in 1977 researchers transposed the technique designed to measure esophageal pressures by using a minimally compliant hydraulic capillary infusion system (Arndorfer pump). Thanks to this technique (16,17), the normal and abnormal functions of the SO could be comfortably studied in humans by the endoscopic sphincter of Oddi manometry (ESOM) (17–19).

METHODS USED IN ENDOSCOPIC SPHINCTER OF ODDI MANOMETRY

Two very different methods, with their respective advantages and disadvantages, are in common use today. One of these uses indwelling or *in situ* microtransducers, the other a capillary infusion system.

A 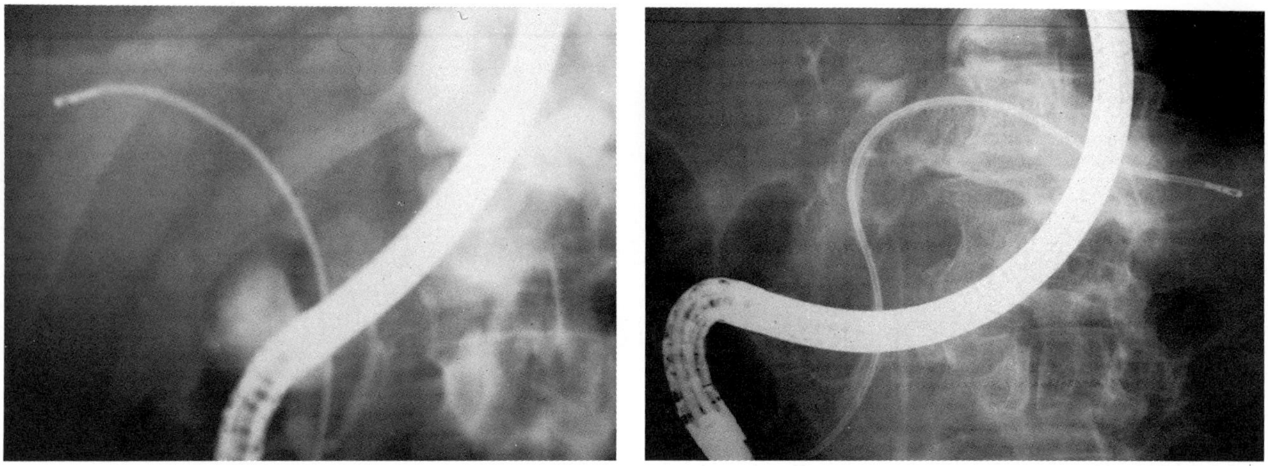 B

FIG. 8.1. A: Triple lumen catheter in bile duct at ERCP. **B:** Triple lumen catheter in pancreatic duct at ERCP.

In Situ Transducer Manometry

This method was the first to be used (14) and was derived from a technique used to measure coronary artery blood pressure. This method is widely used in Japan (20–22). With the commercialization of the Arndorfer triple-lumen catheter, we no longer use this system.

Because it directly records the pressure by transforming the distortion applied to a piezo resistive plaque (wheatstone bridge principle) into an electric signal, this method is more sensitive from a theoretical standpoint. However, its marked sensitivity may be a drawback (e.g., respiratory movements and arterial pulsation interfere with the intraductal recording). The quality of the recording of phasic waves depends on "duodenal silence," which is difficult to achieve without an anticholinergic drug (Figs. 8.1, 8.2).

Perfused Catheter Technique

The signal recorded here results from the variations of resistance in the flow of a column of liquid driven through catheters by a pneumohydraulic pump. Most investigators use a triple-lumen catheter (Arndorfer) of 1.7 mm in external diameter and 0.5 mm in internal diameter. This allows its insertion through the operating channel of all duodenoscopes used for ERCP. A fourth catheter is attached to the endoscope, and its mouth opens very close to the extremity of the endoscope (duodenal pressure used as zero reference). These four catheters are perfused at a constant rate of 0.25 ml/min by an Arndorfer pneumohydraulic infuser (Figs. 8.3, 8.4).

The three recording orifices of the triple-lumen catheter are spaced at intervals of 2 mm, which allows the determination of the direction of the phasic wave con-

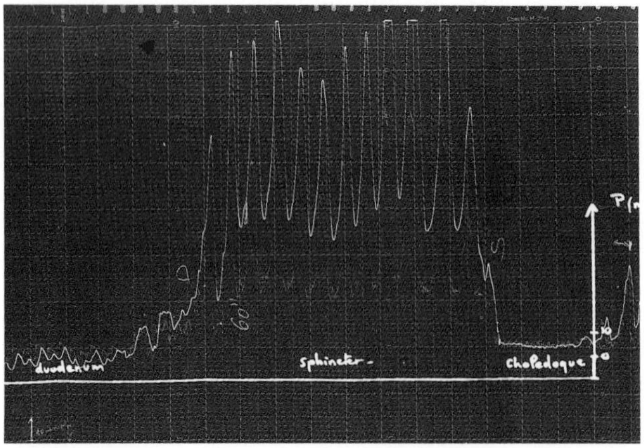

FIG. 8.2. Recording obtained during ESOM with morphine stimulation. This response is abolished by nalaxone, atropine derivatives and nitroglycerine.

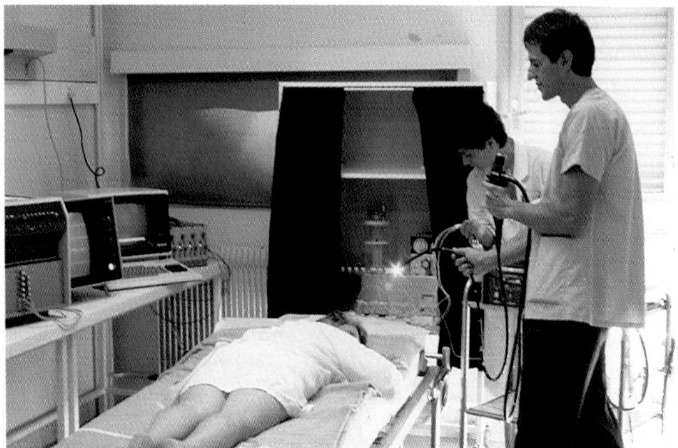

FIG. 8.3. Appearance of procedure room and set up for performing ESOM.

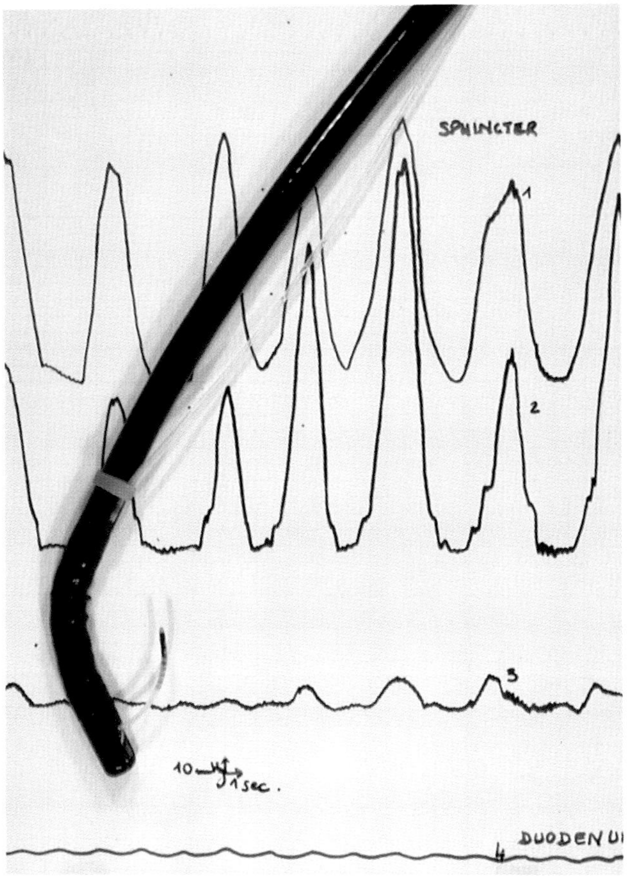

FIG. 8.4. Phasic contractions of the SO, upper 3 tracings produced baseline activity seen on lower tracing.

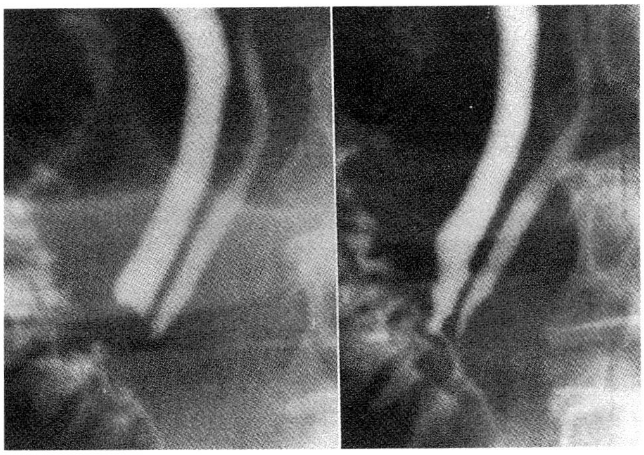

FIG. 8.5. Dynamic sphincter function seen during contraction and relaxation phases. This action prevents reflux of gastrointestinal contents in ducts.

tractions to be recorded. This recording is achieved by a pressure transducer connected to amplifiers, which transform pressure variations into electrical signals visualized on a monitor and/or paper.

The *disadvantages* of this technique, compared to the previous method, are the following: (A) It has lower sensitivity related to the length of the column of water and its small diameter (23). Recording of the pancreaticoduodenal and bilioduodenal gradients with the two methods in the same patient showed that the perfused catheter technique often underestimates them (*personal unpublished data*). (B) It is impossible to differentiate SO hypertonicity owing to spasm from inextensibility (organic stenosis of the SO). However, administration of an antispasmodic (glucagon, amyl nitrite) can overcome this problem. (C) This technique is more difficult and time consuming (because of flushing of the hydraulic system) and has a higher purchase cost.

The *advantages* of perfused catheter technique over *in situ* transducer manometry follow: (A) The catheters are cheaper than the electronic transducers, which are fragile and expensive. (B) The perfused catheter technique provides a better recording of the phase wave contractions: The lower sensitivity probably explains why the tracings have fewer artifacts. The sphincter area is rapidly identified, thanks to the three recording points, because the area of the phase wave contraction is often short and may occur at only one orifice. When this segment is sufficiently long, the direction of the waves can be determined.

STUDIES IN NORMAL SUBJECTS BY ESOM

Functional Anatomy of the SO (24) (Fig. 8.5)

The common bile duct (CBD) and the main pancreatic duct (MPD) join shortly before reaching the duodenal lumen. Thus, the common duct is often very short. An ampulla of Vater (clearly visible in Fig. 8.6) is rarely

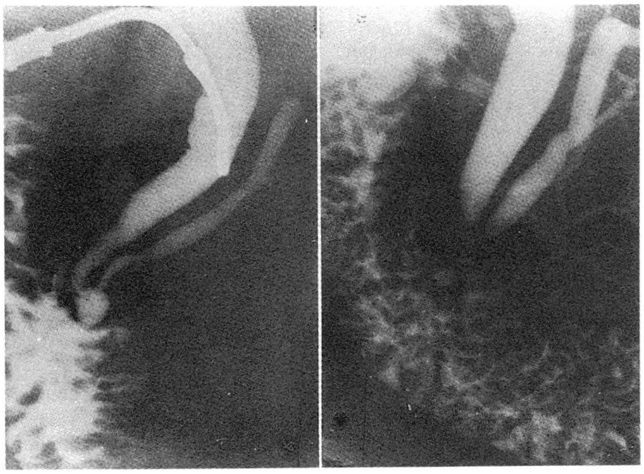

FIG. 8.6. Another example of sphincter function demonstrating contraction and relaxation. The ampullary region is identified radiographically.

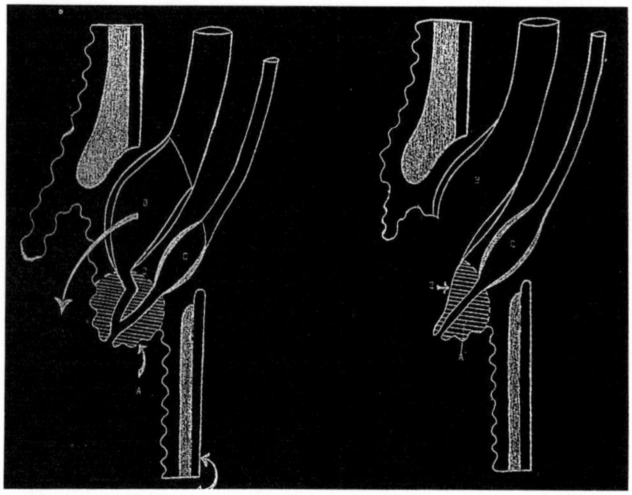

FIG. 8.7. Left: Contraction phase with prominent ampulla bulging into the duodemus (arrow). **Right:** Appearance of sphincter after sphincterotomy.

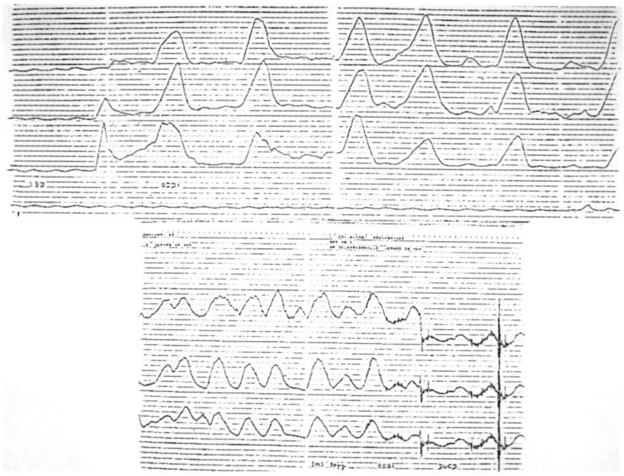

FIG. 8.8. Contraction of sphincter of Oddi following somatostatin injection. Note the frequency and amplitude of contractions.

seen during ERCP (as demonstrated previously by the insertion of a dental film behind the duodenopancreatic unity after surgical detachment) (25) (Figs. 8.6, 8.7).

We, like Hand (26) believe that there is only one muscular layer at this level that functions as a single sphincter, but we maintain the separation into three sphincters for linguistic convenience. The three are the common papillary sphincter, the biliary sphincter, and the pancreatic sphincter.

The *common papillary sphincter,* which surrounds the common duct, is usually short. Caroli (27,28) compared it to a microprostate because it contains a mixture of ramified glands and a few muscular fibers that probably originate from the duodenal muscular layer. Like the prostate, it is not contractile and loses its flexibility and extensibility with age. This may account for the increase in size of the upper ducts with age. Its physiologic role is nonexistent, but its pathophysiologic role is very important.

The biliary sphincter (sphincter cholecosus proprius) surrounds the biliary infundibulum. Although Boyden divides it into several subunits (6), it holds no interest for the physiologist or the physician. This funnel, located between the noncontractile part of the CBD and the ampulla of Vater (when it is there), was often mistaken for the ampulla of Vater. It is ventriculelike, displaying alternative phases of contractions (systoles) and relaxations (diastoles). These movements were well described by Caroli in 1940 (27,28) and by Torsoli (29). It is at this sphincter level that one records an area of high pressure and phasic wave contractions. We have shown (*unpublished data*) that the long-acting somatostatin analog (Sandostatin) can produce marked contractions of the SO (Figs. 8.8, 8.9, 8.10). These contractions, however, are not visible to the endoscopists.

Although the importance of the *pancreatic sphincter (sphincter pancreaticus proprius)* has been minimized by traditional anatomists, ESOM confirms its existence and efficacy. Physiologic duodenobiliary refluxes are often reported, especially in newborns or

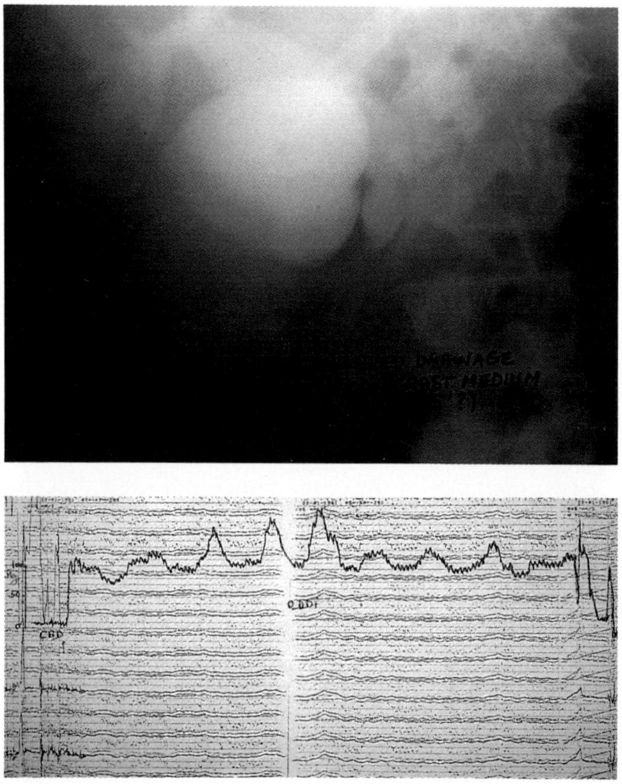

A

B

FIG. 8.9. A: Radiograph showing spasm of SO following somatostatin injection. **B:** Increased basal pressure and frequency of contractions of the sphincter following somatostatin.

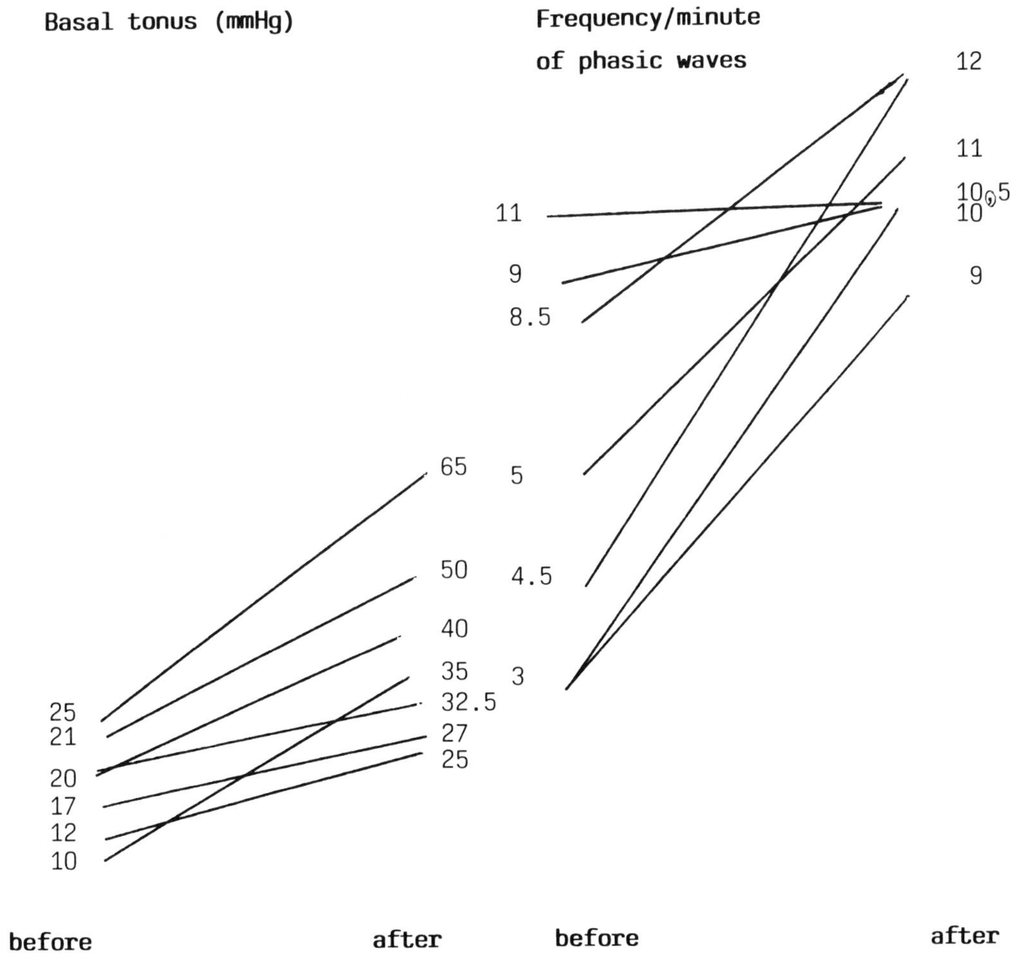

FIG. 8.10. Principal manometric parameters before and after 50 μg Sandostatin in seven healthy volunteers.

during anesthesia with curare (30,31). However, we never came across any duodenopancreatic reflux apart from the pathologic situations. On the other hand, systolic contractions of the pancreatic infundibulum are clearly defined during ERCP. Its anatomic and physiologic importance is inversely correlated with that of the common sphincter. Figure 8.5 shows that the spasm of this sphincter prevents biliopancreatic reflux.

Is the SO a Peristaltic Pump?

Certain authors believe that the SO is filled with bile between two phasic contractions and that it expels its contents into the duodenum by a systolic contraction (milking action). Watts and Dunphy (32) were the first to propose this hypothesis, and it seems to be confirmed in the opossum, which has a voluminous preduodenal SO of 3 cm (18,33). Nevertheless, this theory, advocated by certain authors (18), seems incompatible with the volume of the SO cavities in humans: ampulla of Vater (usually small or nonexistent) and biliary infundibulum (34). Daily practice of ERCP has shown neither spasmodic spurts of bile nor rhythmic contractions of the papilla or the biliary infundibulum. Yet the lower part of the biliary infundibulum bulges under the duodenal mucosa because of a muscular "duodenal window" (Fig. 8.7).

Recently an appealing "nutcracker" hypothesis of this rhythmic activity was put forward. The rhythmic contractions appear to sweep the micocrystals of cholesterol or other debris that may obstruct the SO lumen (35,36).

The SO as a Resistor

This theory, nicely described by Glisson (2), was taken up again by Claude Bernard (3), Oddi (9), Ivy (37), and many authors. Basal SO pressure participates in preventing reflux from the duodenum and interrupts the biliary and pancreatic flow. During interprandial phases, this allows the gallbladder to fill. How does this SO resistance cease during the meal? A local reflex accounts for the fact that any increased pressure that occurs within the biliary tract has an inhibitory effect on the basal SO pressure (38,39).

Recent Contribution to the Understanding of the Physiologic Role of the SO in the Upper GI Tract Function

Important physiologic studies have recently allowed us to understand better the integration of the SO function into gastrointestinal physiology either during or between meals.

A remarkable study of this function during meals by Lanzini et al. (40) enables us, finally, to understand why the gallbladder often empties so incompletely after a Boyden meal during oral cholecystography. This occurs because the gallbladder acts like a bellow that evacuates part of its contents but also concomitantly receives bile from the liver that collides with the tonic closure of the SO. Thus, there are continuous *bellow movements* that alternately empty and fill the gallbladder.

Interruption of bile evacuation through the SO may also harmonize the biliopancreatic secretory mixture with the intermittent gastric emptying. At meal time, when there is increased liquid influx because of liver and pancreatic secretions and gallbladder contraction, the SO harmonizes and coordinates biliopancreatic flow with the passage of gastric chyme through the pylorus (35).

Several recent studies of the SO function between meals have allowed us to integrate SO motility with the classical interdigestive migrating motor complex (MMC) of the GI tract. The SO does not remain closed continuously during the night but opens intermittently. Thus, a little bile and pancreatic juice come through the papilla when it is hit by the "motor activity front" of the MMC. Hence, a secretory component is added to the motor element, which is called the housekeeper of the digestive tract (41–44). This fasting bile flow is related to periodic gallbladder contractions that also occur in the fasting state and is correlated with the MMC. This has been demonstrated by studies in dogs (45), in opossums (46,47), and even in humans (48).

Current Knowledge of the Neurohormonal Regulation of the SO Function

For a long time, surgeons wanted to cut nerves (especially the vagus nerve) in order to induce hypotonicity of the SO, thus preventing a postcholecystectomy syndrome. Numerous experimental studies disagree with this approach (9,49,50). On the other hand, we have already mentioned a possible locoregional reflex (38,39): An extensive dissection of the cystic duct near the CBD may explain why some favor (9) and others oppose (51) postcholecystectomy bile duct dilatation. Hormonal regulation of the SO seems far better documented than the role of the nervous system. A recent general review (52) describes physiologic action of these different hormones. Hormones can act either directly on muscular receptors or indirectly through neurotransmitters: The role of nonadrenergic and noncholinergic (NANC) inhibitory receptors seems increasingly well established, as in several other gastrointestinal sphincters (53,54). Thus, CCK-PZ may contract the SO by its direct action on the muscular fiber. This action can be shown when the nerves are paralyzed by tetrodotoxin (thus the same "denervation syndrome of the SO" proposed by Geenen et al. (17) when one encounters a paradoxic response to CCK). The second action is inhibitory and is predominant because it masks the first one. It occurs through NANC receptors, with VIP as the neurotransmitter (54). The role of gastrin seems limited (17), whereas secretin initially increases basal pressure and phasic activity, which subsequently decrease rapidly (55). Glucagon has an inhibitory effect (56) that seems pharmacologic, whereas physiologic inhibitory effects are essentially due to CCK and VIP. Excitatory effects seem to implicate an excitatory neural pathway, including opiate, serotoninergic, and cholinergic neurons triggered by motilin (57). Motilin is located in the duodenal and CBD mucosa and may be the "housekeeper hormone" because its plasma concentrations are maximal during phase 3 of the MMC.

Contribution of ESOM to SO Pharmacology in Humans

It should be noted that pharmacologic doses of CCK-OP, caerulein, and glucagon used as antispasmodics during ERCP are widely used today. We have studied (*unpublished data*) the effect of pharmacologic doses of a long-acting somatostatin analog, Sandostatin (octreotide, Sandoz). Figures 8.8 and 8.9 show the main results that indicate that this peptide hormone, which is known for its widespread inhibitory effects, has a stimulatory effect on the SO. A recent general review of SO pharmacology (58) mentions the spasmogenic effect of morphine (abolished by naloxone) and pethidine (Fig. 8.2), and the antispasmodic effect of atropine, butylscopolamine, and nitroglycerin derivatives. The more recent drugs that may have a therapeutic role in dyskinesia of the SO are hymecromone (58), nifedipine (59), and tiropramide (60). In this particular case, measurements with microtransducers are sufficient to confirm the markedly increased choledochoduodenal gradient.

TABLE 8.1 *Etiologies of benign SO stenosis*

Secondary	— Cholelithiasis (>90%)	
	— Others	· Parasites (Hydatidosis, Distomiasis)
		· Iatrogenous (Surgery, ES)
		· Senile

CONTRIBUTIONS TO THE DIAGNOSIS OF DYSFUNCTION OF THE SPHINCTER OF ODDI

Benign (organic) stenosis and dyskinesias (spasm) of the SO are currently brought together under the term of dysfunction of the SO. We prefer to separate them, because the latter term has not become a fully established clinical entity (61,62). On the other hand, it seems impossible today to deny the existence of an organic stenosis of the SO. Moreover, their diagnosis and treatment seem relatively well codified. Indeed, in the past, some surgeons made this diagnosis too often (63) during gallstone surgery.

Certain inflammatory states of the SO, established by preoperative radiomanometry, have been reported to disappear, probably owing to drainage with a T-tube (64). However, other cases of odditis have been shown to heal with scar tissue, leading to fibrotic stenosis well described by De Valle and Donovan (65). Table 8.1 shows the main etiologies of these benign stenoses of the SO. The diagnosis is based on the characteristics of pain, clinical and/or biochemical cholestasis, the increased CBD caliber, the analysis of the x-ray images of the SO during surgery or ERCP, and the prolonged emptying time of the CBD (< 45 minutes) during ERCP if the patient is cholecystectomized. In these cases the ESOM is definitely useful but does not seem indispensable. Endoscopic sphincterotomy is imperative and is usually associated with good results and few accidents (19). The problem of dyskinesia of the SO, however, is quite different (66). As we wrote 10 years ago (67), ESOM represents tremendous progress, and knowledge of its uses has indeed expanded considerably during these 10 years. What is its advantage in this area? The following are two different clinical situations encountered in practice.

Unexplained Biliary-Type Pain or Acalculous Biliary Colic

Two subgroups should be differentiated: cholecystectomized patients, who are more commonly encountered, and noncholecystectomized patients (in whom the diagnosis is more difficult to establish). Both subgroups suffer this painful syndrome suggestive of a biliary colic (right upper quadrant pain, dorsal radiation, and so on). In the cholecystectomized patient, an ERCP should of course exclude residual biliary disease (such as retained CBD stones and organic stenosis of the SO). The existence of such a syndrome is not illogical, and by analogy with the irritable bowel, we have proposed the name "irritable SO syndrome" for it (67).

ESOM may detect signs of varying significance (Table 8.2). Increased basal pressure of the SO is the most widely accepted diagnostic criterion if the pressure is higher than three standard deviations (generally > 40 mgHg). Other manometric criteria are less widely accepted. The logical treatment when the diagnosis has been confirmed and when the antispasmodic drugs do not have the expected effect is endoscopic sphincterotomy (ES). Disappearance of all signs after ES may be considered the gold standard of this diagnosis. Many researchers have attempted to make this procedure less invasive. Unfortunately, none of the suggested diagnostic criteria have proved to be accurate or specific. A critical review of these procedures may be found elsewhere (61,67,68). The two most recent procedures, quantitative cholangioscintigraphy and fatty meal ultrasound, are not very convincing (19,68). Data from the Milwaukee group (69) suggest that the ESOM remains the best method.

Idiopathic Recurrent Acute Pancreatitis (IRAP)

Three functional syndromes can be defined: hypotonia of the SO, spastic pancreatic duct sphincter, and pancreas divisum.

Hypotonia of the SO (SO Incompetence)

Necrotic acute pancreatitis has been attributed to SO hypotonia by certain surgeons; we have rejected this on the basis of numerous arguments (30,31).

Spastic Pancreatic Duct Sphincter

Repeated pain suggestive of pancreatitis may be accompanied by increased pancreatic enzymes but is

TABLE 8.2. *Manometric signs of SO dysfunction*

Increased choledochoduodenal gradient
Increased basal pressure
Tachyoddia (high rate of phasic contractions)
Abnormal propagation of phasic contractions
Paradoxical SO response to CCK

clinically less serious than pancreatitis. A spasm of the pancreatis SO has often been invoked. Three studies have evaluated this syndrome with ESOM (70–72). One of them describes the same four disorders reported with the biliary SO (Table 8.2). In this case, dilatation of the pancreatic SO with a balloon has been suggested (73), sometimes preceded by an endoscopic septectomy (pancreatic ES following biliary ES). Nevertheless, these procedures seem dangerous (73) and have been shown to be associated with acute pancreatitis in 62% of cases (72). Such a procedure unfortunately caused severe pancreatitis in one of our patients, so we are strictly opposed to this technique.

On the other hand, conventional sphincterotomy (Fig. 8.7) leaves only a short pancreatic sphincter (2–4 mm) whose contractile strength is markedly reduced. This has also been reported by Geenen et al. (17), who were able to cure 10 of 13 patients who presented with IRAP and increased basal SO pressure. In case of failure, surgical septectotomy may be justified.

Pancreas Divisum: ESOM of the Caroncula Minor

The responsibility of the pancreas divisum in the IRAP is controversial. Our experience suggests that it has a limited yet certain role. Only two groups, to our knowledge, have recorded pressure in the caroncula minor (74,75). These preliminary studies seem very interesting.

LIMITATIONS OF ESOM

In spite of its considerable contributions for patients and healthy people over the past 10 years, this technique has not become widespread. Why is it restricted to a limited number of centers? In France, for example, where more than 50 groups perform ERCP and SE routinely, fewer than five perform ESOM! This reflects its limitations. We shall analyze the reasons and attempt to propose some solutions.

ESOM Is Not a Simple Procedure

ESOM cannot be compared to manometry of the esophagus. It is more difficult than ERCP, which does not always require deep catheterism and is not hampered by duodenal contractions. We find it preferable to work in the dark and to anesthetize the oropharynx well. However, failures do occur with ESOM and are not often reported in papers: This gives the false impression that the technique is easy, which can discourage beginners who have difficulty with it.

Need for Standardizations

ESOM depends on a wide variety of equipment and techniques. Microtransducers or perfused catheters are both used, and we have indicated the advantages of both. The former is easier to use for detecting a gradient, whereas the latter is imperative if the functioning of the SO is to be studied. With respect to the perfused catheter method, it is necessary to standardize the parameters. This has already been advocated by A. Torsoli with the initiation of an International Club of ESOM investigators. These parameters include the same internal and external diameters, the same infusion rate of degazeified water, identical premedication, the same patient position, and the same criteria for interpreting the tracings. This effort should be pursued.

ESOM Requires a Control Group

It is very difficult to set up a control group. Corazziari et al. (76) have insisted on the difficulties and errors in using readings by different investigators. It is thus acknowledged that comparisons between centers are questionable and make it necessary for each center to establish its own control group. Normally this control group should include healthy volunteers, but few centers have done this (77). Although ESOM is associated with very low morbidity, complications can occur (78,79), which makes it difficult to obtain permission from ethical committees. Patients with suspected biliopancreatic disorders but with normal ERCP are eligible for this control group in our opinion.

ESOM Is Used in Disorders That Are Not Clearly Defined

Dyskinetic disorders of the SO remain a controversial clinical concept. Their frequency is difficult to evaluate, and no epidemiologic study has been undertaken. In the least questionable subgroup of cholecystectomized patients, a very interesting study by Bar-Meir et al. (80) showed that these disorders are infrequent.

It is noteworthy that the acalculous biliary pain syndrome has given rise to other hypotheses leading to various therapeutic options, all of which proved to be satisfactory for the physicians in question. Some of these hypotheses, for instance, are the role of microlithiasis (81) and the role of an obstacle at the neck of the gallbladder or cystic duct (82).

Finally, Steinberg compares pain resulting from SO dyskinesia to undetermined chest pain. These conditions are explored during pain-free periods. It would be advantageous to dispose of provocative factors, as in esophageal or coronary disorders (such as the possibilities of increased intraductal pressure by infusion of saline through a catheter inserted above the SO and pharmacologic agents such as morphine).

In conclusion we believe that over the past 15 years ESOM has contributed tremendously to our knowledge of normal and abnormal crossing of the SO and that it deserves to be more widely performed. Despite its current limitations, ESOM remains the gold standard as a diagnostic tool in SO dysfunction.

ACKNOWLEDGMENTS

I would like to acknowledge the following persons: Dr. R. Dumas for recording the SO pressures and Dr. Alan Harris, Dr. C. Grimaldi, Ms. M. J. Manara, and Ms. Marie Scherer for their editorial contributions.

REFERENCES

1. Oddi R. D'une disposition à sphincter spéciale de l'ouverture du canal cholédoque. *Arch Ital Biol* 1887;8:317–22.
2. Glisson F. Anatomia Hepatitis. *Apud A Leers* 1681;175–6.
3. Bernard C. *Mémoire sur le pancréas*. Paris: Baillière, 1856.
4. Bernard C. Memoir on the pancreas and on the role of pancreatic juice in digestive processes, particularly in the digestion of neutral fat. *Monographs of the Physiological Society*, vol 42. New York: Academic Press, 1985.
5. Hendrickson WF. A study of the musculature of the entire extrahepatic biliary system, including that of the duodenal portion of the common bile duct and sphincter. *Johns Hopkins Hosp Bull* 1898;9:221–32.
6. Boyden EA. The anatomy of the choledocoduodenal junction in man. *Surg Gynecol Obstet* 1957;104:641–52.
7. Floquet J, Laurent J, Plenat F, Watrin B. Is the sphincter of Oddi a reality in man? In: Delmont J, ed. *The sphincter of Oddi*. Basel: Karger, 1977;21–4.
8. Velasco Suarez C. Structure of the major duodenal papilla. *Mt Sinai J Med (NY)* 1982;49:31.
9. Oddi R. Sulla tonicita dello sfintere del coledoco. *Archivio per le scienze mediche* 1888;12:333–9.
10. Bergh GS. The effect of food upon the sphincter of Oddi in human subjects. *Am J Dig Dis* 1942;9:40–3.
11. Galmiche JP, Gislon J, Bonfils S. Postoperative biliary manometry. In: Delmont J, ed. *The sphincter of Oddi*. Basel: Karger, 1977;61–5.
12. Ono K. Surgery of the sphincter of Oddi. *Modern handbooks of surgery*. suppl. Tokyo: Nakayama-shoten, 1976.
13. Ono K, Ozawa M, Hada R. Surgery of the sphincter of Oddi in cholelithiasis in Asians. In: Delmont J, ed. *The sphincter of Oddi*. Basel: Karger, 1977;201–5.
14. Vondrasek P, Eberhardt G, Classen M. Endoscopic semi-conductor manometry. *Int J Med* 1974;3:188–92.
15. Nebel OT. Manometric evaluation of the papilla of Vater. *Gastrointest Endosc* 1975;21:126–28.
16. Geenen JE, Hogan WJ, Dodds WJ, Stewart ET, Arndorfer RC. Intraluminal pressure recording from the human sphincter of Oddi. *Gastroenterology* 1980;78:317–24.
17. Geenen JE, Hogan WJ, Dodds WJ. Sphincter of Oddi. In: Sivak MV, ed. *Gastroenterologic endoscopy*. Philadelphia: Saunders, 1987:735–51.
18. Toouli J. Sphincter of Oddi motility. *Br J Surg* 1984;71:251–56.
19. Delmont J, Dumas R, Grimaldi C. Fonctionnement physiologique et dysfonctionnement du sphincter d'Oddi (sténose oddienne bénigne et dyskinésie). *Gastroenterol Clin Biol* 1988;12:455–8.
20. Tanaka M, Ikedas S, Nakayama F. Non operative measurement of pancreatic and common bile duct pressures with a microtransducer catheter and effects of duodenoscopic sphincterotomy. *Dig Dis Sci* 1981;26:545–52.
21. Tanaka M, Ikeda S, Matsumoto S, Yoskimoto H, Nakayama F. Manometric diagnosis of sphincter of Oddi spasm as a cause of post cholecystectomy pain and the treatment by endoscopic sphincterotomy. *Ann Surg* 1985;202:712–9.
22. Kazuichi O, Yasuro Y, Kenichi I. Endoscopic measurement of papillary sphincter zone and pancreatic main, ductal pressure in patients with chronic pancreatitis. *Gastroenterology* 1986;91:409–18.
23. Hagenmuller P, Ossenberg FW, Classen M. Duodenoscopic manometry of the common bile duct. In: Delmont J, ed. *The sphincter of Oddi*. Basel: Karger, 1977;72–6.
24. Delmont J. Le sphincter d'Oddi: anatomie traditionnelle et anatomie fonctionelle. *Gastroenterolol Clin Biol* 1979;3:157–65.
25. Barraya L, Pujol-Soler R, Yvergneaux JP. La région oddienne. Anatomie millimétrique. *Presse Med* 1971;79:2527–34.
26. Hand BH. Anatomy and function of the extra-hepatic biliary system. *Clin Gastroenterol* 1973;2:3–29.
27. Caroli J. Contribution to the study of the functioning of Oddi's sphincter. In: Delmont J, ed. *The sphincter of Oddi*. Basel: Karger, 1977;48–51.
28. Caroli J, Porcher G, Pequignot G, Delatre M. Contribution of cine-radiography to study of the function of the human biliary tract. *Am J Dig Dis* 1960;5:677–96.
29. Torsoli A. Physiology of the human sphincter of Oddi. *Endoscopy* 1988;20:166–70.
30. Delmont J, Vedel JP, Alemanno J. Pancréatite aiguë et reflux bilio-et duodéno-pancréatique. *Gastroenterol Clin Biol* 1980;4:223–26.
31. Delmont J, Vedel JP, Faure X, Vauban G, Harris A. Does incompetence of the sphincter of Oddi exist? Can it account for certain cases of acute pancreatitis? In: Hollender LF, ed. *Controversies of acute pancreatitis*. Berlin, Heidelberg: Springer-Verlag, 1982;1–6.
32. Watts J, Dunphy JE. The role of the common bile duct in biliary dynamics. *Surg Gynecol Obstet* 1966;122:1207–81.
33. Becker JM, Moody FG, Zionmeister AR. Effect of gastrointestinal hormones on the biliary sphincter of the opossum. *Gastroenterology* 1982;1300–7.
34. Toouli J. Sphincter of Oddi motility. *Br J Surg* 1984;71:251–256.
35. Schulze-Delrieu K. Oddities of sphincter contractions. *Gastroenterology* 1986;90:2030.
36. Traynor OJ, Dozois RR, Dimagno EP. Canine interdigestive and post-prandial gallbladder motility and emptying. *Am J Physiol* 1984;246:G246–G432.
37. Sandblom P, Voegtlin WL, Ivy AC. The effect of cholecystokinin on the choledochoduodenal mechanism (sphincter of Oddi). *Am J Physiol* 1935;133:175–80.
38. Thune A, Thornell E, Svanvik J. Reflex regulation of flow resistance in the feline sphincter of Oddi by hydrostatic pressure in the biliary tract. *Gastroenterology* 1986;91:1364–9.
39. Grace PA, Pitt HA. Cholecystectomy alters the hormonal response of the sphincter of Oddi. *Surgery* 1987;102:186–94.
40. Lanzini A, Jazrawi RP, Northfield TC. Simultaneous quantitative measurements of absolute gallbladder storage and emptying during fasting and eating in humans. *Gastroenterology* 1987;92:852–61.
41. Van Berger Hene Gouwen GP, Hofmann AF. Nocturnal gallbladder storage and emptying in gallstone patients and healthy subjects. *Gastroenterology* 1978;75:879–88.
42. Dimagno EP, Hendricks JC, Go VLW, Dozois RR. Relationships among canine fasting pancreatic and biliary secretions, pancreatic duct pressure, and duodenal phase III motor activity—Boldyreff revisited. *Dig Dis Sci* 1979;24:689–93.
43. Vantrappen G, Peeters TL, Janssens J. The secretory component of the inter-digestive migrating motor complex in man. *Scand J Gastroenterol* 1979;14:663–7.
44. Scott RB, Strasberg SM, El-Scharkawy TY, Diament NE. Fasting canine biliary secretion and the sphincter of Oddi. *Gastroenterology* 1984;87:793–804.

45. Itoh Z, Takahashi T. Periodic contractions of the canine gallbladder during the interdigestive state. *Am J Physiol* 1981; 240:G183–9.
46. Coelho JCU, Gouma DJ, Moody FG, Schlegel JF. The effect of feeding on myoelectric activity of the sphincter of Oddi and gastrointestinal tract in the opossum. *Dig Dis Sci* 1986; 31:202–7.
47. Takahashi I, Kern MK, Dodds WJ, et al. Contraction pattern of opossum gallbladder during fasting and after feeding. *Am J Physiol* (*Gastrointest Liver Physiol* 13) 1986;250:G227–35.
48. Marzio L, Neri M, Capone F, et al. Gallbladder contraction and its relationship to interdigestive duodenal motor activity in normal human subjects. *Dig Dis Sci* 1988;33:540–4.
49. Hopton D, White TT. Effect of hepatic and celiac vagal stimulation on common bile duct pressure. *Dig Dis Sci* 1971;16:1905–1101.
50. Tansy MF, Salkin LM, Innes DL, Martin JS, Landin WE, Kendall FM. The occlusive competence of the duodenal orifice of the canine pancreatic duct. *Surg Gynecol Obstet* 1977;144:865–8.
51. Mueller PR, Ferrucci JT, Simeone JF, et al. Post cholecystectomy bile duct dilatation: myth or reality? *Am J Roentgenol* 1981;136:355–8.
52. Sarles JC. Hormonal control of sphincter of Oddi. *Dig Dis Sci* 1986;31:208–12.
53. Alumets J, Fahrenkrug J, Hakanson R, et al. A rich VIP nerve supply is characteristic of sphincters. *Nature* 1979;280:155–6.
54. Wiley JW, O'Dorisio TM, Owyang C. Vasoactive intestinal peptide mediates cholecystokinin-induced relaxation of the sphincter of Oddi. *J Clin Invest* 1988;81:1920–4.
55. Carr-Locke DL, Gregg JA, Chey WY. Effects of exogenous secretin on pancreatic and biliary ductal and sphincteric pressures in man demonstrated by endoscopic manometry and correlation with plasma secretin levels. *Dig Dis Sci* 1985;30:909–17.
56. Rey JF, Corallo J, Lombart J, Pangtay-Tea J. The use of endoscopic manometry to demonstrate the effect of glucagon on the sphincter of Oddi. In: Picazo J, ed. *Glucagon in gastroenterology and hepatology*. Lancaster: MTP, 1982;99–113.
57. Behar J, Biancani P. Effects and mechanisms of action of motilin on the cat sphincter of Oddi. *Gastroenterology* 1988;95:1988–1105.
58. Staritz M. Pharmacology of the sphincter of Oddi. *Endoscopy* 1988;20:171–4.
59. Deschamps JP, Ottignon Y, Miguet JP, Carayon P. Action de la nifedipine sur le fonctionnement du sphincter d'Oddi: resultats préliminaires. *Gastroenterol Clin Biol* 1986;10:279.
60. Trabucchi E, Baratti C, Centemero A, Rizzitelli E, Colombo R. Controlled study of the effects of tiropramide on biliary dyskinesia. *Pharmacotherapeutica* 1986;9:541–50.
61. Steinberg WM. Sphincter of Oddi dysfunction: a clinical controversy. *Gastroenterology* 1988;95:1409–15.
62. Delmont J, Ljunggren B, Faure X, Vedel JP. Functional disorders of the sphincter of Oddi: a clinical reality? In: Classen M, Geenen J, Kawai K, eds. *The papilla Vateri and its diseases*. Baden-Baden: Witzstrock, 1979;57–65.
63. Hepp J. Oddites imaginaires et sphincterotomies abusives. *Ann Chir* 1966;20:343.
64. Delmont J. An attempt to collate. In: Delmont J, ed. *The sphincter of Oddi*. Basel: Karger, 1977;240–55.
65. Del Valle D Jr, Donovan R. Choledocooditis retractil cronica: concepto clinico-quirurgico. *Archos argent Enferm Appar Dig* 1926;1:141.
66. Geenen JE, Hogan WJ, Dodds WJ, Toouli J, Venu RP. The efficacy of endoscopic sphincterotomy after cholecystectomy in patients with sphincter-of-Oddi dysfunction. *N Engl J Med* 1989;320:82–7.
67. Delmont J, Henry JF, Vedel JP, Vauban G, Sieurat P. Kritik studien von dyskinesia von Oddi sphincter. In: Barthelheimer H, ed. *Die kranken gallenwege*. Baden-Baden: Witzstrock, 1980;140–6.
68. Darweesh RMA, Dodds WJ, Hogan WJ, et al. Efficacy of quantitative hepatobiliary scintigraphy and fatty-meal sonography for evaluating patients with suspected partial common duct obstruction. *Gastroenterology* 1988;94:779–86.
69. Hätsbacka J, Järvinen H, Kilivaasko E. Turenen MT. Results of sphincteroplasty in patients with spastic sphincter of Oddi. *Scand J Gastroenterol* 1986;21:516–20.
70. Guelrud M, Siegel JH. Hypertensive pancreatic duct sphincters as a cause of pancreatitis. *Dig Dis Sci* 1984;29:225–31.
71. Toouli J, Roberts-Thomson IC, Dent J, Lee J. Sphincter of Oddi motility disorders in patients with idiopathic recurrent pancreatitis. *Br J Surg* 1985;72:859–63.
72. Guelrud M, Mendoza S, Viera L. Does somatostatin prevent acute pancreatitis after pancreatic duct sphincter hydrostatic balloon dilatation? *Gastrointest Endosc* 1987;33:148.
73. Kozarek RA. Balloon dilation of the sphincter of Oddi. Endoscopy 1988;20:207–10.
74. Staritz M, Hutteroth T, Meyer Sum Buschenfelde K. Pancreas divisum and pancreatitis. *Gastroenterology* 1986;91:525–6.
75. Satterfield ST, McCarthy JH, Geenen JE, et al. Clinical experience in 82 patients with pancreas divisum: preliminary results of manometry and endoscopic therapy. *Pancreas* 1988;3:248–53.
76. Corazziari E, Habib FI, Biliotti D, et al. Reading error and time variability of sphincter of Oddi recording. *Ital J Gastroenterol* 1986;18:343–7.
77. Funch-Jensen P, Krause A, Ravnsbaek J. Endoscopic sphincter of Oddi manometry in healthy volunteers. *Scand J Gastroenterol* 1987;22:243–9.
78. Albert MB, Steinberg WM, Irani SK. Severe acute pancreatitis complicating sphincter of Oddi manometry. *Gastrointest Endosc* 1988;34:342–5.
79. King CE, Kalvaria I, Sininsky CA. Pancreatitis due to endoscopic biliary manometry. *Gastroenterology* 1988;94:A227 (abst).
80. Bar-Meir S, Halpern Z, Bardan E, Gilat T. Frequency of papillary dysfunction among cholecystomized patients. *Hepatology* 1984;4:328–30.
81. Delchier JC, Benredji P, Preaux AM. The usefulness of microscopic bile examination in patients with suspected microlithiasis: a prospective evaluation. *Hepatology* 1986;6:118–22.
82. Rhodes M, Lennard TWJ, Farndon JR, Taylor RMR. Cholecystokinin (CCK) provocation test: long-term follow-up after cholecystectomy. *Br J Surg* 1988;75:951–3.

CHAPTER 9

Pancreatic Disorders: Inflammatory, Congenital, and Malignant

ACQUIRED PANCREATITIS

Whatever the etiology or associated cause of pancreatitis (Table 9.1), the acute phase varies in severity and presentation from the mild edematous to the necrotizing and fatal hemorrhagic forms. The role of ERCP in acute pancreatitis is limited or restricted, because manipulation of an inflamed pancreas is *usually* considered a contraindication (see Table 2.2). It is thought that injection of contrast during an acute episode may exacerbate symptoms and accelerate the pathophysiologic processes.

The *exceptions* to this rule (pancreatitis—contraindications for ERCP) include: biliary or gallstone pancreatitis when urgent ERCP, sphincterotomy, and removal of an obstructing stone may reverse the deteriorating cardiopulmonary function, renal failure, and acidosis that complicate severe pancreatitis (1–9) and ERCP to define a fistulous tract responsible for pancreatic ascites or pleural effusions and either facilitate surgical intervention (10–14) or provide endoscopic drainage.

If the patient's survival is not endangered and his or her condition progressively improves, an urgent ERCP may be postponed or delayed until he or she stabilizes, begins to ingest solids, passes flatus, and resumes activities. This approach is prudent and can avoid unnecessary complications of misadventures. Knowledge of the etiology of pancreatitis allows physicians to decide if and when to perform ERCP. If the etiology is clear (for example, alcohol abuse, viral infection, medications, toxins, steroids, or trauma) (15–26), an ERCP is usually not necessary unless symptoms persist or recur. If gallstones are found, and if the patient presents with cholestasis or obstructive symptoms suggesting common bile duct stones, an ERCP should be performed to confirm their presence. The decision to perform a sphincterotomy depends on the age of the patient, the presence or absence of cholelithiasis, the state of the gallbladder (performing ES in a patient with an intact gallbladder is discussed in Chapter 10), and the potential risks of surgery. This subject will be discussed later in this chapter.

The primary role of ERCP in the workup and evaluation of patients presenting with pancreatitis is to define the morphology of the pancreatic duct system and the presence of stones (usually biliary), strictures, or other obstructive phenomena, including dysfunction of the sphincter at one end of the spectrum and neoplasia at the other end. The results of ERCP will ultimately determine the type of therapy the patient might undergo. Obviously, if a patient has familial hyperlipidemia or chronically uses steroids for hypersensitiv-

TABLE 9.1. *Etiology of pancreatitis*

Cholelithiasis Ethanol abuse	} <90% of all cases
Idiopathic	
Abdominal operations (direct or indirect trauma)	
Hyperlipidemia	
Pancreatic duct injection (post-ERCP)	
Trauma	
Hypercalcemia (metastatic and metabolic disorders)	
Pregnancy	
Peptic ulcer (penetration)	
Obstruction (stone disease; stenosis)	
Pancreas divisum	
Organ transplantation	
End-stage renal failure	
Hereditary (familial pancreatitis)	
Scorpion bite	
Drugs—diuretics, steroids, chemotherapeutic agents, anti-HIV agents	
Miscellaneous: hypoperfusion (shock), viral infections (mumps, etc.), *Mycoplasma pneumoniae* infection, intraductal parasites (fascioliasis, ascariasis, clonorchiasis)	

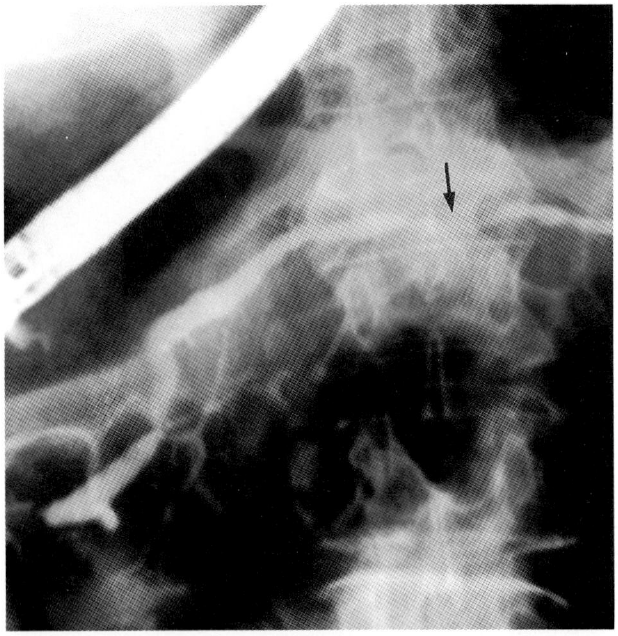

FIG. 9.1. A pancreatogram demonstrating irregularity or beading of the main pancreatic duct in the body of the gland with narrowing at the junction of the body and tail (*arrow*) in a patient presenting with recurrent episodes of pancreatitis. Dilatation of the duct in the head is apparent, and narrowing of the duct at the sphincter was consistent with a hypertensive sphincter. The patient experienced symptoms each time she took medication containing steroids for her allergy.

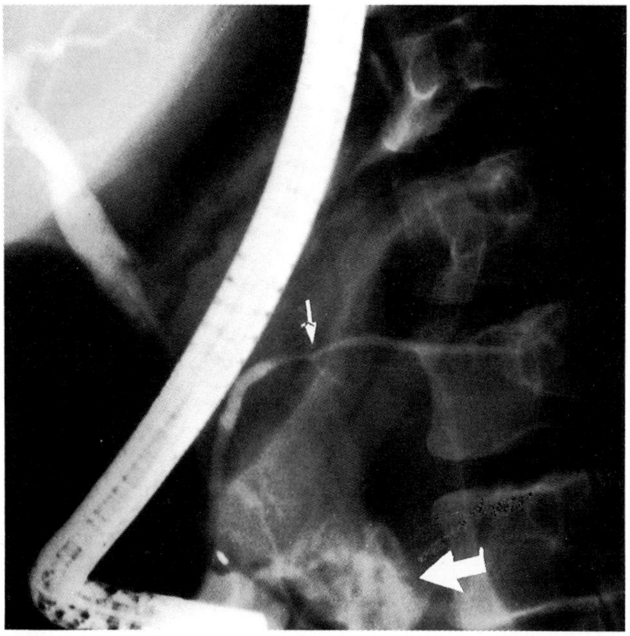

FIG. 9.2. A pancreatogram demonstrating narrowing in the body of the gland (*small arrow*) and irregularity of the uncinate system with parenchymal filling (*large arrow*) in a patient with a recent history of recurrent episodes of acute pancreatitis and hyperlipidemia.

ity and allergic reactions and experiences recurrent episodes of pancreatitis, an ERCP will be helpful in defining the ductular system to determine whether irreversible changes have occurred. If there are chronic changes affecting the pancreatic ducts, a more intensive approach to the management of these conditions (e.g., aggressively reducing blood lipid levels or withdrawing steroids) will be necessary because mechanical therapy—endoscopic or surgical—is not indicated unless, for example, a hypertensive sphincter is proved to be responsible for the symptom complex. This latter

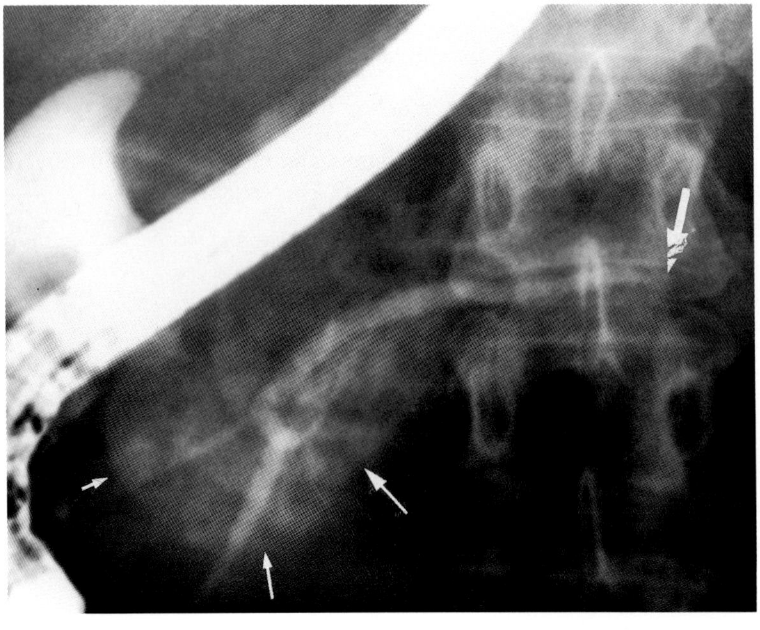

FIG. 9.3. A pancreatogram obtained in a patient with persistent symptoms secondary to acute pancreatitis. Note parenchymal filling in the head of the gland (*small arrows*) caused by overfilling because of a stricture at the junction of the body and tail (*large arrow*).

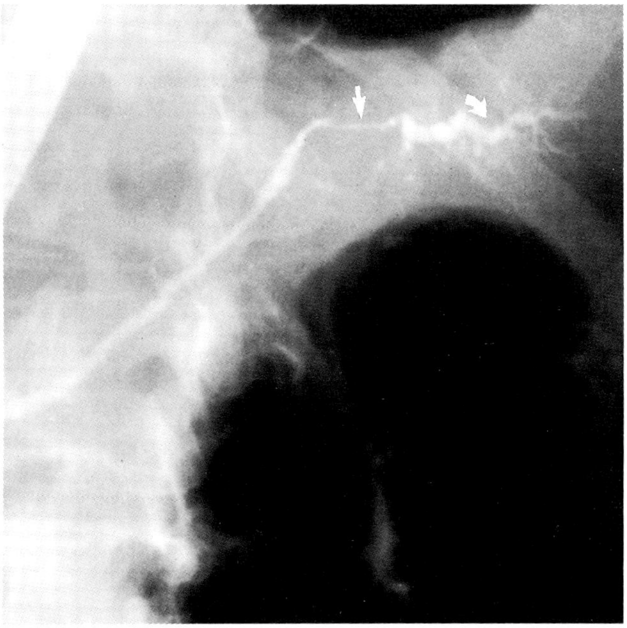

FIG. 9.4. This pancreatogram was completed in a patient following a recurrent episode of pancreatitis and demonstrates beading of the main duct in the tail of the gland (*curved arrow*) and a stricture distal to these changes (*straight arrow*).

syndrome should be confirmed by manometric studies before embarking on mechanical therapeutic techniques. Even if the ducts appear normal on ERP, a more intensive approach to establishing the etiology

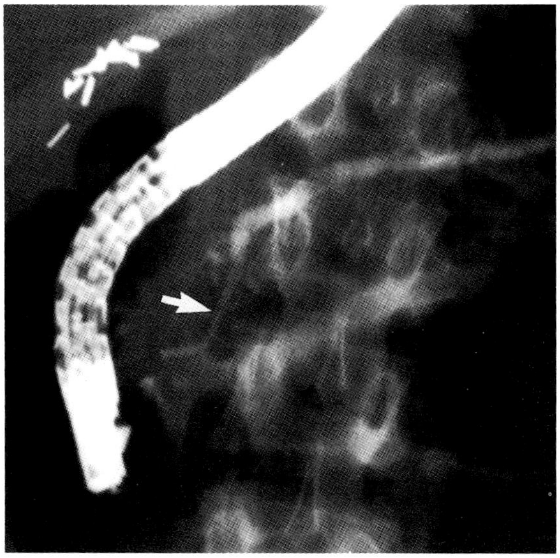

FIG. 9.5. This ERCP demonstrates a pancreatogram in a patient with recurrent pancreatitis, status post cholecystectomy. Narrowing of the duct in the head of the gland (*arrow*) and irregularity of the main and secondary ducts is suggestive of subacute, or subclinical, pancreatitis. Patients with this entity may develop fulminant pancreatitis following ERCP. Distinguishing them from other patients is difficult if not impossible.

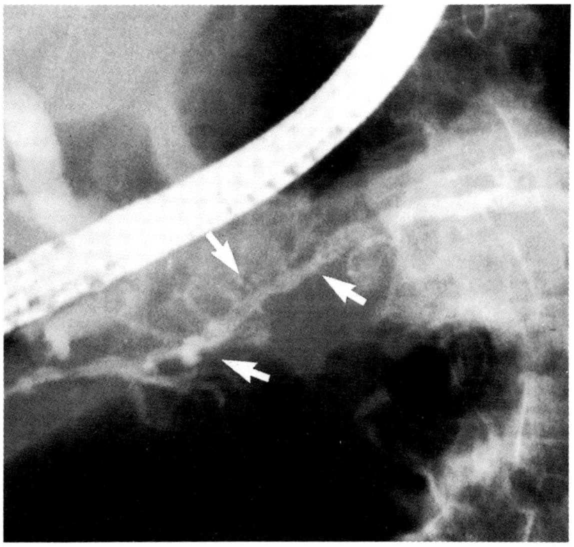

FIG. 9.6. Irregularity of the major and secondary ducts in the head of the gland (*arrows*). These findings are subclinical because these changes are usually reversible.

and providing medical treatment is recommended to avoid debilitating attacks and progression to chronic disease.

Subclinical (Subacute) Pancreatitis

Acute changes of pancreatic duct morphology usually appear as beading or narrowing of the main duct on ERCP, which, by definition, should be reversible (27,28) (Figs. 9.1–9.4). These findings may also involve the secondary radicals of the pancreatic duct (Figs. 9.5–9.8) as found in subclinical, or subacute, pancreatitis. This terminology identifies that group of patients who do not demonstrate morphologic changes of chronic disease but who may be at risk during the performance of ERCP, sphincterotomy, or manipulation of the papilla or ducts. Patients who develop severe pancreatitis—sometimes leading to necrotizing pancreatitis and phlegmon formation (29,30)—after manipulation of the papilla (palpation, probing, or sphincterotomy) or subsequent to the performance of ERCP seem to have a preexisting condition, subclinical pancreatitis. This category of disease, which represents a potential catastrophe when ERCP or ES is attempted or performed, is probably the cause of symptoms for which the patient is being evaluated. Unfortunately, there are no definitive signs of findings to alert the endoscopist to this preexisting condition. Still, despite a high index of suspicion, a post-ERCP complication cannot be prevented or avoided, and, if an ERCP is indicated, it must be performed. The resultant reaction to manipulation in these patients is entirely unpredictable, and it is only after ERCP or an attempted ERCP that this entity is confirmed; unfortunately, this is when the patient manifests symptoms of postprocedure pancreatitis. It is my opinion that severe post-ERCP-ES pancreatitis occurs only in patients with this preexisting condition. Defining and recognizing this entity are important priorities for reducing the frequency and severity of post-ERCP pancreatitis. This group of patients who present with persistent symptoms of pain, abnormal chemistries (i.e., transiently elevated transaminases and amylases), and an equivocal CT scan (in other words, patients with nonspecific but suspected disease) develop severe pancreatitis after ERCP, an attempted ERCP, or sphincterotomy, *even if contrast is never injected into the pancreatic duct*. The acute ductular changes of pancreatitis occuring after ERCP are usually reversible, and, if there are no other recurrent or ongoing inflammatory events, the duct morphology should appear normal or near normal on subsequent ERCPs. When the condition exists, the pancreatic duct often appears normal on pancreatography because ductal abnormalities are usually reversible or may be randomly

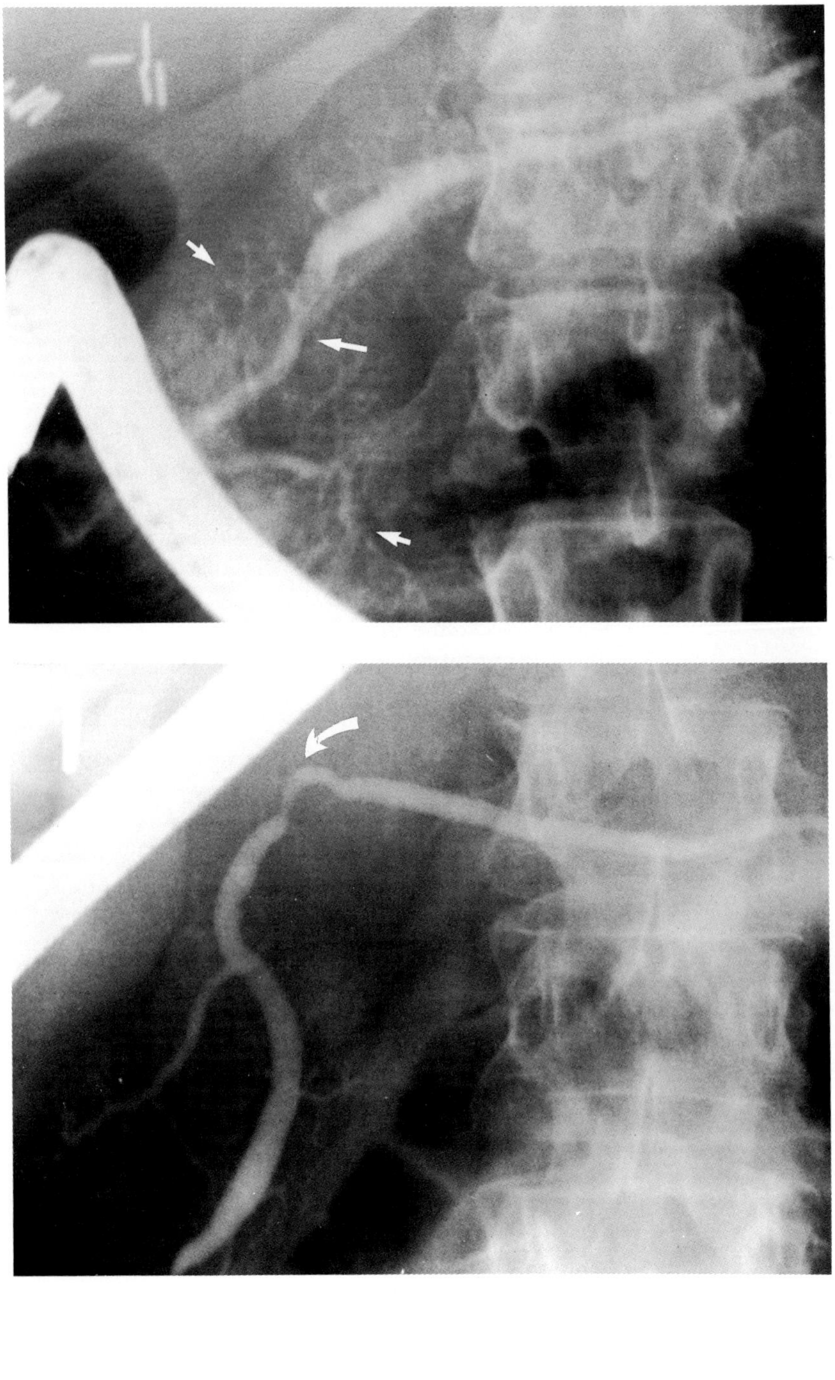

FIG. 9.7. A: Irregularity of the main pancreatic duct in the head of the gland and of the secondary radicals is demonstrated on this ERCP (*arrows*). Narrowing of this segment of the duct is present, and parenchymal filling of the pancreas has occurred. These findings are consistent with subacute or subclinical pancreatitis. **B:** Early changes of the secondary branches in the head of the gland and a rigid, narrowed area at the genu (*arrow*).

A
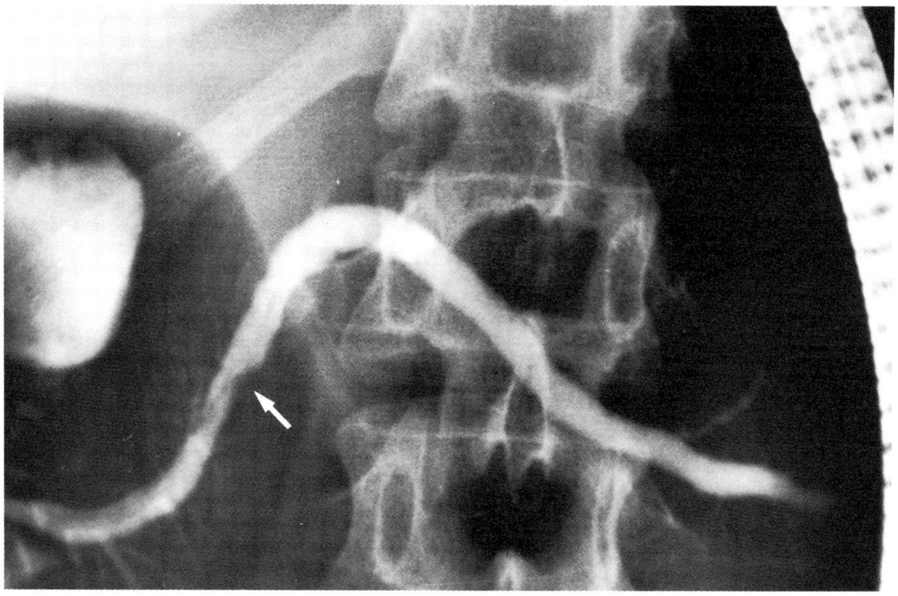

B
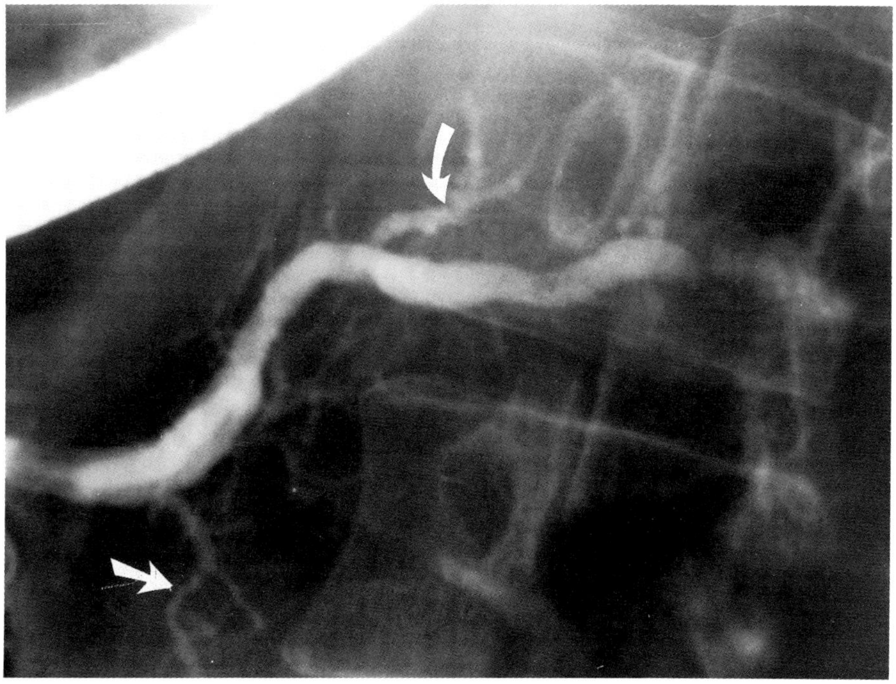

FIG. 9.8. Dilatation of the main pancreatic duct with an irregular area in the head of the gland (*arrow*) and irregularity of the secondary radicals in a patient with subclinical pancreatitis. **B:** Ectasia of secondary radicals in the uncinate process (*straight arrow*) and body of the pancreas (*curved arrow*) in a patient with recent pancreatitis.

abnormal. This paucity of findings creates a perplexing situation for the clinician, who feels compelled to establish a definitive diagnosis. As our appreciation of this condition increases we may be able to alter the severe post-ERCP course by minimizing trauma and manipulation of the papilla. Using the newer nonionized contrast solutions (which have been recommended in patients with contrast sensitivity) may be helpful, but further studies are needed to corroborate a possible association between contrast sensitivity, subclinical, and post-ERCP pancreatitis (31–34). Glucagon and bolus injections of somatostatin, although promising, have not proven effective in aborting or preventing pancreatitis, and recommendations for their use cannot be made (35–36).

Chronic Pancreatitis

The ductular morphology in chronic pancreatitis varies from the less obvious changes of strictures and beading

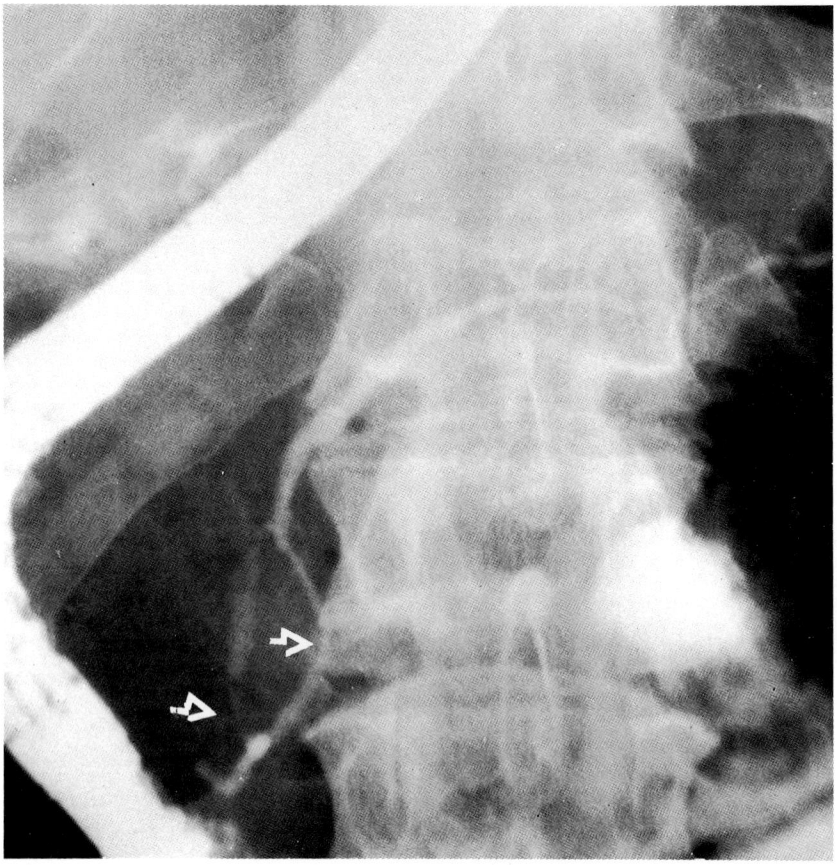

FIG. 9.9. A pancreatogram obtained in a patient with chronic pain and steatorrhea. The patient had a history of heavy alcohol ingestion for years. Narrowing of the main duct in the head is noted (*arrow*), and incomplete filling of the accessory duct is shown (*arrow*), the latter owing to strictures. Because of the patient's symptoms of exocrine dysfunction, pancreatic enzyme replacement was instituted resulting in clinical improvement.

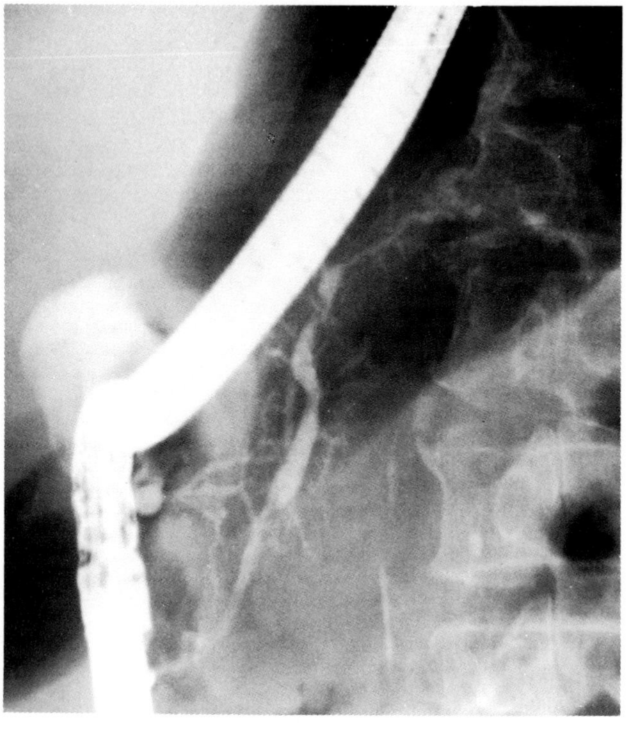

FIG. 9.10. This pancreatogram demonstrates areas of stricturing and dilatation of the main pancreatic duct in an elderly patient with evidence of exocrine dysfunction. Pancreatic enzyme replacement was instituted and resulted in improvement of symptoms. The differential diagnosis would include diffuse carcinomatosis, but there is no evidence of extravasation of contrast into a tumor. More importantly, all the secondary radicals fill, which is an important consideration when entertaining the diagnosis of cancer. When cancer is present, the secondary radicals may be absent because of the presence of tumor.

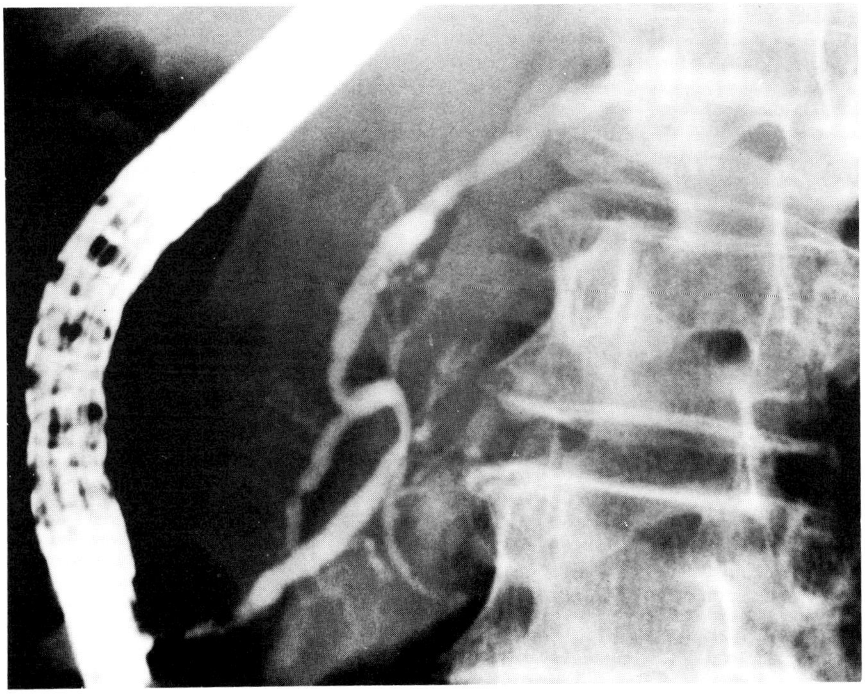

FIG. 9.11. Beading of the duct and irregularity throughout the main duct. The secondary branches are also irregular. These diffuse changes are consistent with inflammatory disease.

(Figs. 9.9, 9.10), which can also be associated with pain and exocrine dysfunction, to the classically dilated, tortuous main pancreatic duct, corresponding ectatic side branches, and the occasional finding of stones or mucous plugs within the ducts (Figs. 9.11–9.14).

Differentiation of benign disease, inflammatory disease, and neoplasia is difficult without definitive findings or histology (37–52). Of course, obtaining histologic evidence is paramount to the diagnosis, but it is not always possible. An attempt should be made to advance an endoscopic cytology brush through any pancreatic duct stricture or to get percutaneous biopsies. Unfortunately, tissue samples obtained in this fashion are scanty and often not diagnostic. One must then move to a second-tier strategy, which would incorporate more invasive radiologic techniques. A high-resolution CT scan with guided biopsies (53–57) may provide tissue for confirmation, but what if the biopsy is negative? Cytologic examination of pancreatic juice obtained after secretory stimulation requires time, fastidious collection techniques, and a skilled examiner. Another, more definitive technique, endoscopic ultrasound (EUS), is assuming a major role in differentiating between neoplasia and benign disease and is most helpful in establishing the diagnosis and staging the disease. However, tissue diganosis is not available with EUS, and more aggressive techniques are necessary.

Careful evaluation of the pancreatogram will enable the endoscopist to interpret the findings with a high degree of certainty. Of course, the endoscopist, who is usually a clinician, must consider all the information presented in the database before rendering an opinion. A history of recurrent pain associated with alcohol and/or substance abuse is certainly confirmatory and supportive for chronic pancreatitis. However, the association of chronic pancreatitis and cancer is well

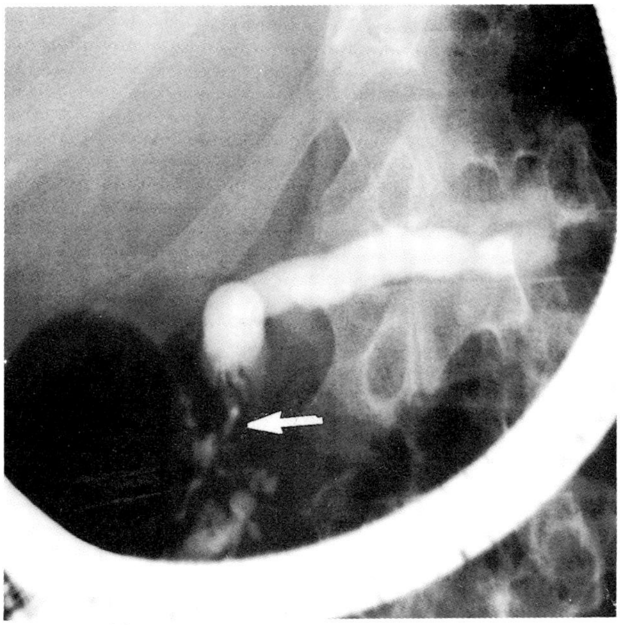

FIG. 9.12. Dilatation of the main pancreatic duct and a stricture in the head of the gland near the sphincter (*arrow*). Note beading of the uncinate radicals consistent with chronic disease.

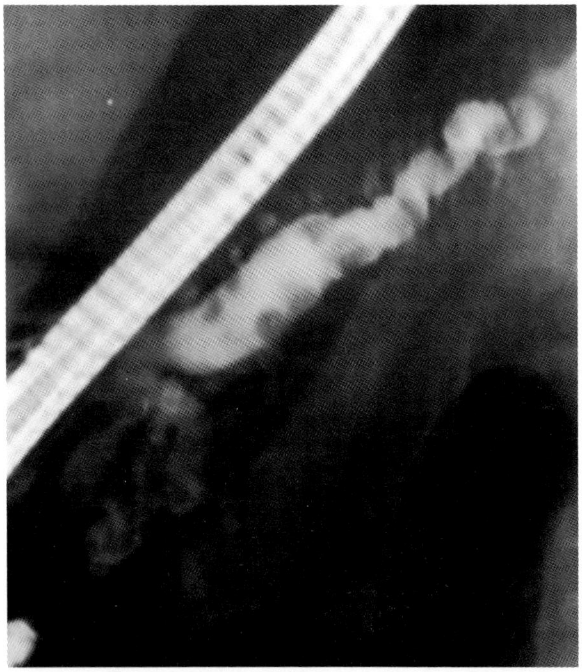

A

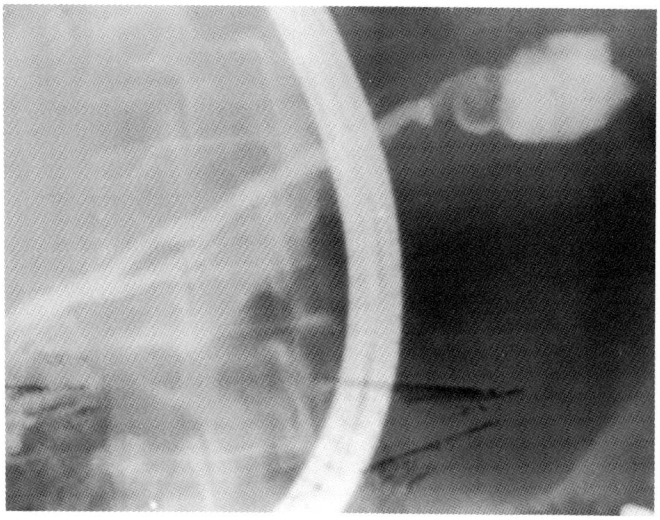

B

FIG. 9.13. A: A classic pancreatogram of chronic pancreatitis showing a dilated, tortuous main duct containing stones or protein plugs (lucencies in duct) and blunted, dilated secondary radicals. **B:** A pancreatogram that demonstrates two significant findings associated with chronic disease: a ring defect (*arrow*) in the body of the pancreas and a communicating pseudocyst of the tail. A ring may interfere with drainage of pancreatic secretions and contribute to pain or other symptoms. The development of a pseudocyst supports this concept.

known (58,59). The most important and distinguishing findings are alluded to and described in the accompanying figures. Dilated secondary radicals (Figs. 9.13, 9.14) and opacification of these secondary radicals in or near strictures (Figs. 9.10, 9.11) are important findings and are critical to confirming the diagnosis of inflammatory disease. Absence of opacification of secondary pancreatic duct radicals may be confirmatory evidence of a tumor if an adequate volume of contrast has been injected to rule out underfilling and if disruption of the pancreatic duct with extravasation of contrast outside the main duct is seen. The latter is usually pathognomonic for neoplasia.

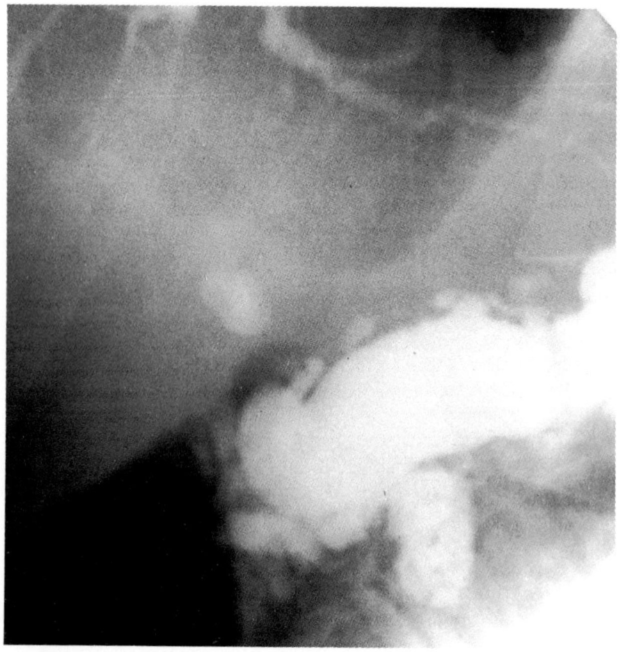

FIG. 9.14. A markedly dilated main pancreatic duct with blunted, dilated secondary radicals consistent with chronic pancreatitis.

It is incumbent upon the endoscopist-clinician to collate all the information in the database before making a specific conclusion. One has to consider the clinical information, scanning data, and the findings on ERCP. If the question of malignancy is raised and the diagnosis is unclear or equivocal, one may recommend more invasive studies, including an exploratory laparotomy unless the patient's age, risk factors, and life expectancy preclude surgery.

Chronic Pancreatitis—Stenosis of Bile Duct

Morphologic changes of the bile duct that are associated with chronic pancreatitis have been previously described (60–70). In approximately 80% of the general population, the bile duct traverses the head of the pancreas enroute to the duodenum. Disease processes affecting the head of the pancreas with resultant fibrotic changes can affect the bile duct by encasing it, ultimately producing cholestasis. This fibrotic process, associated with chronic pancreatitis, then encroaches

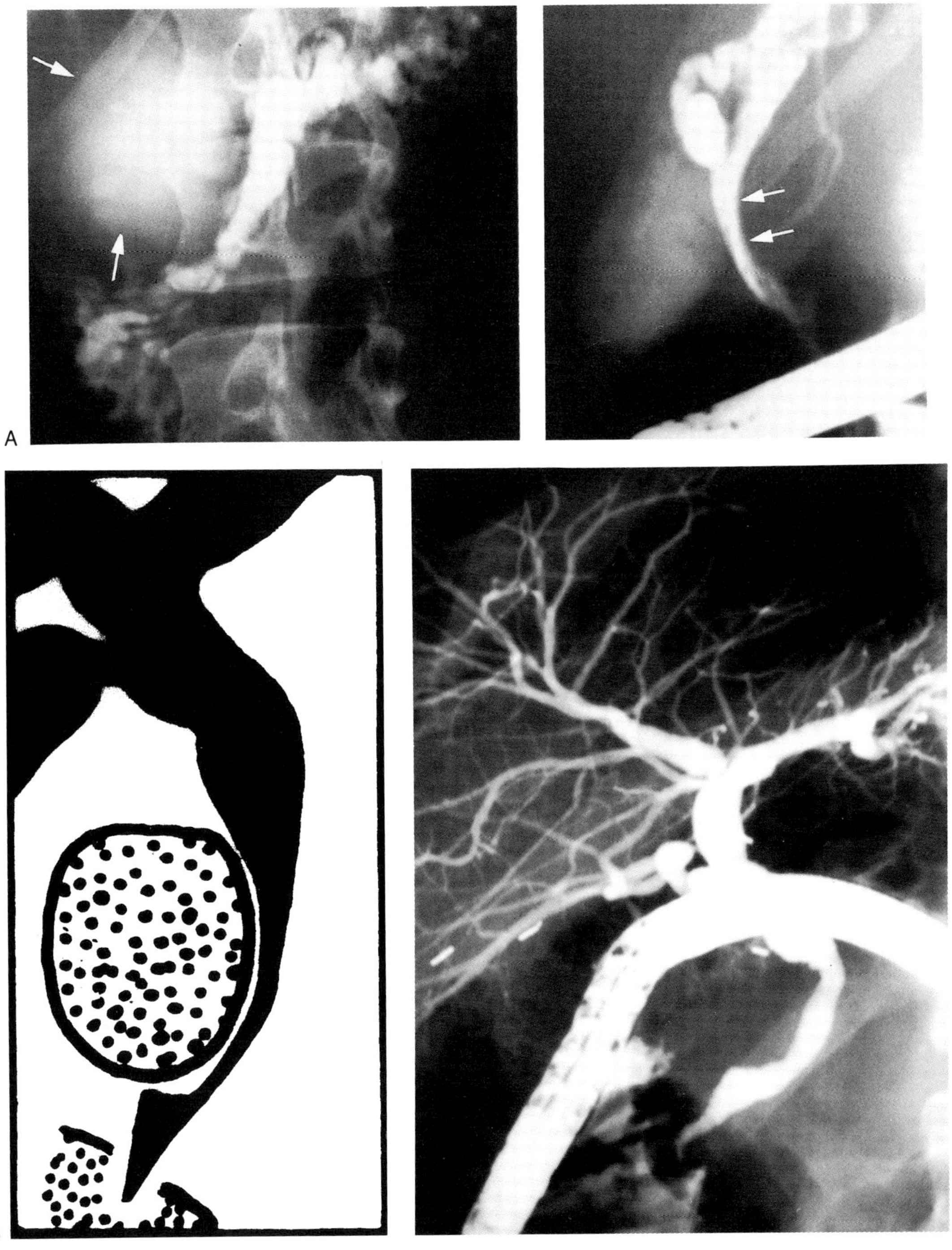

FIG. 9.15. A: Left: A tortuous, dilated pancreatic duct. Note the blush (*arrows*) as a pseudocyst is filled. **Right:** In this ERCP, which was performed on the same patient, the biliary tree is opacified. Note displacement of the distal bile duct secondary to a pseudocyst (*arrows*). **B: Left:** A pseudocyst displacing the distal common bile duct. (From ref. 60, with permission.) **Right:** A defect of the distal common bile duct similar to the artist's illustration.

upon the bile duct, producing a stenotic segment of the distal common duct and, usually, proximal dilatation of the biliary tree (Figs. 9.15–9.19). Transient, fluctuating, or intermittent cholestasis and jaundice occur as a result of an acute-on-chronic episode of pancreatitis. In other words, when there is status quo, no cholestasis is present, even with fibrosis. However, if the person ingests alcohol, or if acute-on-chronic pancreatitis is precipitated by another toxic or causative agent, recrudescent inflammatory changes, especially edema, compress the bile duct and produce cholestasis and jaundice. Eventually, when a firm, chronic, fi-

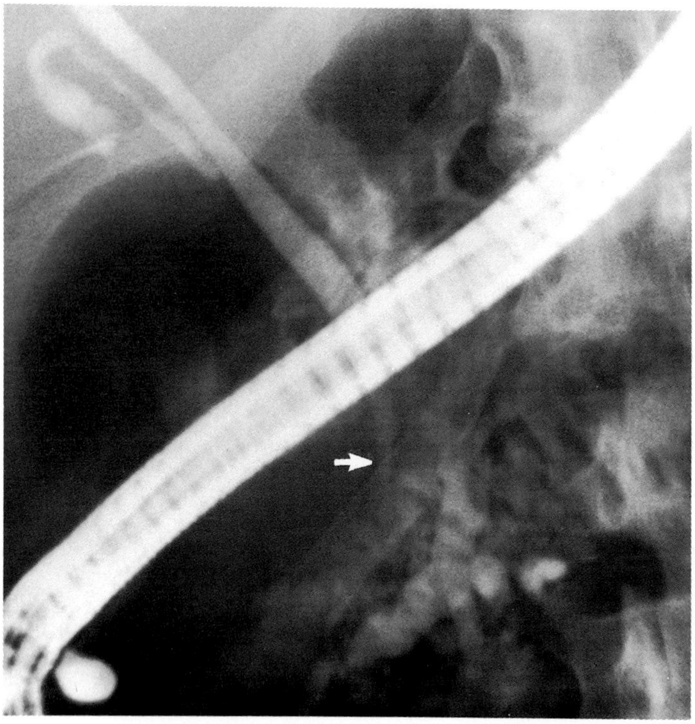

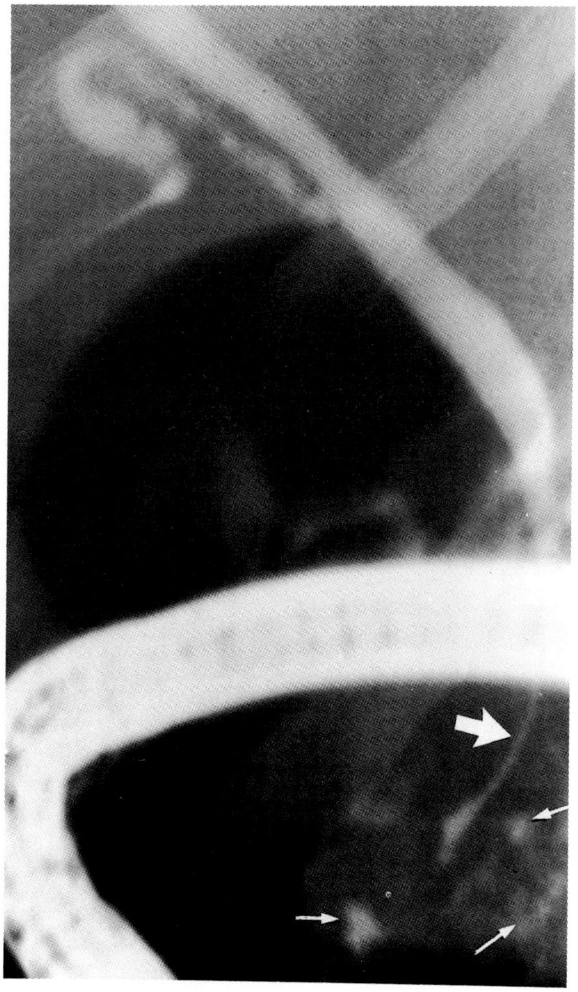

FIG. 9.16. Left: Filling of both duct systems. The pancreatic duct is segmented and tortuous, with filling only in the head. Note the tapered, distal common bile duct, which is affected by fibrosis secondary to pancreatitis (*arrow*). The smooth, tapered stricture should be benign. Minimal dilatation of the bile duct is found. **Right:** An enlarged version of the same bile duct stricture (*large arrow*) and pancreatic calcifications (*small arrows*).

brotic process compresses the bile duct more permanently and completely, cholestasis and jaundice become worse. Decompression of the biliary tree is mandatory at this stage of irreversibility. Despite attempts at endoscopic decompression of the biliary tree associated with chronic pancreatitis (Fig. 9.20), endotherapy has not been as successful in treating this chronic, fibrotic, benign process as in treating malignant pancreatic disease or benign and malignant strictures primarily affecting the bile duct. In my experience, most patients with chronic pancreatitis treated with endotherapy continue to complain of pain after a stent is inserted into the bile duct. Although results reported by other endoscopists may be more encouraging (71), I recommend a more permanent surgical alternative for the management of pain and cholestasis if the patient has an unsatisfactory response to an endoprosthesis. Definitive surgical procedures should be directed toward the management of the obstructive process affecting both duct systems, such as a combined choledochojejunostomy and pancreaticojejunostomy (72–90) (Figs. 9.21, 9.22).

Pseudocysts

Pseudocysts of the pancreas, for the most part, do not communicate with the main pancreatic duct and are better appreciated by ultrasound, CT scan, or endoscopic ultrasound than by ERCP. An ERCP may be performed, however, to outline the ductular morphology, especially if endoscopic therapy or surgery is being considered (91–98). In other words, the surgeon may request a "road map" of the duct system in order to plan an appropriate operation.

For communicating pseudocysts, an ERCP may be performed, but cautiously because of the potential for infection (99–103). Because endoscopic therapy can be provided for some communicating pseudocysts, I recommend that the patient be placed on prophylactic antibiotics, usually a cephalosporin and/or aminoglycoside, and that diluted contrast material be used and injected slowly with as little pressure as necessary to provide an adequate study. Adhering to these precau-

Text continues on page 136.

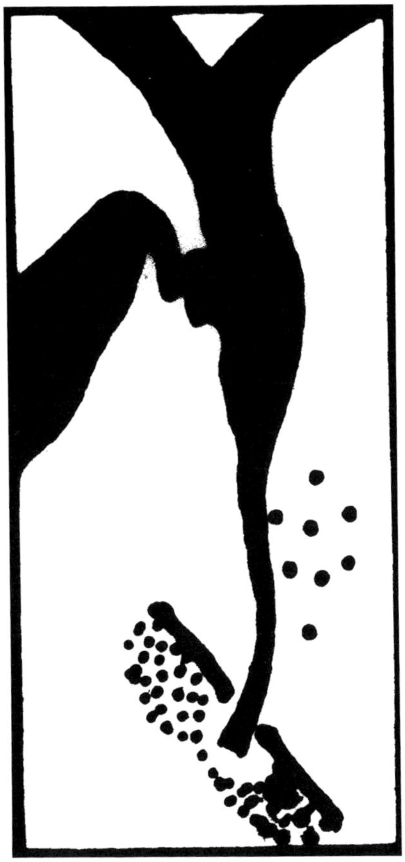

FIG. 9.17. A long, tapered distal common bile duct, similar to the radiograph in Fig. 9.16 Right, affected by fibrosis. Calcific densities are also illustrated. (From ref. 60 with permission.)

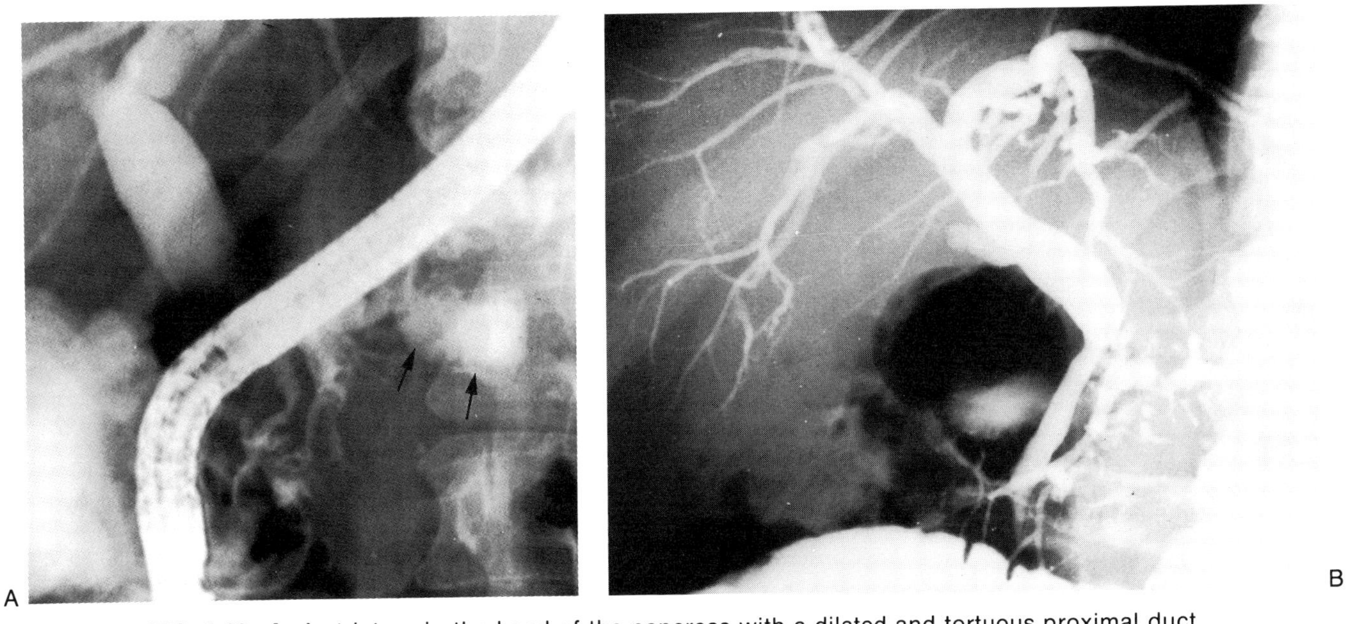

FIG. 9.18. A: A stricture in the head of the pancreas with a dilated and tortuous proximal duct (seen under the endoscope and over the spine). A pseudocyst is seen filling the inferior margin of the pancreatic duct (*arrows*). Note the dilated bile duct and the smooth, tapered distal bile duct secondary to chronic pancreatitis. **B:** On this ERCP, the pancreatogram is consistent with chronic disease with strictures and stenoses. The distal common bile duct is rigid and fixed secondary to fibrosis.

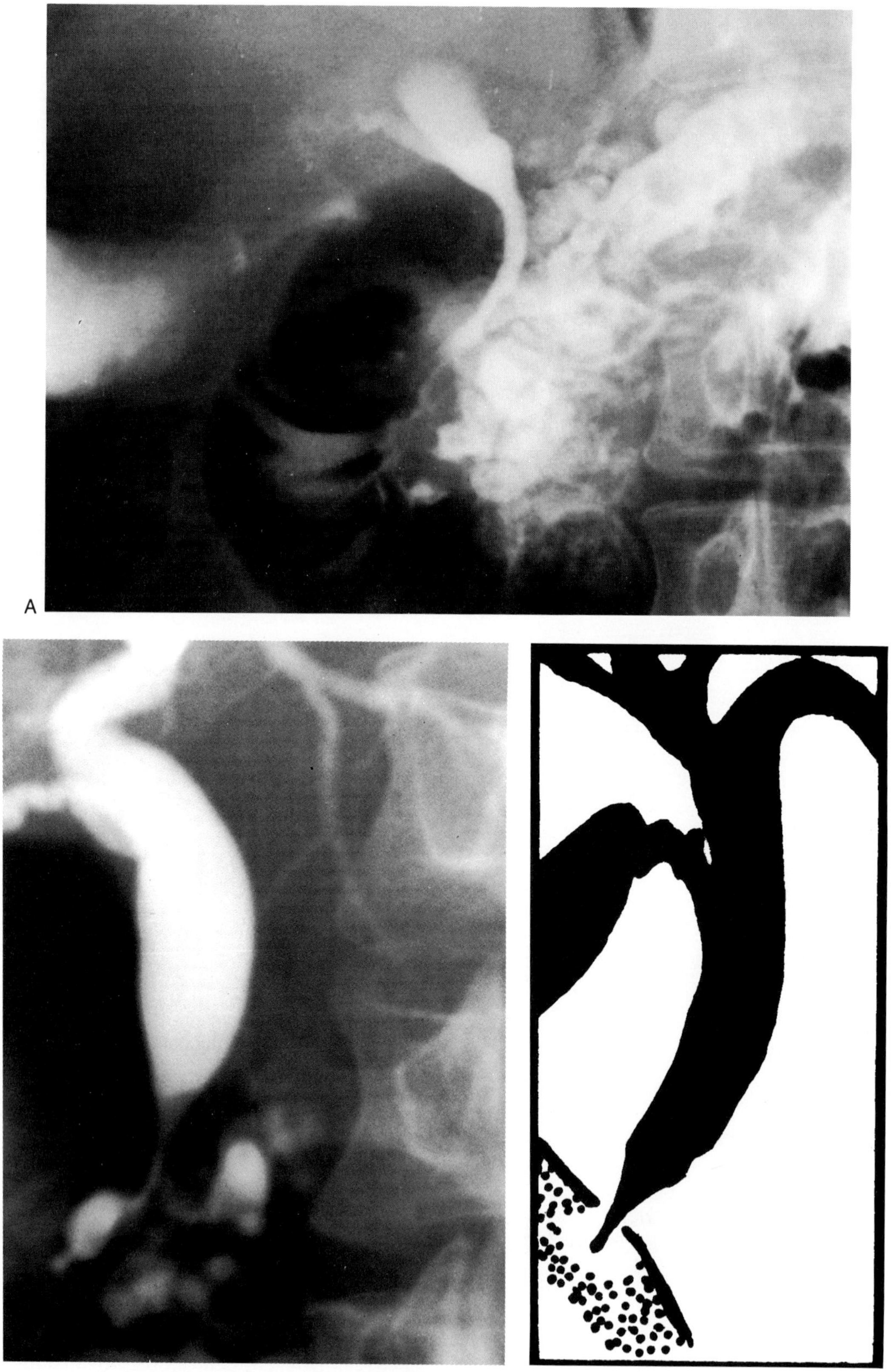

FIG. 9.19. A: A pancreatogram demonstrating profound changes of chronic pancreatitis exemplified by a dilated, tortuous main duct, dilated secondary and tertiary radicals, and lucent filling defects in the duct. A smoothly tapered distal common duct is a consequence of chronic pancreatitis, similar to Fig. 9.18B. **B: Left:** A smooth stricture of the distal common bile duct secondary to chronic pancreatitis. Note calcifications of the pancreas and incomplete filling of the pancreatic duct in the head of the gland. **Right:** A smooth stricture of the distal common bile duct found in chronic pancreatitis. (From ref. 60, with permission.)

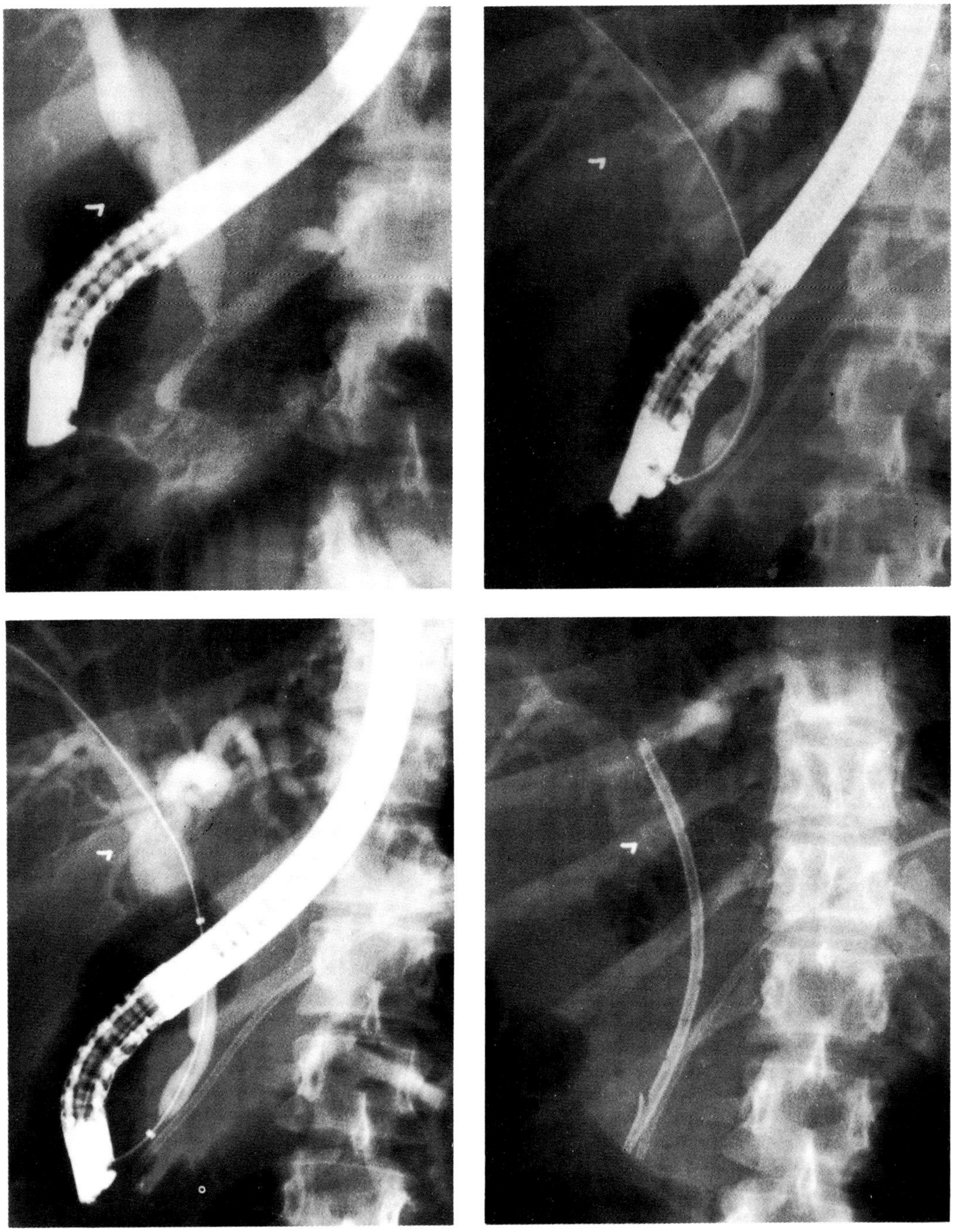

FIG. 9.20. Top left: Filling of the common bile duct demonstrating a smooth, tapered distal duct secondary to chronic pancreatitis. Note the presence of contrast, which is seen in the pancreatic duct near the spine. **Top right:** A prosthesis in the pancreatic duct. A balloon catheter is used to dilate the bile duct stricture. Note the waist of the balloon, which forms as contrast is injected for dilatation. **Bottom left:** The balloon is nearly fully dlstended. Again, the prosthesis is seen in the pancreatic duct. **Bottom right:** A prosthesis in the bile duct and another in the pancreatic duct.

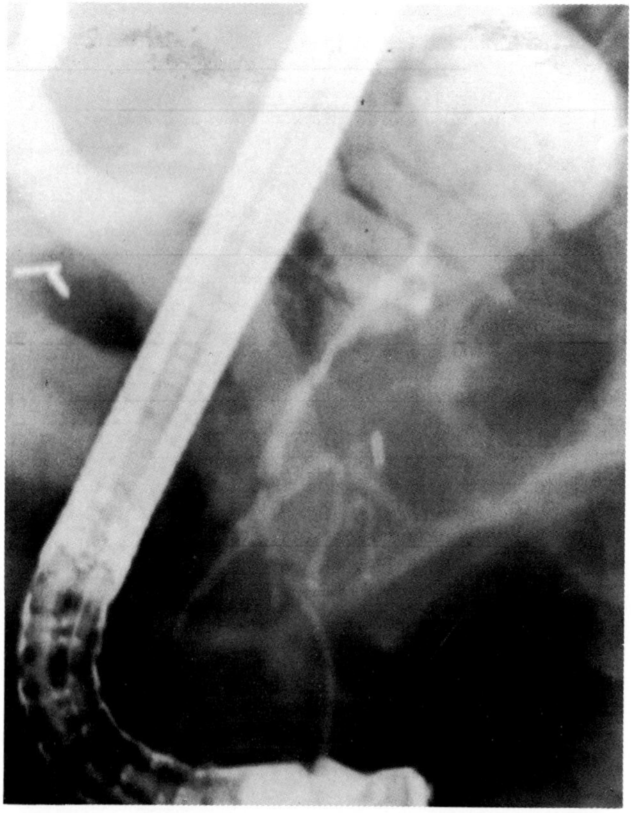

FIG. 9.21. An ERCP performed in a patient who had previously undergone a pancreaticojejunostomy and who presented with recurrent pain. The bile duct appears slightly dilated, but no other abnormality is seen. The pancreatic duct demonstrates beading and irregularity of the duct in the head, but there is no dilatation. Contrast readily flows into the jejunum, indicating that there is a patent enterostomy.

Text continued from page 132.
tions enables one to provide a valuable ductogram and to avoid potential complications (Figs. 9.23–9.25).

Placement of prostheses through the main duct to decompress the pancreas is an optional therapeutic maneuver for the experienced endoscopist. Endoscopic drainage of obstructing pseudocysts that encroach upon the stomach and duodenum is a therapeutic option available to some endoscopists and is described in references 104 through 107.

Pancreatic Duct Ectasia, Chronic Pancreatitis, and Pain

The classic radiologic finding of duct ectasia associated with chronic pancreatitis is usually pathognomonic for exocrine dysfunction and corroborates the clinical history of malabsorption and steatorrhea. Endoscopic therapy in this situation, sphincterotomy or insertion of a prosthesis, is usually not effective, although selected patients may respond (108). In a sense, the gland is burned out. The dilated main pancreatic duct and its radicals result from chronic, diffuse inflammatory changes affecting most, if not all, of the gland, and these changes are not a result of distal stenosis (sphincter). If a patient presents with clinical evidence of exocrine dysfunction and pain that are unresponsive to enzyme supplementation (109–115) or celiac axis blockade (116–119), a definitive surgical procedure can be recommended (72–90). The clinician and patient must be aware, however, that long-term results of surgery in patients with these problems are
Text continues on page 139.

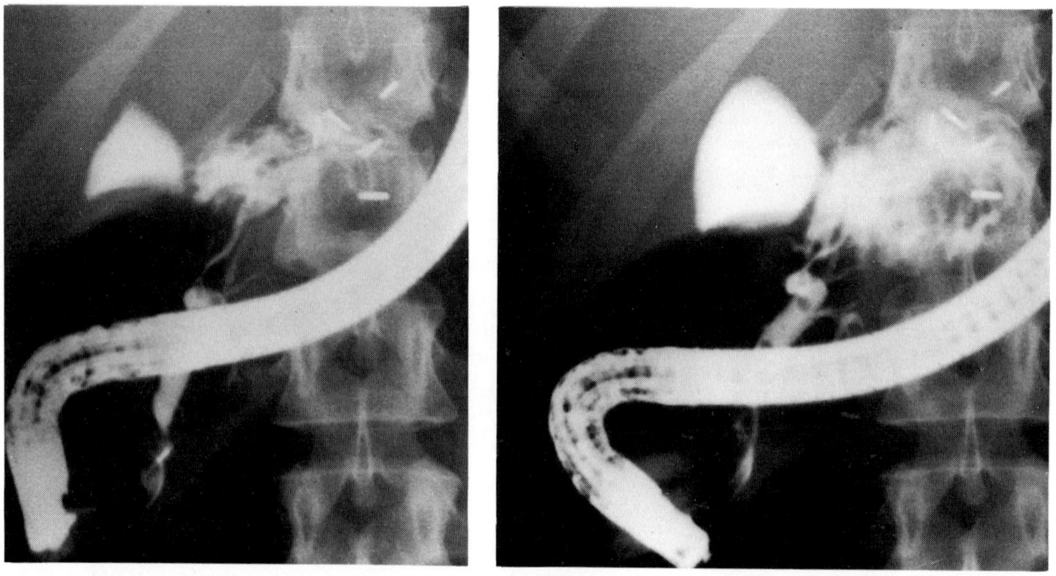

FIG. 9.22. Left: A pancreatogram from a patient who had previously undergone a pancreaticojejunostomy, demonstrating narrowing of the duct at the sphincter. Retrograde flow of contrast into the jejunum is seen, but narrowing of the duct is noted. **Right:** More filling of the jejunum has been accomplished, but a definite stricture of the pancreatic duct at the anastomosis is confirmed, which will require a repeat surgical procedure.

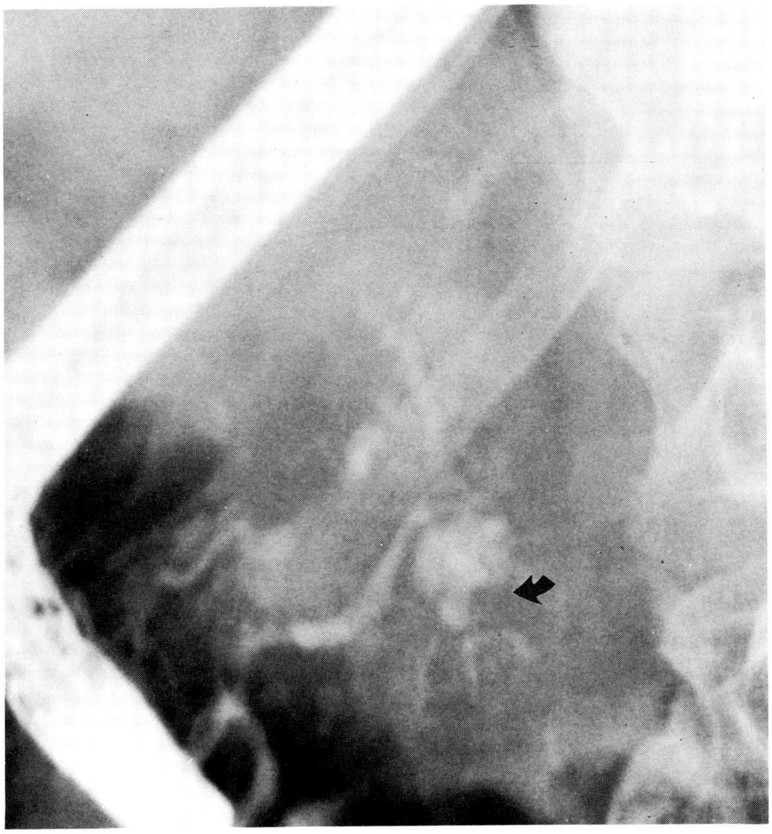

FIG. 9.23. Filling of a small cyst (*arrow*) on the inferior margin of the main pancreatic duct on this pancreatogram obtained in a patient with recurrent pancreatitis. Beading and stricturing of the main pancreatic duct, which is faintly opacified, is appreciated.

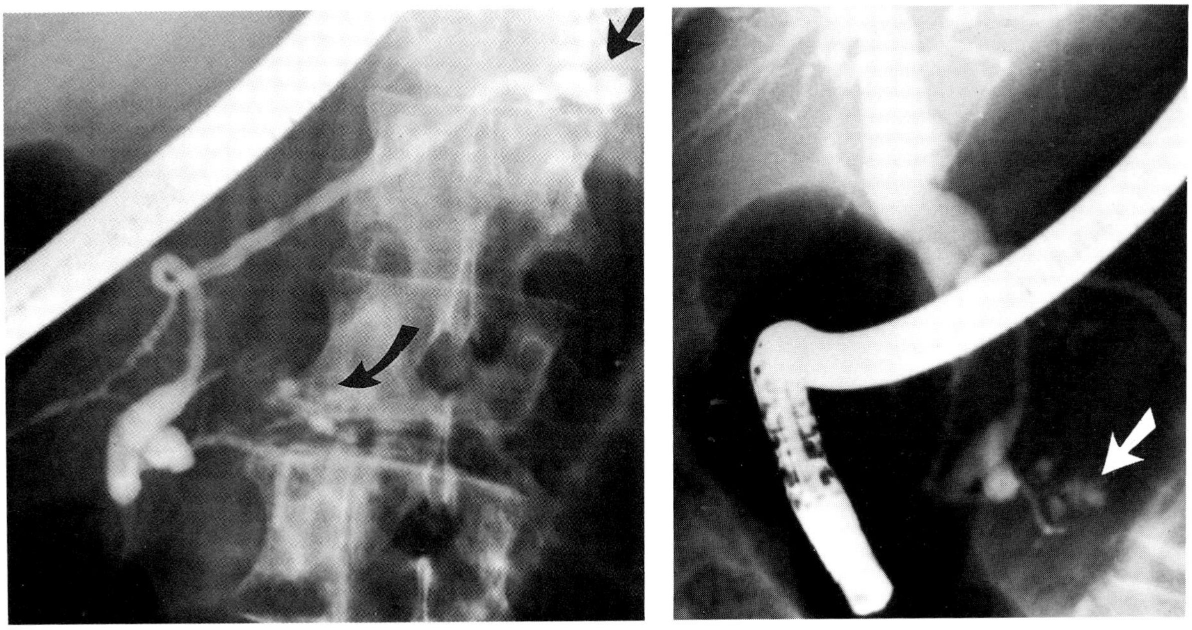

FIG. 9.24. Left: A pancreatogram showing cystic changes in the uncinate process (*curved arrow*) and tail (*straight arrow*) in a patient with recurrent subclinical pancreatitis. **Right:** Small cysts are seen more clearly after rotating the patient, separating the duct from the spine (*arrow*).

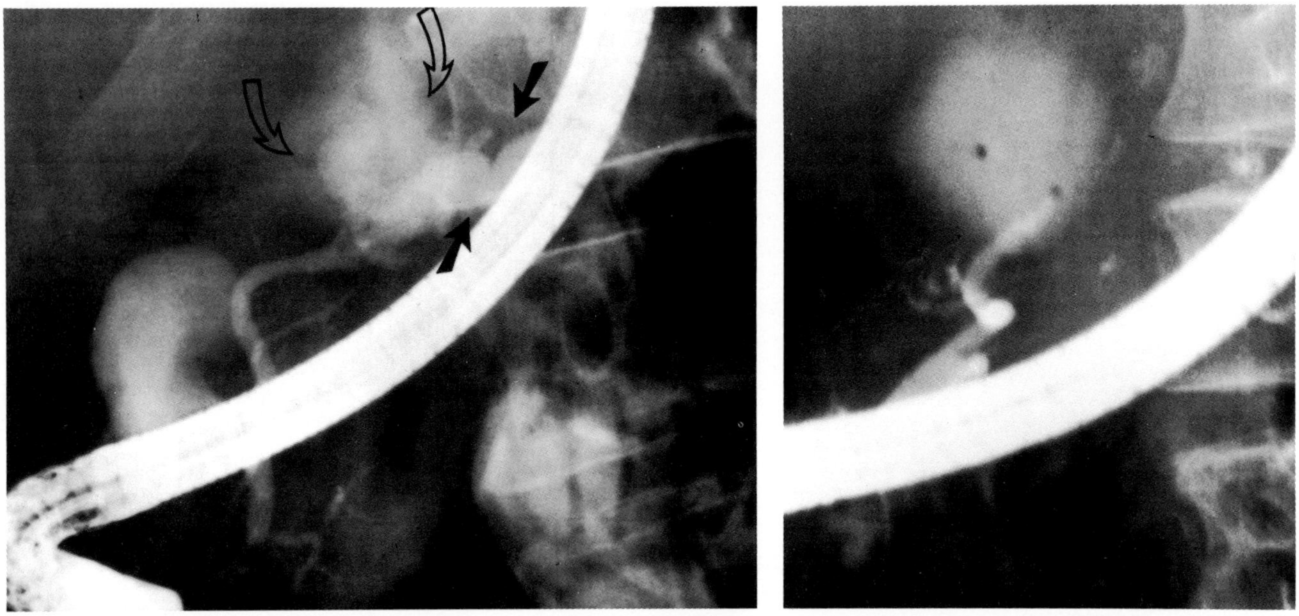

A B

FIG. 9.25. A: A pancreatogram showing filling of a communicating pseudocyst (*open arrows*) of the main pancreatic duct in the body of the gland. The closed arrows identify the dilated pancreatic duct proximal to a stricture. **B:** A pancreatogram that demonstrates a stricture in the body of the gland and a communicating pseudocyst.

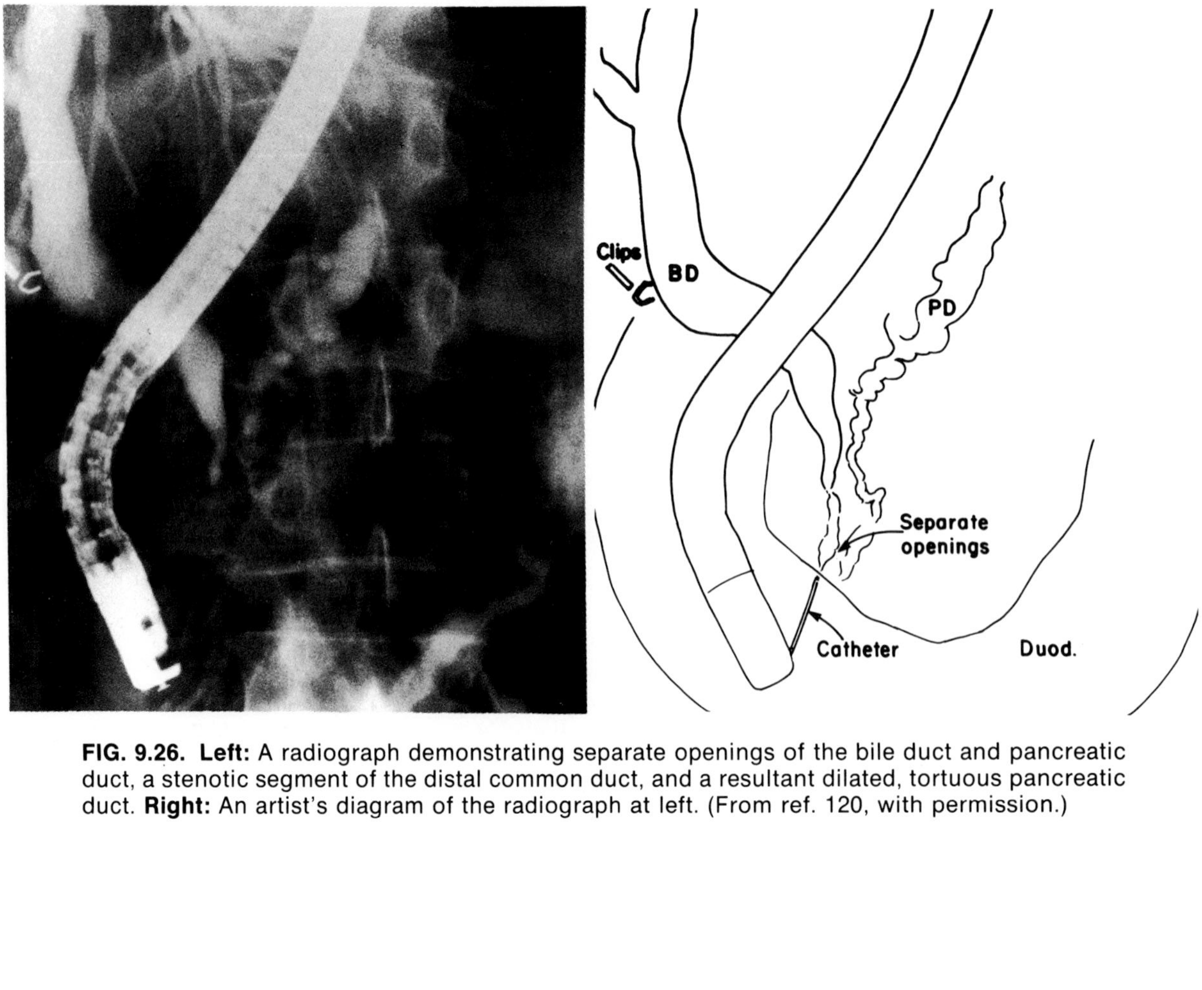

FIG. 9.26. Left: A radiograph demonstrating separate openings of the bile duct and pancreatic duct, a stenotic segment of the distal common duct, and a resultant dilated, tortuous pancreatic duct. **Right:** An artist's diagram of the radiograph at left. (From ref. 120, with permission.)

Text continued from page 136.
only reasonably good and that approximately 60% to 70% of patients undergoing various surgical procedures have sustained relief.

Separate Channel Openings of the Bile Duct and Pancreatic Duct: The Association in Alcohol-Induced Pancreatitis

Alcohol-associated pancreatitis is a seemingly more common occurrence in patients who have the anatomic finding of separate channel entry of the bile duct and pancreatic duct into the duodenum (120–125) than in patients with a common channel. In our index paper (120), we described ERCP findings in 58 patients with chronic alcohol abuse with and without induced pancreatitis and found that 86% of patients with acute-on-chronic pancreatitis had separate openings (Figs. 9.26, 9.27). It is postulated that, like alcohol-related sensitivity and pancreatitis associated with pancreas divisum, both these conditions (divisum and separate openings) are distinguished by a coexisting hyperplasia of the pancreatic duct epithelium and that symptoms related to pancreatitis are a manifestation of a hypersecretory state associated with this condition (hyperplasia) (126,127). It is my contention, contrary to previous knowledge and belief, that separate duct openings rather than a common channel are the main finding in patients with alcohol-induced pancreatitis. This is certainly the explanation for the difficulty endoscopists experience in opacifying both duct systems routinely at ERCP. A channel shared by both duct systems is less common in the general population, which is fortuitous because this latter anatomic arrangement is largely responsible for gallstone pancreatitis (128).

The thought that duodenal-pancreatic reflux, which might occur after alcohol ingestion resulting from relaxation of its sphincter, is responsible for pancreatitis

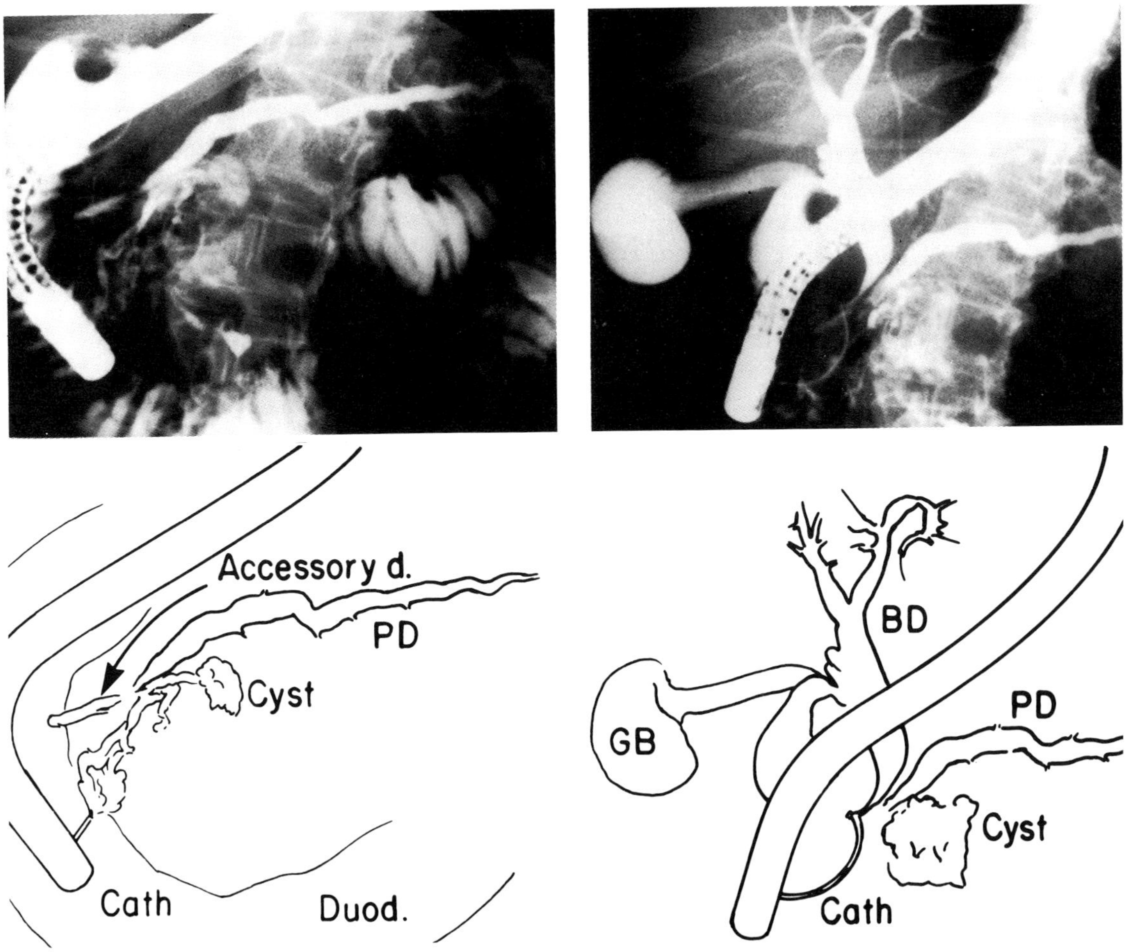

FIG. 9.27. Top left: An ERCP illustrating a dilated pancreatic duct and distal strictures of both the main and accessory ducts. **Bottom left:** An artist's illustration defining the radiograph. **Top right:** An ERCP from the same patient that shows a dilated bile duct and a tapered distal common bile duct, which is secondary to pancreatitis. Separate openings are demonstrated. **Bottom right:** An artist's illustration of the radiograph above it. (From ref. 120, with permission.)

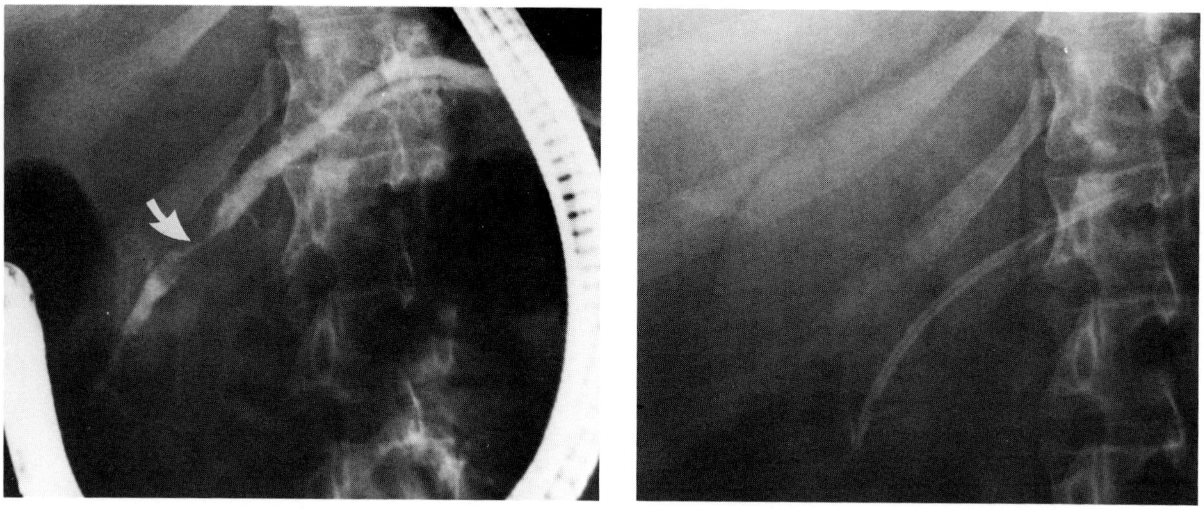

FIG. 9.28. Left: A stricture in the head of the gland (*arrow*). The patient had experienced recurrent episodes of pain, probably owing to a hypertensive sphincter. **Right:** A 7Fr prosthesis has been placed into the pancreatic duct, providing decompression. The patient's symptoms were immediately relieved. The patient will return within 6 months for removal of the stent, and an endoscopic sphincterotomy will be considered.

has not been proved, whereas the separate channel hypothesis appears logical and acceptable. Although spasm of the sphincter has also been postulated to occur after alcohol ingestion contributing to pancreatitis, this theory lacks support. In support of the separate channel theory, we postulate that, after alcohol ingestion, pain and symptoms of pancreatitis, which occur in these preexisting conditions, result from a hypersecretory state induced by humoral stimulation and are not related to local, sphincteric reactions to alcohol (127,128).

Idiopathic Pancreatitis

ERCP findings of strictures of the pancreatic duct in patients presenting with a history of *nonalcoholic* recurrent pancreatitis (due to stone disease, trauma, idiopathic, or unknown causes) (Table 9.1) provide significant and essential information for assisting in the management of the affected patient. It is in these patients that the author (129) and others (71,130) have applied endoscopic decompression techniques, insertion of stents, since 1983. Figures 9.28 through 9.30

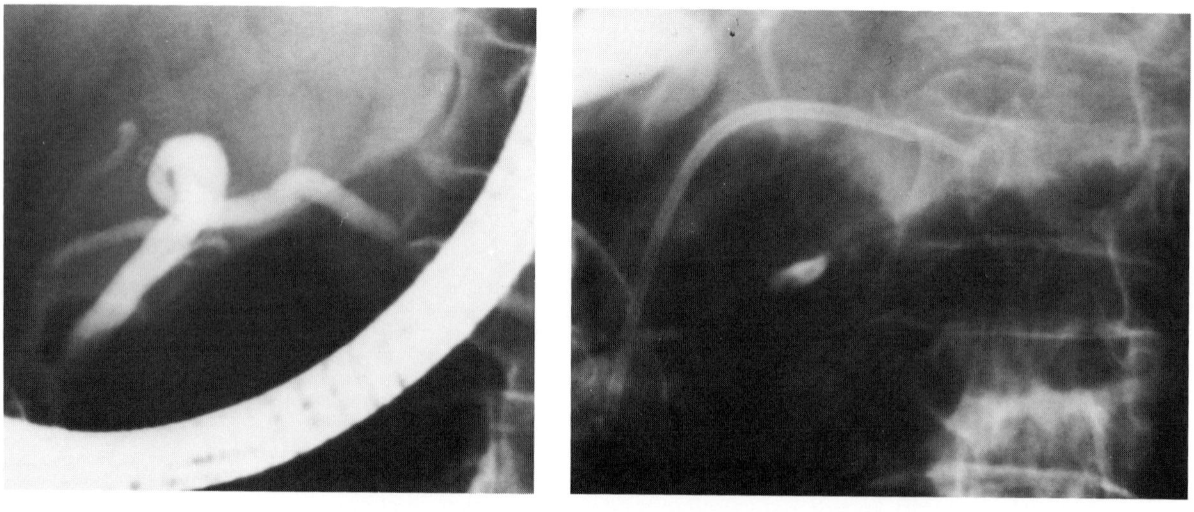

FIG. 9.29. Left: A loop variation in this patient was responsible for pancreatitis. **Right:** A 7Fr stent was inserted into the pancreatic duct for decompression and the patient's symptoms were relieved. Again, the patient will return in 4 to 6 months for either a sphincterotomy and stent exchange or definitive surgery.

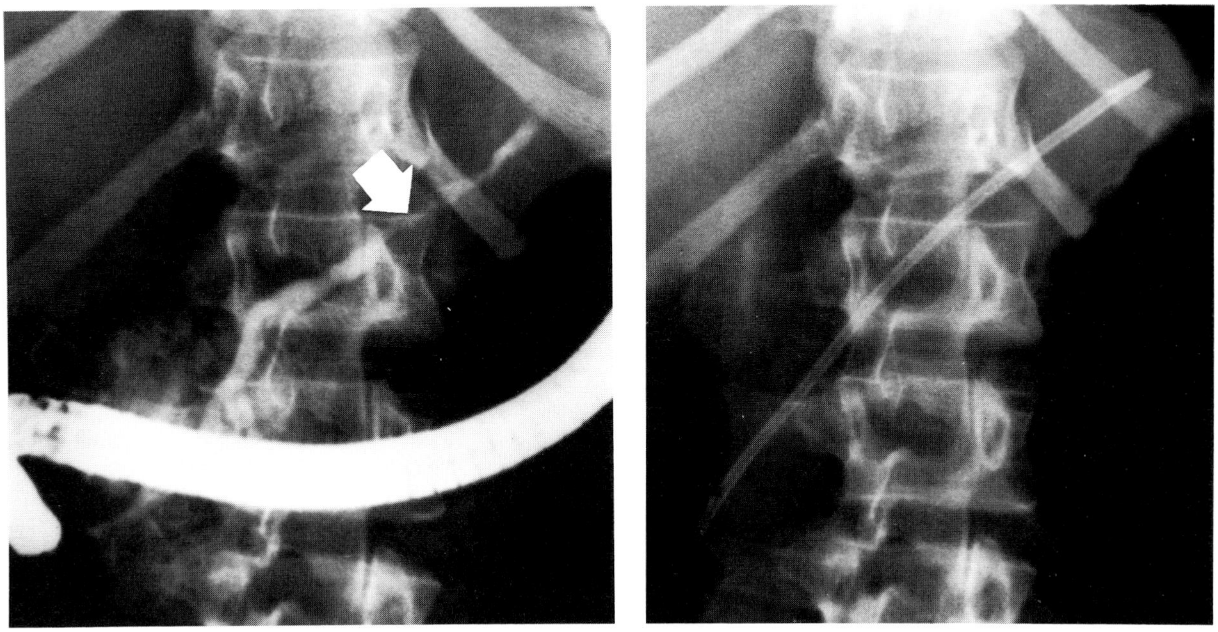

FIG. 9.30. Left: A stricture in the tail of the gland (*arrow*). The patient experienced recurrent pain as a result of pancreatitis. **Right:** A long 7Fr stent was placed in the duct for decompression. The patient's symptoms were relieved, and she will return later for more definitive treatment.

are examples of idiopathic strictures which were treated with prostheses. My colleagues and I have reported our early experience treating patients endoscopically for recurrent, idiopathic pancreatitis, and the results of endotherapy have been gratifying (131). Because our ongoing trial is prospective but not randomized, results of therapy are determined by using the patient as the control. It is our opinion that endoscopic decompression is a viable prognostic and therapeutic alternative in this patient population, and, if the patient responds to endoscopic drainage (i.e., the presenting symptoms improve), he or she may be a good candidate for further endoscopic treatment such as sphincterotomy or for surgical decompression (131). Results of endoscopic treatment are presented in Chapter 12. Much remains to be learned in this field, and we look forward to controlled, randomized trials and, based on past experience, their long-term results. We have been gratified by the long-term results accumulated in our own prospective trials and anticipate the same results in controlled trials.

Gallstone (Biliary) Pancreatitis

Pancreatitis resulting from impaction or passage of gallstones into the ampulla is thought to be a transient problem. The severity of gallstone pancreatitis, however, varies from mild to severe and may be fatal (128,132). The majority of patients with this entity have an intact gallbladder and cholelithiasis, but a small number of patients have undergone cholecystectomy (Table 9.2). In addition to pancreatitis, these patients frequently experience recurrent symptoms of cholestasis or cholangitis because of common bile duct stones.

The etiology is the same in both groups (cholecystectomized patients and those with intact gallbladders): A stone passing into the distal common bile duct produces intermittent obstruction to the pancreatic duct. A sequence of events inciting and leading to pancreatitis has been postulated, but pancreatitis is most likely due to an impacted stone in a common channel (Fig. 9.31–9.33), in which both the bile duct and the pancreatic duct enter into the ampulla through the same orifice, in concert with reflux of *infected* bile into a partially obstructed pancreatic duct (131). Infected bile is thought to be the essential component in the pathogenesis of gallstone pancreatitis because it contains bacterial amidase, a potent proteolytic enzyme.

TABLE 9.2. *Gallstone pancreatitis: endoscopic treatment*

Number of patients	53
Males	22
Females	31
Age range	22–91 years
Mean age 65.5 years	
Previous cholecystectomy	41 (71%)
Mean hospital stay	4.5 days
Emergency surgery	0
Deaths	0

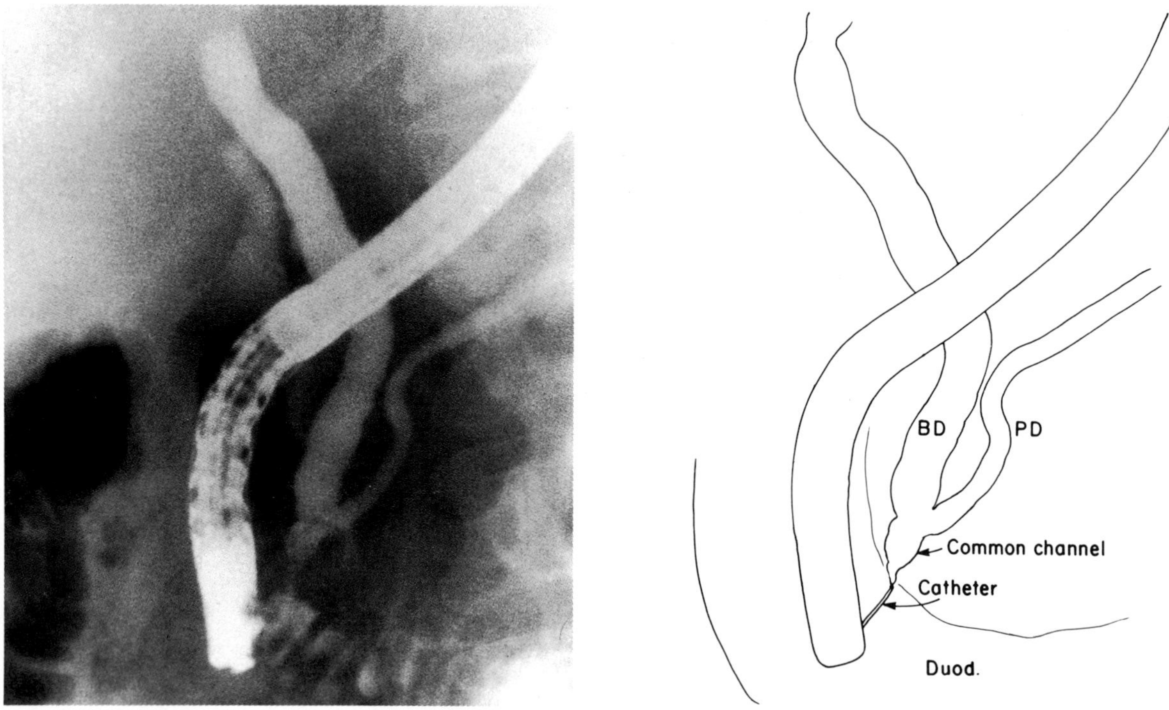

FIG. 9.31. Left: A common channel. **Right:** An illustration of the common channel.

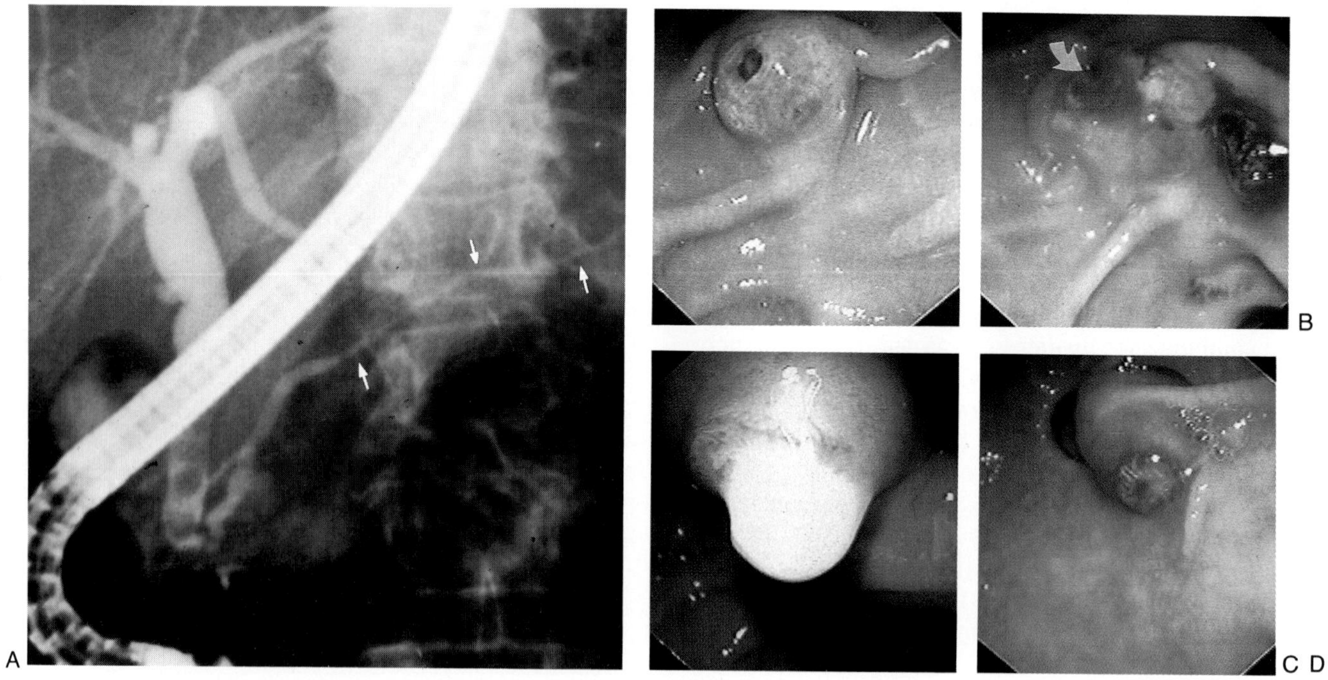

FIG. 9.32. A: This ERCP shows stones in the distal CBD, a common channel, and narrowing of the pancreatic duct in the body and tail of the gland secondary to recurrent pancreatitis (*arrows*). After sphincterotomy and stone extraction, the patient's symptoms and recurrent pancreatitis were relieved. **B: Left:** A pigmented gallstone impacted in the papillary orifice in a patient presenting with gallstone pancreatitis. **Right:** After a sphincterotomy (*arrow*), the stone was released, and the pancreatitis subsided. **C:** A videoendoscopic picture of a large, white stone impacted in the papilla. The patient presented with cholangitis and pancreatitis. The stone is probably pancreatic in origin. **D:** A papilla, which appears inflamed, probably from the recent passage of a stone.

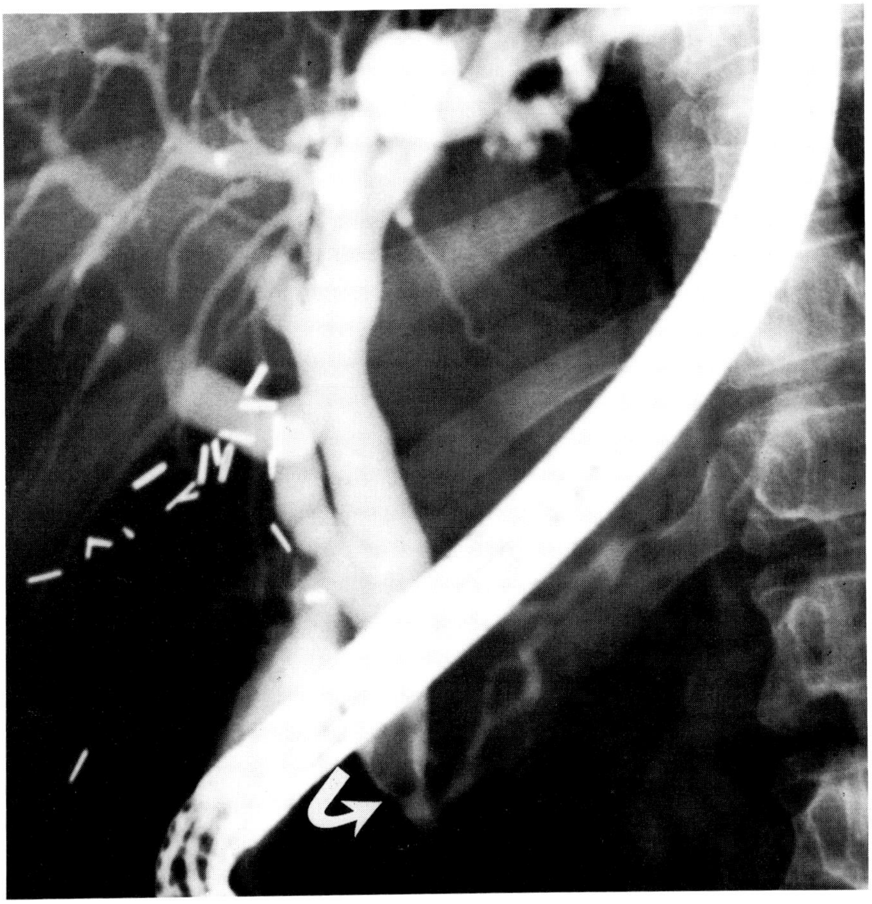

FIG. 9.33. An ERCP demonstrating a common channel, a retained common duct stone (arrow), and narrowing of the pancreatic duct (a consequence of pancreatitis). The patient recovered from sphincterotomy and stone extraction without further incident. Note the long cystic duct remnant.

In the obstructed duct, the infected bile containing bacterial amidase initiates an enzyme cascade, resulting in the production of lecithin and lysolecithin and ultimately leading to tissue destruction (132). There is currently no prophylactic or therapeutic antagonist available to either prevent or reverse this enzyme cascade and tissue destruction. Despite the proposed antisecretory effects of somatostatin, this biological has been only significantly effective when used prior to pancreatic injury (35,36,133). Serious complications, varying from phlegmon and pseudocyst formation to the adult respiratory distress syndrome (ARDS) and death, may ensue. Many affected patients require close observation, monitoring, and supportive care, and hospitalization may be prolonged because of the slow recovery and intercurrent problems associated with this disorder. Although randomized trials using a variety of treatment modalities have been reported, supportive care appears to be the most predictable (134–144).

As previously intimated, gallstone pancreatitis is often transient and self-limiting. The offending stone has been found in the stools of affected persons, having passed spontaneously in 85% to 95% (145). Both Acosta and Kelly independently reported this observation, confirming that gallstone pancreatitis is caused by an offending stone that, in most cases, passes through the sphincter into the duodenum and ultimately into the stool (146,147). In the meantime, most patients recover spontaneously, leaving the issue of definitive treatment to random therapy, speculation, or emergent intervention (148,149).

There is disagreement among surgical experts as to the necessity and timing of surgery for exploration of the common bile duct in the patient presenting with gallstone pancreatitis (150–152). There is no argument among surgeons regarding the performance of cholecystectomy for the treatment and *prevention* of gallstone pancreatitis (153); rather, there is universal agreement for this operation, usually performed electively after full recovery. Regarding common bile duct exploration, most surgeons believe that an urgent operation is not necessary. The offending stone usually passes spontaneously, and most patients improve with conservative management, making surgery unnecessary; also, common bile duct stones are rarely found at laparotomy, so an operation does not justify the high risk. Emergency surgery is associated with an unacceptable morbidity and mortality, which, again, does not justify the operation.

Dr. H. Stone has been an advocate of emergency surgery, and his results with surgical sphincterotomy, although not optimal at the outset, have supported his advocacy of surgery (154). Despite his favorable reports, many surgeons disagree with early surgical intervention, advising a "watch and wait" attitude, and ultimately recommend cholecystectomy.

On the other hand, endoscopists have been very successful in the emergency treatment of gallstone pancreatitis (155). Most patients who have been treated by endoscopic techniques were accepted for treatment because they were seriously ill and clinically deteriorating despite excellent supportive care provided in the intensive care unit or because no other alternative treatment was available and surgery was rejected because of high risk. Fortunately, in most reports, the morbidity of endoscopy is much lower than surgery, and mortality has been very low and acceptable (155,156). These results were confirmed by a prospective trial of endoscopy that emphasized the efficacy of endoscopy in high-risk patients (157–159); all the more reason not to operate on these patients when an experienced endoscopist is available.

Physicians often ask when ERCP should be performed in patients presenting with acute pancreatitis. The acceptable answer to this question is qualified (160). If the etiology of pancreatitis is known—for example, alcohol, prescription drug intolerance or reaction, substance abuse, hyperlipidemia, or gallstones—and the offending substance is removed, one can wait for clinical improvement (normal vital signs, return of peristalsis with passage of flatus, and tolerance of diet) before considering the procedure. In general, if pancreatitis results from a metabolic or nonmechanical cause, ERCP can be performed electively if the primary care physician needs a baseline pancreatogram, especially if pancreatitis is a recurrent problem. If pancreatitis is a single event, however, ERCP can be postponed or ruled out. On the other hand, if pancreatitis is thought to be due to stone disease, I perform an ERCP *electively* when the patient is stable. However, if the patient is deteriorating, becomes stuperous or comatose, and requires vasopressors and mechanical life support, I recommend that an *emergency* ERCP with planned sphincterotomy be undertaken. Of course, a complete informed consent, which includes all anticipated risks and probable outcome, must be explained in detail to the next of kin and accepted before undertaking the procedure. As previously mentioned, the performance of ERCP and ES in seriously ill patients with gallstone pancreatitis has been safely performed with few complications and low mortality. *To recapitulate, ERCP can be performed electively in a patient recovering or having recovered from pancreatitis who is asymptomatic and is tolerating diet. Emergency ERCP and ES are performed in patients with stone disease who are deteriorating and not responding to life-saving measures.*

I have performed ES on 53 occasions in patients with gallstone pancreatitis (Table 9.2). Minimal morbidity and no mortality have resulted from the procedure (ERCP and ES) in my experience, confirming the experience of others in utilizing a safe procedure for disease that may otherwise be fatal.

Prophylactic Sphincterotomy for Gallstone Pancreatitis—Medical Cholecystectomy?

Prophylactic sphincterotomy is another therapeutic category in the management of gallstone pancreatitis, as reported in reference 161. Because elective cholecystectomies are often performed for gallstone pancreatitis as a prophylactic measure (obviously, eliminating the source or probable cause of the inciting stone would eliminate the syndrome), I have occasionally performed a sphincterotomy (ostensibly separating the bile duct from the pancreatic duct) in an attempt to prevent gallstone pancreatitis in patients with cholelithiasis and recurrent pancreatitis (Table 9.3). This prophylactic sphincterotomy has been performed in high-risk patients with comorbid diseases such as cardiac disease and pulmonary disease who were considered at risk for surgery or cholecystectomy but who could undergo an elective endoscopic procedure (Fig. 9.34). Although the numbers are small and the disease, by natural history, may not occur again, no further episodes of pancreatitis have occurred in this group of patients. Significantly, in these patients, the severity of the index episode was so intense (though they survived) that their referring physicians believed that, because these patients could not undergo surgery (cholecystectomy), a less invasive procedure (sphincterotomy) might avoid future, life-threatening occurrences. Therefore, after obtaining a careful but fully descriptive informed consent, the procedure was undertaken. To reiterate, no complications occurred, and there have been no recurrent attacks of gallstone pancreatitis subsequently in a seven-year follow-up. In fact, follow-up of some of these patients has confirmed that the gallbladders are now either free of stones or that the numbers and sizes of stones are reduced. These findings support the hypothesis that sphincterotomy allows for either spontaneous passage of gallstones or endogenous dissolution (162). This

TABLE 9.3. *Prophylactic sphincterotomy for gallstone pancreatitis (medical cholecystectomy)*

Number of patients	15
Males	11
Females	4
Mean age	59 years
Age range 43 to 83 years	
COPD	5
ASHD	10
Complications	0
Surgery	0
Deaths	0

A 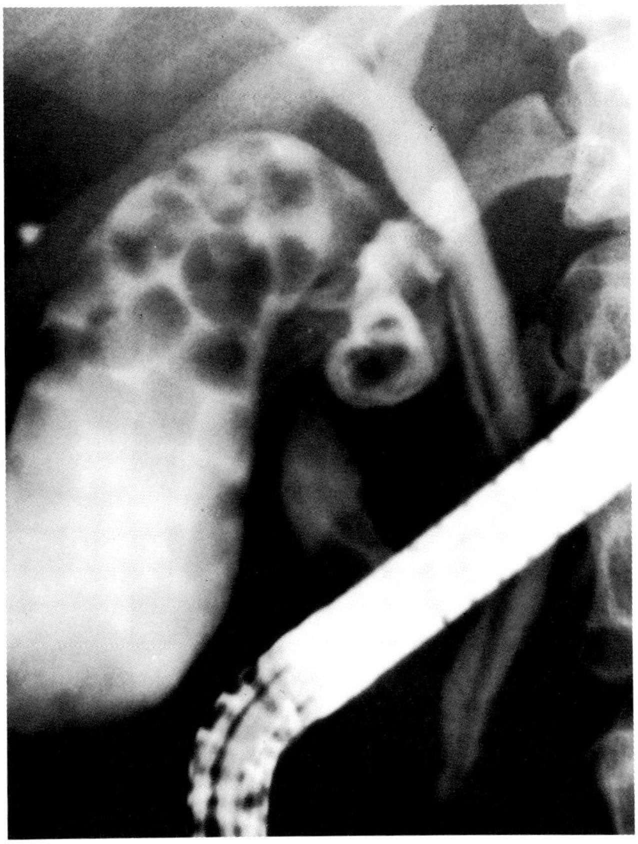

FIG. 9.34. **A:** An ERCP in a patient with recurrent pancreatitis. No common duct stone was found, but cholelithiasis and a common channel were confirmed. The patient was feeble and had other comorbid conditions, so a sphincterotomy was performed. No further episodes of pancreatitis recurred after a 9-month follow-up. **B:** Prophylactic sphincterotomy—medical cholecystectomy. **Left:** A common channel, stones in the bile duct and gallbladder, and evidence of pancreatitis. **Middle:** After a sphincterotomy, a balloon is used to remove the common duct stones. **Right:** Many of the gallbladder stones will assumedly pass from that organ into the duodenum through the sphincterotomy, preventing further episodes of pancreatitis.

B 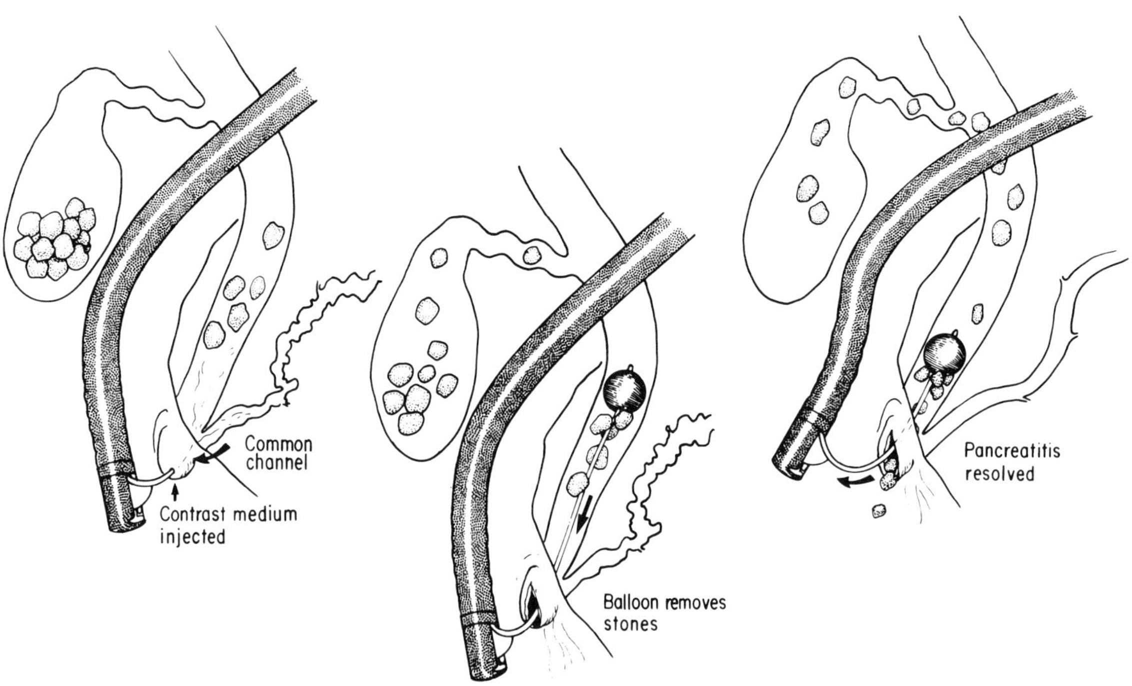

medical endoscopic approach to the management of gallstone pancreatitis is rather bold, but this area is fertile for research and presents researchers with an opportunity to compare cholecystectomy to prophylactic sphincterotomy. In addition, long-term follow-up of patients with intact gallbladders after ES remains a high priority. The effect of ES on cholecystitis is also of great interest and is being studied as well (162–164). Whether the widespread acceptance and performance of laparoscopic cholecystectomy will affect these ongoing studies will be interesting to watch, because comparative studies of these techniques are needed. The endoscopic approach utilizing sphincterotomy may eventually become moot with the advent of the surgical laparoscopic cholecystectomy procedure; but one must keep in mind the fact that general anesthesia is required for laparoscopic cholecystectomy which may exclude candidates at risk.

MALIGNANT PANCREATIC DISEASE

Is pancreatic cancer a surgical disease? At the present time, no. Although patient survival from carcinoma of the pancreas is dismally low, the search for a marker or reliable screening test that may lead to earlier detection of this dreaded disease continues (165–173). The hope is that earlier detection, diagnosis, and treatment will lead to a possible cure, although nothing has yet had a positive effect on survival. In fact, the disease is so aggressive in most individuals that the smallest periampullary pancreatic tumor subsequently presents as metastatic disease in 4 to 6 months, and survival rarely exceeds 1 year.

One may then ask, "Why bother with detection and treatment if the prognosis is so poor?" Perhaps the most rational answer is that aggressive diagnosis and treatment may detect a curable, nonpancreatic, periampullary tumor. Admittedly, this is a rare occurrence. Fewer than 5% of patients who present with findings consistent with carcinoma of the pancreas are found at surgery to have adenocarcinoma of the bile duct, periampullary neoplasms, or cystadenocarcinoma of the pancreas (174,175). Therefore, resection and cure are unlikely in most patients. Patients who have undergone bypass surgical procedures for a presumptive diagnosis of carcinoma of the pancreas (although the surgeon reported a rockhard pancreatic mass at laparotomy, carcinoma was never confirmed histologically) but who survived many years obviously did not have carcinoma but probably had chronic or focal pancreatitis.

Some physicians and surgeons managing patients with carcinoma of the pancreas have stated publicly that because the prognosis of this disease is so poor and because therapy has not altered survival, they would rather not do anything since "no one dies from itching." Although this statement is true, most of us working with such patients believe that palliation is humane and should be provided, if possible, to allow the patient to return to a near-normal life-style and to spend precious time comfortably with family and friends while preparing for the inevitable. Skeptics and nihilists may disagree with the last statement, but an approach to the evaluation and management of such incurable patients, offering a *surgical* alternative to palliation is presented in Chapter 12.

TABLE 9.4. *Workup of cholestasis*

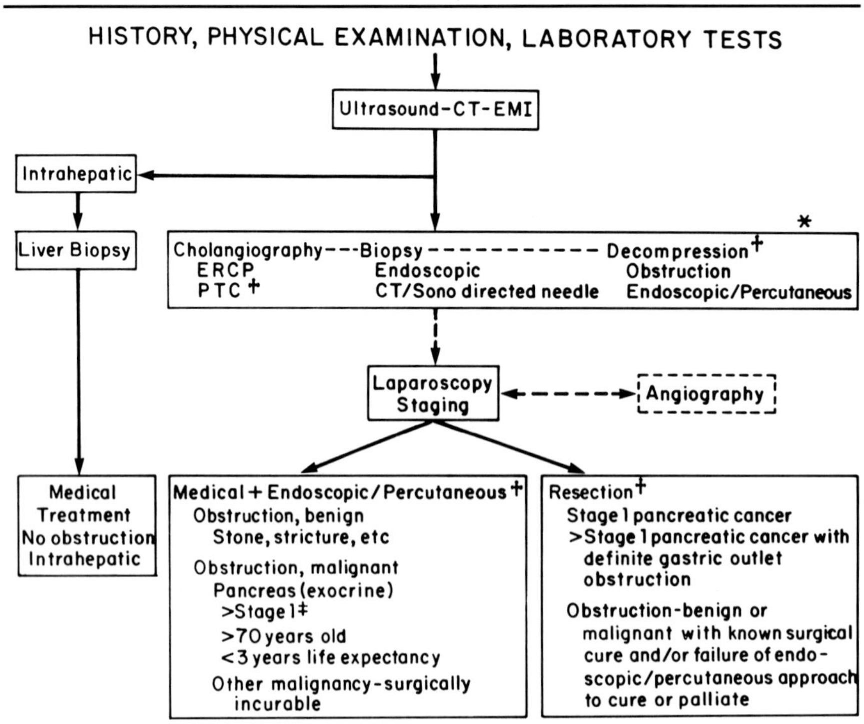

* Cholangiography + biopsy (endoscopic) + decompression desirable as single, initial procedure; directed needle biopsy may precede or follow cholangiography or accompany laparoscopy, in extrahepatic disease.

+ Normal coagulation

‡ From American Joint Committee on Cancer: Manual for Staging of Cancer 1983

The workup and evaluation of patients presenting with cholestasis and/or jaundice should be expeditious and exact. This algorithm is similar to the one in Table 2.2, but Table 9.4 considers the critical issue of staging a patient with a malignancy of the biliary tree or pancreas (176–181). After an initial comprehensive evaluation of the patient (history, physical examination, and laboratory and radiology tests), cholangiography should be performed either endoscopically or radiographically, cytology or biopsies should be obtained,

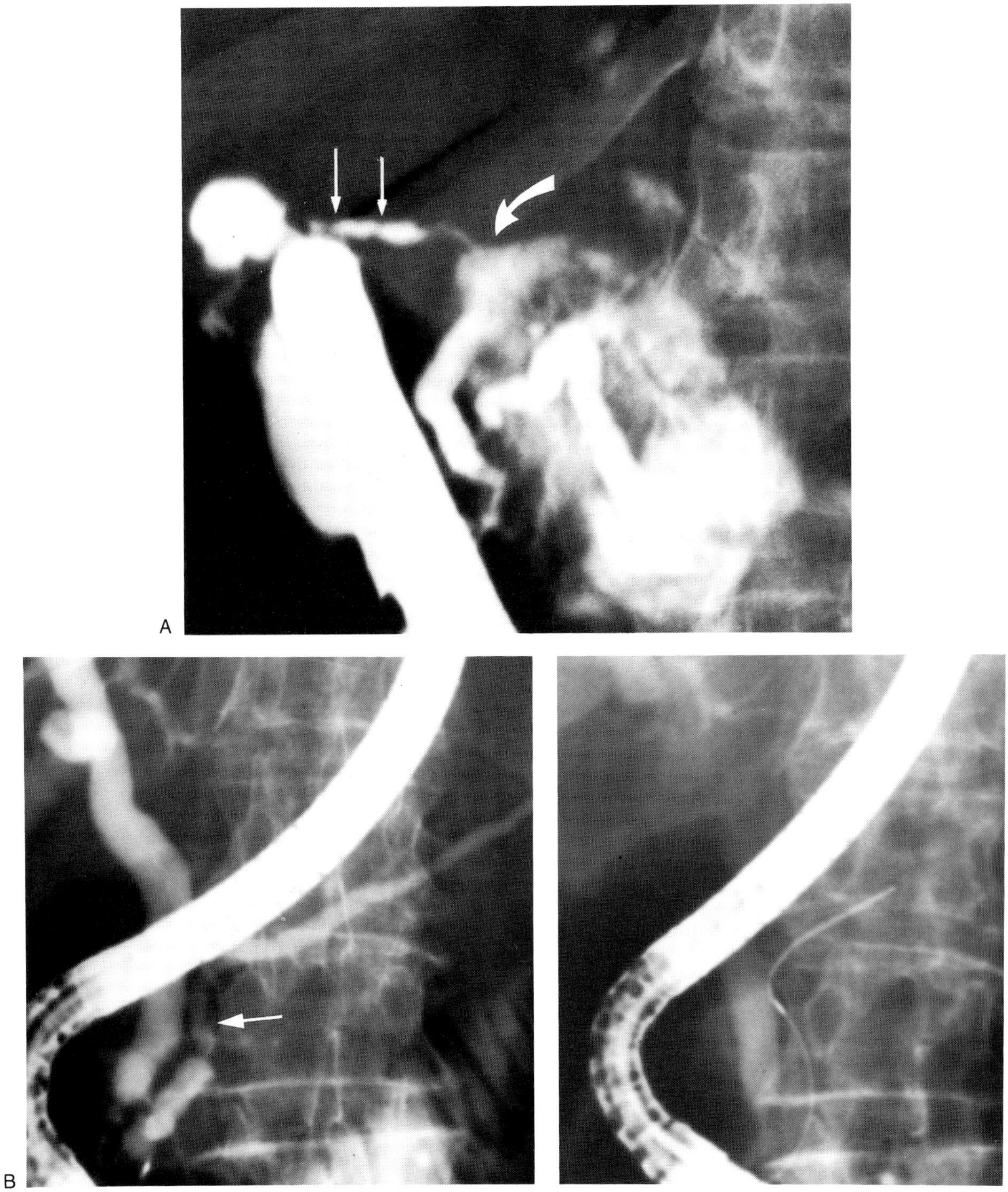

FIG. 9.35. A: An ERCP, consistent with carcinoma of the pancreas, showing a cutoff of the pancreatic duct. Extravasation of contrast into the parenchyma of the head of the gland is noted. Filling of the biliary tree is limited to the distal bile duct, which is also cutoff (*large arrow*). Filling of a contracted gallbladder and scirrhous changes of the cystic duct suggest tumor involvement of the cystic duct (*small arrows*). **B: Left:** A stricture in the pancreatic duct just proximal to the ampulla (*arrow*). **Right:** A cytology brush is advanced through the stricture to obtain tissue.

and decompression should be initiated by placement of either a percutaneous or endoscopic prosthesis (182). This can be accomplished in only 1 to 2 days, which is a positive factor for hospital costs.

The most critical decision in evaluating and treating a patient with a pancreatic neoplasm is staging the lesion for resectability (183). It has been my experience and that of others that angiography and CT are not reliable for staging patients with pancreatic lesions. Until recently, however, these were the only tests utilized. Two procedures, laparoscopy and EUS, are proving to be more sensitive and definitive, in my opin-

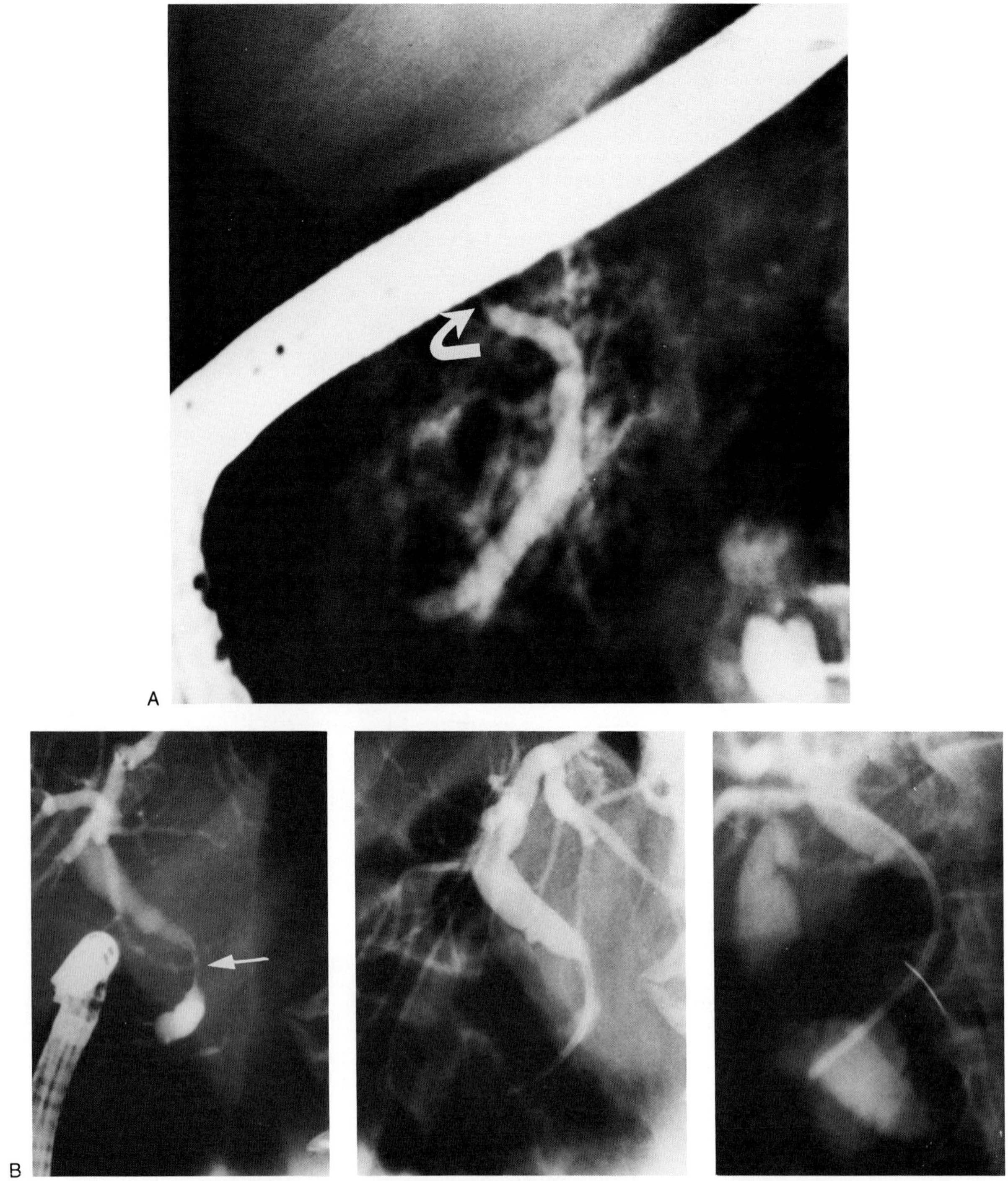

FIG. 9.36. A: Partial filling of the pancreatic duct with a tight stricture (*arrow*). Extravasation of contrast material into the tumor is appreciated. **B: Left:** A "double duct" with a prominent stricture of the bile duct (*arrow*). **Middle:** A stent has been placed into the bile duct. **Right:** With the patient supine and the fluoroscope used for guidance, a needle is placed into the area of stricture for aspiration biopsy.

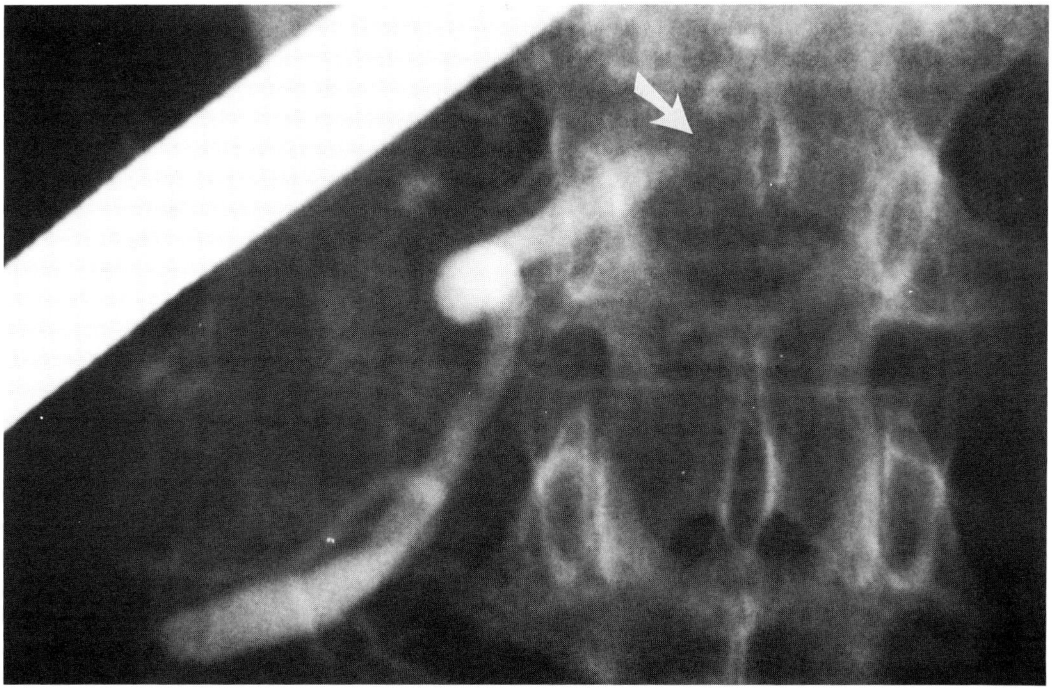

FIG. 9.37. Retrograde filling of the pancreatic duct with a high-grade stricture at the body and tail (*arrow*). Note filling of the side branches of the duct system in the head of the gland, confirming obstruction proximally.

ion, but are underutilized because of lack of availability (184–188). At laparoscopy, metastatic nodules of the liver, peritoneum, or mesentery can be identified and selectively biopsied, providing tissue for analysis. Laparoscopy is comparable to laparotomy in staging disease without invading the abdomen. Recovery from laparoscopy is rapid, and the patient usually returns to normal activity in 24 hours. If metastatic disease is

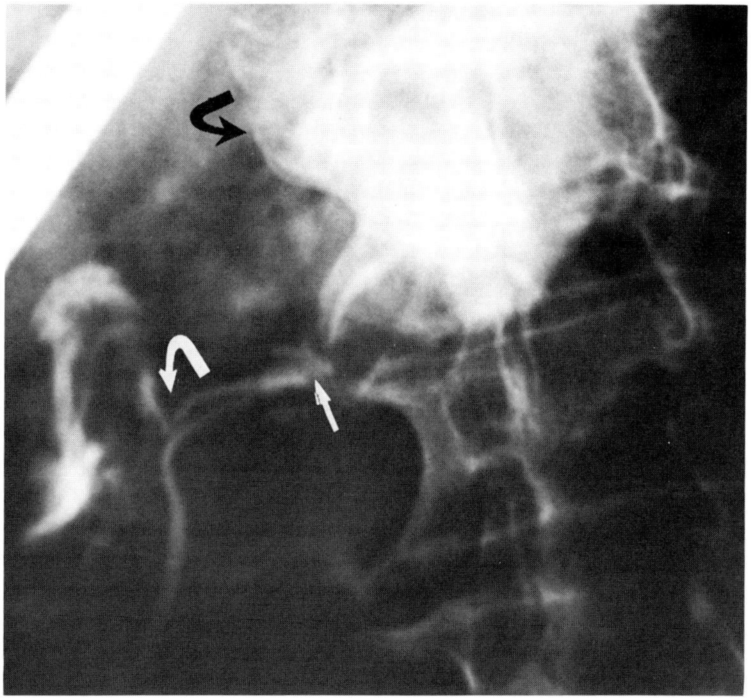

A

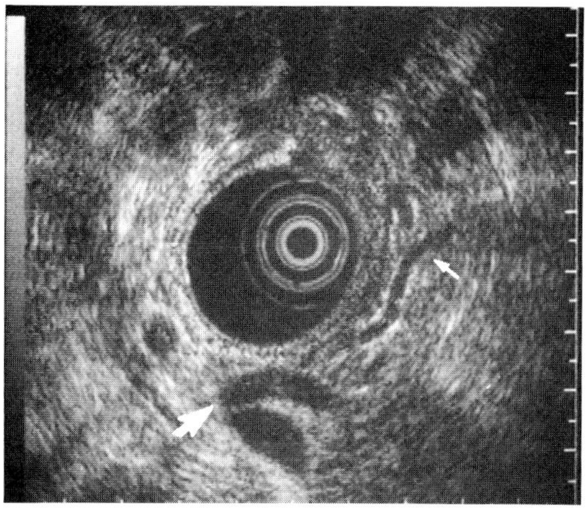

B

FIG. 9.38. A: Retrograde filling of the pancreatic duct. No dilatation of the distal duct is observed (*straight arrow*) at the junction of the accessory duct. Filling of the accessory duct is seen, with contrast entering the duodenum (*curved white arrow*). Filling of a cystic structure is seen over the spine (*black arrow*). An endoscopic ultrasound was performed and was consistent with inflammatory disease but not a tumor. As discussed in the text, distinguishing neoplasia from pancreatitis is difficult not only by pancreatography but also at laparotomy. **B:** An endoscopic ultrasound examination of the patient showing a fibrotic, dilated pancreatic duct in the tail (*small arrow*) and a normal splenic artery and vein (*large arrow*). (Courtesy of Dr. Harry Snady).

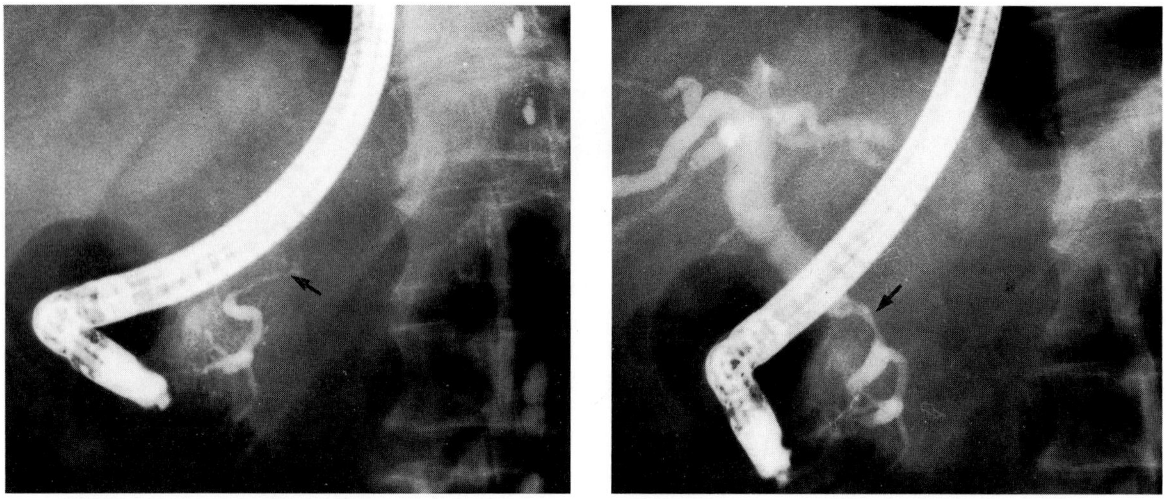

FIG. 9.39. Left: Filling of the pancreatic duct is presented and demonstrates a cutoff at the genu. Note filling of the secondary radicals and the parenchyma owing to increased volume and pressure of injection resulting from the stricture. No filling of secondary radicals is noted near the stricture (*arrow*), which is suggestive of a tumor. **Right:** A cholangiogram taken from the same patient that shows a corresponding stricture of the distal common duct (*arrow*), which is consistent with a tumor.

found, thus ruling out resection, and if biliary decompression has been provided, no further therapy is necessary. The patient can return home more quickly to spend valuable time with his or her family.

Percutaneous biopsies by either CT or ultrasound guidance are also very helpful and safe (189,190). The results are dependable in experienced hands, and confirmation of histology is provided in nearly 70% of patients, again obviating the need for surgery. Morbidity associated with percutaneous biopsy techniques is low, and mortality is nil. This underutilized technique should be more actively promoted.

The most confirmatory examination currently available for staging of pancreatic or biliary cancer is certainly endoscopic ultrasound. Dr. Harry Snady, a colleague with whom I have worked closely in evaluating and staging patients with pancreatic carcinoma, has supplied the figures used in this section to illustrate

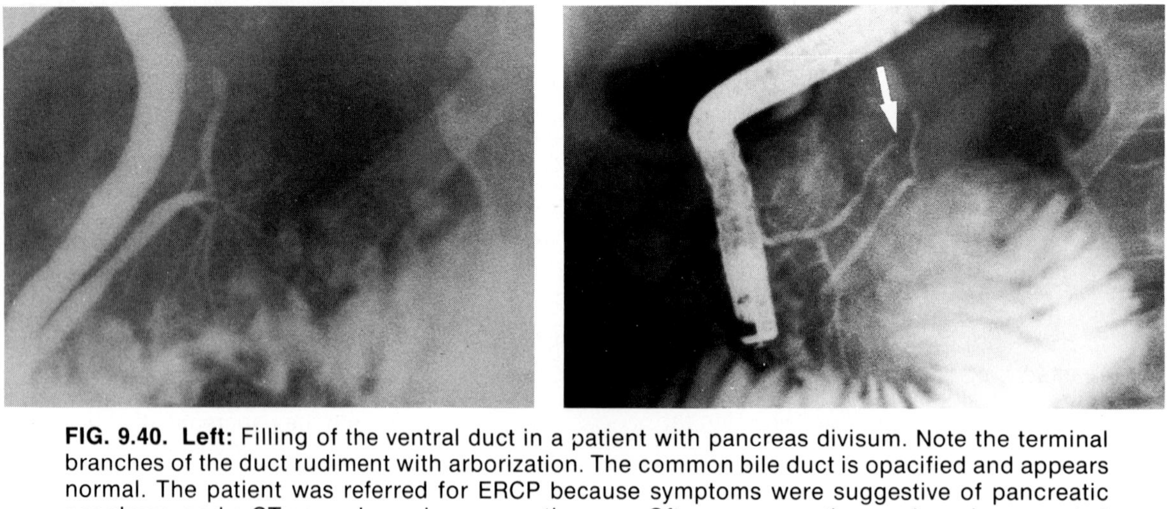

FIG. 9.40. Left: Filling of the ventral duct in a patient with pancreas divisum. Note the terminal branches of the duct rudiment with arborization. The common bile duct is opacified and appears normal. The patient was referred for ERCP because symptoms were suggestive of pancreatic neoplasm, and a CT scan showed a pancreatic mass. Often a pancreatic neoplasm is suspected in patients presenting with vague symptoms. The index of suspicion increases when the pancreatogram demonstrates a stricture of the pancreatic duct. The experienced endoscopist and radiologist direct their attention to ductular branching, which is consistent with pancreas divisum, to avoid a false-positive diagnosis of cancer. It is imperative to attempt cannulation of the minor papilla and to opacify the dorsal duct to determine pancreas divisum and rule out tumor. **Right:** On cannulation of the dorsal duct through the minor papilla, a cutoff of this duct is seen (*arrow*), consistent with a pancreatic neoplasm. Note the absence of filling of the secondary radicals. At surgery, cancer was confirmed.

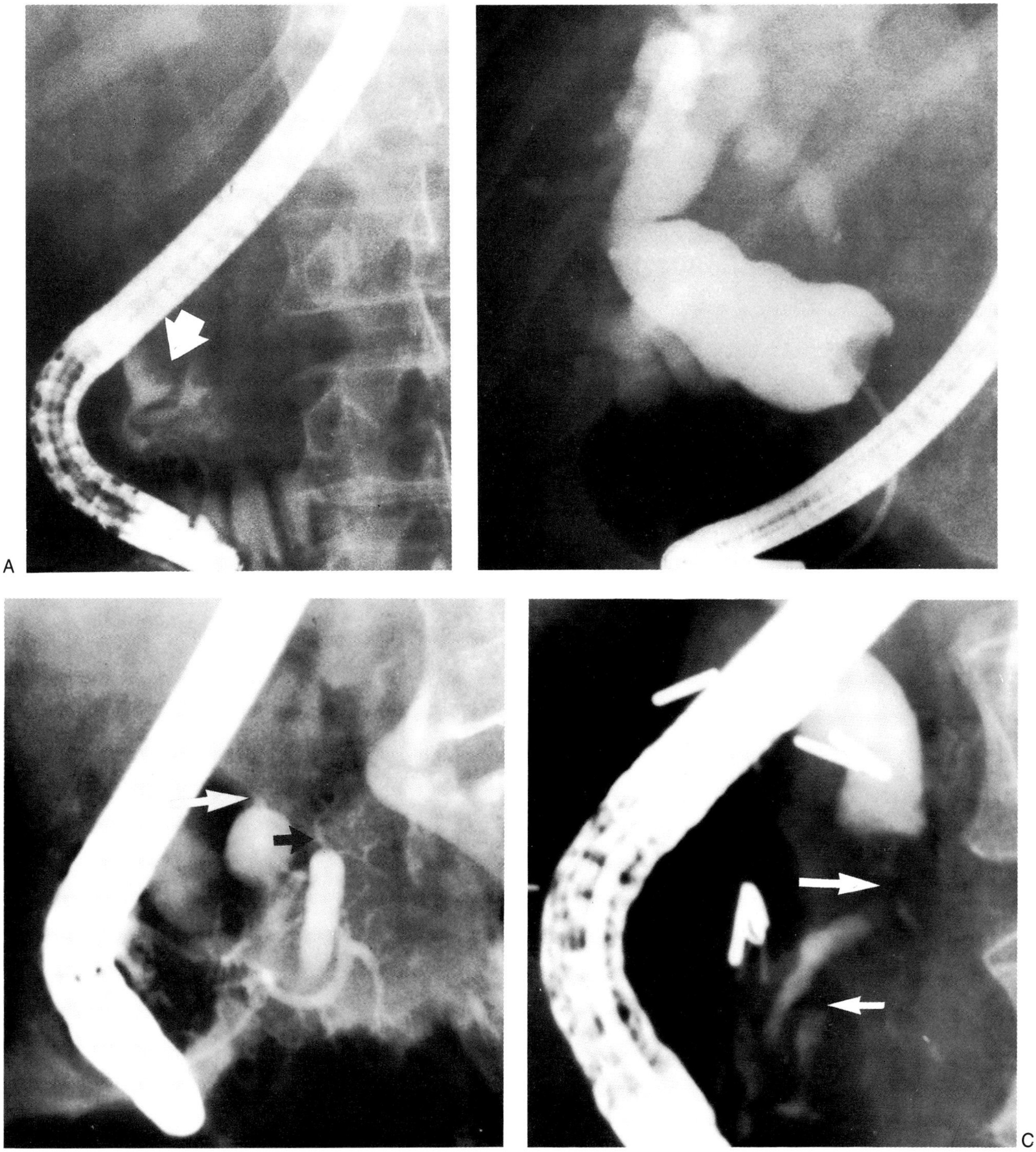

FIG. 9.41. A: Left: An ERCP showing the classic double duct sign. Both the pancreatic duct and the bile duct are interrupted by a tumor (*arrow*). **Right:** The biliary tree is opacified using a catheter-guidewire system, confirming a high-grade obstruction and dilatation of the proximal ducts. **B, C:** The double duct sign. The large arrow in each radiograph identifies the stricture of the bile duct, and the small arrow the corresponding stricture of the pancreatic duct.

the sensitivity of this new modality. EUS offers the primary physician a less invasive but accurate staging tool, and its further development and availability will provide information previously supplied only by surgery.

We can now utilize modalities that provide accurate assessment, staging, and tissue without subjecting the patient to "exploratory" laparotomy. *No one need ever suggest that exploratory surgery be performed to prove a diagnosis of malignancy of the bile duct or*

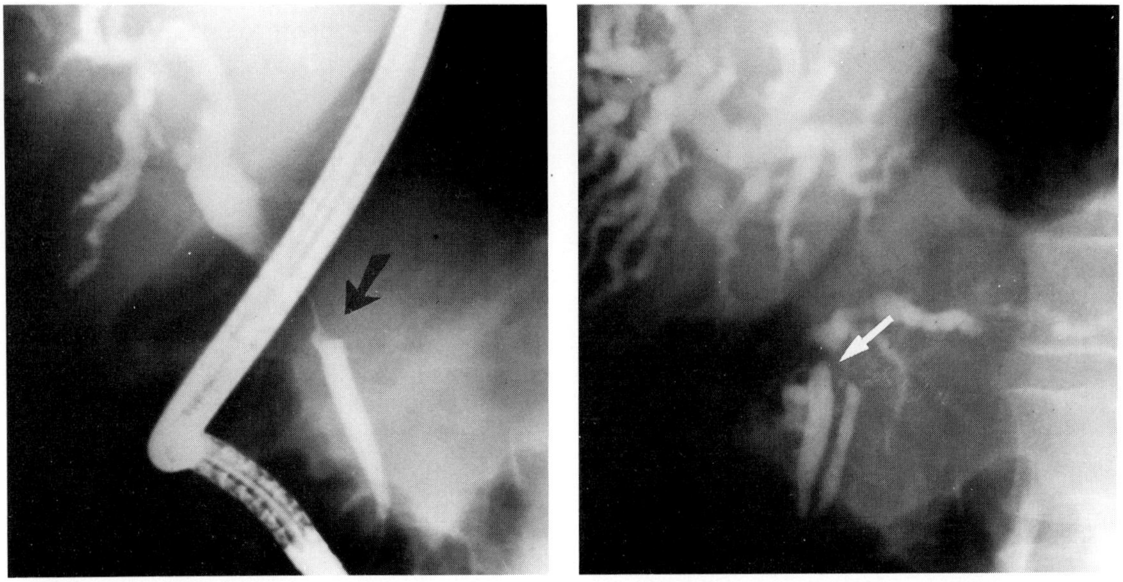

FIG. 9.42. Left: A cholangiogram obtained at ERCP that shows a high-grade stricture of the lower common bile duct and poststricture dilatation. Note the masslike effect, producing an overhanging margin (*arrow*) and tight stricture. **Right:** Opacification of the pancreas demonstrating a corresponding stricture, double duct (*arrows*), and postobstruction dilatation of the pancreatic duct.

pancreas or to provide tissue when laparoscopy, endoscopic ultrasound, and endoscopic and percutaneous biopsies are available.

In general, histologic proof of a malignant lesion of the pancreas is rarely provided at laparotomy if there is no obvious metastatic disease. Most surgeons do not attempt direct biopsies of a pancreatic mass, so the positive yield at laparotomy is less than 25%. This yield rises to about 80% *if there are metastatic nodules* (175). The latter results, then, help to explain why laparoscopy is just as effective as laparotomy. If laparoscopy is negative for metastatic disease, percutaneous biopsies should be attempted before considering laparotomy. Because the prognosis for pancreatic car-

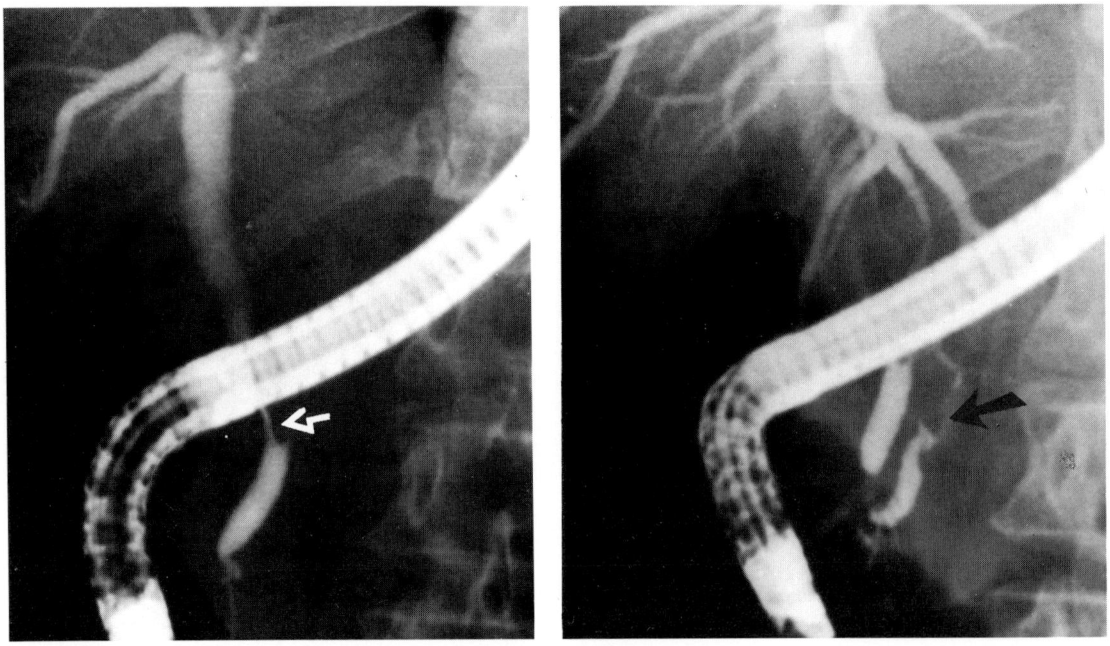

FIG. 9.43. Left: A cholangiogram showing a high-grade stricture (*arrow*) in the lower common bile duct and dilatation of the proximal bile duct. **Right:** Completion of the ERCP and selective cannulation of the pancreatic duct. Note the high-grade stricture and narrowing of the duct corresponding to the stricture of the bile duct (*arrow*).

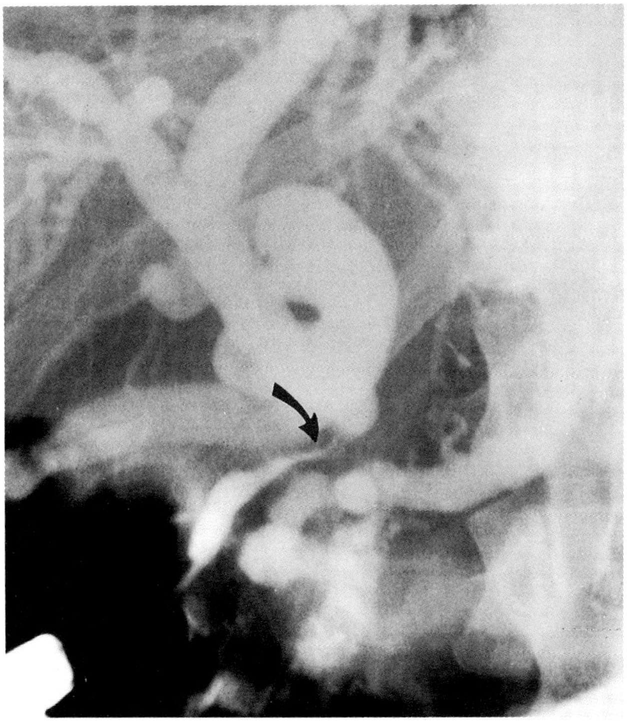

FIG. 9.44. A dilated, tortuous pancreatic duct. Diffuse changes are present. A high-grade stricture of the bile duct also is seen (*arrow*). These findings are compatible with neoplasia at surgical resection. This proved to be inflammatory at surgical exploration.

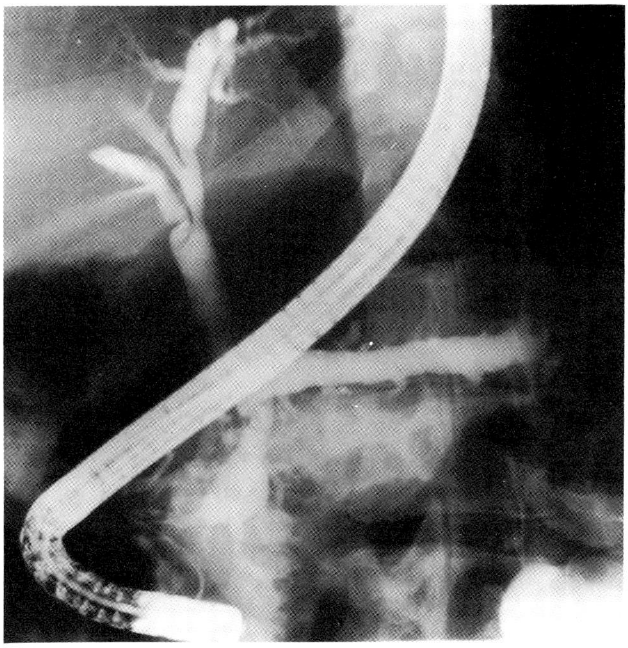

FIG. 9.45. This is an ERCP demonstrating a dilated, tortuous pancreatic duct in a patient with chronic pancreatitis. Note the dilatation of the secondary and tertiary radicals, with no absence or loss of radicals of the pancreatic duct. A smooth stricture of the distal common bile duct is present, and dilatation of the duct accompanies the stenosis. No neoplasm was confirmed in this patient.

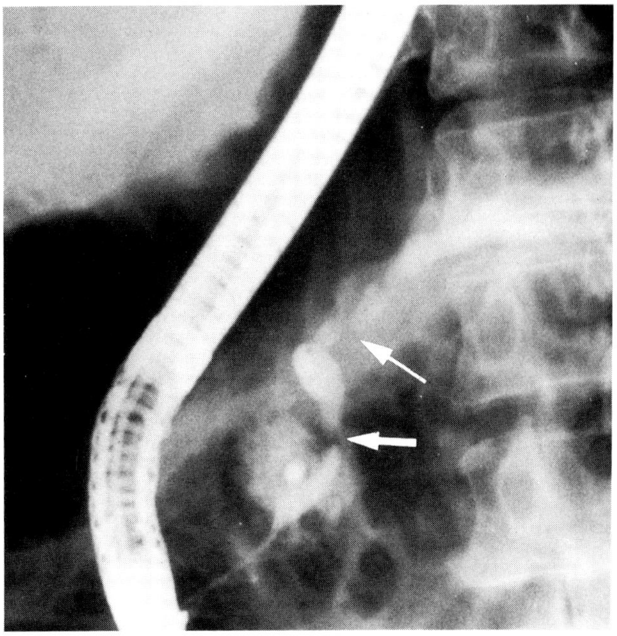

FIG. 9.46. An ERCP demonstrating disruption of the pancreatic duct (*arrows*) with alternating areas of strictures and dilatation in an elderly patient with "senile pancreatitis." This finding has been referred to as a "string of pearls."

cinoma is so poor (191), and because 91% of patients usually benefit from endoscopic or percutaneous decompression techniques (192,193), surgical intervention and bypass are obviated.

Which morphologic changes seen on pancreatography are suggestive of or compatible with carcinoma? First, a stricture, or cutoff (Figs. 9.35–9.41), is suggestive of carcinoma until ruled out by biopsy or surgical

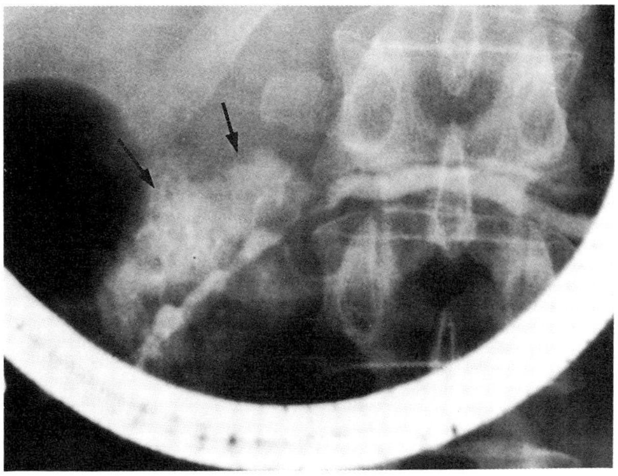

FIG. 9.47. A "string of pearls" sign in the head of the gland in a patient with pancreatitis. Note extravasation of contrast into the parenchyma of the gland (*arrows*). The difference between neoplasia and inflammation is demonstrated in this case as all the secondary radicals are present, which rules out neoplasia in most cases.

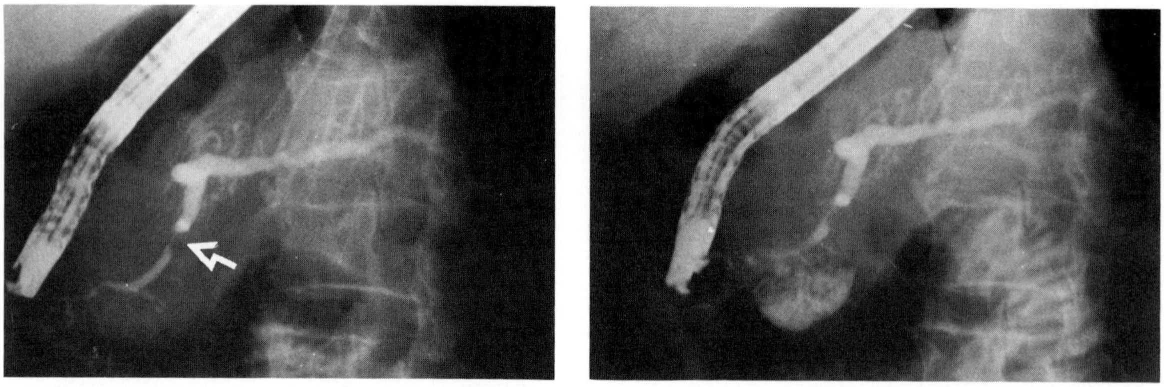

FIG. 9.48. Left: Filling of the pancreatic duct with dilatation of the gland. A stricture (*arrow*) is noted in the head of the gland where there is an absence of secondary branches. **Right:** This ERCP shows disruption of the pancreatic duct and filling of the parenchyma consistent with tumor. Note that some secondary branches are absent in the affected area, despite overfilling of the duct.

excision. In most cases, the main pancreatic duct is affected by a high-grade stricture, and proximal (the sphincter being distal) dilatation of the duct is often found if contrast can be injected beyond the stricture (Figs. 9.42, 9.43).

It is usually difficult to differentiate cancer from chronic pancreatitis because the pancreatograms are very similar (194–198) (Figs. 9.44–9.47). Filling of the side branches during pancreatography is considered a differentiating point; that is, the side branches usually are ectatic (dilated) in chronic pancreatitis. In cancer, however, these side branches may be absent or less obvious, having been destroyed by the cancer (Figs. 9.48, 9.49). This finding is illustrated in Fig. 9.49, in which the duct appears scirrhous and thin rather than dilated, but the side branches are affected. Of course, this rule doesn't always apply because the morphology of the dilated pancreatic duct proximal to a malignant stricture appears similar to that found in chronic pancreatitis (i.e, ectatic secondary branches). This finding, destroyed side branches, can be relied on with a high degree of certainty if the cannula was inserted deeply into the duct and a large volume of contrast material was injected to eliminate false-positive conclusions from inadequate injection volume. Another important finding on the pancreatogram, which is path-

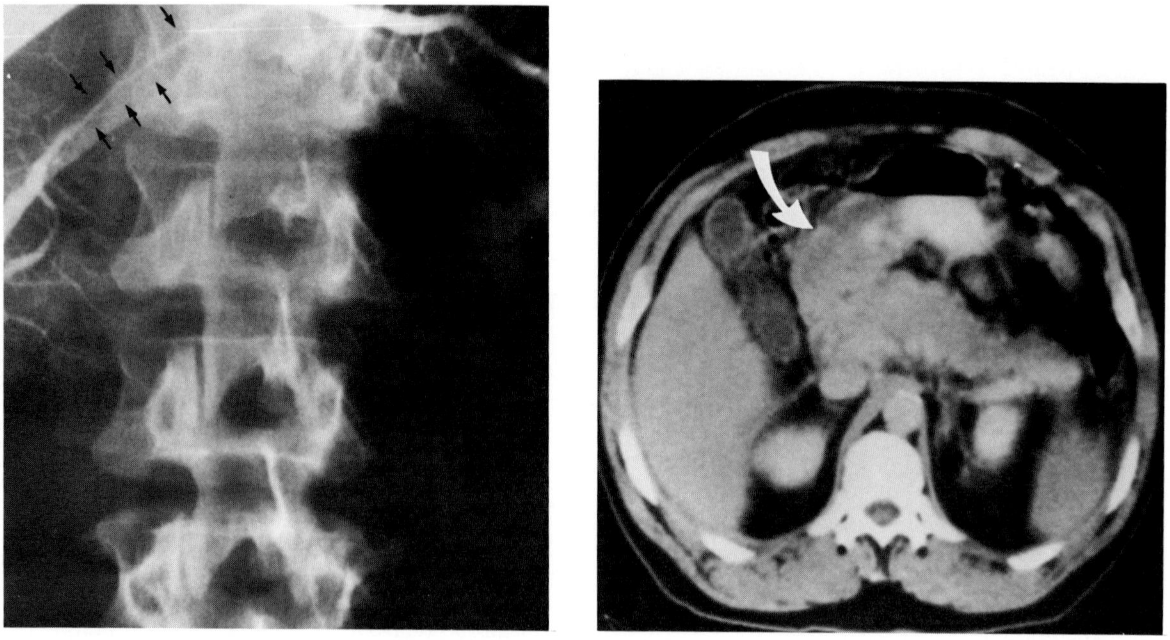

FIG. 9.49. Left: Filling of the pancreatic duct and most of the secondary branches, except in the section outlined by arrows. **Right:** A CT scan of the same patient shows a mass in the head of the pancreas (*arrow*) corresponding to the section in which the side branches are absent.

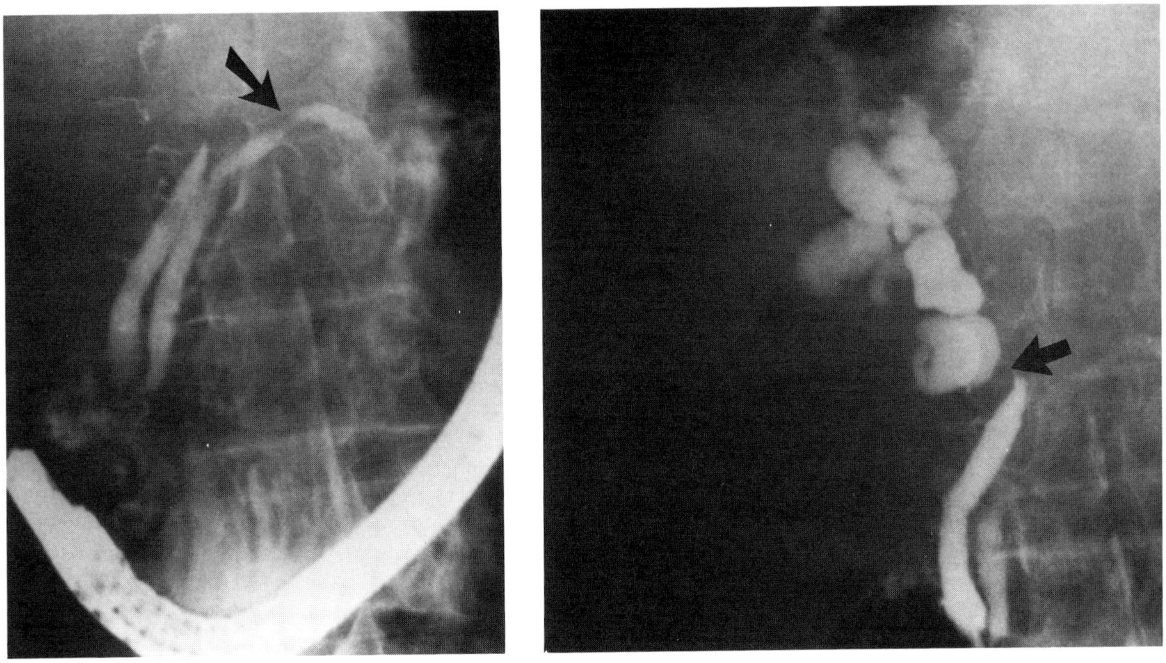

FIG. 9.50. Left: An ERCP consistent with carcinoma showing a high-grade stricture of the bile duct. Even though the pancreatic duct appears uninvolved, a stricture of the proximal pancreatic duct is apparent (*arrow*) and dilatation of the duct is seen proximal to that stricture. **Right:** Dilatation of the bile duct proximal to the stricture (*arrow*). Filling of the proximal duct was accomplished after advancing a catheter-guidewire assembly through the stricture.

ognomonic for carcinoma, is disruption of the duct and extravasation of contrast, especially in an area where side branches are absent. Figure 9.50 demonstrates a dilated pancreatic duct, ectatic secondary branches, and an abrupt cutoff of the main duct as well as absence of secondary branches. This pancreatogram was obtained in a patient who had previously undergone a subtotal gastrectomy.

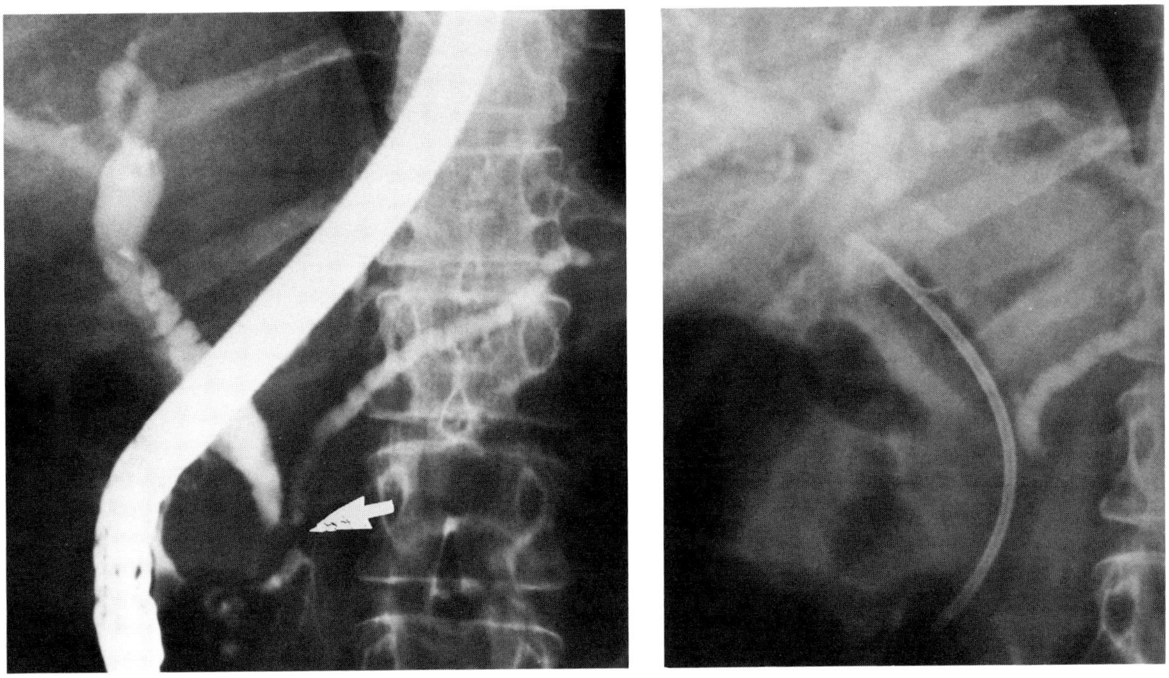

FIG. 9.51. Left: A small lesion of the pancreatic duct and a corresponding stricture of the bile duct (*arrow*). Despite the absence of a mass on CT scan, this lesion produced profound cholestasis and was unresectable. **Right:** A radiograph showing the presence of a stent in the bile duct. Note air in the biliary tree following placement of a large-caliber prosthesis.

Subtle changes on the pancreatogram must be carefully studied after appropriate films are taken, especially in patients presenting with a history compatible with cancer. Often, the clinical presentation of anorexia, weight loss, and jaundice, which are nonspecific but still consistent with an occult neoplasm, necessitate the performance of an ERCP. To further confuse the less experienced clinician, the CT scan and sonogram may not demonstrate a pancreatic mass, yet dilated intrahepatic ducts are usually present (199–204). Whether the ducts are dilated or not, an ERCP should be performed when the clinical presentation supports the indications (Fig. 9.51). Findings at ERCP are often consistent with carcinoma of the pancreas: Even if no mass is seen on a CT scan, at surgery, a lesion may be found and may be unresectable. This is another example of the frustration and futility in evaluating and treating patients with carcinoma of the pancreas. EUS has already begun to enlighten clinicians and has been helpful in selecting patients who appear resectable (fewer than 10%) (191). It is becoming more evident that CT scans are not as reliable as EUS in staging pancreatic neoplasms.

ERCP findings are not always clearly diagnostic and may require other complimentary studies and/or surgery for confirmation. Such a diagnostic problem is shown in Fig. 9.52. The radiograph on the left shows a high-grade stricture affecting the bile duct, producing proximal dilataiion of the biliary tree. The pancreatogram demonstrated irregularity of the pancreatic duct, and extravasation of contrast into the parenchyma was noted. There was no filling of the secondary branches of the pancreas. Although these findings were consistent with a neoplasm, this diganosis was not completely supported by EUS. The endoscopic ultrasound confirmed a hypoechoic mass extending up the bile duct, and lymph nodes were present near the gallbladder. These findings were suggestive of a tumor; however, of greater significance, the portal vein was uninvolved, and the patient, who was only 45 years old, was explored for resectability (Fig. 9.53). No evidence of cancer was found at surgery. Endoscopic ultrasound is valuable in staging pancreatic and periampullary lesions, providing information not available with other techniques. Hopefully, as experience accumulates with this technique, EUS will be predictive and more sensitive for resectability.

Finally, pancreatography is helpful in defining the anatomy of a suspected cystic mass of the pancreas. Figure 9.54 illustrates a cystic mass containing lucencies that constitute the solid portion of a cystadenocarcinoma (205,206). Figure 9.55 is an endoscopic picture of gelatinous material seen exuding from a duodenal mass found in a patient with a cystadenocarcinoma. Aspiration of the material and cytologic examination are suggested prior to surgery. This lesion

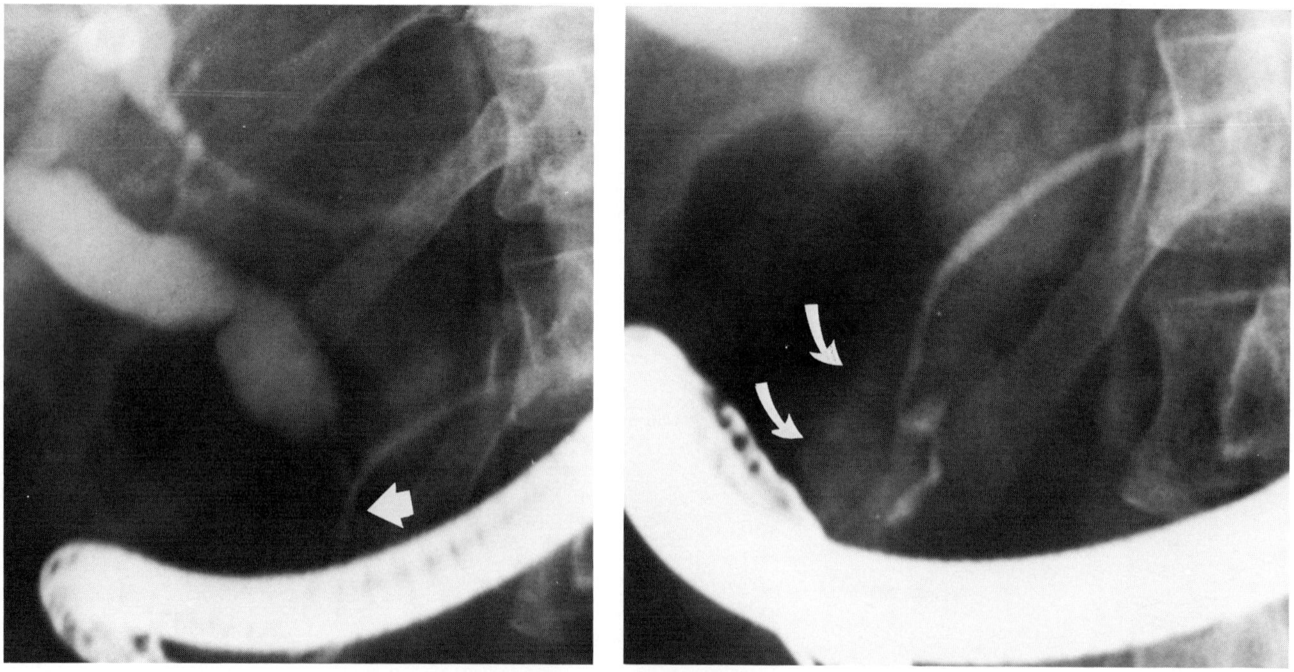

FIG. 9.52. Left: An ERCP that demonstrates a high-grade stricture of the bile duct (*arrow*) and proximal dilatation. A slender pancreatic duct is seen. **Right:** Irregularity of the duct in the head of the gland, with beading. Acinar filling in the head of the gland is noted (*arrows*), but there is no filling of the secondary radicals. The patient underwent endoscopic ultrasound as an aid in defining the lesion (See Fig. 9.53).

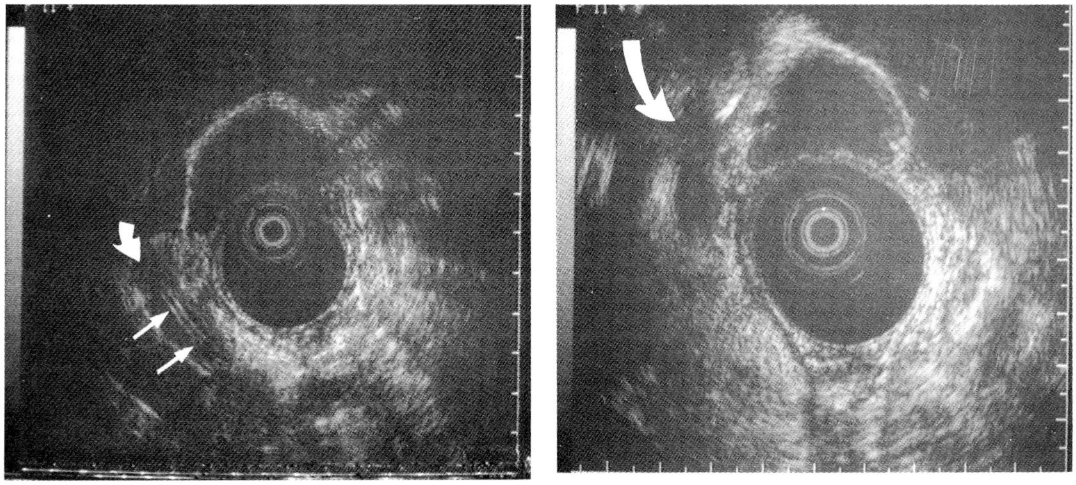

A

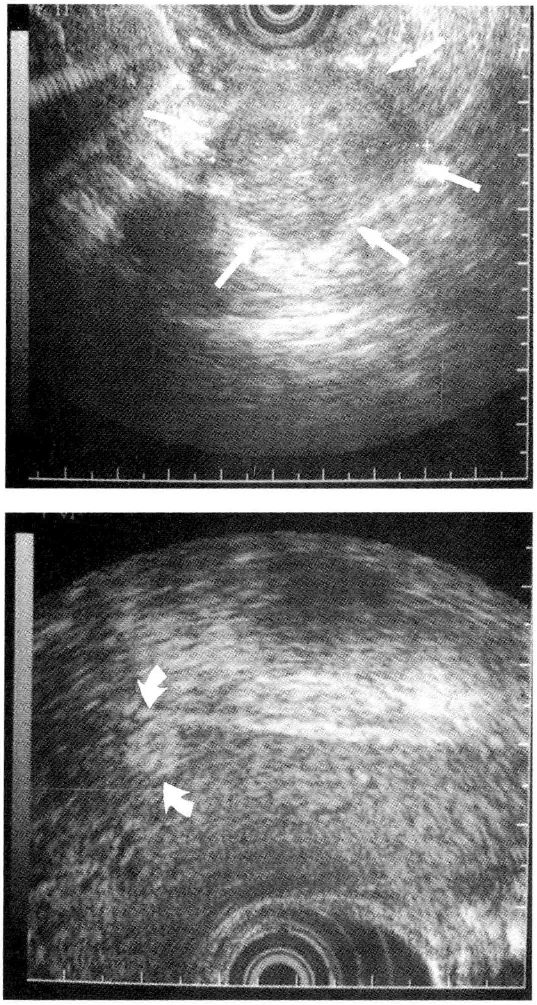

B

FIG. 9.53. A: Left: An endoscopic ultrasound of the patient described in Fig. 9.52. A hypochoic mass extends up the bile duct (*large arrow*), and a stent is in the bile duct (*small arrows*). **Right:** Another view of the endoscopic ultrasound examination of the same patient, showing enlarged lymph nodes (*arrow*). The adjacent structure is the gallbladder. **B: Top:** An endoscopic ultrasound showing a large (4.2 cm) mixed echoic mass (*large arrows*) in the uncinate process of the pancreas. The mass is consistent with a carcinoma. **Bottom:** A 7 mm hyperechoic nodule (*arrows*) in the left lobe of the liver, consistent with a metastatic nodule. These figures were supplied by Dr. Harry Snady, who reports this occurrence as the first metastatic nodule he has found in the left lobe.

is slow growing, so a complete resection is usually possible. The prognosis is therefore far better than that for adenocarcinoma.

Ancillary information gathered during the workup of patients is helpful in determining the diagnosis of cancer of the pancreas. The patient's presentation, symptoms, and history of initial onset (usually heralded by a flulike syndrome several weeks or months before clinical presentation, followed by anorexia, weight loss, back pain, epigastric discomfort associated with meals, and possible diabetes) are supportive evidence when cancer is suspected.

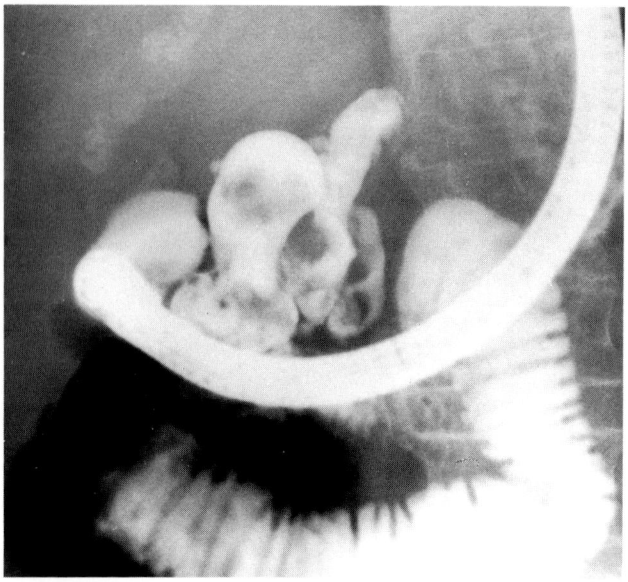

FIG. 9.54. A classic example of a cystadenocarcinoma in a patient in whom a mass was noted on CT scan. Note the lucencies in the cystic structure, representing the solid component of the tumor.

Other tests that corroborate the initial impression of cancer of the pancreas include the findings obtained by sonography and CT scan and endoscopic findings (compression of the posterior wall of the stomach, rigidity of the gastric antrum, stenosis of the pylorous, rigidity of the first and second portions of the duodenum with friability, incomplete distensibility, ulcerations, and occasionally invasion of the duodenal mucosa with submucosal edema and masslike findings). Occasionally, tumor erosion into the duodenum and an exophytic lesion are appreciated endoscopically (Fig. 9.55).

Contrast radiographs (barium ingestion) are rarely needed in the evaluation of patients with a suspicion of carcinoma of the pancreas because the barium remains in the gastrointestinal tract too long and obscures other examinations. An upper gastrointestinal series is helpful only when gastric outlet obstruction is suspected, but an endoscopic examination and a good physical examination demonstrating a succussion splash will confirm obstruction without the patient having to ingest barium.

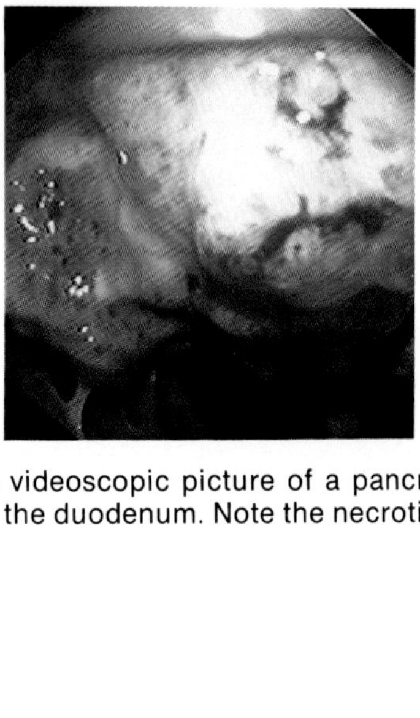

FIG. 9.55. A videoscopic picture of a pancreatic tumor eroding into the duodenum. Note the necrotic tissue and mass effect.

The algorithm alluded to (Table 9.4) differentiates between nonsurgical and surgical treatment of malignant obstruction. As shown, nonsurgical treatment is suggested for benign obstruction, for pancreatic tumors greater than stage 1 (from the American Joint Committee on Cancer *Manual for Staging of Cancer*), for patients over 70 years of age, and for patients whose life expectancy is estimated to be less than 3 years. It is also suggested if the malignancy is deemed incurable. Surgery is suggested for a pancreatic mass less than stage 1 (which is an assumption that such a lesion is resectable) or greater than stage 1 with definite gastric outlet obstruction. If biliary obstruction is present, whether benign or malignant, surgery is recommended if the obstruction could *not* be decompressed by other nonsurgical means. Adherence to these guidelines is cost effective, because more than 90% of patients presenting with pancreatic neoplasms can and should be treated nonsurgically. In previous publications we estimated that annual savings to the health care delivery system in the United States could approach 519,376 days of hospitalization when nonsurgical techniques, especially endoscopic, are employed in the evaluation and treatment of pancreatic neoplasms (207).

Interestingly, a prospective, randomized study from the United Kingdom indirectly confirmed our estimates of cost savings, supporting our conclusion that endoscopic decompression offers a distinct economic advantage over percutaneous decompression techniques, both of which were found to be superior to surgical decompression, especially when the results of all modalities were compared in patients with a poor prognosis and short survival (208). If patients survived more than 6 months, the economic benefits were dissipated because the stented patients were required to return to hospital for stent exchange. But there was a distinct advantage of endoscopy over surgery both in cost effectiveness and in functional status of short-term survivors. Because of the requirements of stent exchange in long-term survivors, repeat hospitalization was necessary, eroding the economic advantages. We have amended our recommendations for surgical intervention in the management of obstructive jaundice, especially carcinoma of the pancreas, because of the results of a study by Neff et al. (209), which evaluated and assessed the combined disciplines of percutaneous decompression and surgical bypass. These newer recommendations are reiterated in Chapter 12.

In summary, in 1991, *carcinoma of the pancreas is not considered a surgical disease*. If nonsurgical in-

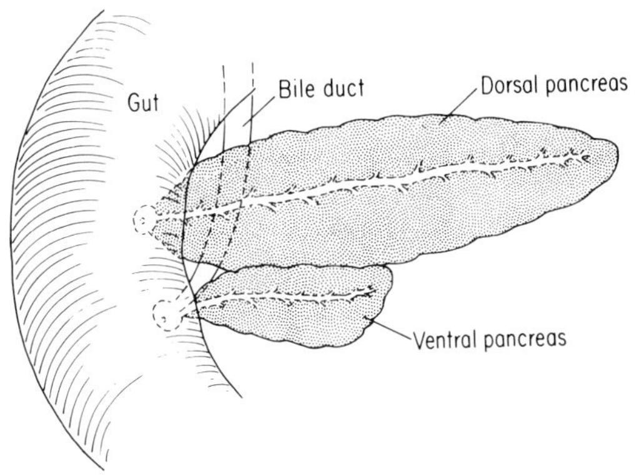

FIG. 9.56. The pancreas in the seventh and eighth weeks of gestation. Note the separate ventral and dorsal systems.

tervention is unsuccessful or unavailable or if gastric outlet obstruction coexists, surgical palliation is recommended as an alternative because resection and extirpation of the tumor usually is not possible.

CONGENITAL VARIANTS AND PANCREATITIS

The most common congenital variant of the pancreas is certainly pancreas divisum (210–215). Pancreas divisum has been reported to occur in 5% to 10% of the population. In our treatment experience, this variant occurs predominantly in women, most commonly in the second to fourth decades of life. If our series of 65 patients, the age range was 17 to 70 years, with a mean age of 35. The variation occurs when the pancreatic buds fail to fuse during the seventh to eighth weeks of gestation, resulting in separate ventral pancreatic duct and dorsal pancreatic duct systems (Fig. 9.56). In this situation, the majority of secretions drain through the minor papilla because the dorsal duct functions as the major duct and empties through this structure. The ventral pancreatic duct, on pancreatography, appears as a rudiment of the duct and can be easily confused as a stricture. Branching of this duct is commonly found, and this distinguishing feature differentiates between the congenital variant and neoplasia (Figs. 9.57–9.64). In the early experience of ERCP, the finding of an abrupt termination of the ventral pancreatic duct seen on pancreatography (which was correctly identified as Wirsung's duct) was falsely interpreted to be compatible with carcinoma, especially when the CT scan demonstrated enlargement of the head of the pancreas (216), until we began to recognize and appreciate the congenital variation of pancreas divisum. The distinguishing characteristic of pancreas divisum, which is appreciated when filling the ventral duct, is the presence of side branches or arborization of the rudimentary ventral duct. However, pancreas divisum is confirmed definitively only after cannulating the minor papilla and opacifying the dorsal duct. The reader is

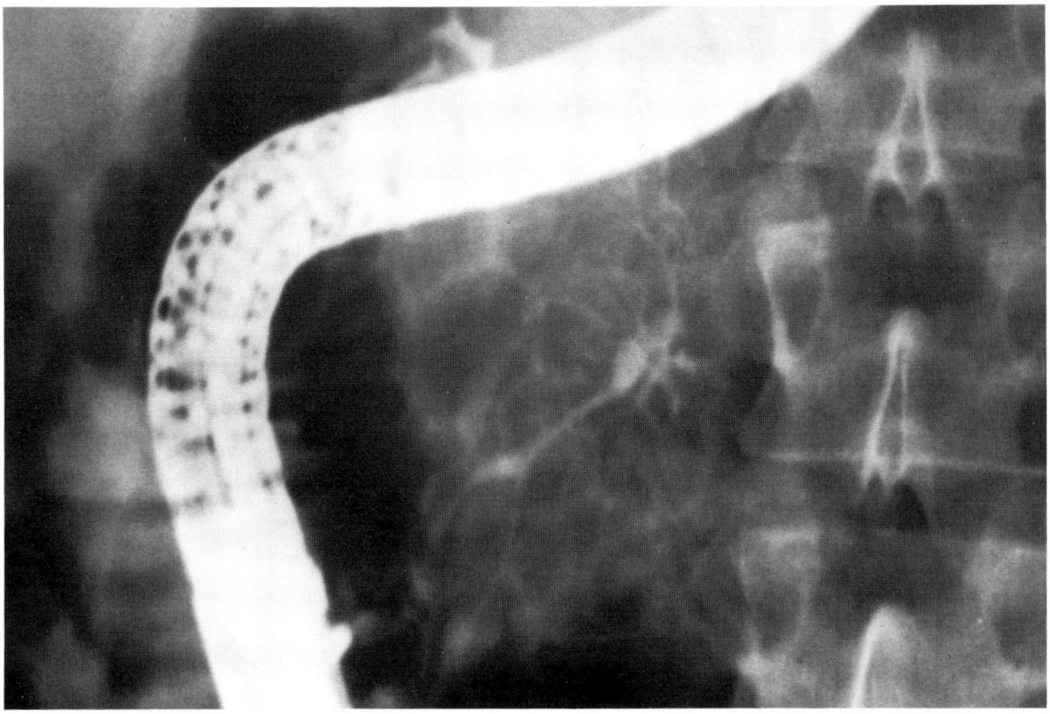

FIG. 9.57. The rudimentary ventral pancreatic duct with branching of the terminal portion. Rigidity of this duct with dilatation of the proximal portion suggests pancreatitis of this structure.

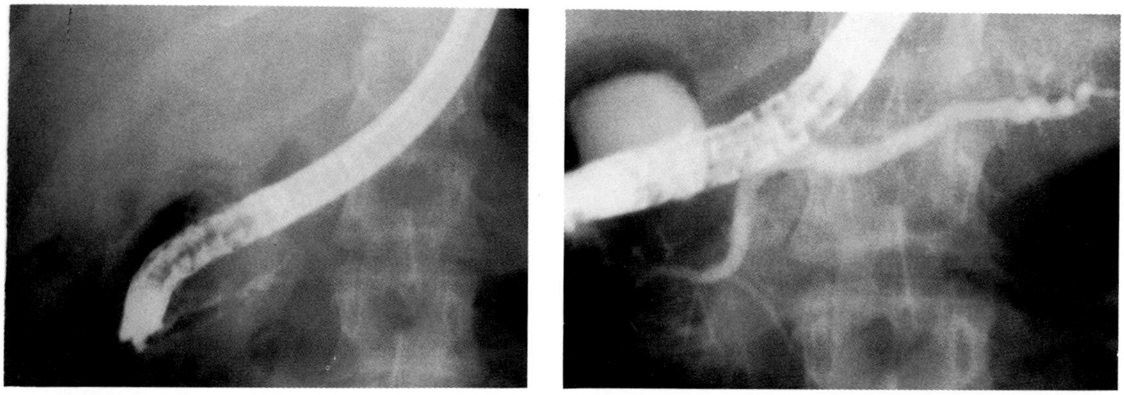

FIG. 9.58. Left: Opacification of the ventral, rudimentary pancreatic duct. **Right:** Opacification of the dorsal pancreatic duct showing dilatation of the duct and evidence of pancreatitis with a tortuous segment in the tail and dilated secondary branches.

advised to review radiographs that are illustrative for pancreas divisum, especially those characteristic findings seen on opacifying the ventral duct. As indicated earlier in this chapter, cancer involving the pancreatic ducts usually destroys side branches, whereas in pancreas divisum, the side branches are present. This should alert the endoscopist that cannulation of the minor papilla and opacification of the dorsal duct are necessary for the diagnosis. Figures 9.57 through 9.64 are examples of the appearance of the ventral, rudimentary duct and the separate dorsal duct, which is opacified through the minor papilla.

The etiology of pain experienced by some people with pancreas divisum is attributed to the incapacity of the minor papilla and its sphincter to accommodate the pancreatic juices flowing at maximum stimulation (210,217–220). Therefore, most patients report an exacerbation of symptoms occuring either with meals or shortly after a meal corresponding to the maximum secretory flow. Why the symptoms of pancreatitis occur unpredictably and at any time in a person with this variation remains unclear. Interestingly, many patients report an association of symptoms with the ingestion of alcohol. However, alcoholic pancreatitis

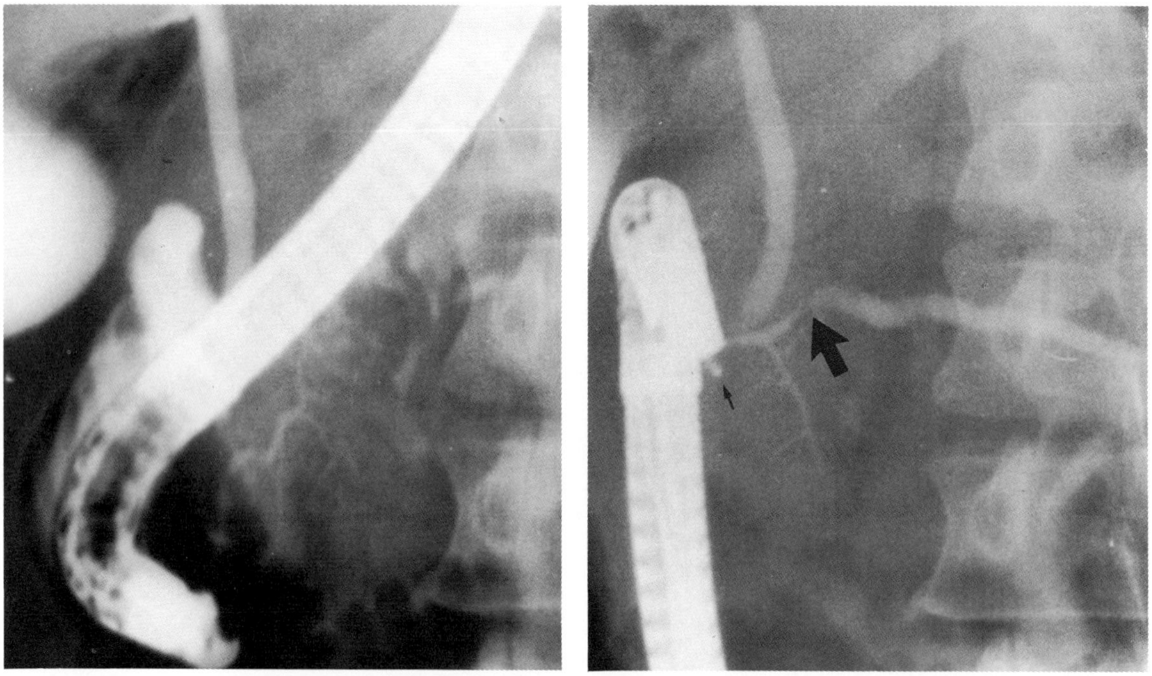

FIG. 9.59. Left: A ventral, rudimentary pancreatic duct, which shows branching of the secondary radicals. **Right:** The cannulation technique for opacifying the dorsal pancreatic duct using a needle-tip catheter (*small arrow*). Note the stricture (*large arrow*) and the dilated proximal segment of the dorsal duct.

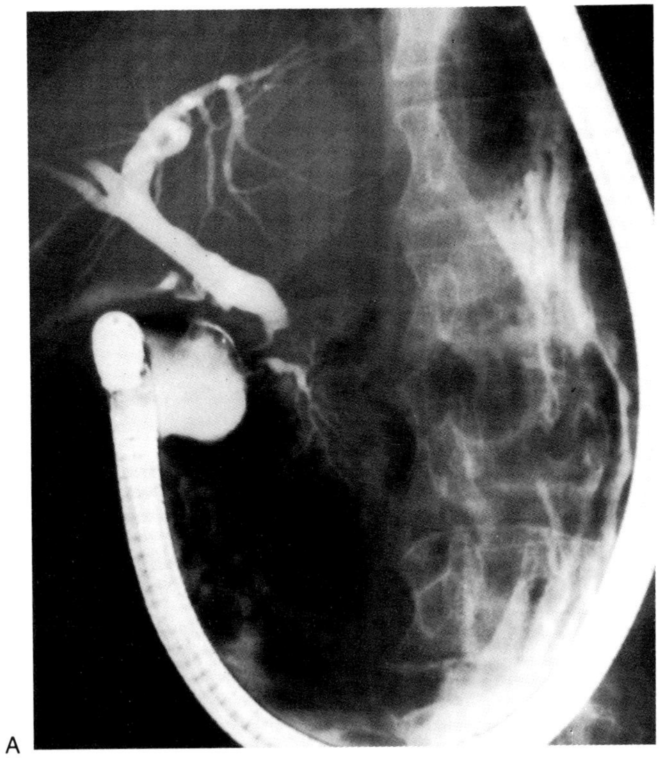

FIG. 9.60. A: A pancreatogram showing opacification of the ventral pancreatic duct and branching of the duct, which clearly rules out a possible neoplasm. There is narrowing of the distal common bile duct and dilatation of the biliary tree present. Abnormalities of the bile duct are not uncommon in patients with pancreatitis and pancreas divisum because inflammatory disease produces encasement of the bile duct with stenosis, just as with pancreatitis in patients with the usual or normal anatomy. **B: Left:** A deformity of the distal common bile duct (*arrow*). **Right:** After opacification of the dorsal duct of pancreas divisum, the bile duct deformity is seen to correspond to a loop of the dorsal duct of pancreas divisum (*arrow*).

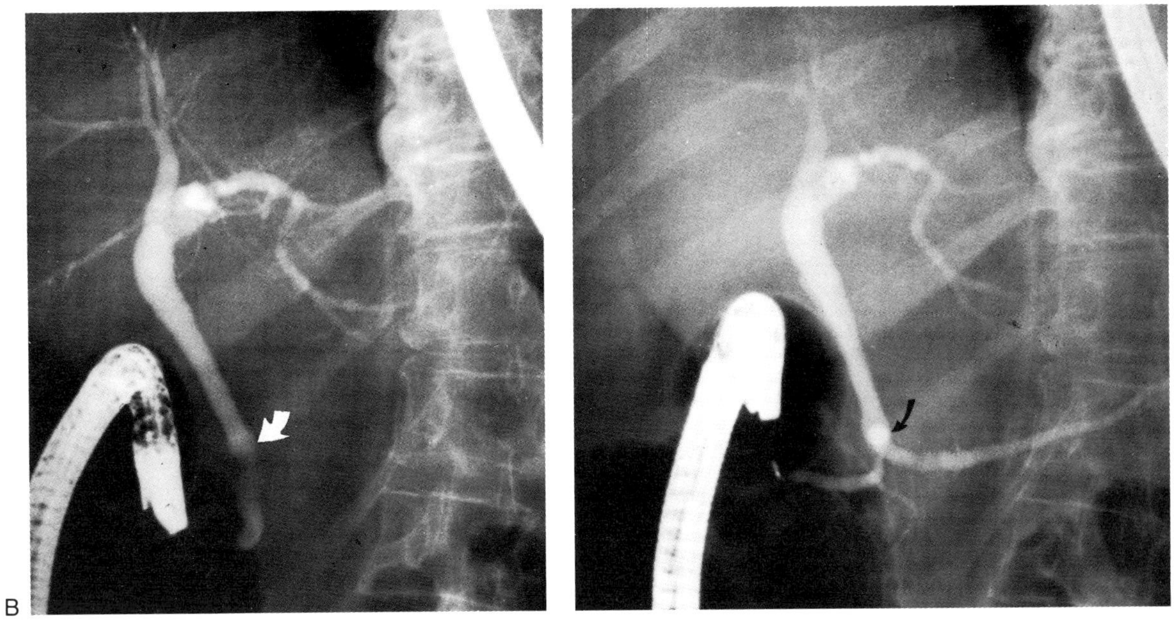

has not been commonly associated with this congenital variation, probably because *pain accompanies alcohol ingestion, thus deterring the patient from drinking*. Incidently, separation of the pancreatic duct and bile duct openings into the duodenum (papilla) has been thought to be a predisposition to pancreatitis associated with alcohol abuse (see the section on separate channel openings) (120). Pain experienced by patients with pancreas divisum on ingestion of alcohol may be a prognosticator in determining which person or persons may develop pancreatitis secondary to alcohol ingestion, a point better appreciated by our knowledge of the anatomy and dysfunction of separate openings of the bile duct and pancreatic duct (i.e., pancreas divisum).

Confirmation of this anatomic variation is established after performance of pancreatography. When the ventral duct is opacified and found to represent a short segment with branching, the endoscopist is then compelled to selectively cannulate the minor papilla in an attempt to opacify the dorsal duct system and confirm divisum. This formidable task has been accom-

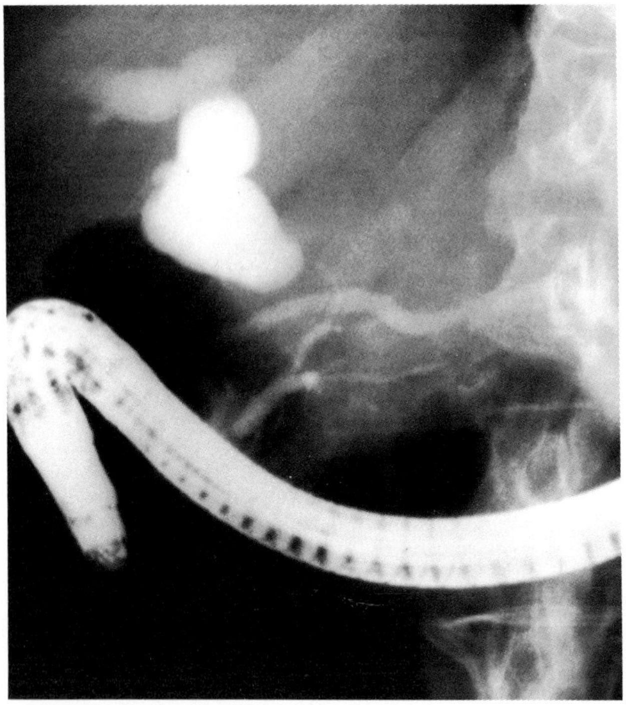

FIG. 9.61. An example of the functional, or incomplete, pancreas divisum as connoted by the communication of the rudimentary ventral system with the dorsal system. Once again, dilatation of the bile duct is appreciated and is secondary to recurrent pancreatitis and fibrosis.

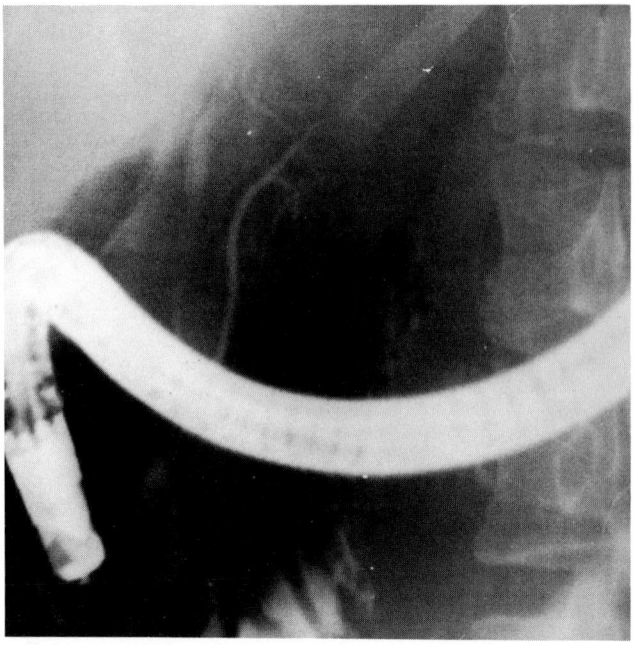

FIG. 9.62. A long ventral segment of the pancreatic duct. Branching of this duct allows one to rule out a neoplasm with a high degree of certainty.

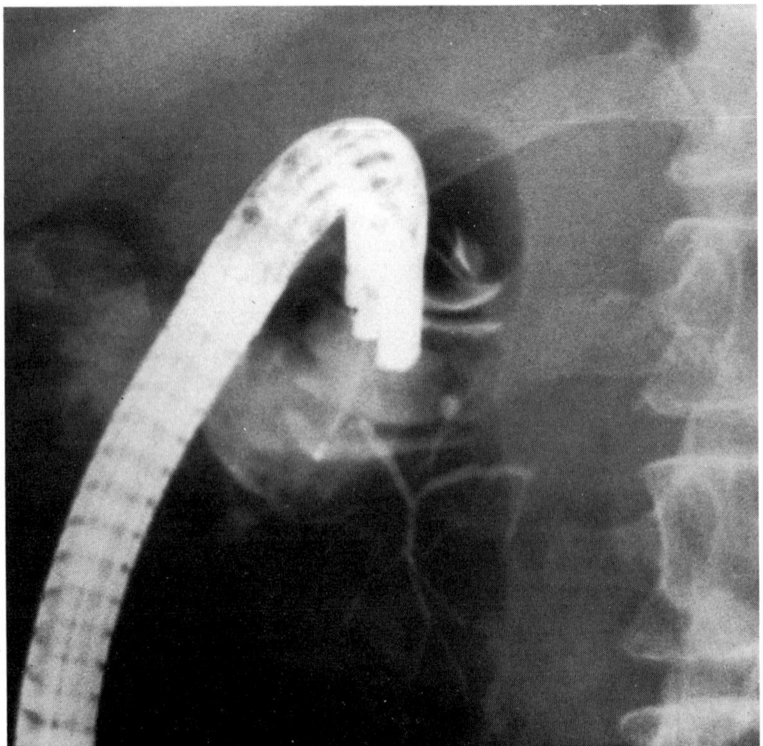

FIG. 9.63. Cannulation and opacification of the ventral duct system of the pancreas. In this case, the duct is located in a more inferior direction than usual.

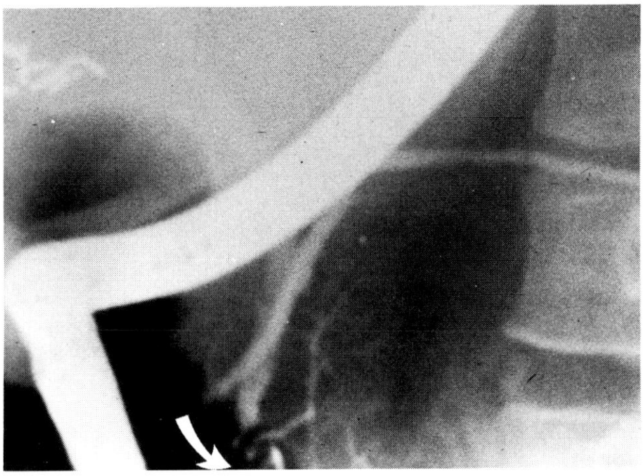

FIG. 9.64. Pancreas divisum, with separate openings of the ventral duct and bile duct arising from the major papilla (*arrow*). After selective cannulation of the minor papilla, the dorsal duct is opacified.

plished more readily with the availability of a needle-tip catheter, which permits the operator to opacify the dorsal duct system (221). Thus, opacification of the dorsal duct system from the origin of the minor papilla confirms the impression of pancreas divisum. In my experience, manipulation of the minor papilla is often facilitated by insertion of a guidewire, providing access to the dorsal duct and easing placement of dilating catheters and dilating balloons and insertion of prostheses. I have had great success with a 7Fr dilating catheter, which tapers to 5Fr at the tip. Through it, a standard 0.035″ guidewire can be inserted through the minor papilla and into the duct itself. Other accessories are currently available for specific cannulation of the minor papilla and dilatation of its orifice. These accessories include a thin-caliber guidewire, usually 0.018″ to 0.025″ in diameter, which is inserted through a series of dilating catheters ranging from 3Fr to 7Fr. Although these small guidewires are usually soft and flimsy, one made by Wilson-Cook has a flexible tip attached to a sturdy monofilament body and can be used effectively for small structures such as the minor papilla.

Pancreatitis, or symptoms related to pancreatitis, may be associated with a normal-appearing dorsal pancreatic duct. Subtle changes in the morphology of the duct may provide evidence of the existence of pancreatitis even though the duct is not dilated and does not portray the classic morphologic picture of pancreatitis (Figs. 9.65–9.72). Some patients do have a dilated pancreatic duct and develop ectasia of the secondary and tertiary radicals, findings consistent with chronic pancreatitis. However, in my experience, symptoms of pancreatitis and response to therapy have been similar in patients with dilated ducts and with ducts that appear normal in contour and configuration.

When should therapy be provided for patients with pancreas divisum? Should therapy be provided at all? Patients who present with unremitting pain and dietary restrictions and intake respond to endoscopic decompression techniques. Using the patient as the control, the endoscopist may place a prosthesis into the dorsal duct to provide drainage. A careful assessment of the patient's response should be carried out, and

Text continues on page 166.

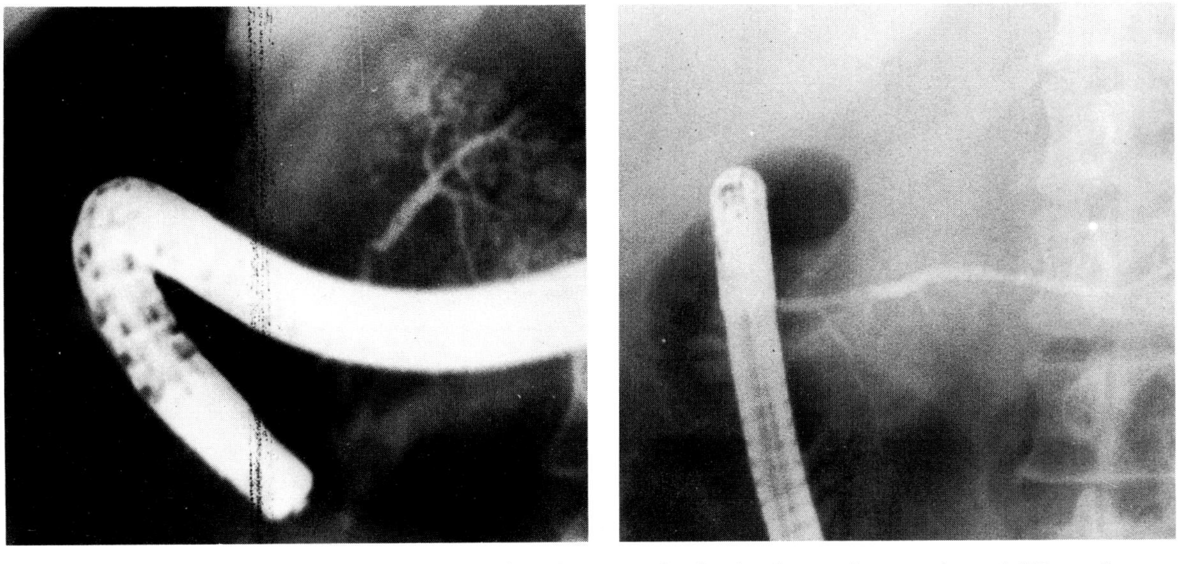

FIG. 9.65. Left: A pancreatogram showing the ventral arborization and parenchymal filling of the pancreatic duct. The branching connotes benignity. **Right:** Opacification of the dorsal duct of pancreas divisum.

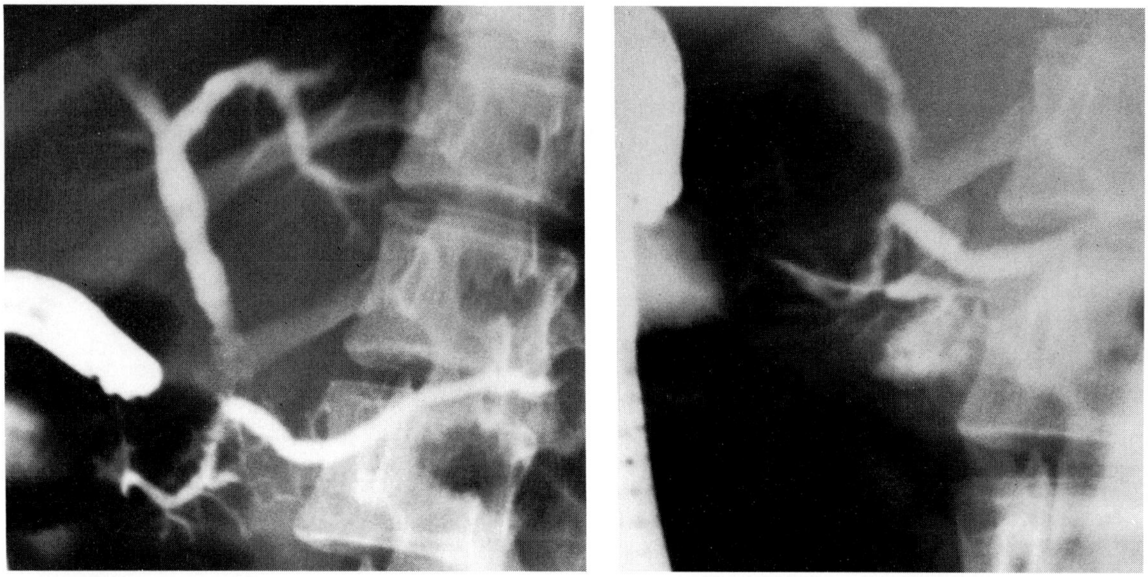

FIG. 9.66. Left: A pancreatogram obtained in a patient who previously underwent surgical sphincterotomies of both the dorsal and ventral pancreatic ducts for pancreatitis secondary to pancreas divisum. Note the narrowed distal segment of the dorsal duct and the dilatation of the duct proximal to the narrowed segment. **Right:** Overfilling of the duct system with acinarization of the ventral duct system and parenchyma.

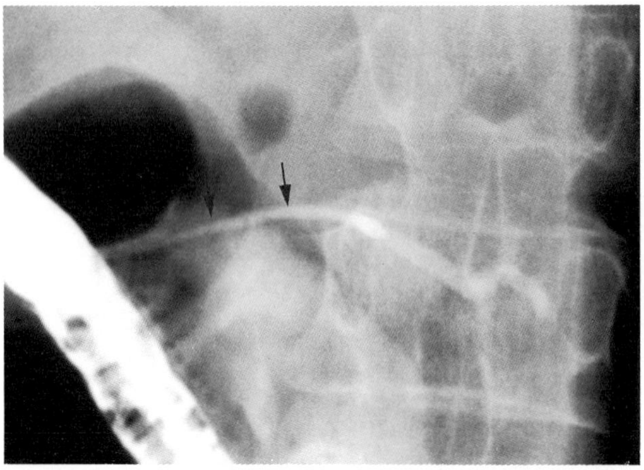

FIG. 9.67. Evidence of pancreatitis of the dorsal pancreatic duct with a long, rigid segment of the distal duct (*arrows*) and proximally dilated duct. Air is noted in the biliary tree secondary to a prior sphincterotomy.

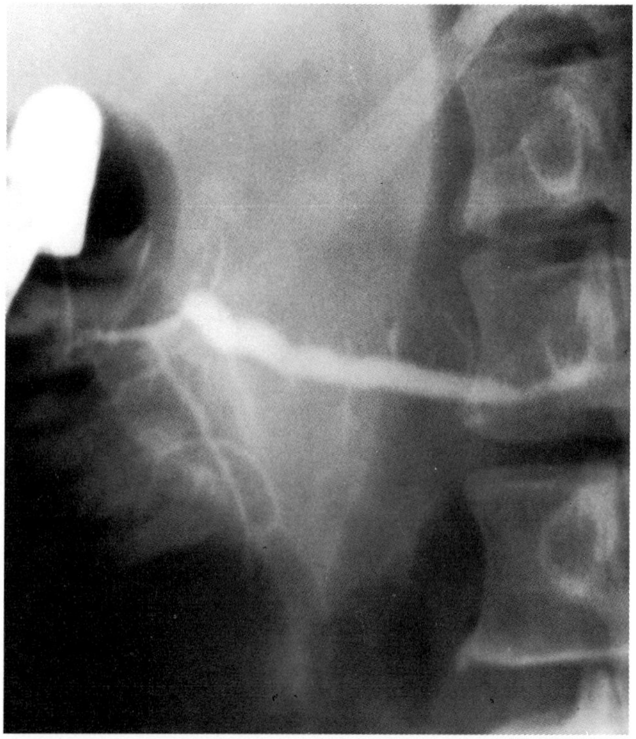

FIG. 9.68. Evidence of pancreatitis of the dorsal pancreatic duct with a tight stricture of the distal duct producing dilatation of the proximal duct.

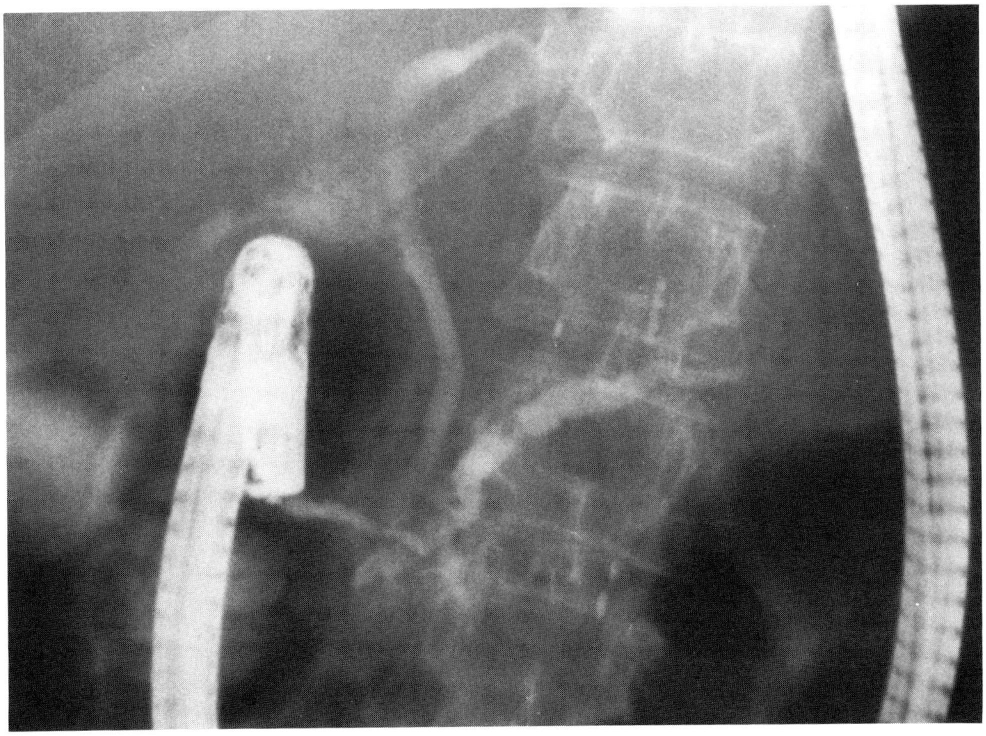

FIG. 9.69. A radiograph consistent with pancreatitis which is confirmed by demonstrating a rigid segment of the dorsal duct (actually the duct of Santorini) in a patient with recurrent symptoms. Because of fibrosis of the ventral duct system, the entire pancreatic duct was opacified through the minor papilla.

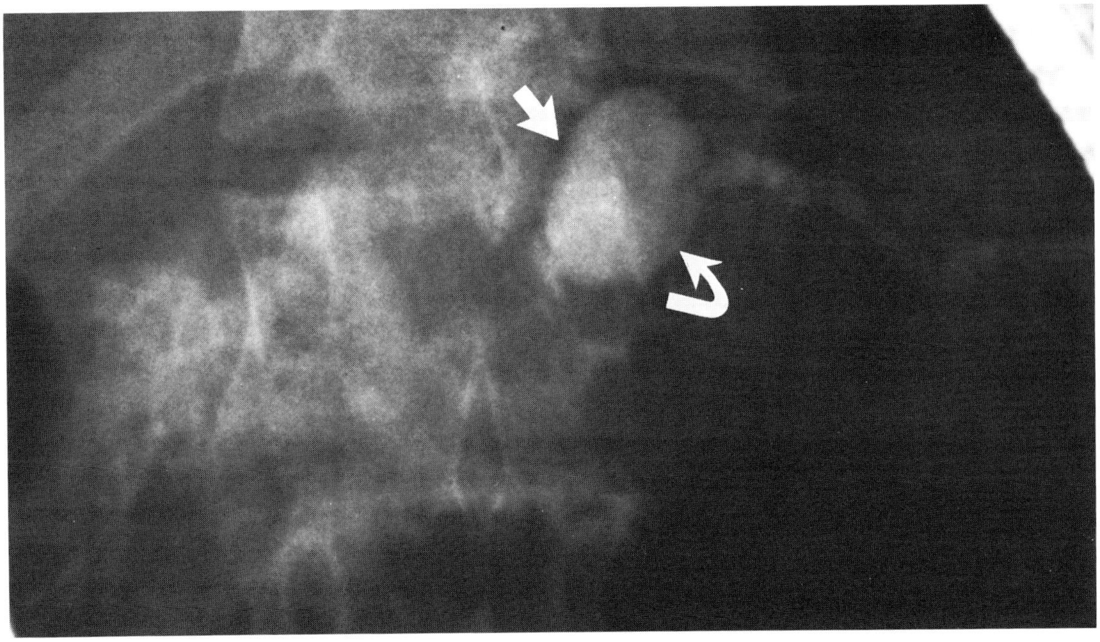

FIG. 9.70. A pancreatogram obtained in a patient with pancreatitis secondary to pancreas divisum. The distal duct is not clearly visualized, but a communicating pseudocyst (*arrows*) is evident in the body of the pancreas, confirming the severity of the patient's symptoms.

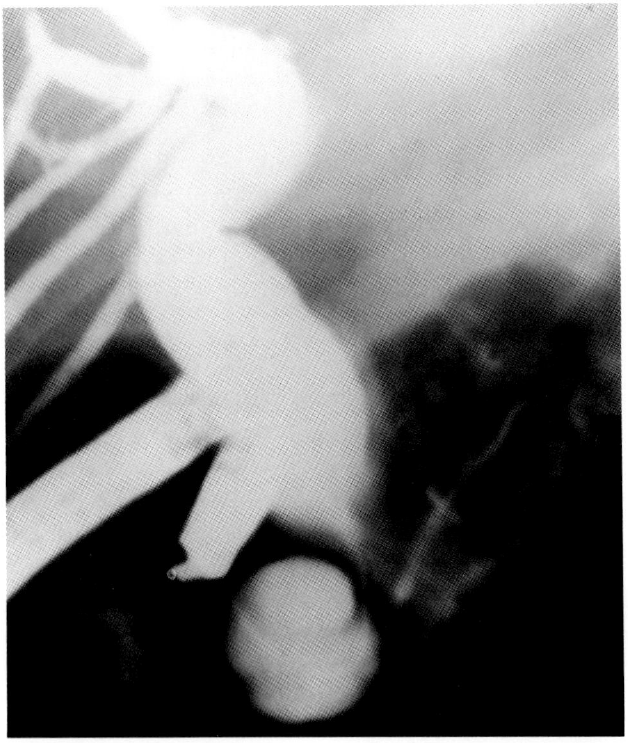

FIG. 9.71. Bile duct dilatation secondary to fibrosis associated with pancreatitis is not uncommon. However, its appearance with pancreas divisum is unusual. Note the ventral duct and branching consistent with this congenital variation. Note also the calcifications in the ventral pancreas.

Text continued from page 163.

follow-up visits or telephone surveys should determine the response of this form of therapy. Long-term data are being analyzed to determine the benefit of such treatment (222). In our experience, patients with pancreas divisum and patients with other congenital variants have benefitted from endoscopic decompression, experiencing relief of symptoms after placement of prostheses (Figs. 9.73–9.76). The duration of this relief is correlated with the time the prosthesis remains in place or patent and functioning. In some patients, the prosthesis migrated from the duct into the duodenum. This migration was heralded by a return of symptoms and intolerance to most foods. Also, if the prosthesis remained in place but became occluded, the patient experienced recurrent symptoms, but to a milder degree. This change in status was contrasted with the period of normalcy provided by the prosthesis and the decompression it provided. Pancreatitis may be indolent and progressive despite the placement of a prosthesis, and we have seen progression of disease as evidenced by further dilatation of the pancreatic duct and its secondary branches after occlusion of the prosthesis (or before occlusion). Surgical intervention in some of these patients revealed evidence of focal pancreatitis and progression of the inflammatory process extending from the sphincter and head of the gland toward the neck, but no further. These progressive changes have been attributed to progression of disease

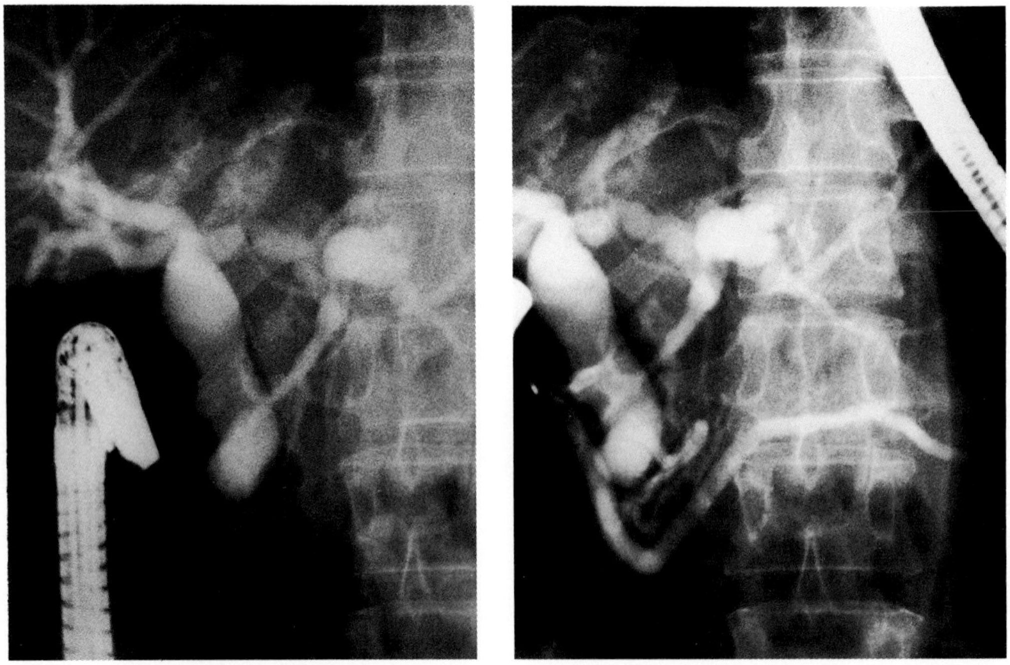

FIG. 9.72. Left: Dilatation of the biliary tree and blunting of the distal common bile duct on this ERCP are consistent with fibrosis secondary to pancreatitis. **Right:** Note that the dorsal pancreatic duct and smaller branches of the duct in the head of the gland are acutely angulated.

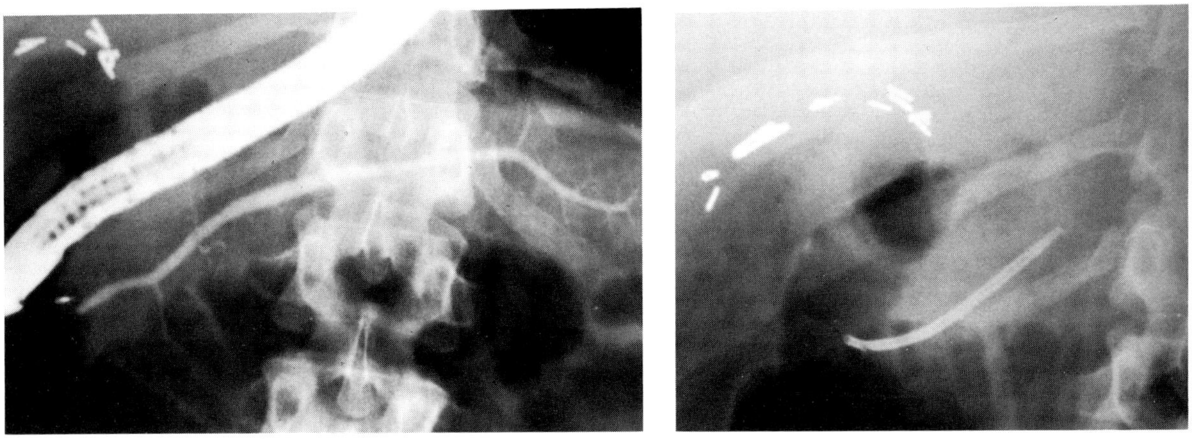

FIG. 9.73. Left: Evidence of pancreatitis. **Right:** Placement of a prosthesis.

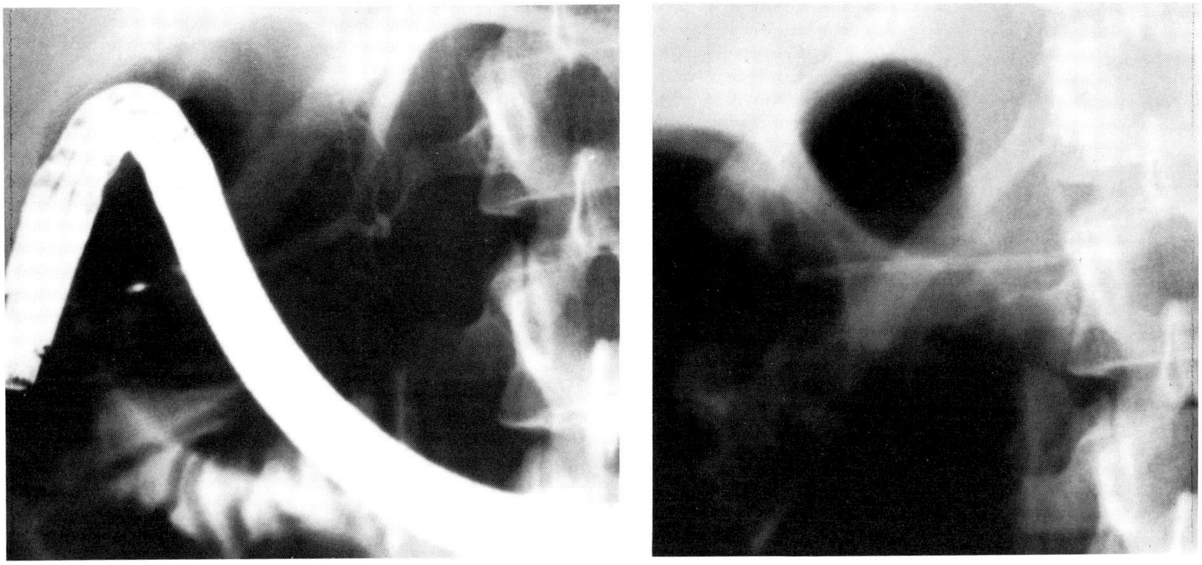

FIG. 9.74. Left: A pancreatogram showing pancreatitis. **Right:** Placement of a prosthesis.

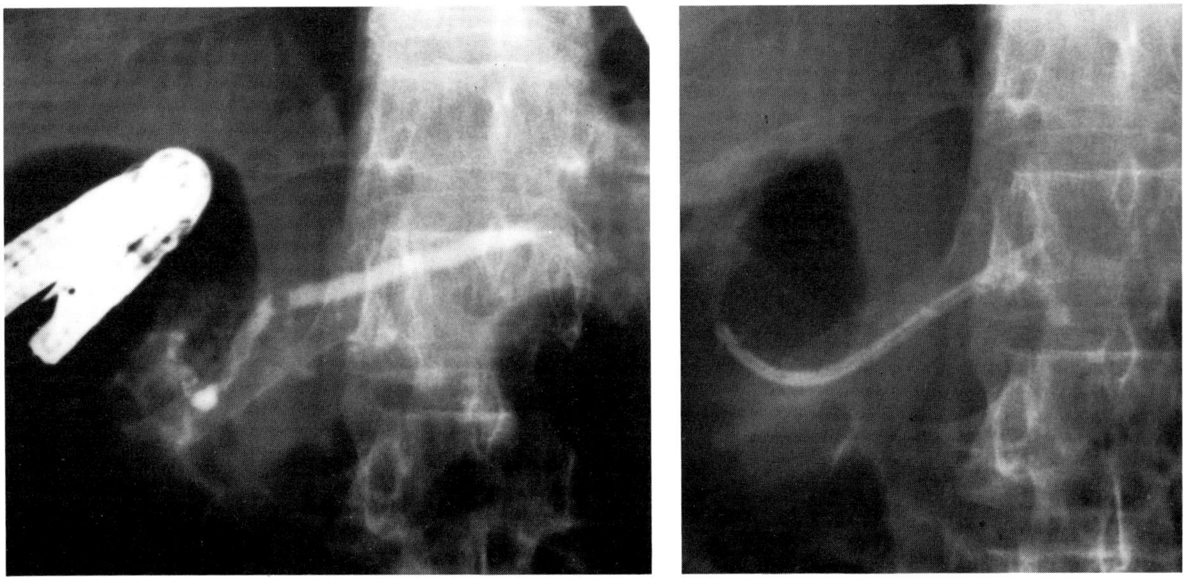

FIG. 9.75. Left: Another example of pancreatitis. **Right:** A prosthesis.

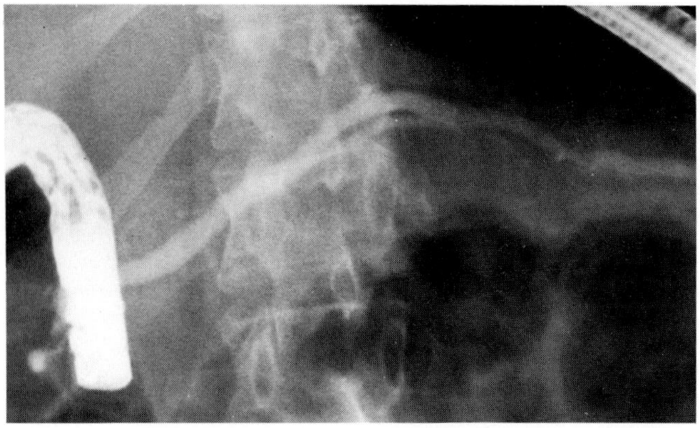

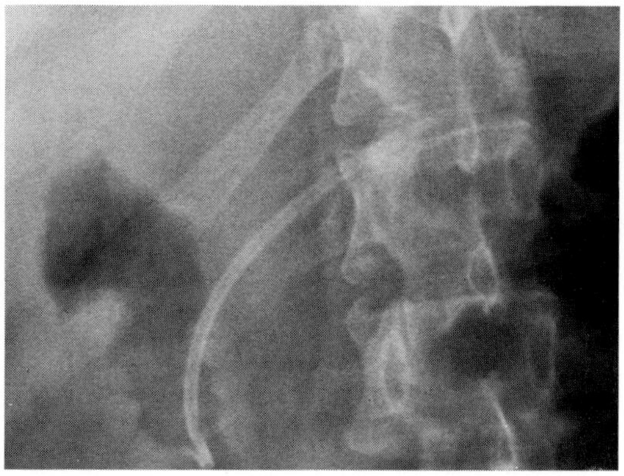

FIG. 9.76. Left: A pancreatogram that presents evidence of pancreatitis. **Right:** Placement of a prosthesis.

rather than to the prosthesis, and, over a long follow-up period, patients who had morphologic progression of disease continued to remain asymptomatic while drainage or decompression was provided.

Specific surgical procedures have been designed for decompression of the dorsal pancreatic duct in patients with pancreatitis secondary to pancreas divisum. More commonly, sphincterotomy or sphincteroplasty of the minor papilla is performed. However, other procedures have been devised, such as precise mucosa-to-mucosa anastomoses of the pancreatic duct to jejunum, which requires resection of the tail of the pancreas (222–229). The spleen is usually left *in situ*. In the latter procedure, a small-caliber stent is advanced by the surgeon from the duodenum through the sphincter and length of the dorsal pancreatic duct through the anastomosis to the anterior abdominal wall, where it is left under the skin for duct access. At an appropriate time, if the patient is symptomatic or if a diagnostic study is indicated, the catheter can be se-

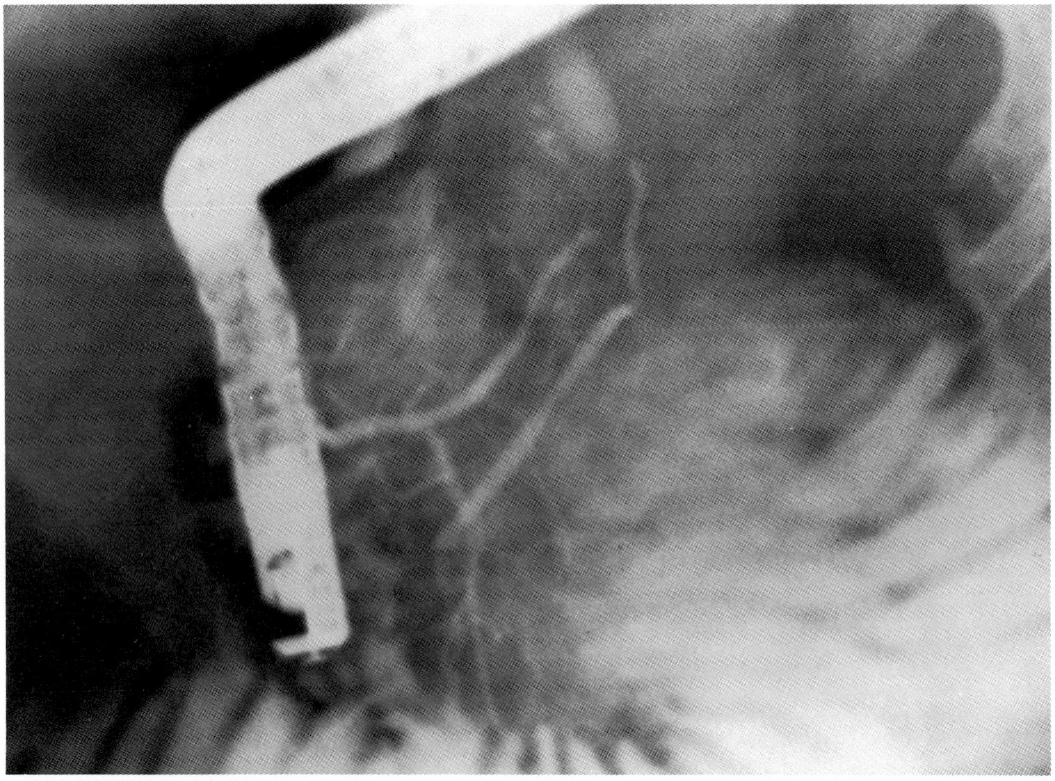

FIG. 9.77. A pancreatogram demonstrating an abrupt cutoff of the ventral duct of a pancreas divisum. Opacification of the dorsal duct also revealed a cutoff of this duct (*arrow*), which was consistent with carcinoma.

lectively injected with contrast, providing a pancreatogram that can be helpful for determining appropriate drainage of the pancreatic duct. Other surgical procedures performed for this disease include a modified pylorus-sparing Whipple's procedure. The extent of surgery is unpredictable for each patient, and in our series, some required two or three operations. To the extreme, one patient ultimately underwent a total pancreatectomy because of progressive symptoms and unremitting pain.

The management of patients with pancreas divisum is therefore not yet optimal, and difficult at best because of the subjective complaints associated with minimal objective findings. It is indeed a sad commentary that some patients may undergo several surgical procedures and even a Whipple's procedure or total pancreatectomy for a benign process. These perplexing problems have prompted many authorities in the field to dissuade clinicians from treating patients with pancreas divisum and symptoms suggestive of pancreatitis unless there is objective, morphologic evidence of pancreatitis (i.e., dilated duct with tortuous side branches). Unless controlled trials are undertaken, various treatment modalities will be untested by statistical analysis and left to anecdotal conclusions, which are inexact and not totally objective.

A perplexing problem facing the endoscopist and clinician in the evaluation of a patient with pancreas divisum is the difficulty in interpreting the pancreatogram exactly and objectively to rule in the presence of divisum and to rule out carcinoma (230,231). If a patient presents with symptoms compatible with pancreatitis or tumor, noninvasive studies such as US or CT scans may be inconclusive or suggest fullness of the head of the pancreas compatible with either diagnosis (216). A pancreatogram obtained in a patient with pancreas divisum demonstrates incomplete filling of the ventral portion of the pancreas, and, if this is interpreted by an inexperienced endoscopist or radiologist, the initial impression could be misinterpreted as a stricture compatible with carcinoma. In this situation one must take several radiographs of the duct system using high-resolution equipment. Such radiographs should demonstrate branching of the ventral duct, which is compatible with pancreas divisum. Most importantly, when the ventral duct has been opacified and the differential diagnosis includes a pancreatic tumor, selective opacification of the dorsal duct should be attempted through the minor papilla. Therefore, I recommend that an attempt be made to opacify the pancreatic duct system through the minor papilla to confirm the presence of pancreas divisum. Accomplishing this task should eliminate the diagnosis of carcinoma and determine the diagnosis of pancreas divisum. Figure 9.77 demonstrates the coexistence of pancreas divisum and carcinoma. I have found this association in four patients and advocate that a complete examination of the pancreatic duct system be accomplished at each ERCP for a conclusive diagnosis.

REFERENCES

1. Brady PG. Endoscopic retrograde cholangiopancreatography. Its role in diagnosis and therapy of pancreatitis. *Postgrad Med* 1986;253–6, 259–61.
2. Neuhaus H, Classen M. Endoscopy in the diagnosis and treatment of acute obstructive pancreatitis. *Bildgebung* 1987–89;56:42, 45–6, 48.
3. Neoptolemos JP, Carr-Locke DL, London N, Bailey I, Fossard DP. ERCP findings and the role of endoscopic sphincterotomy in acute gallstone pancreatitis. *Br J Surg* 1988;75:954–60.
4. Neoptolemos JP, Carr-Locke DL, London NJ, Bailey IA, James D, Fossard DP. Controlled trial of urgent endoscopic retrograde cholangiopancreatography and endoscopic sphincterotomy versus conservative treatment for acute pancreatitis due to gallstones. *Lancet* 1988;89, 2:979–83.
5. Brake DH, Fry WJ. Ductal drainage for chronic pancreatitis. *Surgery* 1989;105:131–40.
6. Ranson JH. Endoscopy for gallstone pancreatitis. *Gastroenterology* 1989;97:1592–3.
7. Scholmerich J, Gross V, Johannesson T, et al. Detection of biliary origin of acute pancreatitis. Comparison of laboratory tests, ultrasound, computed tomography, and ERCP. *Dig Dis Sci* 1989;34:830–3.
8. Sugawa C, Lucas CE. The case for preoperative and intraoperative ERCP in pancreatic trauma (editorial). *Gastrointest Endosc* 1988;34:145–7.
9. Nealon WH, Townsend CM Jr, Thompson JC. Preoperative endoscopic retrograde cholangiopancreatography (ERCP) in patients with pancreatic pseudocyst associated with resolving acute and chronic pancreatitis. *Ann Surg* 1989;209:532–8.
10. Hayward SR, Lucas CE, Sugawa C, Ledgerwood AM. Emergent endoscopic retrograde cholangiopancreatography. A highly specific test for acute pancreatic trauma. *Arch Surg* 1989;124:745–5.
11. Cooper CB, Bardsley PA, Rao SS, Collins MC. Pleural effusions and pancreatico-pleural fistulae associated with asymptomatic pancreatic disease. *Br J Dis Chest* 1988;82:315–20.
12. Ellenbogen KA, Cameron JL, Cocco AE, Gayler BW, Hutcheon DF. Fistulous communication of a pseudocyst with the common bile duct: demonstration by endoscopic retrograde cholangiopancreatography. *Johns Hopkins Med J* 1981; 149:110–1.
13. McPherson GA, Collier NA, Lavender JP, Blumgart LH. The role of HIDA scanning in the assessment of external biliary fistulae. *Surg Gastroenterol* 1984;3:77–80.
14. Izbicki JR, Wiler DK, Waldner H, Rueff FL, Schweiberer L. Thoracic manifestations of internal pancreatic fistulas: report of five cases. *Am J Gastroenterol* 1989;84:265–71.
15. Pancreatitis from oral contraceptives. [Editorial]. *Br Med J* 1973;3:688.
16. Mallory A, Kern F Jr. Drug-induced pancreatitis: a critical review. *Gastroenterology* 1980;78:813.
17. Dobrilla G, Felder M, Chilovi F. Medication-induced acute pancreatitis. *Schweiz Med Wochenschr* 1985;115:850.
18. Bennett IL Jr, Cary FH, Mitchell GL Jr, Cooper MN. Acute methyl alcohol poisoning: a review based on experience in an outbreak of 323 cases. *Medicine* 1953;32:431.
19. Dressel TD, Goodale RL, Arneson MA, Borner JW. Pancreatitis as a complication of anticholinesterase insecticide intoxication. *Ann Surg* 1978;189:199.
20. Haber CJ, Meltzer SJ, Present DH, Koerelitz BI. Nature and course of pancreatitis caused by 6-mercaptopurine in the treatment of inflammatory bowel disease. *Gastroenterology* 1986;91:982.
21. Northrup WF III, Simmons RL. Pancreatic trauma. A review. *Surgery* 1972;71:27.

22. Bess MA, Edis AJ, van Heerden JA. Hyperparathyroidism and pancreatitis. Chance or a causal association? *JAMA* 1980; 243:246.
23. Hochgelernt EL, David DS. Acute pancreatitis secondary to calcium infusion in a dialysis patient. *Arch Surg* 1974;108:218.
24. Gallagher S, Sankaran H, Williams JA. Mechanisms of scorpion toxin-induced enzyme secretion in rat pancreas. *Gastroenterology* 1981;80:970.
25. Lashner BA, Kirsner JB, Hanauer SB. Acute pancreatitis associated with high-concentration lipid emulsion during total parenteral nutrition therapy for Crohn's disease. *Gastroenterology* 1986;90:1039.
26. Feldstein JD, Johnson FR, Kallick CA, Doolas A. Acute hemorrhagic pancreatitis due to mumps. *Ann Surg* 1974;180:85.
27. Brambs HJ, Ruckauer K, Scholmerich J, et al. ERCP in acute pancreatitis. A preliminary report. *Dig Surg* 1988;5:156.
28. Axon ATR. Minimal change pancreatitis. In: Mitchell CJ, Kelleher J, eds. *Pancreatic Disease in Clinical Practice*. London: Pitman, 1981;399–403.
29. Nordback I, Airo I. Post-ERCP acute necrotizing pancreatitis. *Ann Chir Gynaecol* 1988;77:15–20.
30. Ammann RW, Deyhle P, Butkofer E. Fatal necrotizing pancreatitis after cholangiopancreatography. *Gastroenterology* 1973;63:320–3.
31. Hopper KD, Wegert SJ, Hallgren SE. Renal excretion of endoscopic retrograde cholangiopancreatography injected contrast. A common phenomenon. *Invest Radiol* 1989;24:394–6.
32. Cunliffe WJ, Cobden I, Lavalle MI, Landrum R, Tait NP, Venables CW. A randomized, prospective study comparing two contrast media in ERCP. *Endoscopy* 1987;19:201–2.
33. O'Connor HJ, Ellis WR, Manning AP, Lintott DJ, McMahon MJ, Axon AT. Iopamidol as contrast medium in endoscopic retrograde pancreatography: a prospective randomized comparison with diatrizoate. *Endoscopy* 1988;20:244–7.
34. Rambow A, Staritz M, Manns M, Hutteroth T, Meyer-Zum-Buschenfeld KH. ERCP: which contrast medium is suitable? *Z Gastroenterol* 1988;26:279–82.
35. Ponce J, Garriguss V. Pertejo V, et al. Effect of intravenous glucagon and glucagon (1-21)-peptide on motor activity of sphincter of Oddi in humans. *Dig Dis Sci* 1989;34:61–4.
36. Bordas JM, Toledo V, Mondelo F, Rodes J. Prevention of pancreatic reactions by bolus somatostatin administration in patients undergoing endoscopic retrograde cholangio-pancreatography and endoscopic sphincterotomy. *Horm Res* 1988;29:106–8.
37. Sivak M. Endoscopic retrograde cholangiopancreatography (ERCP). *Cleve Clin Q* 1974;41:93.
38. Stewart ET, Vennes JA, Geenen JE, eds: *Atlas of endoscopic retrograde cholangiopancreatography*. St. Louis: CV Mosby, 1977.
39. Ogoshi K, Niwa M, Hara Y, et al. Endoscopic pancreatocholangiography in the evaluation of pancreatic and biliary disease. *Gastroenterology* 1973;64:210.
40. Nagata A, Homma T, Tamai K, et al. A study of chronic pancreatitis by serial endoscopic pancreatography. *Gastroenterology* 1981;81:884.
41. Jones SN, Lees WR, Frost RA. Diagnosis and grading of chronic pancreatitis by morphological criteria derived by ultrasound and pancreatography. *Clin Radiol* 1988;39:43–8.
42. Braganza JM, Hunt LG, Warwick F. Relationship between pancreatic exocrine function and ductal morphology in chronic pancreatitis. *Gastroenterology* 1982;82:1341–7.
43. Axon ATR, Classen M, Cotton PB, et al. Pancreatography in chronic pancreatitis; international definitions. *Gut* 1984; 25(10):1107–12.
44. Sarner M, Cotton PB. Classification of pancreatitis. *Gut* 1984;5:756.
45. Borgstrom A, Wehlin L. Correlation between serum concentrations of three specific exocrine pancreatic proteins and pancreatic duct morphology at ERCP examinations. *Scand J Gastroenterol* 1984;19:220–7.
46. Schneider MU, Lux G. Floating pancreatic duct concrements in chronic pancreatitis. *Endoscopy* 1985;17:8.
47. Itai Y, Ohhashi K, Nagai H, et al. "Ductectatic" mucinous cystadenoma and cystadenocarcinoma of the pancreas. *Radiology* 1986;161:697.
48. Gilmore IT, Pemberton J, Thompson RPH. Retrograde cholangiopancreatography in the diagnosis of carcinoma of the pancreas. *Gastrointest Endosc* 1982;28:77.
49. Fukomoto K, Nakajima M, Kurakami K, et al. Diagnosis of pancreatic cancer by endoscopic pancreatocholangiography. *Am J Gastroenterol* 1974;60:210–23.
50. Reuben A, Cotton PB. Endoscopic retrograde cholangiopancreatography in carcinoma of the pancreas. *Surg Gynecol Obstet* 1979;148:179.
51. Ralls PW, Halls J, Renner I, Juttner H. Endoscopic retrograde cholangiopancreatography (ERCP) in pancreatic disease. *Radiology* 1980;134:347.
52. Siegel JH. ERCP update: diagnostic and therapeutic applications. *Gastrointest Radiol* 1978;3:311–8.
53. Dekker A. Fine-needle aspiration biopsy in ampullary and pancreatic carcinoma. *Arch Surg* 1979;114:592.
54. Itoh K, Yamanaka T, Kasahara K, et al. Definitive diagnosis of pancreatic carcinoma with percutaneous fine needle aspiration biopsy under ultrasonic guidance. *Am J Gastroenterol* 1979;71:469.
55. Yamanaka T, Kimura K. Differential diagnosis of pancreatic mass lesion with percutaneous fine-needle aspiration biopsy under ultrasonic guidance. *Dig Dis Sci* 1979;24:694.
56. Taylor KJW, Brand MH. Ultrasonic biopsy guidance in the management of patients with pancreatic cancer. *J Clin Gastroenterol* 1979;1:267.
57. Ferrucci JT, Wittenberg J, Margolis MN, Carey RW. Malignant seeding of the tract after thin-needle aspiration biopsy. *Radiology* 1979;130:345.
58. Wyndner EL, Mabuchi K, Maruchi N, Fortner JG. Epidemiology of cancer of the pancreas. *J Natl Cancer Inst* 1973;50:645.
59. Ammann RW, Knoblauch M, Moeher P, et al. High incidence of extrapancreatic carcinoma in chronic pancreatitis. *Scand J Gastroenterol* 1980;15:395.
60. Siegel JH, Sable RA, Balthazar EJ, Rosenthal WS. Abnormalities of the bile duct associated with chronic pancreatitis. Demonstration by ERCP. *Am J Gastroenterol* 1979;72:259–66.
61. Schulte WJ, LoPorta AJ, Condin RE, Unger GF, Geenen JE, DeCosses JJ. Chronic pancreatitis: a cause of biliary stricture. *Surgery* 1977;82:303.
62. Gregg JA, Carr-Locke DL, Gallagher MM. Importance of common bile duct stricture associated with chronic pancreatitis. Diagnosis by endoscopic retrograde cholangiopancreatography. *Am J Surg* 1981;141:199.
63. Snape WJ, Long WB, Trotman BW, Marin GA, Czaja AJ. Marked alkaline phosphatase elevation with partial common bile duct obstruction due to calcified pancreatitis. *Gastroenterology* 1976;70:70.
64. Yadegar J, Williams RA, Passaro E Jr, Wilson SE. Common duct stricture from chronic pancreatitis. *Arch Surg* 1980; 115:582–6.
65. Wisloff F, Jakobsen J, Osnes M. Stenosis of the common bile duct in chronic pancreatitis. *Br J Surg* 1982;69:52–4.
66. Prinz RA, Aranha GV, Greenlee HB, Kruss DM. Common duct obstruction in patients with intractable pain of chronic pancreatitis. *Am Surg* 1982;48:373–7.
67. Eckhauser FE, Knol JA, Strodel WE, Achem S, Nostrant T. Common bile duct strictures associated with chronic pancreatitis. *Am Surg* 1983;49:350–8.
68. Gadacz TR, Lillemoe K, Zinner M, Merrill W. Common bile duct complications of pancreatitis evaluation and treatment. *Surgery* 1983;93:235–42.
69. Stahl TJ, Allen MO, Ansel HJ, Vennes JA. Partial biliary obstruction caused by chronic pancreatitis. An appraisal of indications for surgical biliary drainage. *Ann Surg* 1988;2070:26–32.
70. Wilson C, Auld CD, Schlinkert R, Hasan AH, et al. Hepatobiliary complications in chronic pancreatitis. *Gut* 1989;30:520–7.

71. Geenen JE. ASGE distinguished lecture. Endoscopic therapy of pancreatic diseases: a new horizon. *Gastrointest Endosc* 1988;34:386.
72. Prinz RA, Aranha GV, Greenlee HB. Combined pancreatic duct and upper gastrointestinal and biliary tract drainage in chronic pancreatitis. *Arch Surg* 1985;120:361–6.
73. Ammann RW, Aovbiantz A, Largiader F, Schueler G. Course and outcome of chronic pancreatitis. Longitudinal study of a mixed medical-surgical series of 245 patients. *Gastroenterology* 1984;820–8.
74. Proctor HJ, Mendes OC, Thomas CG Jr, Herbst CA. Surgery for chronic pancreatitis:drainage versus resection. *Ann Surg* 1979;89:664.
75. White TT, Hart MJ. Pancreaticojejunostomy versus resection in the treatment of chronic pancreatitis. *Am J Surg* 1979; 138:129.
76. Taylor RH, Bagley RH. Ductal drainage or resection for chronic pancreatitis. *Am J Surg* 1981;141:28.
77. White TT, Slavotinek AH. Results of surgical treatment of chronic pancreatitis. Report of 142 cases. *Ann Surg* 1979; 189:217.
78. Frey CF, Child CG, Fry W. Pancreatectomy for chronic pancreatitis. *Ann Surg* 1976;184:403.
79. Braasch JW, Vito L, Nugent FW. Total pancreatectomy for end-stage chronic pancreatitis. *Ann Surg* 1978;188:317.
80. Priestley JT, Remine WH, Barber KW Jr, Gambill EE. Chronic relapsing pancreatitis: treatment by surgical drainage of the pancreas. *Ann Surg* 1965;161:838.
81. Arnesjo B, Ihse I, Kugelberg C, Tyler U. Pancreaticojejunostomy in chronic pancreatitis. An appraisal of 29 cases. *Acta Chir Scand* 1975;141:139.
82. Warshaw AL, Popp JW Jr, Schapiro RH. Long term patency, pancreatic function, and pain relief after lateral pancreaticojejunostomy for chronic pancreatitis. *Gastroenterology* 1980; 79:289.
83. Rossi RL, Heiss FW, Braasch JW. Surgical management of chronic pancreatitis. *Surg Clin North Am* 1985;65:79.
84. Travero LW, Tompkins RK, Uttea PT, Longmire WP. Surgical treatment of chronic pancreatitis. Twenty-two years experience. *Ann Surg* 1979;290:312.
85. Ammann RW, Largiader R, Akovbiantz A. Pain relief by surgery in chronic pancreatitis? Relationship between pain relief, pancreatic dysfunction, and alcohol withdrawal. *Scand J Gastroenterol* 1979;14:209.
86. Prinz RA, Greenlee HR. Pancreatic duct drainage in 100 patients with chronic pancreatitis. *Ann Surg* 1981;194:313.
87. Holmberg JT, Isaksson G, Ihse I. Long-term results of pancreaticojejunostomy in chronic pancreatitis. *Surg Gynecol Obstet* 1985;160:339.
88. Prinz RA, Aranha GV, Greenlee HB. Redrainage of the pancreatic duct in chronic pancreatitis. *Am J Surg* 1986;151:150.
89. Greenlee HB. The role of surgery for chronic pancreatitis and its complications. *Surg Annu* 1983;15:283–305.
90. Rutledge PL; Warshaw AL. Persistent acute pancreatitis. A variant treated by pancreatoduodenectomy. *Arch Surg* 1988; 123:597–600.
91. Cooperman AM, Sivak MV, Sullivan BH Jr, Hermann RE. Endoscopic pancreatography. Its value in preoperative and postoperative assessment of pancreatic disease. *Am J Surg* 1975;129:38.
92. Kolars JC, Allen MO, Ansel H, Silvis SE, Vennes JA. Pancreatic pseudocysts; clinical and endoscopic experience. *Am J Gastroenterol* 1989;84:259–64.
93. O'Connor M, Kolars J, Ansel H, Silvis S, Vennes J. Preoperative endoscopic retrograde cholangiopancreatography in the surgical management of pancreatic pseudocysts. *Am J Surg* 1986;151:18–24.
94. Sugawa C, Walt AJ. Endoscopic retrograde pancreatography in the surgery of pancreatic pseudocysts. *Surgery* 1979;86:639.
95. Cooperman AM. Chronic pancreatitis. *Surg Clin North Am* 1981;61:71.
96. Martin EW, Catalano P, Copperman M, Hecht C, Carey LC. Surgical decision-making in the treatment of pancreatic pseudocysts: internal versus external drainage. *Am J Surg* 1979;138:821.
97. Ravel HR, Aldrete JS. Analysis and forty-five patients with pseudocysts of the pancreas treated surgically. *Surg Gynecol Obstet* 1979;148:735.
98. Warshaw A, Rattner DW. Timing of surgical drainage for pancreatic pseudocyst-clinical and chemical criteria. *Ann Surg* 1985;202:720.
99. Davis JL, Milligan FD, Cameron JL. Septic complications following endoscopic retrograde cholangiopancreatography. *Surg Gynecol Obstet* 1975;140:365–7.
100. Galvan A, Klotz AP. Is transduodenal pancreatography ever contraindicated? A case report of provoked pancreatitis and pseudocyst. *Gastrointest Endosc* 1973;20:28–30.
101. Siegman-Iora Y, Spinrad S, Rattan J. Septic complications following endoscopic retrograde cholangiopancreatography: the experience in Tel Aviv Medical Center. *J Hosp Infect* 1988;12:7–12.
102. Brandes JW, Scheffer B, Lorenz-Meyer H, Korst HA, Littmann KP. ERCP: complications and prophylaxis. A controlled study. *Endoscopy* 1981;13:27.
103. Classen DC, Jacobson JA, Burke JP, Jacobson JT, Evans RS. Serious Pseudomonas infections associated with endoscopic retrograde cholangiopancreatography. *Am J Med* 1988;84:590–6.
104. Rogers BHG, Ciawel NJ, Seed RW. Transgastric needle aspiration of pancreatic pseudocyst through an endoscope. *Gastrointest Endosc* 1975;21:133–4.
105. Kozarek RA, Brayko CM, Harlan J, Sanowski RA, Cintora I, Kovac A. Endoscopic drainage of pancreatic pseudocysts. *Gastrointest Endosc* 1985;31:322–8.
106. Sahel J, Bastid C, Pellat B, et al. Endoscopic cystoduodenostomy of cysts of chronic calcifying pancreatitis: a report of 20 cases. *Pancreas* 1987;2:447.
107. Buchi KN, Bowers JH, Dixon JA. Endoscopic pancreatic cystogastrostomy using the Nd:YAG laser. *Gastrointest Endosc* 1986;32:112.
108. Siegel JH, Yatto RP. Endoscopic management of chronic pancreatitis. *Gastrointest Endosc* 1981;27:240–1.
109. Graham DY. Pancreatic enzyme replacement. The effect of antacid or cimetidine. *Dig Dis Sci* 1982;27:485.
110. Regan PT, Malagelada JR, DiMagno EP, Glanzman SL, Go VLW. Comparative effects of antacids, cimetidine, and enteric coating on the therapeutic response to oral enzymes in severe pancreatic insufficiency. *N Engl J Med* 1977;297:854.
111. DiMagno EP, Malagelada JR, Go VLW, Moertel CG. Fate of orally ingested enzymes in pancreatic insufficiency. Comparison of two dosage schedules. *N Engl J Med* 1977;296:1318.
112. DiMagno EP. Medical treatment of pancreatic insufficiency. *Mayo Clin Proc* 1970;54:435.
113. DiMagno EP. Controversies in the treatment of exocrine pancreatic insufficiency. *Dig Dis Sci* 1982;27:481.
114. Graham DY. Enzyme replacement of pancreatic insufficiency in man. Relation between in vitro enzyme activities and in vivo potency in commercial pancreatic extracts. *N Engl J Med* 1977;296:1314.
115. Isaksson G, Ihse I. Pain reduction by an oral pancreatic enzyme preparation in chronic pancreatitis. *Dig Dis Sci* 1983;28:97.
116. Bell S, Cole R, Robert-Thomson IC. Coeliac plexus block for control of pain in chronic pancreatitis. *Br Med J* 1980;281: 1604.
117. Leung JWC, Bowen-Wright M, Aveling W, Shorvon PJ, Cotton PB. Coeliac plexus block for pain in pancreatic cancer and chronic pancreatitis. *Br J Surg* 1983;70:730.
118. Madsen P, Hansen E. Coeliac plexus block versus pancreaticogastrostomy for pain in chronic pancreatitis. A controlled randomized trial. *Scand J Gastroenterol* 1985;20:1217.
119. Ballegaard S, Christophersen SJ, Pawids SG, Hesse J, Olsen NV. Acupuncture and transcutaneous electric nerve stimulation in the treatment of pain associated with chronic pancreatitis. A randomized study. *Scand J Gastroenterol* 1985; 20:1249.
120. Yatto RP, Siegel JH. The role of pancreaticobiliary duct anat-

omy in the etiology of alcoholic pancreatitis. *J Clin Gastroenterol* 1984;6:419–23.
121. Sigfusson BF, Wehlin L, Lindstrom CG. Variants of pancreatic duct system of importance in endoscopic retrograde cholangiopancreatography. *Acta Radiol Diagn* 1983;24:113.
122. Millbourn E. On the excretory ducts of the pancreas divisum in many, with a special reference to their relations to each other, to the common duct and to the duodenum. *Acta Anat (Basel)* 150;9:1–34.
123. DiMagno EP, Shorter RG, Taylor WF, Go VLW. Relationships between pancreaticobiliary ductal anatomy and pancreaticobiliary ductal anatomy and pancreatic ductal parenchymal histology. *Cancer* 1982;49:361.
124. Anderson MC, Mehn WH, Methad HL. An evaluation of the common channel as a factor in pancreatic or biliary disease. *Ann Surg* 1960;151:379.
125. Miska SP, Divivedi M. Pancreaticobiliary ductal union. *Gut* 1990;31:1144–9.
126. Volkholf H, Stolte M, Becker V. Epithelial dysplasia in chronic pancreatitis. *Virchows Arch* 1982;392:331–49.
127. Dreiling DA, Greenstein AJ, Bordalo O. The hypersecretory states of the pancreas. Implications in the pathophysiology of peptic ulcer diasthesis. *Am J Gastroenterol* 1973;59:503–11.
128. Opie EL. The etiology of acute hemorrhagic pancreatitis. *Bull Johns Hopkins Hosp* 1901;12:182.
129. Siegel JH. Evaluation and treatment of acquired and congenital pancreatic disorders: endoscopic dilatation and insertion of endoprostheses. *Am J Gastroenterol* 1983;78:696(abstract).
130. Huibregtse K, Schneider B, Vrij AA, Tytgat GNJ. Endoscopic pancreatic drainage in chronic pancreatitis. *Gastrointest Endosc* 1988;34:9.
131. Siegel JH, Pullano WE, Cooperman AM. Endoscopic therapy of acquired pancreatitis: an effective long term modality. 5 year followup. *Am J Gastroenterol* 1987;82:973(abst).
132. Siegel JH, Tone P, Menikeim D. Gallstone pancreatitis: pathogenesis and clinical forms. The emerging role of endoscopic management. *Am J Gastroenterol* 1986;81:774–8.
133. Leuschner U, Ueberla K, Usadel KH. Somatostatin in der Therapie der akuten Pankreatitis. *Z Gastroenterol [Verh]* 1987;22:138.
134. Sarr MG, Sanfey H, Cameron JL. Prospective randomized trial of nasogastric suction in patients with acute pancreatitis. *Surgery* 1986;100:500.
135. Regan PT, Malagelada JR, Go VLW, Wolf AM, DiMagno EP. A prospective study of the antisecretory and therapeutic effects of cimetidine and glucagon in human pancreatitis. *Mayo Clin Proc* 1981;56:449.
136. Soergel KH. Medical treatment of acute pancreatitis. What is the evidence? *Gastroenterology* 1978;76:620.
137. Medical Research Council Multicentre Trial. Morbidity of acute pancreatitis: the effect of aprotinin and glucagon. *Gut* 1980;21:334.
138. Balldin G, Borstrom A, Genell S, Ohlsson K. The effect of peritoneal lavage and aprotinin in the treatment of severe acute pancreatitis. *Res Exp Med (Berl)* 1983;183:203.
139. Goebell H, Amman R, Herfath C, et al. A double-blind trial of synthetic salmon calcitonin in the treatment of acute pancreatitis. *Scand J Gastroenterol* 1979;14:881.
140. Howes R, Zuidema GD, Cameron JL. Evaluation of prophylactic antibiotics in acute pancreatitis. *J Surg Res* 1975;18:197.
141. Ebbehoj N, Friss J, Srendsen LB, Bulow S, Madsen P. Indomethacin treatment of acute pancreatitis. A controlled double-blind trial. *Scand J Gastroenterol* 1985;20:798.
142. Tykka HT, Vaittinen EJ, Mahlberg KL, et al. A randomized double-blind study using CaNa EDTA, a phospholipase A. *Scand J Gastroenterol* 1985;20:5.
143. Mayer AD, McMahoy MJ, Corfield AP, et al. Controlled clinical trial of peritoneal lavage for the treatment of severe acute pancreatitis. *N Engl J Med* 1985;312:299.
144. Goodgame JT, Fischer JE. Parenteral nutrition in the treatment of acute pancreatitis. Effects on complications and mortality. *Ann Surg* 1977;186:651.
145. Goodman AJ, Neoptolemos JP, Carr-Locke DL, Finlay DBL, Fossard DP. Detection of gallstones after acute pancreatitis. *Gut* 1985;26:125.
146. Acosta JM, Pelligrini CA, Skinner DB, et al. Etiology and pathogenesis of acute biliary pancreatitis. *Surgery* 1980;88:118.
147. Kelly TR, Swaney PE. Gallstone pancreatitis: the second time around. *Surgery* 1982;95:571–5.
148. Howard MJ. Gallstone pancreatitis. In: Howard JM, Jordan GL Jr, Reber HA, eds. *Surgical diseases of the pancreas*. Philadelphia: Lea & Febiger, 1987.
149. Mayer AD, McMahon MJ. Gallstones and acute pancreatitis—is the association underestimated? *Br J Surg* 1984;71:905.
150. Ranson JHC. The timing of biliary surgery in gallstone pancreatitis. *Am Surg* 1979;189:654–62.
151. Kelly TR. Gallstone pancreatitis, the timing of surgery. *Surgery* 1980;88:345–9.
152. Osborne DH, Imrie CW, Carter DC. Biliary surgery in the same admission for gallstone-associated pancreatitis. *Br J Surg* 1981;68:758.
153. Moreau JA, Sinsmeister AR, Melton LJ, DiMagno EP. Gallstone pancreatitis and the effect of cholecystectomy: a population-based cohort study. *Mayo Clin Proc* 1988;63:466–73.
154. Stone HH, Fabian TC, Dunlop WE. Gallstone pancreatitis. Biliary tract pathology in relation to time of surgery. *Ann Surg* 1981;194:305.
155. Safrany L, Cotton PB. A preliminary report: urgent duodenoscopic sphincterotomy for acute gallstone pancreatitis. *Surgery* 1981;89:424.
156. Van der Spuy S. Endoscopic sphincterotomy in the management of gallstone pancreatitis. *Endoscopy* 1981;13:25–6.
157. Neoptolemos JP, Hall AW, Finlay DF, et al. The urgent diagnosis of gallstones in acute pancreatitis: a prospective study of three methods. *Br J Surg* 1984;71:230.
158. Neoptolemos JP, Carr-Locke DL, London N, et al. ERCP findings and the role of endoscopic sphincterotomy in acute gallstone pancreatitis. *Br J Surg* 1988;75:954.
159. Neoptolemos JP, London N, Slater ND, et al. Prospective study of ERCP and endoscopic sphincterotomy in the diagnosis and treatment of gallstone acute pancreatitis. *Arch Surg* 1986;121:697–702.
160. Lee MJ, Choi TK, Lai EC, Wong KP, Ngan Hi, Wong J. Endoscopic retrograde cholangiopancreatography after acute pancreatitis. *Surg Gynecol Obstet* 1986;163:354–8.
161. Siegel JH. Endoscopic sphincterotomy: when is it appropriate? In: Barkin JS, Rogers AI, eds. *Difficult decisions in digestive diseases*. Chicago: Yearbook Medical Publishers, 1989.
162. Siegel JH, Safrany L, Ben-Zvi J, Pullano WE, Cooperman A. Duodenoscopic sphincterotomy in patients with gallbladders in situ: report of a series of 1272 patients. *Am J Gastroenterol* 1988;83:1255–8.
163. Halver B. Endoscopic treatment of symptoms from gallbladder stones. Presentation, International Congress of gastroenterology and digestive endoscopy. Rome, 1988.
164. Siegel JH. Controversies, dilemmas, and dialogues. *Am J Gastroenterol* 1989;84:1356.
165. Fitzgerald PJ, Fortner JG, Watson RC, et al. The value of diagnostic aids in detecting pancreas cancer. *Cancer* 1978;41:868.
166. Mackie CR, Moosa AR, Go VLM, et al. Prospective evaluation of some candidate tumor markers in the diagnosis of pancreas cancer. *Dig Dis Sci* 1980;25:161.
167. Bender RA, Weintraub BD, Rosen SW. Prospective evaluation of two tumor-associated proteins in pancreatic adenocarcinoma. *Cancer* 1979;43:591.
168. Podolsky DK, McPhee MS, Alpert E, Warshaw AL, Isselbacher KJ. Galactosyltransferase isoenzyme II in the detection of pancreatic cancer: comparison with radiologic, endoscopic, and serologic tests. *N Engl J Med* 1981;304:1313.
169. Weickmann JL, Olson EM, Glitz DG. Immunological assay of pancreatic ribonuclease in serum as an indicator of pancreatic cancer. *Cancer Res* 1984;44:1682.
170. Kurihara M, Ogawa M, Ohta T, et al. Radioimmunoassay for human pancreatic ribonuclease and measurement of serum immunoreactive pancreatic ribonuclease in patients with malignant tumors. *Cancer Res* 1984;44:2240.
171. Magnani JL, Steplewski Z, Koprowski H, Ginsburg V. Identification of the gastrointestinal and pancreatic cancer-associated antigen detected by monoclonal antibody 19-9 in the sera of patients as a mucin. *Cancer Res* 1983;43:5489.

172. Brockhaus M, Wysocka M, Magnani JL, Steplewski Z, Kaprowski H, Ginsburg V. Normal salivary mucin contains the gastrointestinal cancer-associated antigen by monoclonal antibody 19-9 in the serum mucin of patients. *Vox Sang* 1985;48:34.
173. Lake-Bakaar G, McKavanagh S, Summerfield JA. Urinary immunoreactive trypsin excretion: a noninvasive screening test for pancreatic cancer. *Lancet* 1979;2:878.
174. Malesci A, Evangelists A, Mariani A, et al. CA 19-9 in serum and pancreatic juice: its role in the differential diagnosis of resectable pancreatic cancer from chronic pancreatitis. *Int J Pancreatol* 1988;Suppl 1:S119–23.
175. Tweedle DEF. Peroperative transduodenal biopsy of the pancreas. *Gut* 1979;20:992.
176. Siegel JH, Yatto RP. Approach to cholestasis—an update. *Arch Int Med* 1982;142:1877–9.
177. Siegel JH, Schapiro M, Hughes RW Jr. Endoscopy, obstructive jaundice, and DRG's: the buck stops in the hospital bank account. *Am J Gastroenterol* 1987;82:173–4.
178. Cotton PB, Denyer ME, Kreel L, Husband J, Meire HB, Lees W. Comparative clinical impact of endoscopic pancreatography, grey-scale ultrasonography, and computed tomography (EMI scanning) in pancreatic disease: preliminary report. *Gut* 1978;19:679.
179. Foley WD, Stewart ET, Lawson TL, et al. Computed tomography, ultrasonography, and endoscopic retrograde cholangiopancreatography in the diagnosis of pancreatic disease: a comparative study. *Gastrointest Radiol* 1980;5:29.
180. Moss AA, Federle M, Shapiro HA, et al. The combined use of computed tomography and endoscopic retrograde cholangiopancreatography in the assessment of suspected pancreatic neoplasm: a blind clinical evaluation. *Radiology* 1980;134:159.
181. Simeone JF, Wittenberg J, Ferrucci JT. Modern concepts of imaging of the pancreas. *Invest Radiol* 1980;15:6.
182. Siegel JH. Interventional endoscopy in diseases of the biliary tree and pancreas. *Mt Sinai J Med* 1984;51:535–42.
183. Moosa AR. Pancreatic cancer: approach to diagnosis, selection for surgery and choice of operation. *Cancer* 1982;50:2689.
184. Warshaw AL, Tepper JE, Shipley WU. Laparoscopy in the staging and planning of therapy for pancreatic cancer. *Am J Surg* 1985;151:76.
184a. Hirakawa TH, Fukumoto S, Shimada Y. Pancreatic biopsy under visual control in conjunction with laparoscopy for diagnosis of pancreatic cancer. *Endoscopy* 1989;21:105–7.
185. Nagy AG, James D. Diagnostic laparoscopy. *Am J Surg* 1989;157:490–3.
186. Snady H, Cooperman A, Siegel J. Endoscopic ultrasonography (EUS)—clinical utility and comparison to CT scan and ERCP in the evaluation of obstructive jaundice (OJ) and/or a perpancreatic mass (PM). *Gastrointest Endosc* 1989;35:169(abst).
187. Kaufman AR, Sivak MV. Endoscopic ultrasonography in the differential diagnosis of pancreatic disease. *Gastrointest Endosc* 1989;35:214–9.
188. Tio JL, Tytgat GNJ. Endoscopic ultrasonography in staging local resectability of pancreatic and periampullary malignancy. *Scand J Gastroenterol* 1986;21:135–42.
189. Parsons L, Palmer CH. How accurate is fine-needle biopsy in malignant neoplasia of the pancreas? *Arch Surg* 1989;124:681–3.
190. Kocjan G, Rode J, Lees WR. Percutaneous fine-needle aspiration cytology of the pancreas: advantages and pitfalls. *J Clin Pathol* 1989;42:341–7.
191. Gudjonsson B. Pancreatic carcinoma: diagnosis and therapeutic approach—a word of caution. *J Clin Gastroenterol* 1981;3:301–5.
192. Siegel JH, Snady H. The significance of endoscopically placed prostheses in the management of biliary obstruction due to carcinoma of the pancreas: results of non-operative decompression in 227 patients. *Am J Gastroenterol* 1986;81:634–41.
193. Cotton PB. Nonsurgical palliation of jaundice in pancreatic cancer. *Surg Clin North Am* 1989;69:613–27.
194. Silvis SE, Rohrmann CA, Vennes JA. Diagnostic accuracy of endoscopic retrograde cholangiopancreatography in hepatic, biliary, and pancreatic malignancy. *Ann Intern Med* 1976; 84:438.
195. Mizumoto K, Inagaki T, Koizumi M, et al. Early pancreatic duct adenocarcinoma. *Hum Pathol* 1988;19:242–4.
196. Reuben A, Cotton PB. Endoscopic retrograde cholangiopancreatography in carcinoma of the pancreas. *Surg Gynecol Obstet* 1979;148:179–84.
197. Pomerri F, Pittarello F, Muzzio PC. Pancreatic carcinoma; diagnostic ERCP. *Int J Pancreatol* 1989;3 Suppl 1:S131–6.
198. Siegel JH. Endoscopy and papillotomy in diseases of the biliary tract and pancreas. *J Clin Gastroenterol* 1980;2:337–47.
199. Thomas MJ, Pellegrini CA, Way LW. Usefulness of diagnostic tests for biliary obstruction. *Am J Surg* 1982;144:102–8.
200. Suramo I, Hyvarinen S, Kariralumo M. Gray-scale ultrasonography and jaundice. *Scand J Gastroenterol* 1980;15:705–9.
201. Shimizu H, Ida M, Takayama S, et al. The diagnostic accuracy of computed tomography in obstructive biliary disease: a comparative evaluation with direct cholangiography. *Radiology* 1981;138:411–6.
202. Matzen P, Haubek A, Holst-Christensen J, Lejerstofte J, Juhl E. Accuracy of direct cholangiography by endoscopic or transhepatic route in jaundice—a prospective study. *Gastroenterology* 1981;82:237–41.
203. Gilinsky NH, Bornman PC, Girdwood AH, Marks IN. Diagnostic yield of endoscopic retrograde cholangiopancreatography in carcinoma of the pancreas. *Br J Surg* 1986;73:539–43.
204. Manegold BC. Possibilities and limits of diagnostic and therapeutic ERCP in obstructive jaundice. *Chirurg* 1981;52:423–32.
205. Warshaw AL, Rutledge PL. Cystic tumors mistaken for pancreatic pseudocysts. *Ann Surg* 1987;205:393.
206. Series H, Cambon P, Choux R, et al. Chronic obstructive pancreatitis due to tiny (0.6 to 8 mm) benign tumors obstructing pancreatic ducts: report of three cases.
207. Siegel JH, Pullano W, Kodsi B, Cooperman A, Ramsey W. Optimal palliation of malignant bile duct obstruction: experience with endoscopic 12 French prostheses. *Endoscopy* 1988;20:137–41.
208. Shepherd HA, Royle G, Ross APR, Diba A, Arthur M, Colin-Jones D. Endoscopic biliary endoprosthesis in the palliation of malignant obstruction of the distal common bile duct: a randommized trial. *Br J Surg* 1988;75:1166–8.
209. Neff A, Fankuchen EI, Cooperman AM, et al. The radiological management of malignant biliary obstruction. *Clin Radiol* 1983;34:143–6.
210. Siegel JH, Ben-Zvi JS, Pullano W, Cooperman A. Effectiveness of endoscopic drainage for pancreas divisum: endoscopic and surgical results in 31 patients. *Endoscopy* 1990;22:139–33.
211. Madura JA. Pancreas divisum: stenosis of the dorsally dominant pancreatic duct. A surgically correctable lesion. *Am J Surg* 1986;151:742–5.
212. Delhaye M, Engelholm L, Cremer M. Pancreas divisum: congenital anatomic variant or anomaly? Contribution of endoscopic retrograde dorsal pancreatography. *Gastroenterology* 1985;89:951–8.
213. Mitchell CJ, Lintott DJ, Ruddell SJ, et al. Clinical relevance of an unfused pancreatic duct system. *Gut* 1979;20:1066–71.
214. Cotton PB. Congenital anomaly of pancreas divisum as cause of obstructive pain and pancreatitis. *Gut* 1980;21:105–14.
215. Wagner CW, Golladay ES. Pancreas divisum and pancreatitis in children. *Am Surg* 1988;54:22–6.
216. Soulen MC, Zerhouni EA, Fishman EK, Gayler BW, et al. Enlargement of the pancreatic head in patients with pancreas divisum. *Clin Imaging* 1989;13:51–7.
217. Staritz M, Meyer zum Buschenfeld KH. Elevated pressure in the dorsal part of pancreas divisum: the cause of chronic pancreatis? *Pancreas* 1988;3:108–10.
218. Bernard JP, Sahel J, Giovannini M, Sarles H. Pancreas divisum in a probable cause of acute pancreatitis: a report of 137 cases. *Pancreas* 1990;5:248–54.
219. Hayakawa T, Kondo T, Shibata T, et al. Pancreas divisum. A predisposing factor to pancreatitis? *Int J Pancreatol* 1989; 5:317–26.
220. Heiss FW, Shea JA. Association of pancreatitis and variant ductal anatomy: dominant drainage of the duct of Santorini. *Am J Gastroenterol* 1978;70:158–62.
221. O'Conner KW, Lehman GA. An improved technique for ac-

cessory papilla cannulation in pancreas divisum. *Gastrointest Endosc* 1985;31:13–17.
222. Siegel JH, Cooperman AM, Pullano W, Hammerman H. Pancreas divisum: observation, endoscopic drainage and surgical treatment. *Hepatogastroenterology* [In press].
223. Richter JM, Schapiro RH, Mulley AG, et al. Association of pancreas divisum and pancreatitis, and its treatment by sphincteroplasty of the accessory ampulla. *Gastroenterology* 1981;81:1104–10.
224. Warshaw AL, Richter JM, Schapiro RH. The cause and treatment of the pancreatitis associated with pancreas divisum. *Ann Surg* 1983;198:443–52.
225. Gregg JA, Monaco AP, McDermott WV. Pancreas divisum. Results of surgical intervention. *Am J Surg* 1983;145:488–92.
226. Cooperman M, Ferrara JJ, Fromkes JJ, Carey LC. Surgical management of pancreas divisum. *Am J Surg* 1982;143:107–12.
227. Bragg LE, Thompson JS, Burnett DA. Surgical treatment of pancreatitis associated with pancreas divisum. *Nebr Med J* 1988;73:169–73.
228. Adzick NS, Shamberger RC, Winter HS, Hendren WH. Surgical treatment of pancreas divisum causing pancreatitis in children. *J Pediatr Surg* 1989;24:54–8.
229. Warshaw AL, Richter JM, Schapiro RH. The cause and treatment of pancreatitis associated with pancreas divisum. *Ann Surg* 1983;198:443–52.
230. Brambs HJ, Schutz B, Wimmer B, Hoppee-Seyler P. Pancreas divisum as a possible cause of misinterpretation of ERCP, computed tomography, sonography and MDP. *ROFO* 1986; 144:273–7.
231. Fink AS, Perez de Ayala V, Chapman M, Cotton PB. Radiologic pitfalls in endoscopic retrograde pancreatography. *Pancreas* 1986;1:180–7.

PART III

Therapeutic Endoscopy

CHAPTER 10

Techniques; Biliary and Pancreatic Endoscopic Sphincterotomy: Standard, Wire Guided, Precut, Needle Knife

The development of endoscopic sphincterotomy reported by Kawai et al. in Japan and Classen and Demling in Germany pulled the endoscopist into a newly evolving category of interventional, or therapeutic, endoscopy (1,2). Although endoscopists and gastroenterologists had removed polyps and performed other types of invasive procedures such as liver biopsy and esophageal dilatation, incising the sphincter of Oddi using special accessories that incorporated electrocautery was a great departure from what was then perceived as therapeutic endoscopy. We are indeed grateful to the pioneers of endoscopy, whose foresight helped develop a technique that has ultimately supplanted the established surgical procedure of sphincteroplasty and introduced a unique method for exploration of the common bile duct (3–9).

The technique and method of performing sphincterotomy have changed very little since its initial descriptions, but the accessories used in the procedure have been modified to improve efficacy and safety. For example, shortening the length of the cutting wire of the sphincterotome has directly resulted in a decrease in the frequency of perforation.

Sphincterotomy is performed in sequence after completing the diagnostic ERCP; the sedated patient is positioned on a fluoroscope table in the left lateral recumbent or right oblique position, and a standard diagnostic duodenoscope, which has either a 2.8 mm or 3.2 mm channel, is advanced into the second position of the duodenum. The papilla is then identified and cannulated, and contrast material is injected into the ductular systems. A fluoroscopic image of the procedure is accomplished, and appropriate radiographs are obtained for documentation (10,11). After performing the diagnostic ERCP and confirming the specific indication for which a sphincterotomy is to be performed (e.g., stone or stricture), the endoscopist removes the cannula and inserts the sphincterotome into the duct of intention. In the majority of cases, this duct is the bile duct, and in most cases, sphincterotomy is performed for stone disease. Stone disease is followed in incidence and frequency by stenosis, stricture, and other obstructive lesions, such as cholangiocarcinoma, carcinoma of the pancreas, and ampullary carcinoma (Table 10.1). Prior to ERCP, the patient has undergone evaluation for other intercurrent medical problems that may require special medication or monitoring equipment such as cardiac drugs and prophylactic antibiotics. In addition to routine laboratory studies and coagulation profile, I request 2 units of packed red blood cells on hold or type and screen the patient in advance of the procedure in case a transfusion is necessary. Having the blood typed and/or available is important and avoids unnecessary delays in an urgent situation.

TABLE 10.1. *Indications and contraindications for endoscopic sphincterotomy (ES)*

Indications		Contraindications
Choledocholithiasis	Primary	Coagulopathy
	Recurrent	
	Retained	
Cholangitis		
Pancreatitis		
Cholestasis		
Jaundice		
Stenosis or stricture (distal and proximal)		
Cholangitis		
Pancreatitis		
Cholestasis		
Jaundice		
Tumor		
Cholangitis		
Pancreatitis		
Cholestasis		
Jaundice		

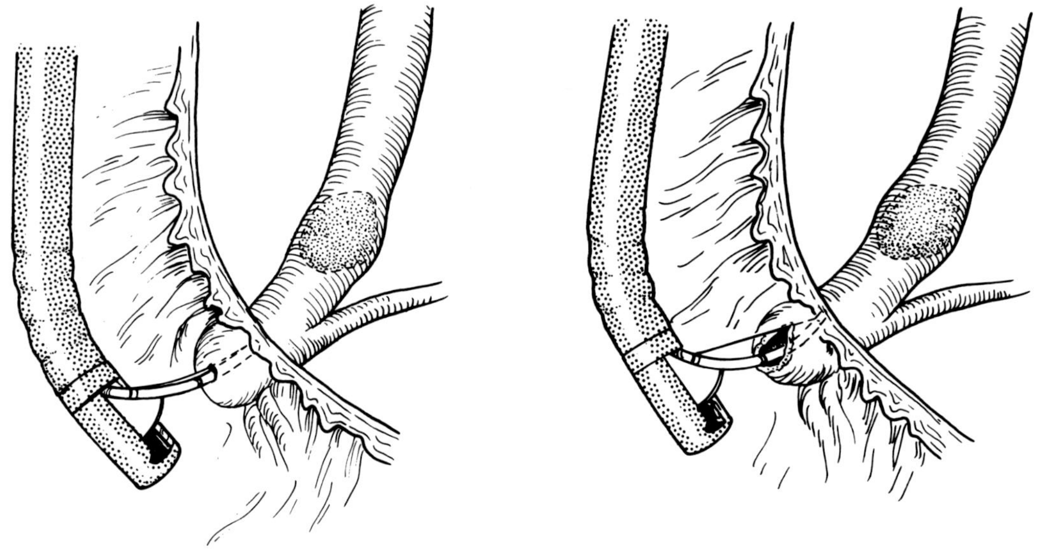

A B

FIG. 10.1. A: Insertion of the sphincterotome into the bile duct. Note the shorter cutting wire of the sphincterotome and the insertion of only one-third of the wire into the duct. Also note that the cutting wire does not extend beyond the intramural portion of the bile duct. **B:** A sphincterotomy incision being performed as a controlled, incremental incision is made.

Figures 10.1 through 10.3 demonstrate the insertion and correct orientation of a standard-type sphincterotome into the bile duct. The sphincterotome is positioned appropriately for completing an adequate incision, transecting the sphincter fibers so that a stone can be removed or can pass spontaneously or a prosthesis can be inserted. The incision is directed along the longitudinal axis of the intramural segment of the common bile duct but is limited to the length of the intramural segment, thus preventing perforation. An

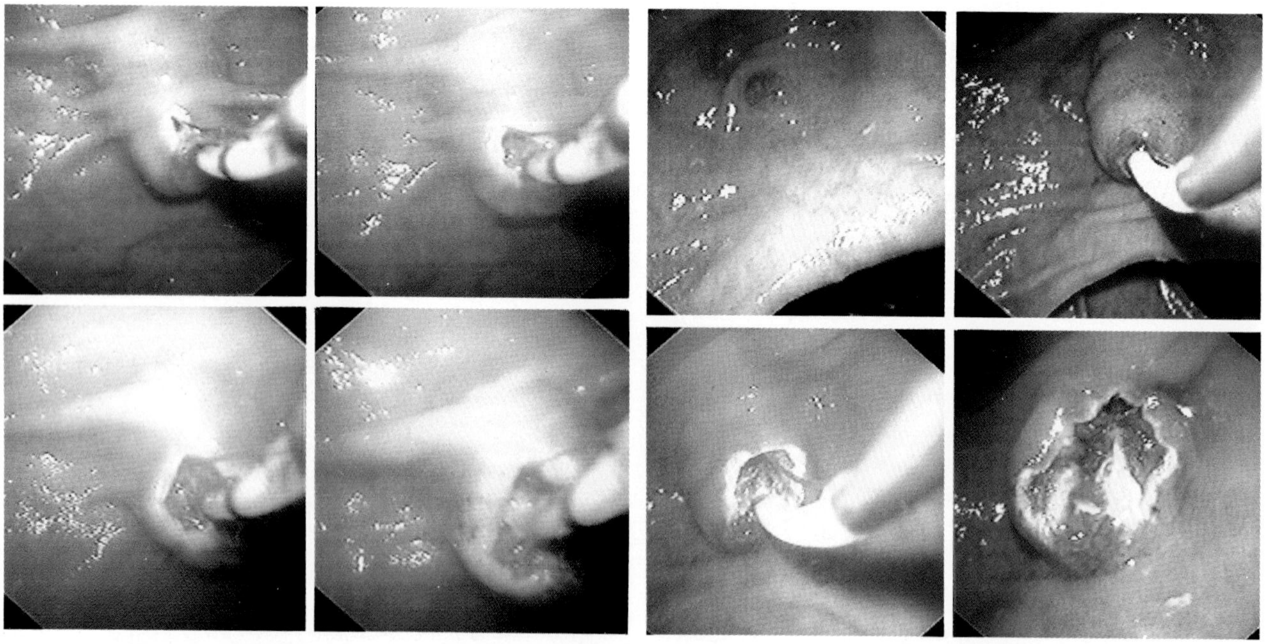

A B

FIG. 10.2. A: Videoendoscopic pictures of the correct insertion of a sphincterotome into the papilla. Note the short length of wire inserted into the duct. These videoendoscopic images demonstrate an incremental, controlled incision. The images illustrate the incision beginning at the top left and proceeding to the bottom right. Smoke is seen while the incision is being made. The smoke results from desiccation of the tissue as cautery current is applied. **B:** A prominent papilla and a periampullary diverticulum. The sphincterotomy incision is shown in sequence.

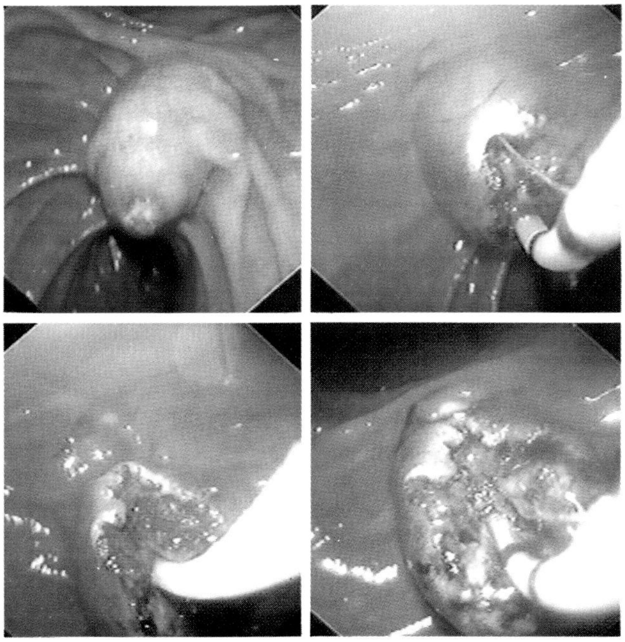

FIG. 10.3. This sequence of video images again illustrates the proper progression of a sphincterotomy incision, beginning at the top and progressing from left to right. This papilla is prominent and has a long intramural segment requiring an incision of approximately 13 mm to achieve complete transection of the sphincter fibers.

improvement in the sphincterotomes, which has enabled the endoscopist to avoid an over-generous incision resulting in retroperitoneal perforation, is the newer sphincterotomes that are constructed with only 20 mm to 25 mm of active wire for insertion into the sphincter. *The technique that permits the safe performance of a sphincterotomy and a precise incision requires free and selective insertion of the sphincterotome through the sphincter into the bile duct, allowing for complete control of this accessory.* Depending on the type of sphincterotome used (Fig. 10.4), the depth of insertion of the catheter will vary. For example, a long-nose sphincterotome (longer lead on the catheter) can be more deeply inserted because the cutting wire is more proximal to the tip of the catheter. The wire length, which must be known to the endoscopist, is identified by most manufacturers with colored markers that identify the length of the wire in millimeters. The midlength of the wire is generally identified on the catheter as a different color, double markings, or a broader marking distinct from the other catheter markings and indicates the half-way mark. The endoscopist can then withdraw the wire to the desired length of the incision, and even if the incision progresses more rapidly than intended, the "zipper" cut, the incision will not exceed the length of the wire inserted into the sphincter and bile duct, thus avoiding a possible perforation.

Endoscopists should familiarize themselves with all accessories and special equipment and have several sphincterotomes readily available and accessible in case one does not perform properly. Sphincterotomes are supposed to be standardized to exit the endoscope correctly oriented to the bile duct, but variations of accessories or the patient's anatomy exist. When ori-

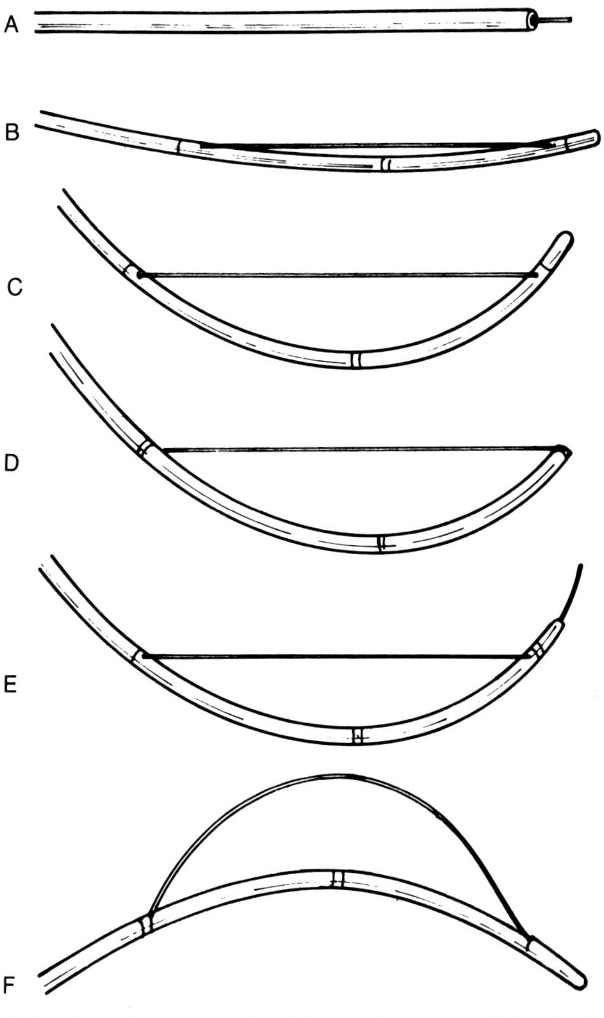

FIG. 10.4. The types of sphincterotomes available to the endoscopist. **A:** Thin wire needle knife. **B:** Standard sphincterotome with the cutting wire relaxed. **C:** Standard sphincterotome with the cutting wire flexed as it should appear during sphincterotomy. **D:** Precut sphincterotome with the cutting wire flexed. Note that the cutting wire of the precut sphincterotome is anchored at the distal tip of the catheter, permitting wire contact to the mucosa on initial insertion of the catheter. **E:** The guidewire extending from the lumen of the distal tip of the sphincterotome. **F:** Push-type sphincterotome used for performing sphincterotomy in patients who have previously undergone a gastric resection, Bilroth II type. Other types of spincterotomes not pictured are tapered sphincterotomes and long-nose sphincterotomes. The latter is advocated by some endoscopists who believe that the long catheter is advantageous because it ensures proper orientation of the sphincterotome in the bile duct.

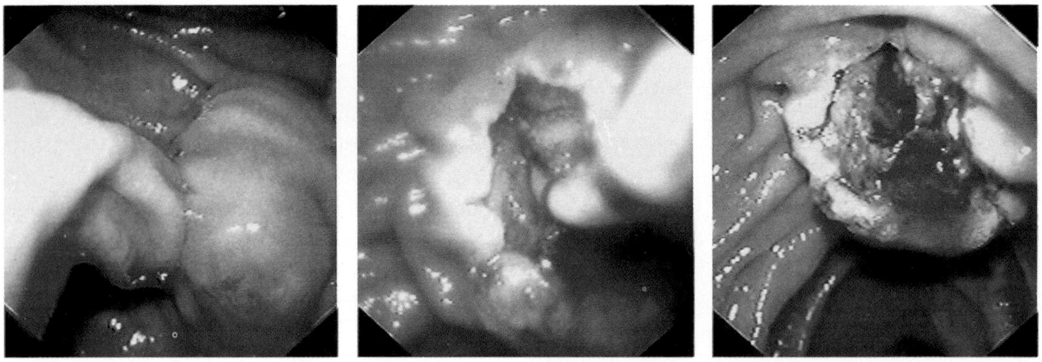

FIG. 10.5. Left: A videoendoscopic image of a prominent papilla during ERCP. **Middle:** A sphincterotomy being performed in the same patient. **Right:** The completed sphincterotomy. Note the generous length of the incision. The red color of the mucosa is the natural color of the bile duct mucosa. The yellow edges of the incision represent fibrous tissue, and these findings are compatible with papillary stenosis.

entation is improper, I advise using another sphincterotome until the orientation is correct. This latter adjustment may require using several sphincterotomes. Some manufacturers produce sphincterotomes that are supposed to be oriented toward the bile duct, whereas others produce rotatable sphincterotomes. I recommend that the endoscopist have several types of sphincterotomes available and in satisfactory working order before beginning the procedure to offer variety, especially in an unpredictable situation.

The length of the incision is critical to the ultimate success of the therapeutic endeavors, that is, satisfactorily relieving obstruction caused by papillary stenosis (Figs. 10.5, 10.6) or ampullary tumors (Fig. 10.7) or accessing the bile duct for removal of a stone. Earlier descriptions of the performance of sphincterotomy for stone disease recommended that the length of the incision approximate the size of the gallstone (4,7,8). I have found it difficult to make this approximation because the incision length cannot always be accurately measured, especially in the presence of edema or a short intramural segment. *The sphincterotomy incision should instead be made through all the sphincter fibers within the intramural segment (lower and upper) regardless of the stone size.* This is accomplished by extending the incision up to, but not through, the major horizontal fold crossing the intramural portion of the bile duct (Figs. 10.8, 10.9). If the incision is made up to or into this landmark, a true sphincterotomy or sphincteroplasty will be accomplished, and resultant stenosis or narrowing of the orifice will be minimal (Fig. 10.10).

A 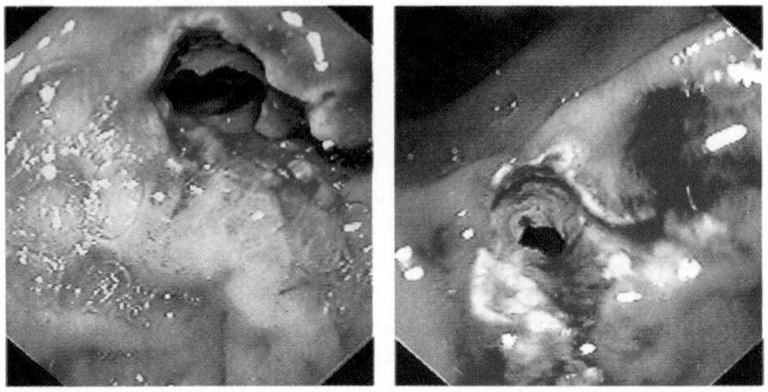 B

FIG. 10.6. A, B: Videoendoscopic images taken after completion of generous sphincterotomy incisions performed in patients with papillary stenosis. Note the presence of fibrous tissue within the incision.

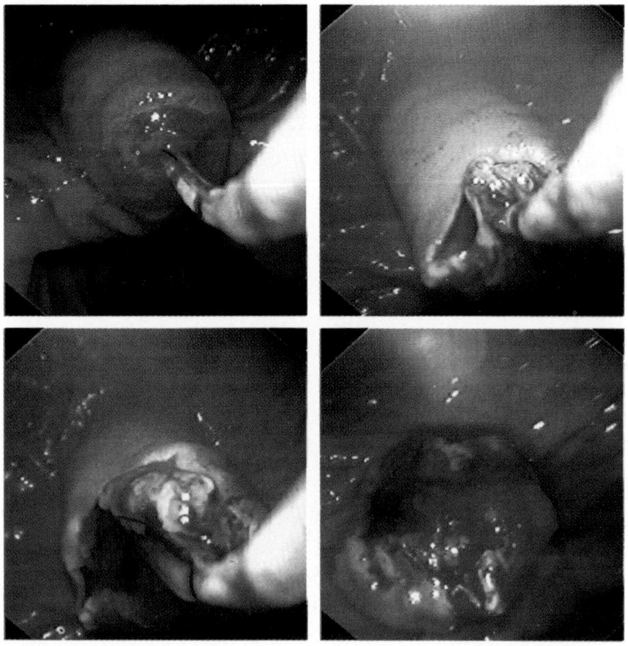

FIG. 10.7. Upper left: The initial examination and evaluation of a prominent papilla and insertion of a sphincterotome. **Upper right:** The progressive performance of a sphincterotomy incision. **Lower left:** Incision. One can appreciate nodular tissue contained within the ampulla. **Lower right:** After the sphincterotomy was completed, tumor tissue (nodular) is more apparent, and, on biopsy, was adenocarcinoma.

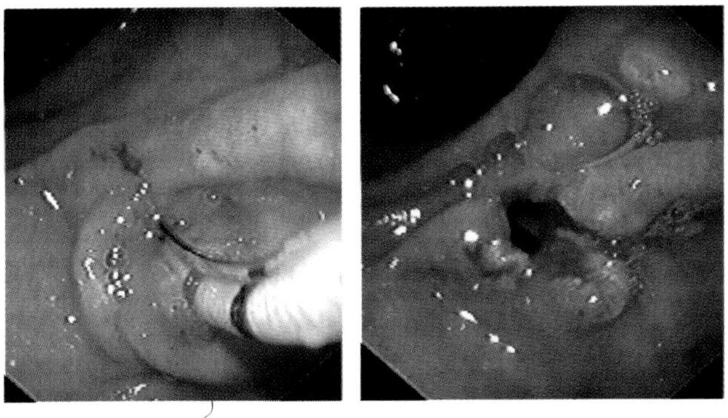

FIG. 10.8. **Left:** A papilla with a short intramural segment and several horizontal folds that make it difficult to decide the length of sphincterotomy incision to be made. **Right:** A photograph obtained after the sphincterotomy incision was made. Note the adequate opening, which resulted from a generous incision that extended into the major horizontal fold.

Occasionally, an endoscopist may encounter more than one horizontal fold (Fig. 10.11). The first fold may represent part of the hood of the papilla, and if the incision extends only to this point, a true sphincterotomy will not be the end result (Fig. 10.12). The endoscopist must approximate the length of the intramural portion of the bile duct; in my experience, this segment is more accurately identified after injection of contrast and filling of the distal common bile duct. After injection of contrast, one can better appreciate these anatomic landmarks, and a complete sphincter-

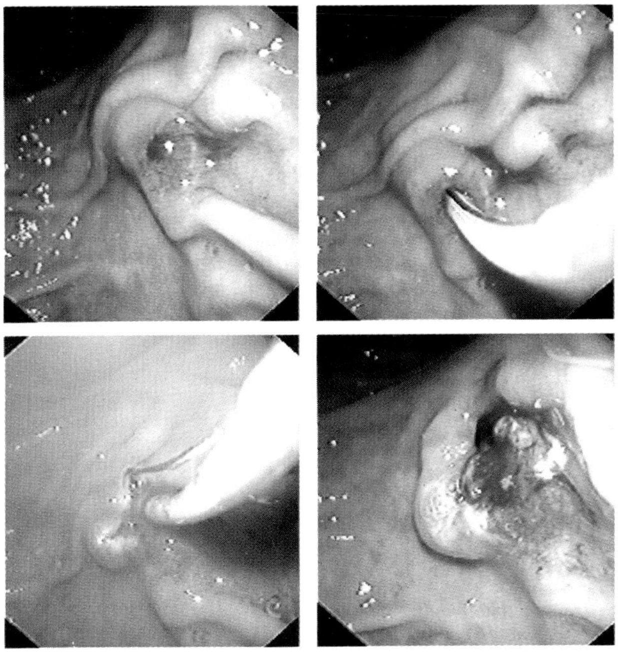

FIG. 10.9. **Upper left:** A papilla prior to insertion of a sphincterotome but after removal of the cannula, which accounts for the reddened papillary orifice. The intramural segment is modest but longer than that seen in Fig. 10.8. Note a horizontal fold crossing the middle of the papilla. **Upper right:** The correct insertion of the sphincterotome and the limited length of wire inserted, which is directed toward 11:00. Again, a horizontal fold traverses the midportion of the papilla. **Lower left:** The incision,with the orientation of the sphincterotome maintained. Note that less wire is inserted into the ampulla as the incision advances up toward the intramural segment. **Lower right:** The completed incision. Note that the incision extended into the major horizontal fold.

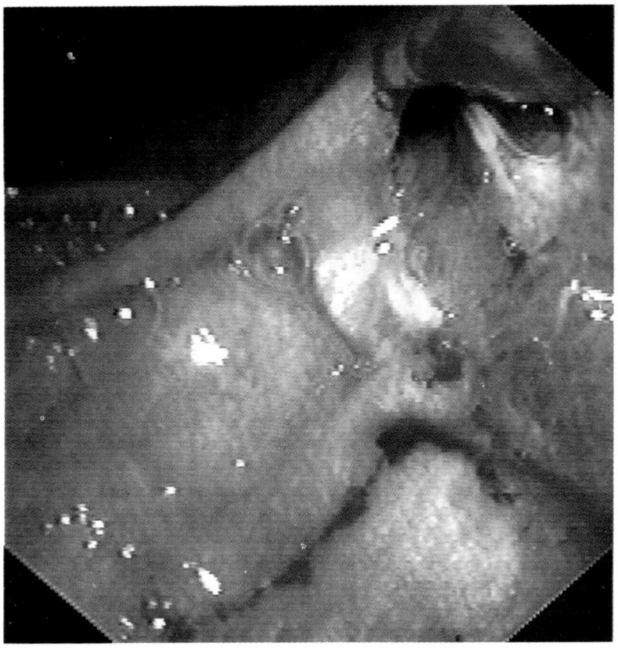

FIG. 10.10. Formation of a complete sphincterotomy. Note that the incision has extended into the horizontal fold and that a wide opening has been established.

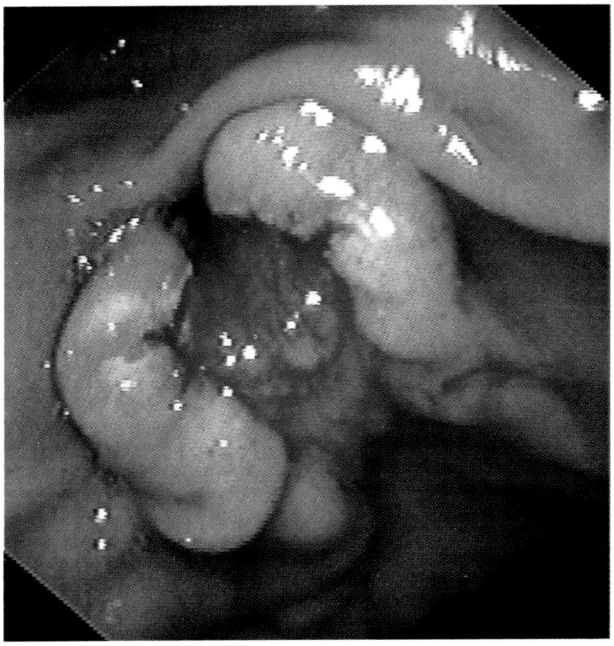

FIG. 10.11. A completed sphincterotomy that was formed by incising a mucosal fold overlying the papilla and extending it upward to the major horizontal fold.

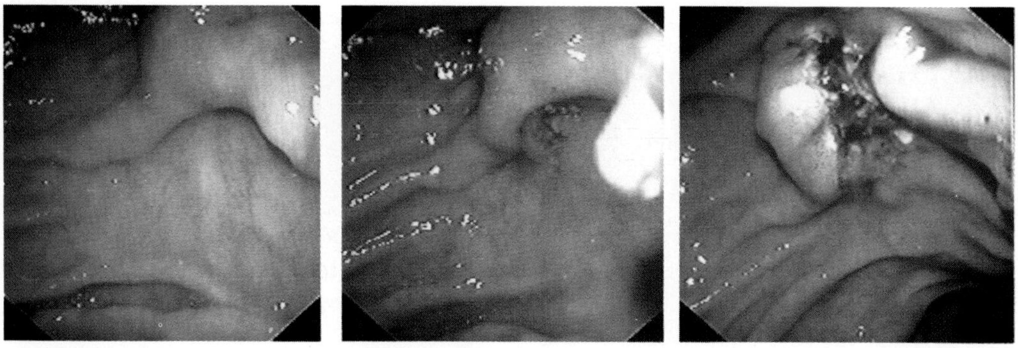

FIG.10.12. **Left:** A papilla with an overhanging fold obscuring the papillary orifice. **Middle:** The papilla after manipulating and moving of the fold using a catheter. **Right:** A completed sphincterotomy. The overlying mucosal fold was actually transected.

otomy can be safely performed. In order to prevent retroperitoneal perforation, the sphincterotomy incision must not extend through the proximal horizontal fold.

After the sphincter fibers have been served, regardless of the length of the incision, removal of a modest-sized stone can be accomplished even though the measured stone size may exceed the size of the incision. A larger stone can be pulled through a smaller sphincterotomy if the sphincter fibers have been transected, because the remaining intramural tissue is more pliable and relaxed and can be stretched when a larger stone is pulled through. This latter maneuver is analogous to the placement of forceps on the head of a neonate for delivery through an episiotomy.

With the current state of the art of mechanical lithotripsy (Chapter 11), there is little danger associated with capturing a stone in a basket and attempting to pull it through a sphincterotomy. If the sphincterotomy does not accommodate the stone and basket, a mechanical lithotriptor can be attached to the basket, the stone ultimately fragmented, and the apparatus removed (12–14). These new accessories have eliminated the formidable task of attempting to extract an impacted stone and basket and reduce the need for patient surgery. In nearly all cases, the basket can be broken when a mechanical lithotripsy apparatus is attached or the stone may be fragmented, permitting the basket to exit through the sphincterotomy.

SPHINCTEROTOMY USING A WIRE-GUIDED/ DOUBLE-LUMEN SPHINCTEROTOME

The success rate for the performance of sphincterotomy has increased with experience. Even in difficult situations, such as papillary stenosis and periampullary diverticula, the rate has improved (15). This has been largely due to improved endoscopes and accessories. One accessory, the wire-guided sphincterotome (Wilson-Cook, Olympus Corporation Microvasive Inc.) has contributed to this success (Fig. 10.13,

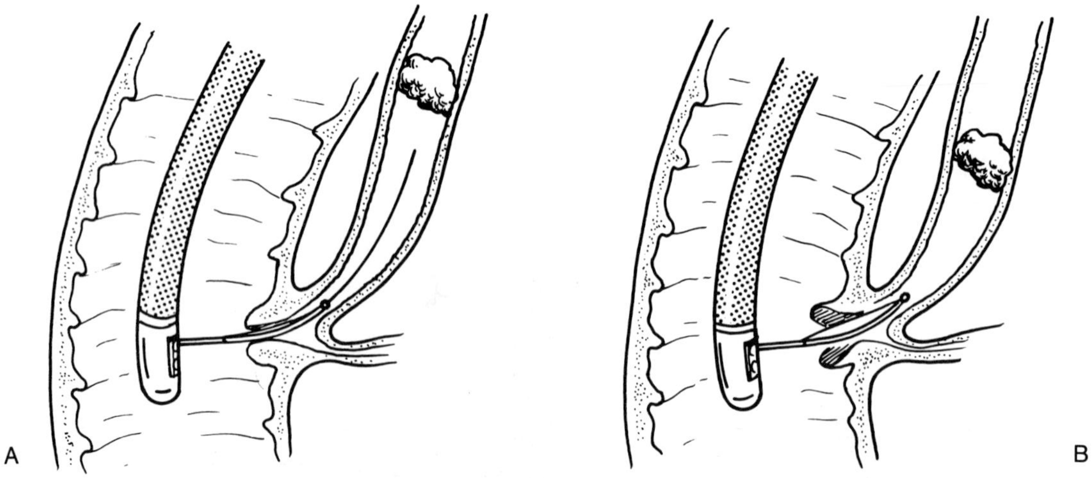

FIG. 10.13. **A:** A wire-guided sphincterotome being passed over the guidewire, which has already been inserted into the bile duct. A stone is visible in the proximal duct. **B:** The guidewire has been removed from the sphincterotome, and a sphincterotomy is being performed. Note the slight flexion applied to the sphincterotome wire as the incision is being made.

10.14). With this technique, a catheter-guidewire assembly is introduced through the sphincter into the bile duct when insertion of a sphincterotome has not been possible. The guidewire technique often facilitates entry into the bile duct (15). Once the guidewire is in place, the special sphincterotome is advanced over it and inserted into the sphincter. If the sphincterotome is a double-lumen type, which is insulated from active electrical power, the sphincterotomy can be performed with the wire in place (16). However, this is qualified, and most endoscopists remove the wire before using electrocautery. Theoretically, there should be no danger to the patient, and there is no danger of explosion from sparking. If the guidewire touches the sphincterotome wire, the sphincterotome wire disintegrates or gives the patient a harmless shock. A recent report described damage to the sphincterotome resulting from tension exerted by the opposed axes of the guidewire and the cutting wire of the sphincterotome (17). The authors of that report recommended removal of the guidewire before applying cautery current, and I support that recommendation because of a few uncomplicated yet definite shock reactions. If the single-lumen wire-guided type of sphincterotome is used (Microvasive Inc.), there is no insulation from the active wire because there is only one channel shared by both the guidewire and the active wire. Therefore, when using this system, the endoscopist should remove the guidewire before applying electrocautery to avoid an electrical short or shock. I am even skeptical of the so-called totally insulated wire because it too may shock. If this wire proves to be safe, I will alter my opinion and recommendation. Once the wire-guided sphincterotome is in place, a sphincterotomy may be performed in the same manner as when using the standard sphincterotome. This accessory has enabled me and my associates to complete a sphincterotomy in a safe manner in difficult situations (15).

The wire-guided sphincterotomy technique should be safer to perform than the precut sphincterotomy or needle-knife precut fistulotomy (18–22). Although the latter two procedures have an implied increased morbidity, their utility is necessary if neither the standard sphincterotome nor the guidewire can be selectively introduced into the papilla. Accessory manufacturers are currently producing thinner wire-guided sphincterotomes that are safer than earlier models. In my opinion, the 7Fr double-lumen sphincterotome, which is a larger caliber catheter containing a braided cutting wire, produces greater thermal energy and may cause more tissue injury. The incidence of postsphincterotomy pancreatitis is slightly higher in my experience with this device than that following sphincterotomy performed with a smaller appliance and a thin mon-

A 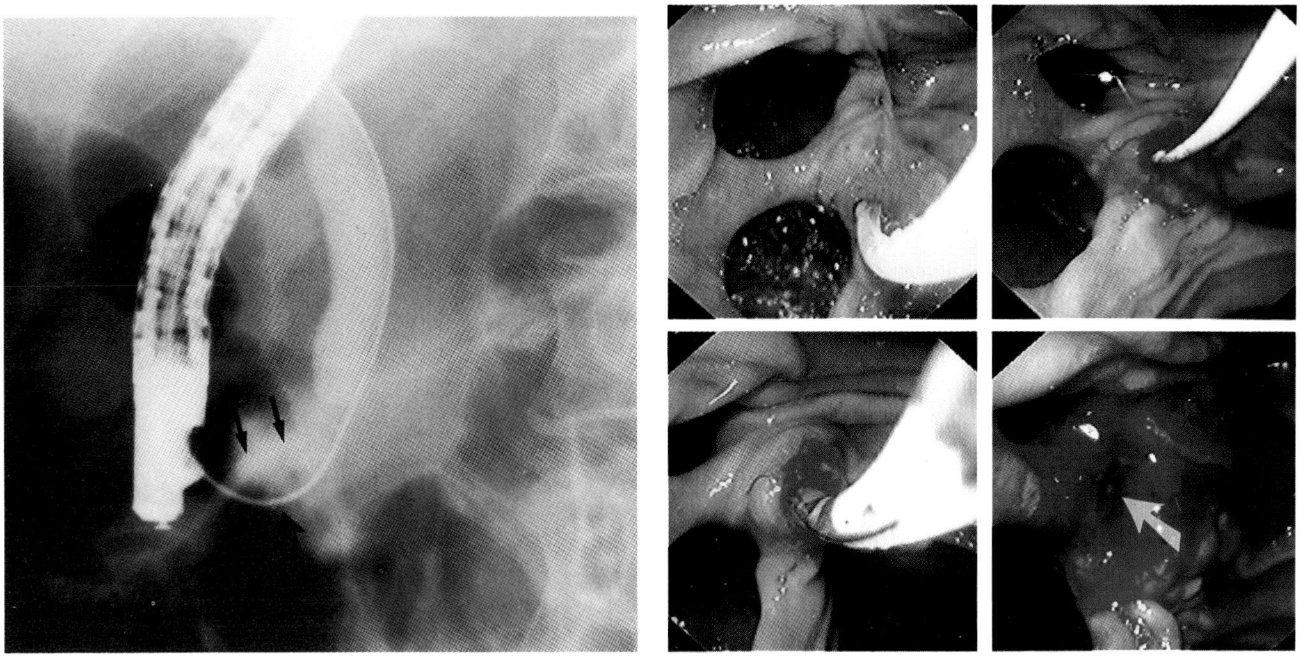 B

FIG. 10.14. A: A guidewire in place in an opacified bile duct. The sphincterotome has been advanced onto the guidewire (*dark arrow, lower*), and the cutting wire of the sphincterotome is identified by the two smaller arrows. **B:** A videoendoscopic sequence demonstrating the performance of a sphincterotomy using a wire-guided sphincterotome in a patient who has multiple periampullary diverticula. **Upper left:** A catheter has been deeply inserted into the bile duct. **Upper right:** The guidewire is in place. **Lower left:** The sphincterotome has been inserted. **Lower right:** The sphincterotomy has been completed. Clotted blood is visible on the sphincterotomy opening (*arrow*). No complications occurred despite the small amount of blood noted.

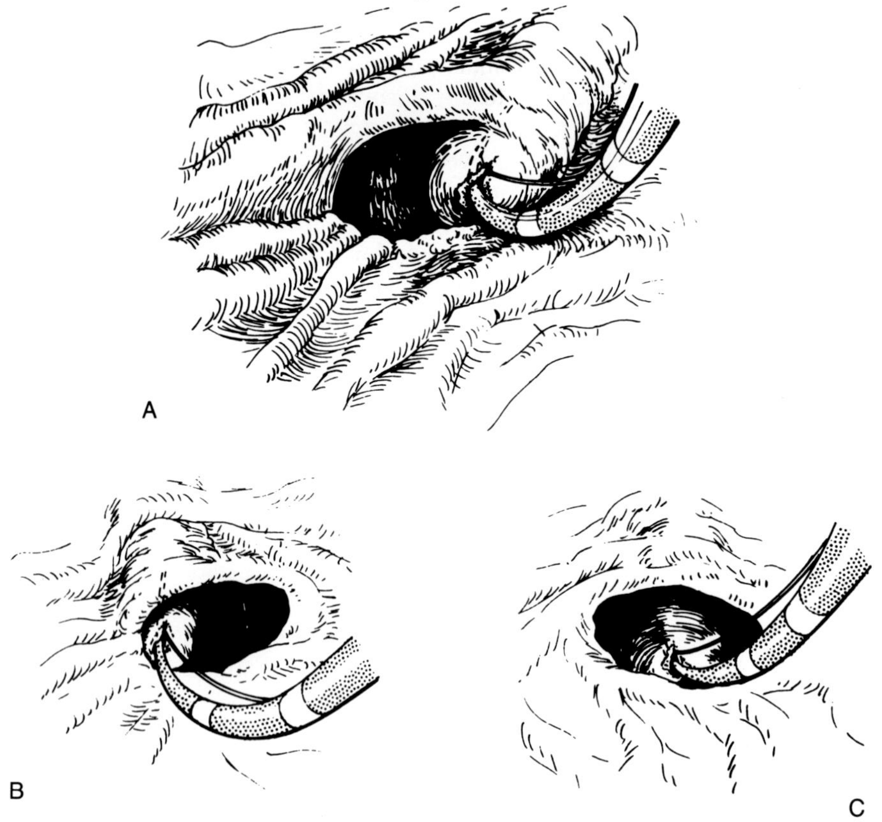

FIG. 10.15. A sphincterotomy. **A:** Periampullary diverticulum located medially. **B:** Diverticulum located laterally. **C:** A pantaloon type in which the papilla is centrally located.

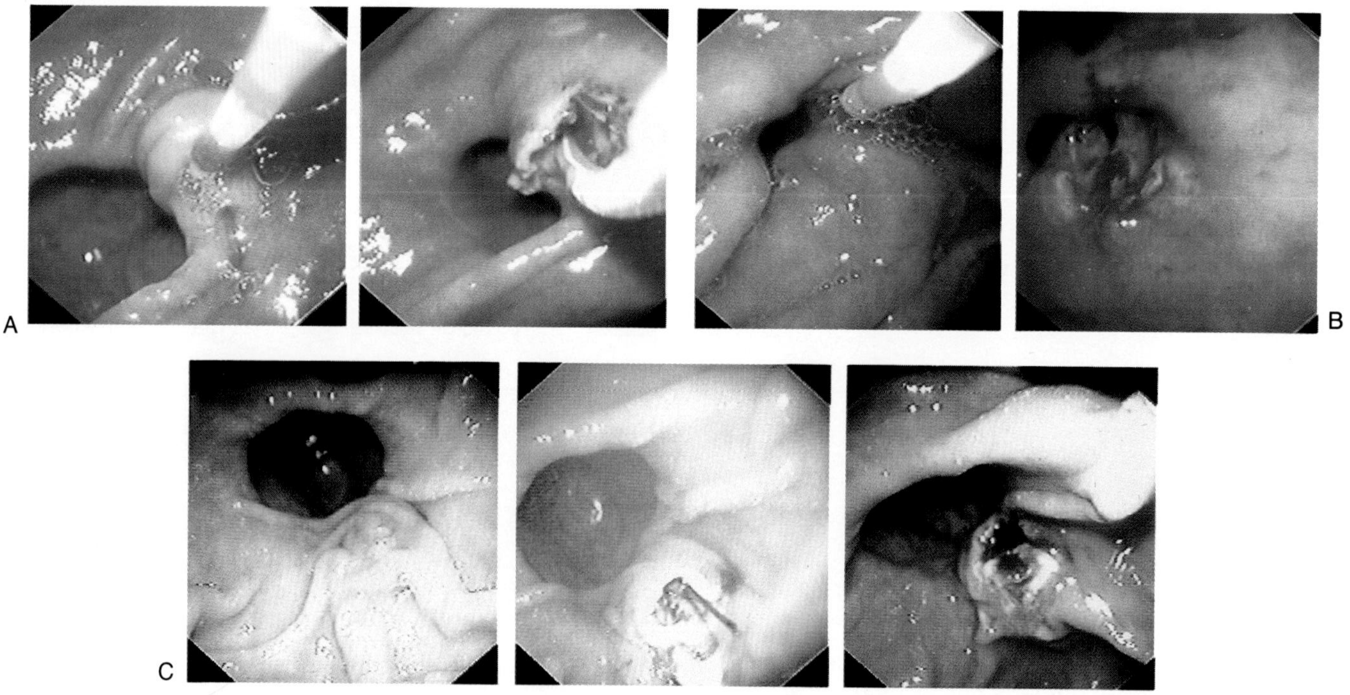

FIG. 10.16. A: The performance of a sphincterotomy in a patient with a medial wall periampullary diverticulum. **Left:** The papillary orifice being cannulated. **Right:** The sphincterotomy being performed. **B: Left:** Cannulation of the papilla, with a medial periampullary diverticulum. **Right:** A generous sphincterotomy. **C: Left:** The papilla visible on the inferior margin of a medial diverticulum. **Middle:** A sphincterotomy being performed. **Right:** A completed generous sphincterotomy.

ofilament cutting wire. I currently use a 6Fr double-lumen sphincterotome, modified by Wilson-Cook, which contains a monofilament wire. A similar style sphincterotome produced by Olympus Corporation is being investigated. I also use a wire-guided, single-lumen sphincterotome made by Microvasive that is performing flawlessly. The incision with these newly modified sphincterotomes is cleaner and is not delayed, and no pancreatitis has occurred. Use of these accessories has been a great benefit to endoscopists and has allowed a higher-than-expected rate of successful sphincterotomies. This accomplishment overshadows the slight increase in risk.

SPHINCTEROTOMY IN SPECIAL SITUATIONS

Periampullary Diverticula

The performance of sphincterotomy in the presence of a periampullary diverticulum may technically be more difficult to complete, but the failure rate in this situation has not been significant (23). Parenthetically, the complication rate for the performance of sphincterotomy in the presence of a periampullary diverticulum has not been significantly greater than the rate for sphincterotomies performed under standard conditions (23). One major reason for these favorable results is the fact that inexperienced endoscopists will not attempt a sphincterotomy in most difficult high-risk situations but instead refer such cases to more experienced endoscopists (Fig. 10.15). Diverticula, which are usually encountered in 18% of our caseload, may pose a technical problem, but complications have increased only minimally with their presence.

Regardless of the location of the papilla on the wall of the diverticulum, the incision extends to the edge of the diverticulum or at least to the point where the sphincterotome is no longer visible. Figure 10.16 is an example of a sphincterotomy being performed in a papilla that is located on the medial wall of the diverticulum. The limiting factors in performing a sphincterotomy in patients with periampullary diverticula may be the extent of the sphincterotomy and the inability to visualize the length of the incision. Similarly, these precautions are observed when performing a sphincterotomy in a patient with a periampullary diverticulum of the lateral wall (Figs. 10.17, 10.18). Again, the incision is carried as far as the visualized portion of

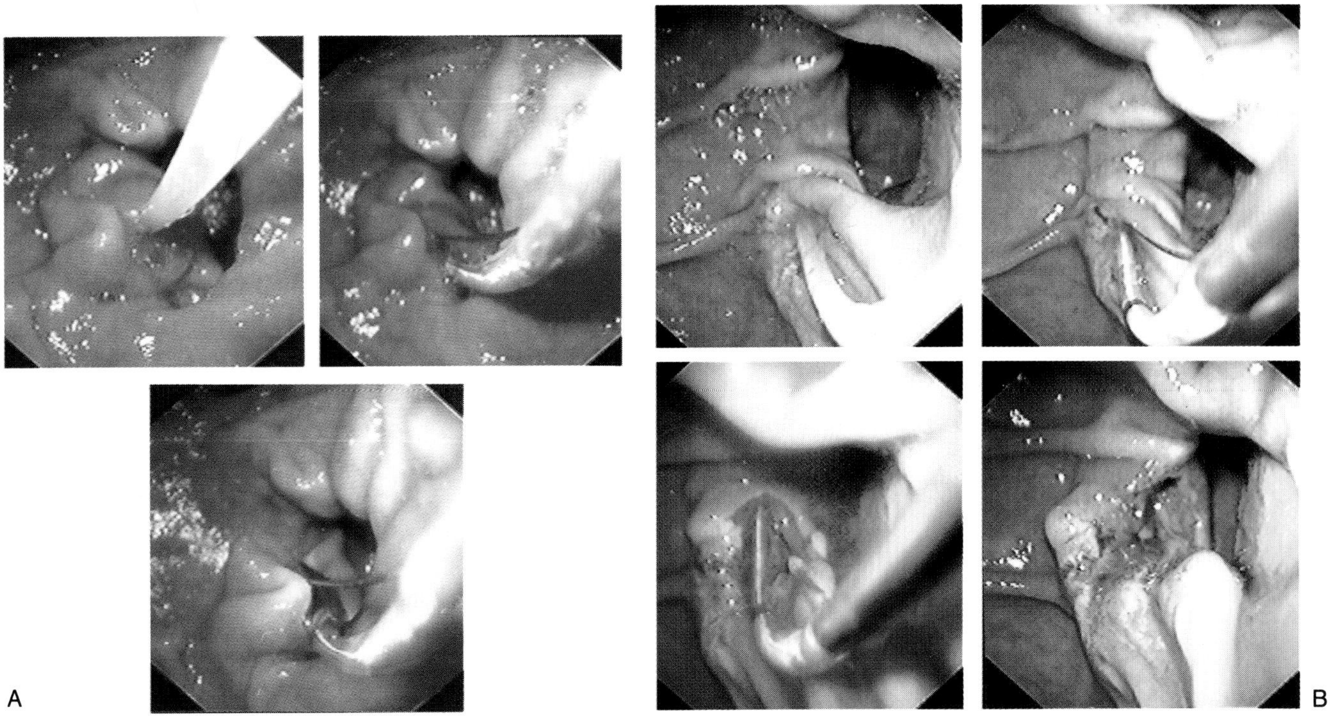

FIG. 10.17. A: The performance of a sphincterotomy in a patient with a lateral periampullary diverticulum. **Top left:** Cannulation of the papilla. **Top right:** The sphincterotome positioned properly for a sphincterotomy. Note the short length of wire inserted. **Bottom:** The sphincterotomy has been completed, and a dry incision has been made to the upper sphincter. The bile duct made up the medial wall of the diverticulum, and the incision was extended as far as possible or as far as the visual limits. **B:** A series of video pictures showing the sequential performance of a sphincterotomy in a patient with a lateral diverticulum. **Upper left:** The cannula has been inserted into the bile duct. **Upper right:** The sphincterotomy is being started. Note the length of wire outside the bile duct, which will avoid injury to the bowel wall. **Lower left:** The sphincterotomy is nearly completed. Note that the distal portion of the wire is used to complete the incision. **Lower right:** The completed incision, which measures 1.3 cm.

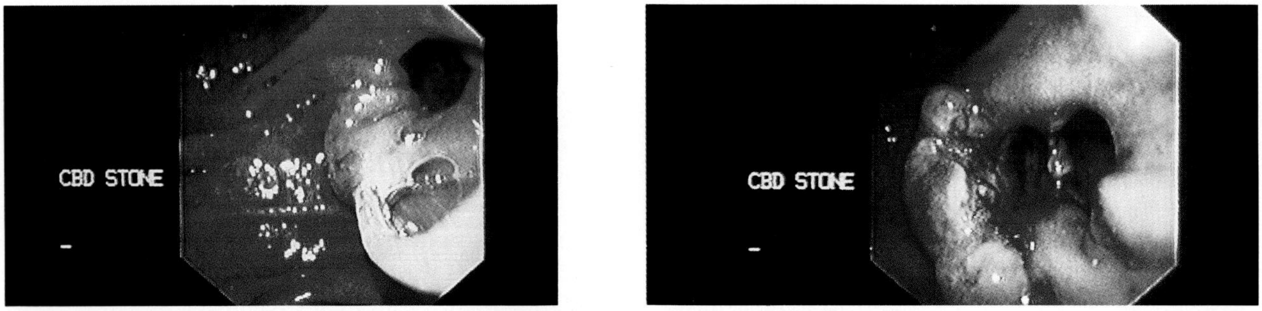

A

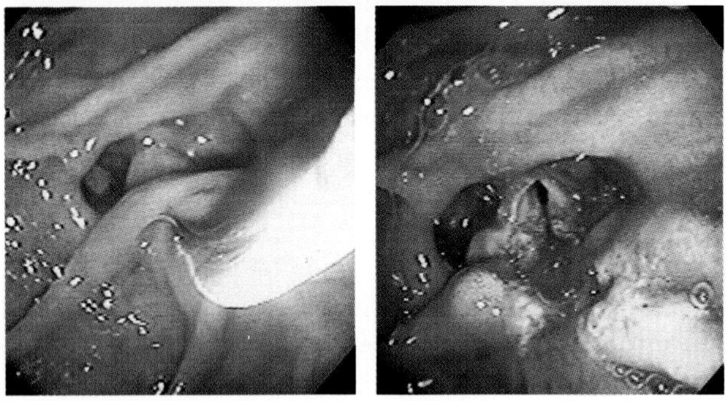
B

FIG. 10.18. **A: Left:** Selective cannulation of the bile duct, which is located medially to a diverticulum (lateral periampullary diverticulum). **Right:** After a very gracious sphincterotomy, only a thin septum of the wall of the diverticulum remains. In this picture, one cannot distinguish the diverticulum opening from the large sphincterotomy. **B: Left:** A sphincterotome is in place in preparation for a sphincterotomy in this example of a central or pantaloon diverticulum. Note the horizontal fold proximal to the bulge of the contrast-filled bile duct. **Right:** The completed sphincterotomy incision, which extended deeply into the diverticulum but only into that portion in which the inferior wall was shared with the bile duct.

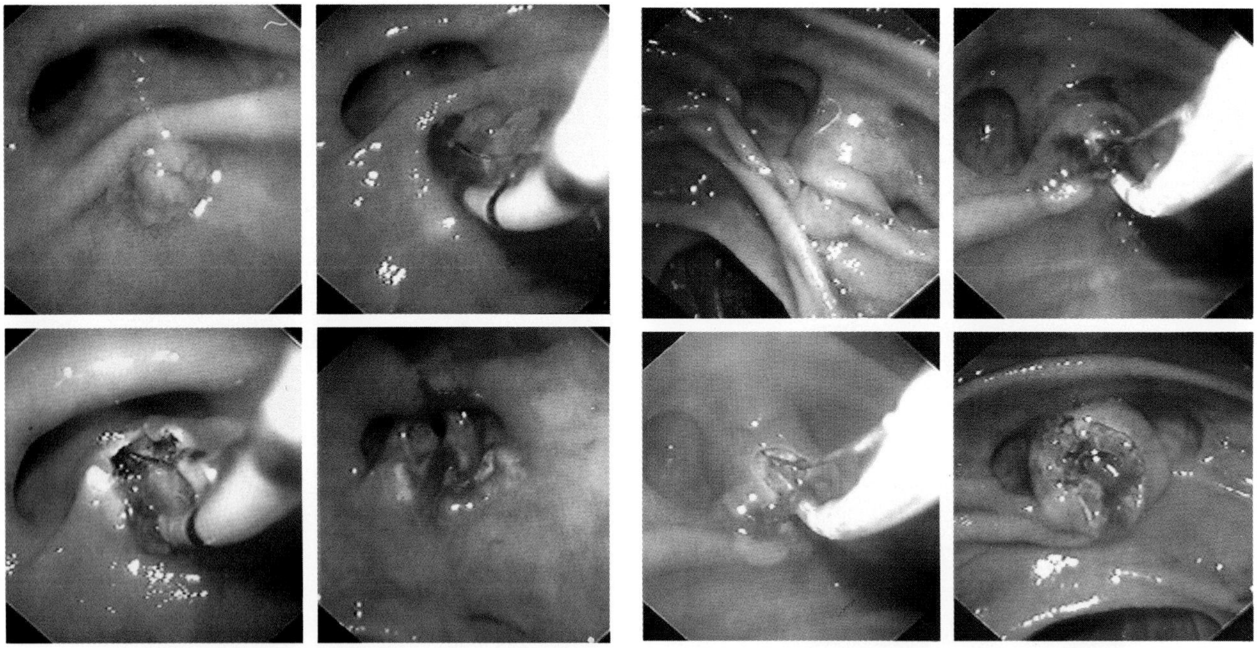
A B

FIG. 10.19. A: A sequence of video images depicting a pantaloon diverticulum, cannulation, and sphincterotomy. **Upper left:** The papilla is located inferior to a fold. The bile duct traverses cephalad between the two holes, which is the landmark necessary to determine the length of the incision. **Upper right:** The sphincterotome has been inserted into the duct, and a short length of wire is left to make contact and to avoid a zipper cut in this risky situation. **Lower left:** The sphincterotomy has extended through the horizontal fold. **Lower right:** The completed sphincterotomy. **B:** Another example of the performance of a sphincterotomy in a pantaloon diverticulum. From top left to bottom right, the sequence progresses with a generous sphincterotomy. Note the short length of wire inserted into the duct to prevent perforation should a zipper cut ensue.

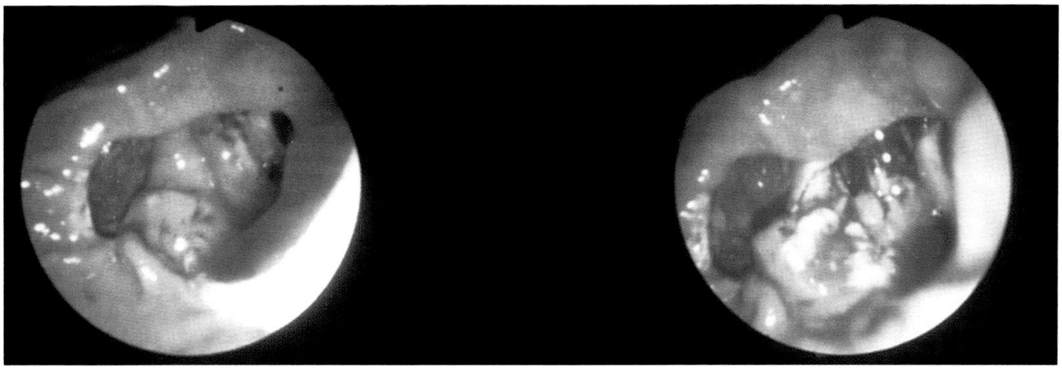

FIG. 10.20. Left: Another example of a pantaloon diverticulum. The opening to the papilla, which is located most inferiorly, is being cannulated. **Right:** After an adequate sphincterotomy, one can appreciate the upper limit of the incision.

the bile duct. The same principle applies to the performance of a sphincterotomy in a pantaloon diverticulum (Fig. 10.19). In this situation, the papilla and bile duct are located in the center of the diverticulum cavity, creating the impression of a double diverticulum. In general, the bile duct is within the partition, and the incision is carried to the uppermost portion of the visualized bile duct (Fig. 10.20).

In my experience, large stones can be removed intact from a bile duct in which the sphincter is contained in (or around) a diverticulum because anatomically, part of the supporting wall of the sphincter is absent, and fewer muscle fibers constitute the sphincter mechanism. Therefore, a stone can either be entrapped in a basket or extracted using an occlusion balloon, and it can be withdrawn more easily from the duct in which an incision has been made through a sphincter contained in a periampullary diverticulum than from an intact bile duct that is not part of a periampullary diverticulum.

Double-Lumen or Wire-Guided Sphincterotome

Safe alternative techniques that allow for the performance of a sphincterotomy in the presence of a periampullary diverticulum when a sphincterotome cannot be selectively or easily inserted have been reported (15,24). One method requires selective cannulation of the bile duct using a catheter-guidewire assembly (Fig. 10.14B). With this technique, a double-lumen or wire-guided sphincterotome is advanced over the guidewire, and the sphincterotomy is performed as previously described. The wire-guided technique is performed in a more controlled fashion, accounting for lower morbidity.

Endoprosthesis—Needle Knife

The author has introduced another safe technique for performing sphincterotomy in patients with periampullary diverticula. This new method requires placing a prosthesis into the bile duct and subsequently using a needle knife to perform the sphincterotomy (24) (Fig. 10.21). This technique permits the endoscopist to perform a sphincterotomy over a prosthesis, which reduces the probability of perforation or misadventure because the prosthesis defines the location and position of the bile duct in or around the diverticulum, and its presence in the duct and intramural portion of the duct provides a guide that can be safely followed.

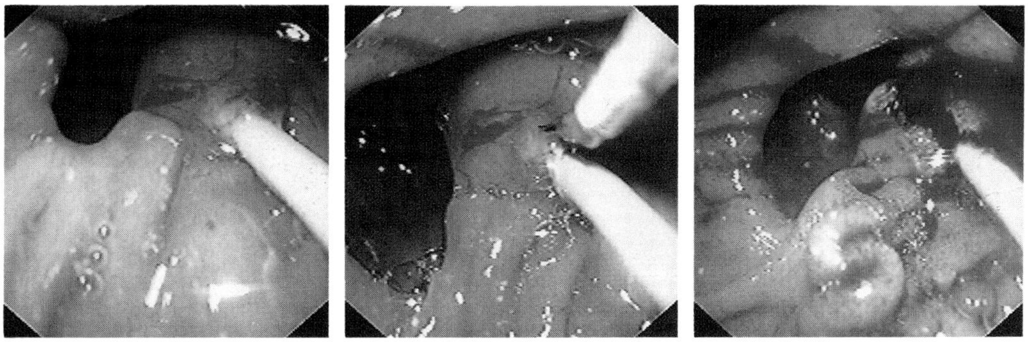

FIG. 10.21. Left: An endoprosthesis exiting from the papilla. A medial periampullary diverticulum is evident. **Middle:** A needle knife poised to begin performing a sphincterotomy. **Right:** The completed incision. Some blood is noted, but the large incision can be identified.

Percutaneous Prosthesis—Needle-Knife or Standard Sphincterotome

In collaboration with others, I described a technique for performing sphincterotomy in patients with periampullary diverticula using a prosthesis that had been advanced percutaneously through the bile duct into the duodenum (25). Again, the principle for this approach is the same as that when an endoprosthesis has been placed; that is, an incision is made over the external or internal prosthesis protecting the duodenal wall. Therefore, if a standard sphincterotomy cannot be performed, I recommend using either of the techniques—insertion of an endoprosthesis (Fig. 10.21) or a percutaneous one—to facilitate sphincterotomy (Fig. 10.22). However, the percutaneous technique is associated with a higher morbidity rate because of the approach through the liver, which requires liver puncture. In experienced hands, the morbidity rate of percutaneous procedures is declining.

Sphincterotomy, Bilroth II Gastrectomy

Performance of sphincterotomy in patients who have undergone gastric resection, Bilroth II, is difficult to accomplish because of the altered anatomy, gastrojejunostomy, created by this operation. A Bilroth I resection, however, in which a foreshortened stomach is present because of the performance of an antrectomy and end-to-end gastroduodenostomy, does not pose a major hindrance to the performance of ERCP or sphincterotomy. Access to the papilla in the Bilroth I patient is straight on as opposed to the Bilroth II anatomy, in which a circuitous route must be followed through the tortuous and redundant afferent limb of the gastrojejunostomy. In the Bilroth II resection, the gastric pouch is anatomosed in an end-to-side fashion with the jejunum creating efferent and afferent limbs (Fig. 10.23). The intention of the endoscopist is to locate the afferent stoma, which is more often the orifice located proximally and posteriorly on the enterostomy. The endoscope is advanced into the afferent limb, which is usually identified by the presence of bile, whereas the efferent limb is usually dry because the patient has been fasting for several hours. As the endoscope is advanced proximally through the afferent limb into the jejunum and duodenum, bile should be more evident. Injury to the bowel wall (perforation) can occur while negotiating the tortuous jejunum, which is due to fixation of the bowel by adhesions or to injury and disruption of the anastomosis. Caution is recommended when advancing the endoscope in patients who have previously undergone gastric resection. If the procedure is unusually painful to the patient or difficult for the endoscopist, the procedure should be aborted in order to avoid misadventure.

I prefer to use the duodenoscope, which is my primary instrument for performing ERCP in patients who have undergone Bilroth II resections (26). But if negotiating the acute angles of the anastamosis with the duodenoscope is too difficult or painful to the patient (sometimes noticed when using the electronic—video—duodenoscopes because the rigid distal tip of the endoscope is longer owing to the placement of the video chip and its components), a forward-viewing instrument, either a gastroscope or pediatric colonoscope, is recommended. Some endoscopists prefer a forward-viewing instrument and have enjoyed great success with that instrument, but I am more comfortable with the duodenoscope because it is longer than the gastroscope (the extra length is necessary in patients who have long and tortuous afferent limbs). Also, it has an elevator for manipulating accessories, which is important to me, and I use it as my primary instrument. Other techniques for negotiating the afferent limb, identifying the papilla, cannulating it, and performing sphincterotomy have been described in various references (27–33). Endoscopists should re-

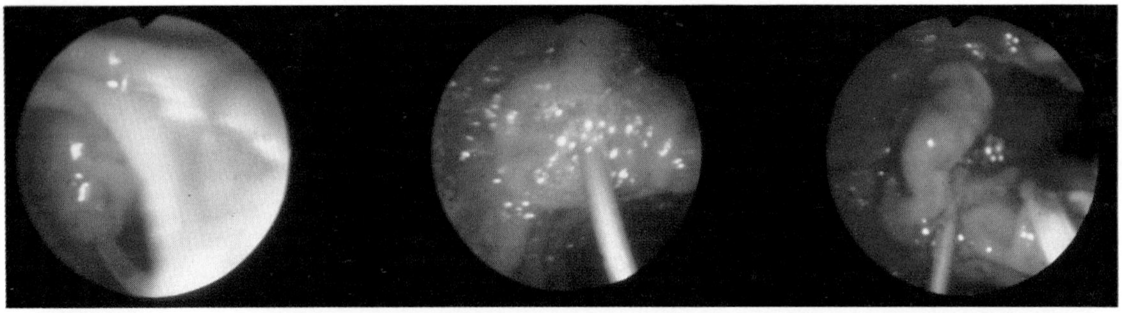

FIG. 10.22. Left: The papilla located within a diverticulum. The cannula was inserted, and a cholangiogram was accomplished. **Middle:** Because the upper limits of the papilla could not be seen and the sphincterotome could not be inserted freely, a percutaneous catheter was placed through the liver, down the bile duct, and into the duodenum. **Right:** After placing the percutaneous drain, the papilla was pushed into the duodenum for a safer approach, the sphincterotome was inserted, and a sphincterotomy was performed.

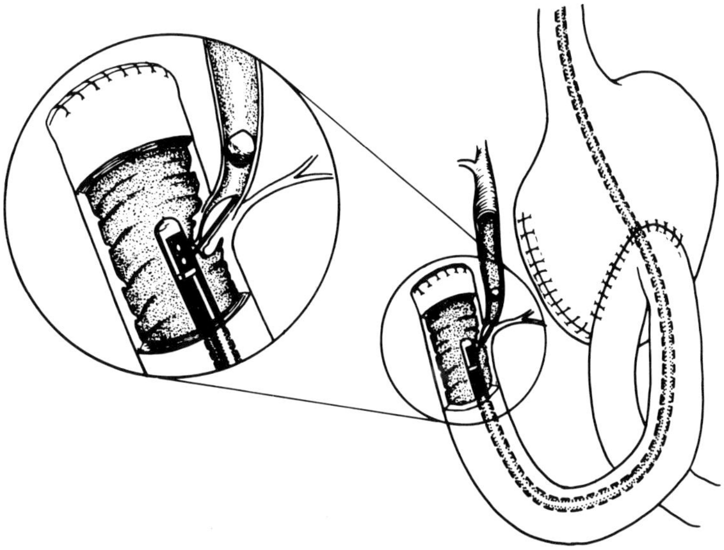

A

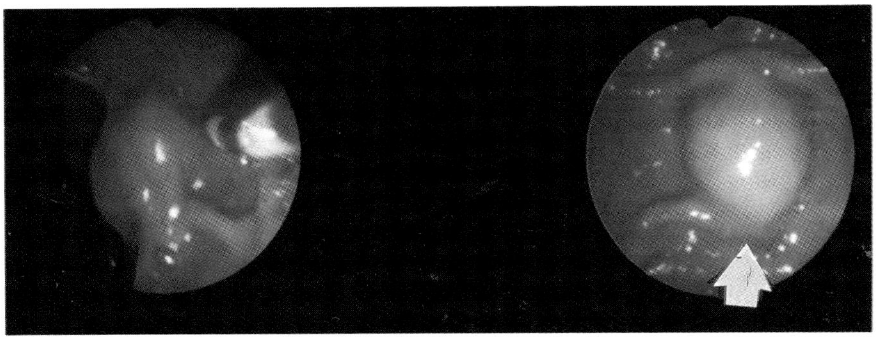

B

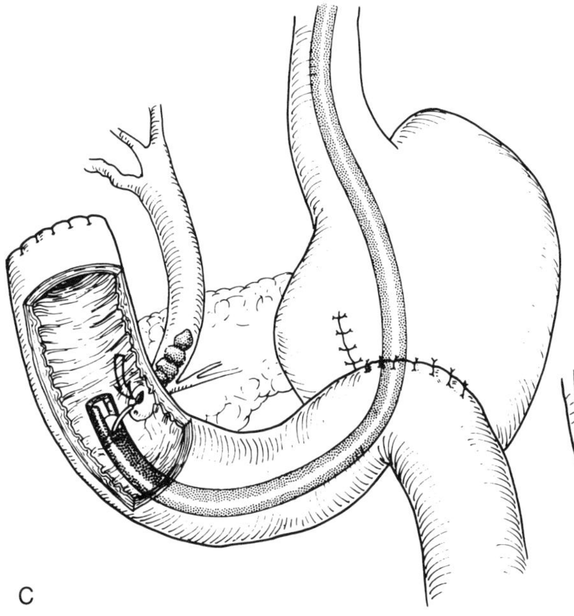

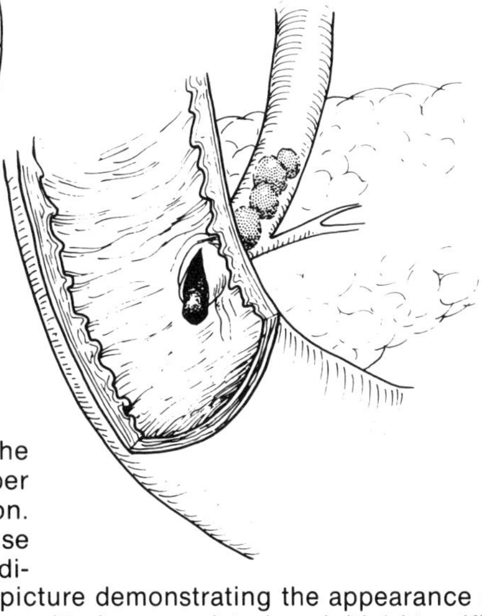

C

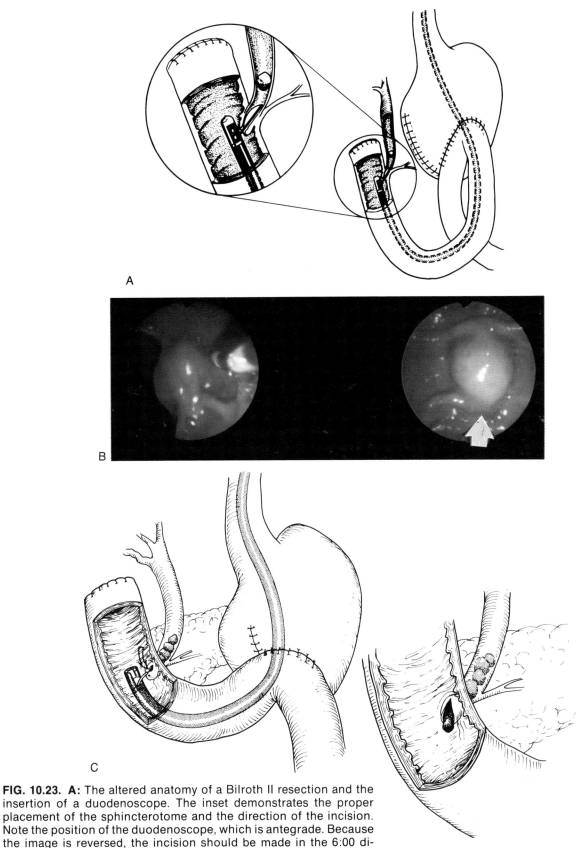

FIG. 10.23. A: The altered anatomy of a Bilroth II resection and the insertion of a duodenoscope. The inset demonstrates the proper placement of the sphincterotome and the direction of the incision. Note the position of the duodenoscope, which is antegrade. Because the image is reversed, the incision should be made in the 6:00 direction. (From ref. 26, with permission.) **B: Left:** An endoscopic picture demonstrating the appearance of the papilla when first approached in a retrograde fashion. The apex of the papilla is appreciated on initial identification of the mound. **Right:** Cannulation of the papilla (*arrow*) is accomplished after rotating the endoscope to visualize the orifice. **C: Left:** The Bilroth II anatomy depicting common bile duct stones. A needle knife is seen creating a fistulotomy-sphincterotomy. **Right:** After completion of the sphincterotomy, the stones are permitted to pass spontaneously.

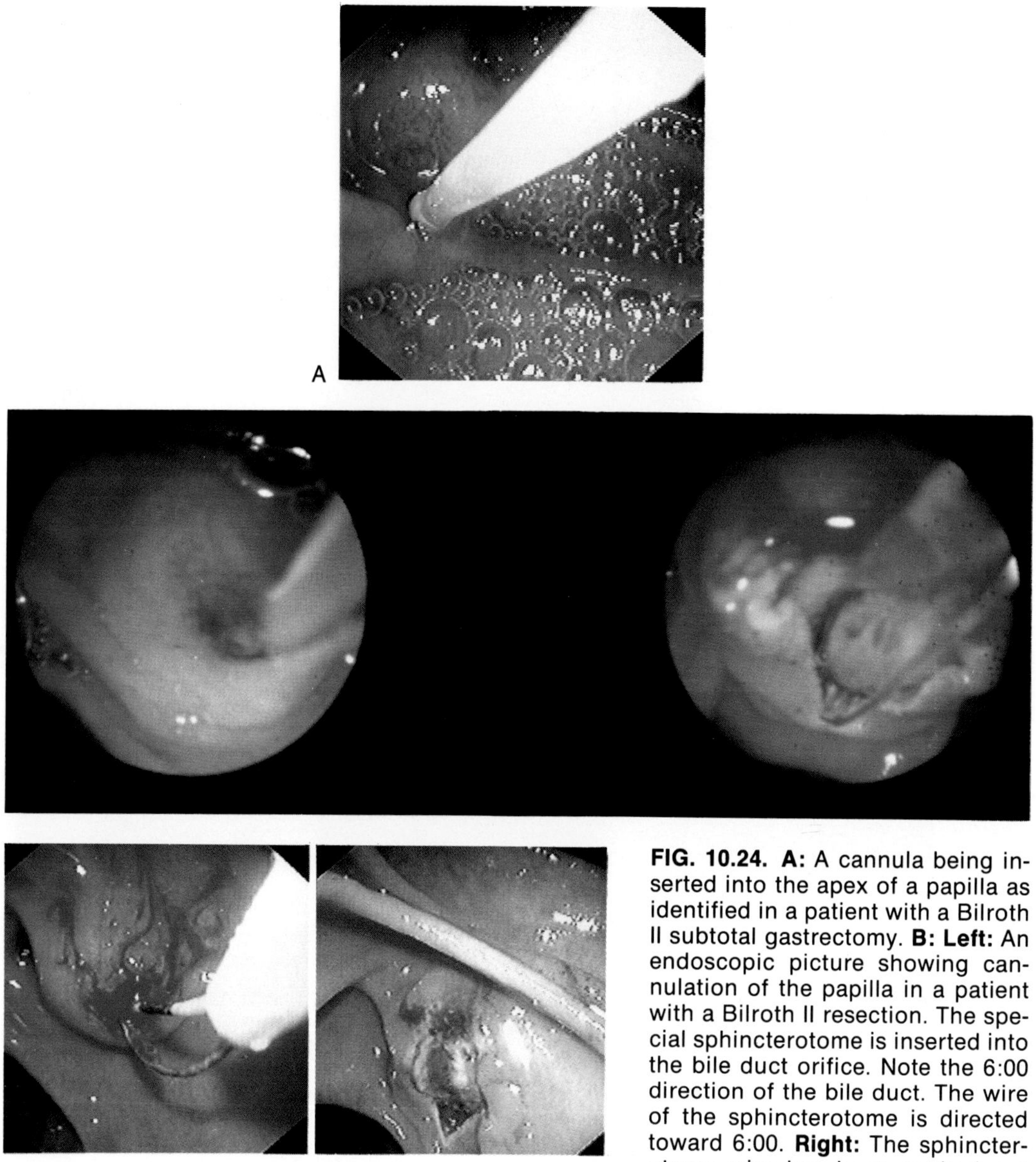

FIG. 10.24. A: A cannula being inserted into the apex of a papilla as identified in a patient with a Bilroth II subtotal gastrectomy. **B: Left:** An endoscopic picture showing cannulation of the papilla in a patient with a Bilroth II resection. The special sphincterotome is inserted into the bile duct orifice. Note the 6:00 direction of the bile duct. The wire of the sphincterotome is directed toward 6:00. **Right:** The sphincterotome wire has been pushed out and bowed downward. The incision is in progress. **C: Left:** Cannulation of the papilla and selective insertion of a Bilroth II sphincterotome in the bile duct. The wire has been pushed out, and, by design, bows downward toward 6:00. **Right:** After the incision, the completed sphincterotomy is visible.

view all the endoscopic techniques and descriptions for approaching the surgically altered stomach to improve proficiency.

In patients with Bilroth II resections, the papilla is located more laterally and inferiorly on the duodenal wall. This orientation is due to the retrograde approach of the endoscope (retrograde from the anastamosis through the jejunum and into the duodenum). The appearance of the papilla can be misleading, and the endoscopist should be completely familiar with the retrograde approach. Optically, the papilla is upside-down or reversed from the usual appearance; the bile duct, in this configuration, should be at the most inferior aspect of the papilla, at 6:00 which is opposite that of routine, antegrade duodenoscopy (Fig. 10.23).

The cannula is advanced and placed at the 6:00 position, and the papilla is palpated in an effort to cannulate the bile duct selectively (Fig. 10.23). The pancreatic duct orifice should be located more superiorly on the papilla, near the center of the mound (similar to its location for standard cannulation).

Because most cannulas, catheters, and sphincterotomes assume an upward curve (toward 12:00), I prefer using a new catheter. A new catheter should exit the endoscope at a less acute angle and make it easier to enter the bile duct, which is located on the inferior margin of the papilla. When I experience difficulty in cannulating the bile duct in Bilroth II patients, I next use a catheter-guidewire assembly, which should be straighter and more rigid and approaches the 6:00 position more readily, or I use either a double-lumen or a special Bilroth II sphincterotome. Again, these accessories are stiffer and can be advanced more readily toward the inferior margin of the papilla.

Bilroth II Accessories—Special Sphincterotome

If cannulation of the papilla has been achieved, the pathology has been defined, and a sphincterotomy is to be performed, I approach its performance in several ways, depending on the degree of difficulty created by the anatomy. First, if a special Bilroth II sphincterotome can be inserted, I will use this accessory. As shown in Figure 10.24, the sphincterotome is introduced into the papilla. This special accessory is a "push-type" instrument (Fig. 10.4F). In other words, when the wire is pushed out of its sheath, it produces a bow, or arc, configuration. When the bow is formed, pressure is exerted against the sphincter while cautery current is applied, and the sphincterotomy is completed (Fig. 10.24). This accessory provides a safe sphincterotomy in this anatomic variation because the incision can be controlled, but despite this, sphincterotomy performed in patients with Bilroth II resections is not quite as safe or as controlled as a sphincterotomy performed in a patient with unaltered anatomy using the pull-type sphincterotome for standard sphincterotomy. The pull-type sphincterotome may be used in Bilroth II situation, but only if it can be rotated toward the 6:00 position, which is difficult indeed. Remember, when performing a sphincterotomy in a patient with a Bilroth II gastrectomy, *the direction of the incision should be downward toward 6:00 and not upward toward 12:00!* Proper orientation is a strict requirement before applying electrocautery current, and the endoscopist must be completely aware of the altered anatomy to prevent misadventures such as perforation or pancreatitis, which are potentially serious consequences of an incision directed toward 12:00.

If the special sphincterotome cannot be inserted into the sphincter, one can invoke several options, which have been described in references 26 through 33, in order to complete the sphincterotomy. Each option has its own risks and complications. A wire-guided sphincterotome and a rotatable sphincterotome, dedicated to the Bilroth II–hemigastrectomy anatomy, are currently available. These accessories permit easier insertion and completion of a sphincterotomy under these postoperative anatomic conditions. More experience and studies are awaited before these accessories receive general approval.

Alternatives For Performing Sphincterotomy in Patients with Bilroth II Resection

Because a Bilroth II wire-guided sphincterotome was not available earlier, endoscopists developed alternative methods for accomplishing sphincterotomy in patients with a Bilroth II resection. One method, which I use routinely, incorporates the combined use of a catheter-guidewire assembly and the subsequent insertion of a 7French endoprosthesis that is inserted into the bile duct prior to performing a sphincterotomy over the prosthesis (Fig. 10.25). After inserting the prosthesis, I use a needle-knife sphincterotome to incise the sphincter, utilizing the prosthesis as a guide and thus minimizing injury to the wall of the duodenum. This procedure has been described in other sit-

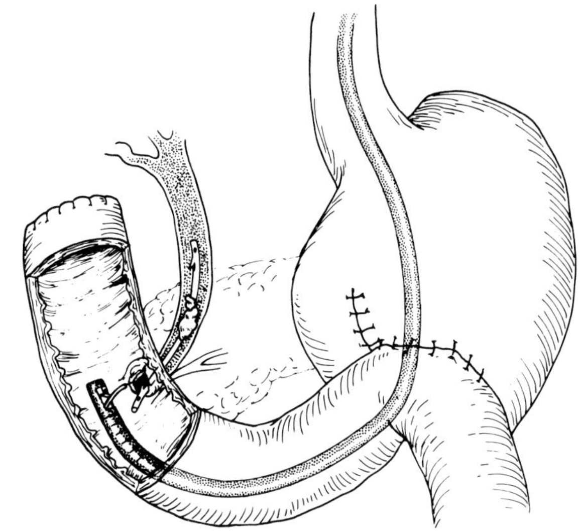

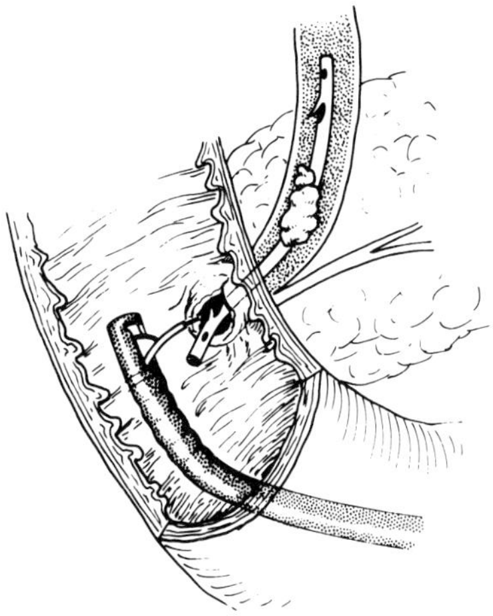

FIG. 10.25. Top: A Bilroth II gastric resection showing the position of the duodenoscope after placement of a prosthesis into the duct. A needle knife is shown beginning the incision over the prosthesis. **Bottom:** A close-up view of the sphincterotomy incision being made over the prosthesis.

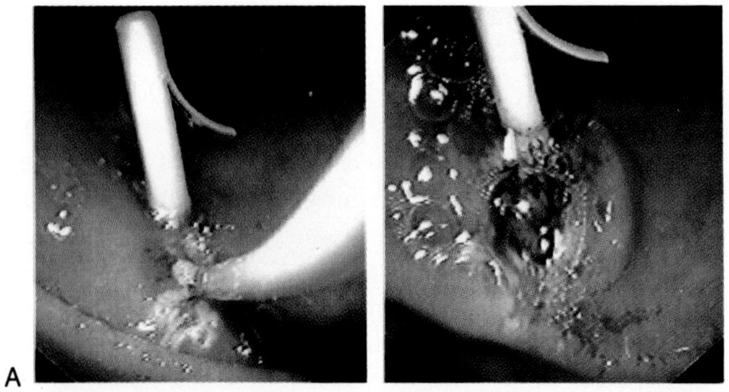

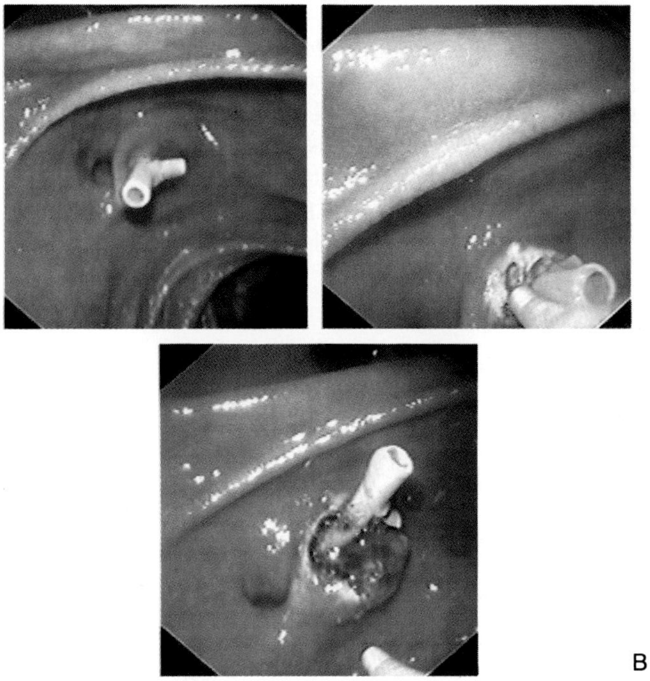

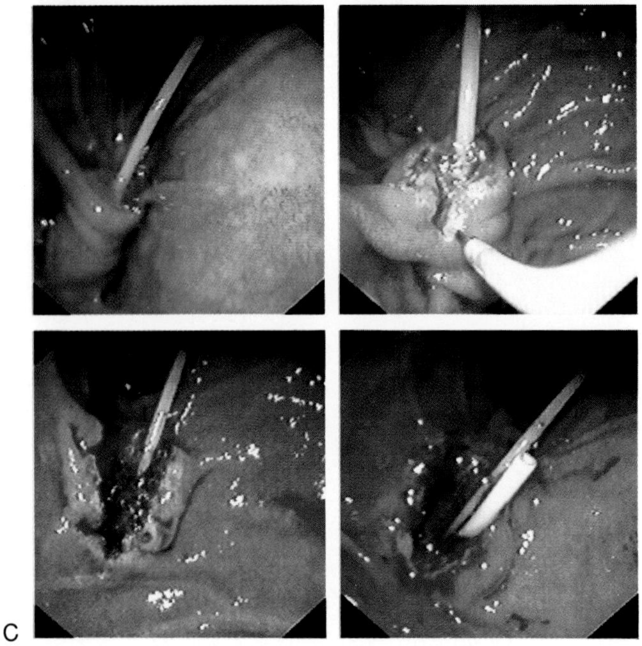

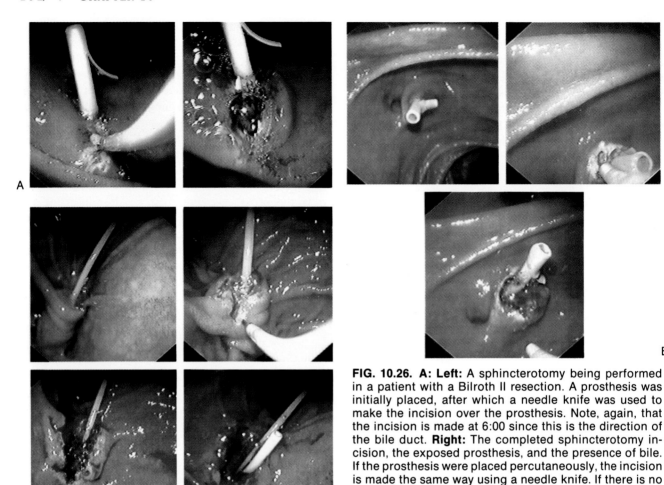

FIG. 10.26. A: Left: A sphincterotomy being performed in a patient with a Bilroth II resection. A prosthesis was initially placed, after which a needle knife was used to make the incision over the prosthesis. Note, again, that the incision is made at 6:00 since this is the direction of the bile duct. **Right:** The completed sphincterotomy incision, the exposed prosthesis, and the presence of bile. If the prosthesis were placed percutaneously, the incision is made the same way using a needle knife. If there is no prosthesis, a needle knife still can be used very carefully. The incision is directed downward from the papillary orifice into the intramural segment or bulge, which represents the bile duct. After penetration of the duct, contrast should be injected to confirm that the bile duct was entered. Completion of the incision can be accomplished using the needle knife or using the Bilroth II sphincterotome. **B: Top left:** The presence of a prosthesis extending from the papilla after placement into the bile duct in a patient who has undergone a Bilroth II gastric resection. **Top right:** The needle knife, seen to the left of the prosthesis, being swept downward toward 6:00. Cautery current is applied. **Bottom:** The sphincterotomy is nearly completed. The needle knife is visible in the lower portion of this video image. Assessment of the length of this incision determined that the incision could be extended another 4 mm to 5 mm. **C: Top left:** A papilla in a patient with a Bilroth II hemigastrectomy who presented with obstructive jaundice. A percutaneous prosthesis had been placed into the duodenum for decompression. **Top right:** A needle knife is being used to make an incision over the stent toward 6:00 (the location of the bile duct). **Bottom left:** The sphincterotomy is complete. **Bottom right:** An endoscopic stent is placed alongside the percutaneous stent, which can be removed now that endoscopic drainage is established.

uations (24). The incision is made downward, beginning at the papillary orifice, orienting the sphincter toward 6:00 (Fig. 10.26). In my experience, fewer complications have occurred with this method. After completing the sphincterotomy, the endoscopist can remove the prosthesis using a basket or snare and can treat the stone or stricture. Obviously, if a stricture is present, the endoscopist may wish to leave the prosthesis in place or to exchange it for a larger one.

Percutaneous Prosthesis

If the endoscopist cannot insert a guidewire, prosthesis, or both to complete the sphincterotomy as previously described, two other options exist. One method is to perform a precut or a full-length sphincterotomy de novo using a needle knife without a prosthesis in place (Fig. 10.23C). The other, safer option is to place a percutaneous prosthesis through the sphincter into the duodenum and to invoke the needle-knife incision over-the-prosthesis technique (Fig. 10.26C) (25,33). Because of the potential for increased complications resulting from the combined percutaneous–over-the-stent sphincterotomy, the endoscopist should discuss this approach with the patient, weighing the risks and alternatives and discussing a possible surgical approach.

Needle-Knife Sphincterotomy

The final option for performing a sphincterotomy in the post–Bilroth II gastrectomy patient is to perform the sphincterotomy de novo using a needle knife with no stent as a guide (21). One must exercise caution in performing this procedure, beginning at or near the papillary orifice and working progressively downward to the apex of the papilla at 6:00. If bile is seen to flow readily from the newly created hole, and, if the operator is more comfortable placing a stent or a Bilroth II sphincterotome to complete the incision, one may do so to minimize risk. However, in my experience few complications have occurred when using carefully controlled strokes with the needle knife. Also, a complete incision can be accomplished safely.

Precut Sphincterotomy

The technique of precut sphincterotomy remains a valid option for performing sphincterotomy or for enhancing selective cannulation of the bile duct when a standard sphincterotome or a guidewire cannot be inserted into the intended duct. The precut sphincterotomy may be necessary for Bilroth II patients, and I continue to use this technique when other options have failed. In my experience, performing a precut is less risky than placing a catheter or guidewire percutaneously, and, if performed as described in reference 19, it can potentiate the completion of the ERCP and sphincterotomy.

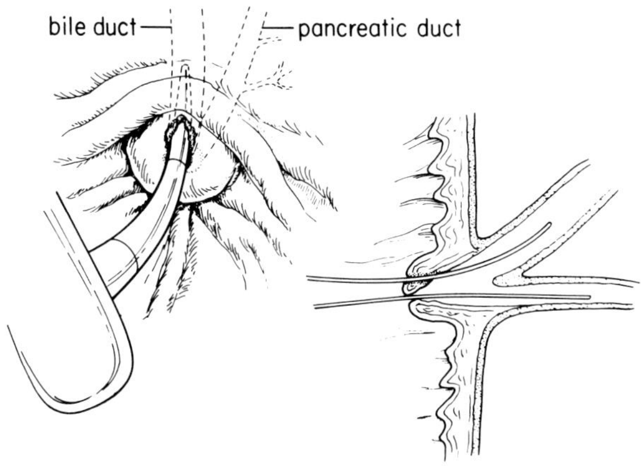

FIG. 10.27. Left: The performance of a precut sphincterotomy. Note that a short length of the sphincterotome is introduced toward the bile duct and that a short incision has been made. **Right:** The papilla as it appears from the side. Note that a guidewire is placed through the precut into the bile duct, whereas, if a precut were not formed, the wire would enter the pancreatic duct. The wire is seen entering the papillary orifice and preferentially entering the pancreatic duct. The precut was necessary to enter the bile duct.

As originally described, a short-nose sphincterotome or a specially designed precut sphincterotome is inserted approximately 5 mm into the papilla (Figs. 10.27, 10.28). The catheter may enter the common channel orifice or even the pancreatic duct, but if the wire is directed toward the bile duct (identified as the prominent intramural segment proceeding toward 12:00), short bursts of cautery current are applied to unroof the ampulla. During the performance of the precut incision, the fluoroscope is used to guide the sphincterotome toward the bile duct and away from the pancreatic duct. After making an incision of about 5 mm, the endoscopist can manipulate the sphincterotome in the direction of the bile duct and can slide it into the duct easily (Fig. 10.29). At that point, if a cholangiogram has not been obtained, contrast can be injected to determine the need for completion of the sphincterotomy. The ampulla can occasionally be unroofed, but the sphincterotome cannot selectively enter the bile duct. A catheter-guidewire assembly can be used to enter the duct, or a needle knife may be used to penetrate the bile duct if it can be identified within the open ampulla. The bile duct is identified by its pale appearance and round configuration. Once it is identified, the bile duct can often be entered using the needle knife (Fig. 10.30).

If it is risky to extend the precut or to use a needle knife, especially when the bile duct is not prominent or bulging, it has been my experience that after 3 to 5 days of healing, a fistula forms, providing access to the bile duct. On repeat ERCP, the bile duct orifice is identified and cannulated with little difficulty, and the incision can be extended if needed.

Endoscopists originally recommended the precut method with caution because they thought that edema formation would result in an increased incidence of pancreatitis. In actual fact, this complication occurs infrequently if the initial incision is begun using cutting current as desiccation and resultant edema is minimized. If performed properly, precut sphincterotomy can be a valuable adjunct to the therapeutic armamentarium. I continue to employ this technique in my approach to performing sphincterotomy without increasing risks, but I have acquired extensive experience and advise caution.

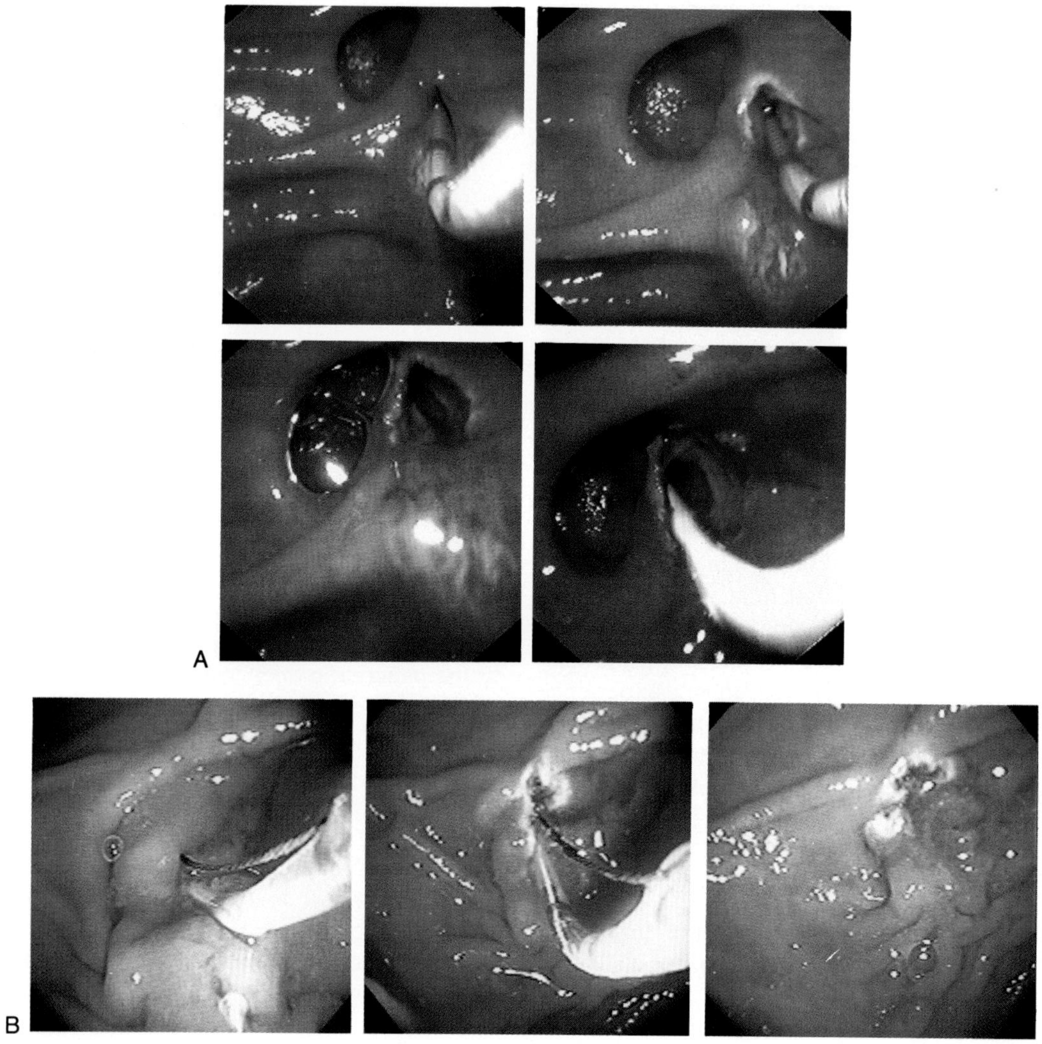

FIG. 10.28. A: Top left: The precut sphincterotome being placed into the papilla, which constitutes the lateral wall of a diverticulum. The sphincterotome could not be deeply inserted into the duct, which required the performance of a precut incision. **Top right:** The precut being performed. **Bottom left:** The sphincterotome was advanced deeply enough to complete the incision. **Bottom right:** After completion of the sphincterotomy, a balloon catheter is placed to retrieve a stone and to calibrate the size of the incision. **B: Left:** The tip of the sphincterotome is placed into the papilla in preparation for application of cautery current. **Middle:** Cautery is being applied to the sphincter. **Right:** The precut incision of 6 mm has been completed.

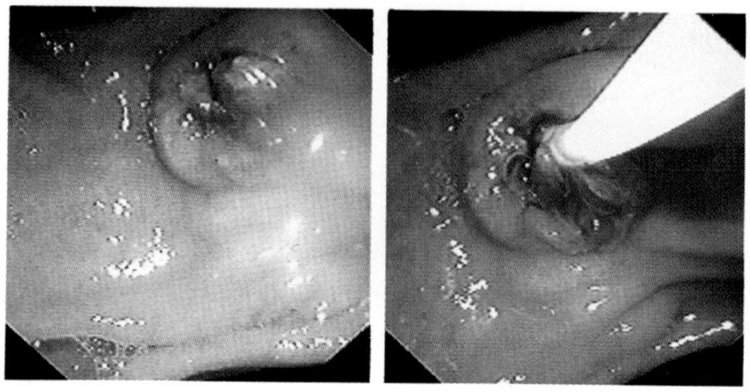

FIG. 10.29. Left: A papilla seen 5 days after using a needle knife to perform a sphincterotomy. **Right:** A catheter is easily inserted into the bile duct of this healed needle-knife sphincterotomy. During the incision phase, the bile duct could not be selectively cannulated despite the large opening created. After healing the tract became more defined and established. A 1.5 cm balloon catheter was pulled through the sphincterotomy to calibrate the opening.

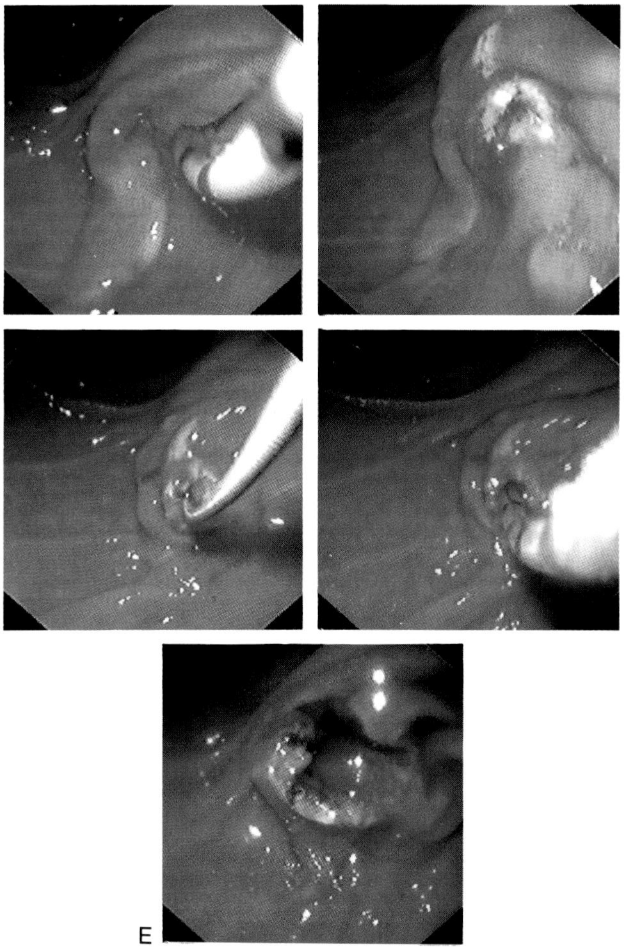

FIG. 10.30. A: A precut sphincterotome is inserted into the papillary orifice. Selective insertion of the sphincterotome was not possible. **B:** The appearance of the sphincter after a short precut incision was made. **C:** A guidewire has been placed into the bile duct to access a wire-guided double-lumen sphincterotome. **D:** The double-lumen sphincterotome is positioned for the final incision. **E:** The final incision, which required a selection of different accessories before achieving the completed sphincterotomy. Little or no edema is present, even after cautery current is applied several times.

TABLE 10.2. *Utilization of the needle-knife sphincterotome for special situations*

Biliary Tree
Impacted stone or obstruction
Distended intramural segment
Endoprosthesis
Difficult cannulation
Normal papilla
Neoplasm
Endoprosthesis
Bilroth II gastrectomy
De novo
Endoprosthesis
Periampullary diverticula
De novo
Endoprosthesis
Choledochocele
Spontaneous fistulas
Extend fistula
Endoprosthesis
Pancreatic Duct
Duct of Wirsung (major papilla)
De novo
Endoprosthesis
Duct of Santorini (minor papilla)
De novo
Endoprosthesis

Needle-Knife Precut Fistulotomy (Table 10.2)

Although the needle knife has been part of our therapeutic armamentarium for a short time, some endoscopists utilized a straight cutting device early in the development of therapeutic sphincterotomy (35–41). I initially used an electrified guidewire to penetrate an intact papilla (21), which was usually prominent or bulging, but other endoscopists used a snare tip or basket tip to accomplish the same thing. Although an earlier version of the needle knife has been available, it contains a thicker cutting wire, the diameter of which is the same as a guidewire. Subsequently, a thin wire needle knife has been introduced that, by its design, minimizes the tissue injury and swelling that is attendant with the other devices (Fig. 10.31).

Caution should be the watch word when using any cautery device in or around the papilla of Vater, but a more cautious and tentative approach is recommended when attempting to open or unroof the papilla itself. Because sphincterotomy using a standard sphincterotome is associated with predictable morbidity and mortality, utilizing other devices in a free style manner may be associated with an increased frequency of complications (20,41,42). Such a procedure should therefore be reserved for experienced endoscopists who have performed a large number of sphincterotomies. However, if there are no alternatives available and all risks are fully explained, one may, by necessity, attempt this type of procedure.

The needle knife can be used to open the ampulla to facilitate entry into the bile duct by cutting either in an upward direction starting at the papilla and working upward toward the apex, as described by Huibregtse (40), or in a downward direction starting from

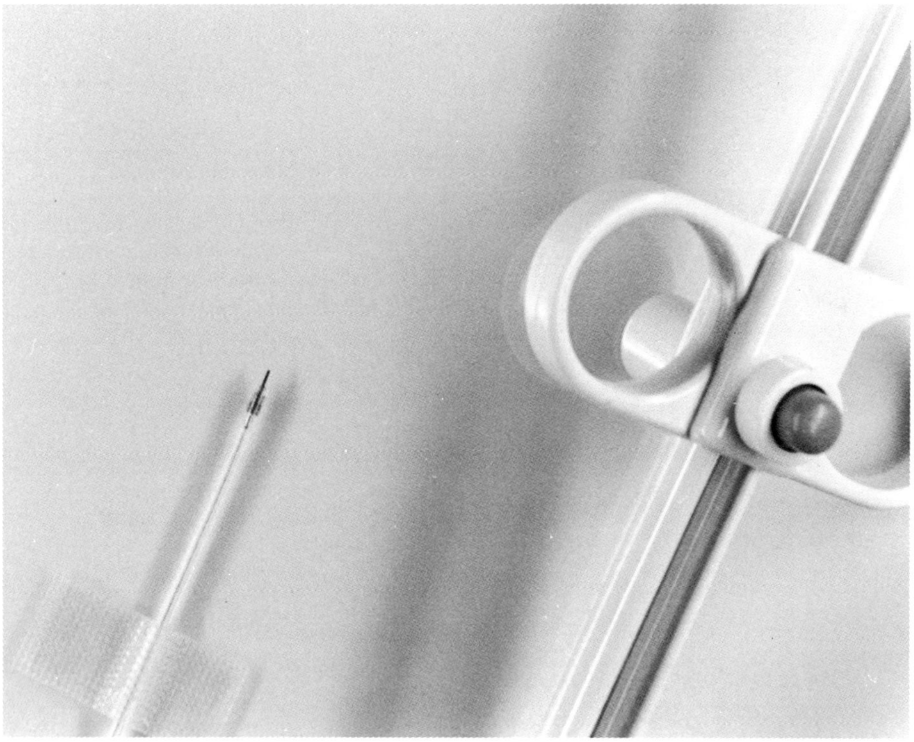

FIG. 10.31. A commercially available needle knife. (See also Fig. 10.4A.)

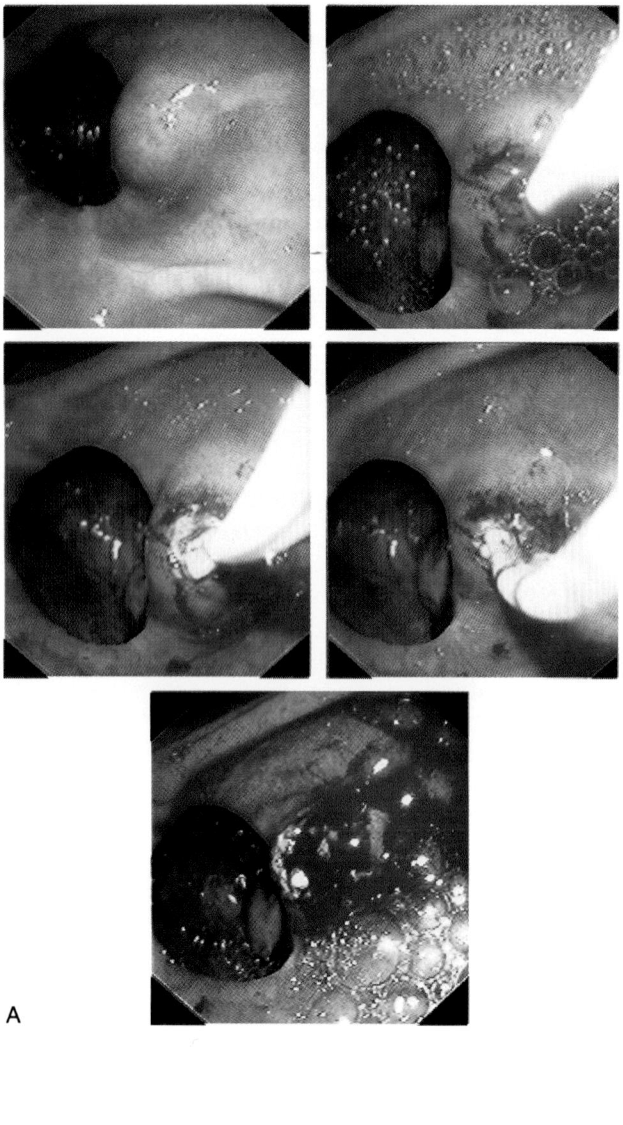

A

FIG. 10.32. A: Top left: The effective use of a needle knife in performing a precut incision. The bile duct is seen as a protuberance on the lateral wall of a diverticulum. The papillary orifice is within the diverticulum and could not be visualized, much less cannulated. **Top right:** The needle knife with the knife extended from the sheath in preparation for making an incision. **Middle left:** The needle knife has been placed against the bulging duct, light pressure applied, and electrical current generated, which penetrates the duodenal mucosa. A small cholesterol stone is seen exiting through the incision inferior to the knife. The incision could be extended superiorly, but the needle knife was removed, and a standard sphincterotome was inserted. **Middle right:** The standard sphincterotome is inserted into the fistula created by the needle knife. **Bottom:** The completed incision, which extended to the top of the mound, or protuberance. Although some bleeding was noted, it stopped spontaneously, and a stone was retrieved using a basket without incurring a complication.

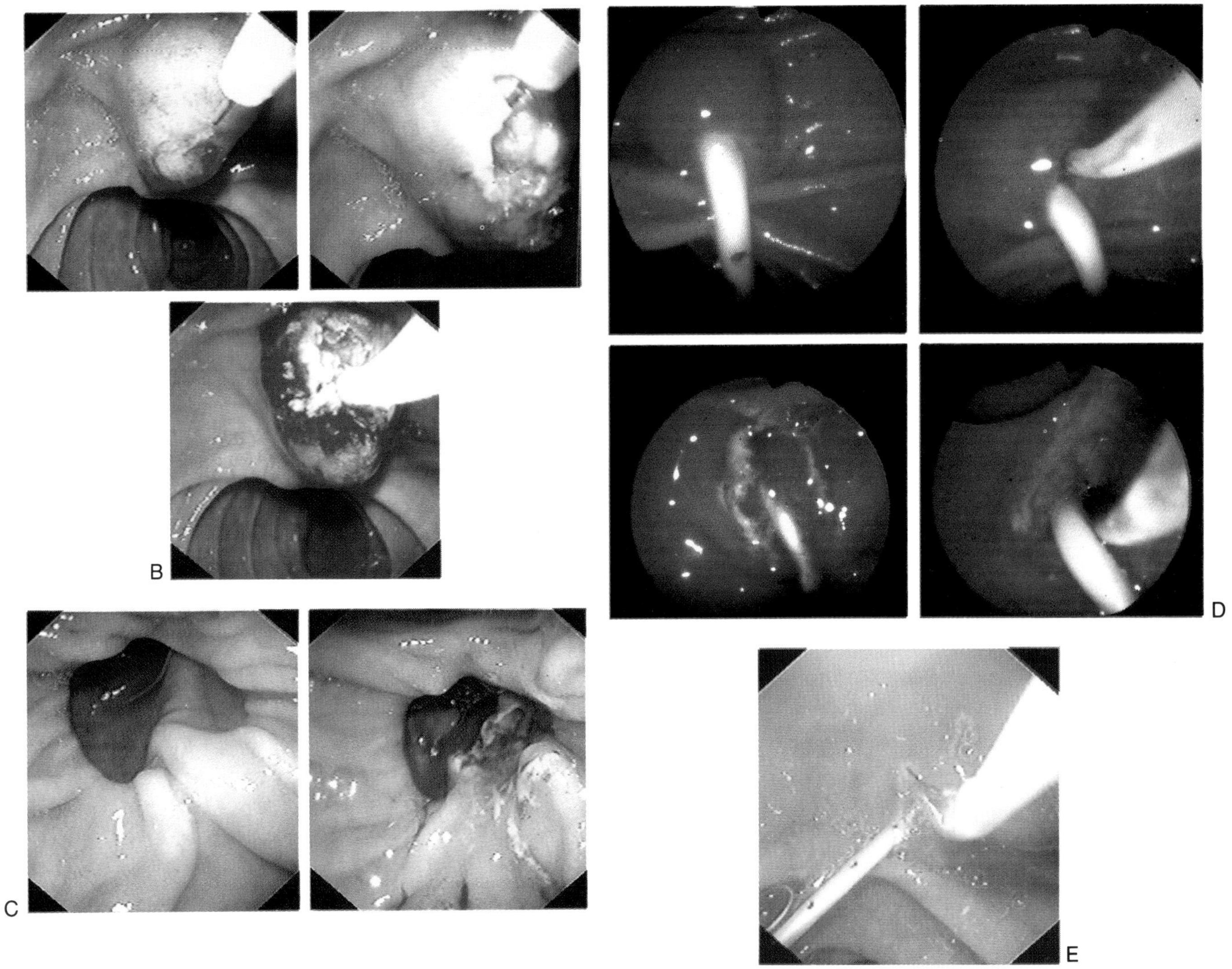

FIG. 10.32. (*Continued*). **B: Left:** A prominent papilla. The needle knife is poised and aligned properly before the incision is begun. **Middle:** The incision is begun using the needle knife in an upward sweep from the papillary orifice. **Right:** The incision is nearly completed, and the bile duct has been selectively entered. The needle knife can be removed and the standard sphincterotome inserted to complete the sphincterotomy. **C: Left:** A pantaloon-type periampullary diverticulum with the papillary orifice located on the inferior internal margin. A cannula could not be inserted, and a guidewire was not successful in entering the bile duct. **Right:** A widely patent sphincterotomy extending deeply into the diverticulum, accomplished using a needle knife. An alternative to this treatment would have been placement of a percutaneous catheter and a sphincterotomy with either a sphincterotome or needle knife. **D: Top left:** An intact papilla through which a percutaneous catheter was advanced into the duodenum. **Top right:** A needle knife is placed at the papillary orifice to facilitate a sphincterotomy, and the incision is started using the stent as a buffer to prevent or reduce injury. **Bottom left:** After the sphincterotomy, the extent of the incision may be appreciated. **Bottom right:** Even with the percutaneous stent in position, a catheter, balloon, or basket can be inserted around it because of the generous incision. This endoscopic photograph shows a basket catheter being inserted along side the stent. **E:** The performance of a sphincterotomy using a standard sphincterotome with a percutaneous catheter already in place.

the midpapilla or apex and working toward the papilla, as I have described (21) (Figs. 10.32–10.35). I prefer to avoid direct contact with the papilla, which may directly injure the pancreas, by initiating the incision above the orifice. This maneuver minimizes the incidence of pancreatitis. Huibregtse's group reported their experience with a large series of patients, and even though they initiate the incision at the papillary orifice directed cephalad, the incidence of pancreatitis was not increased. However, most precut procedures

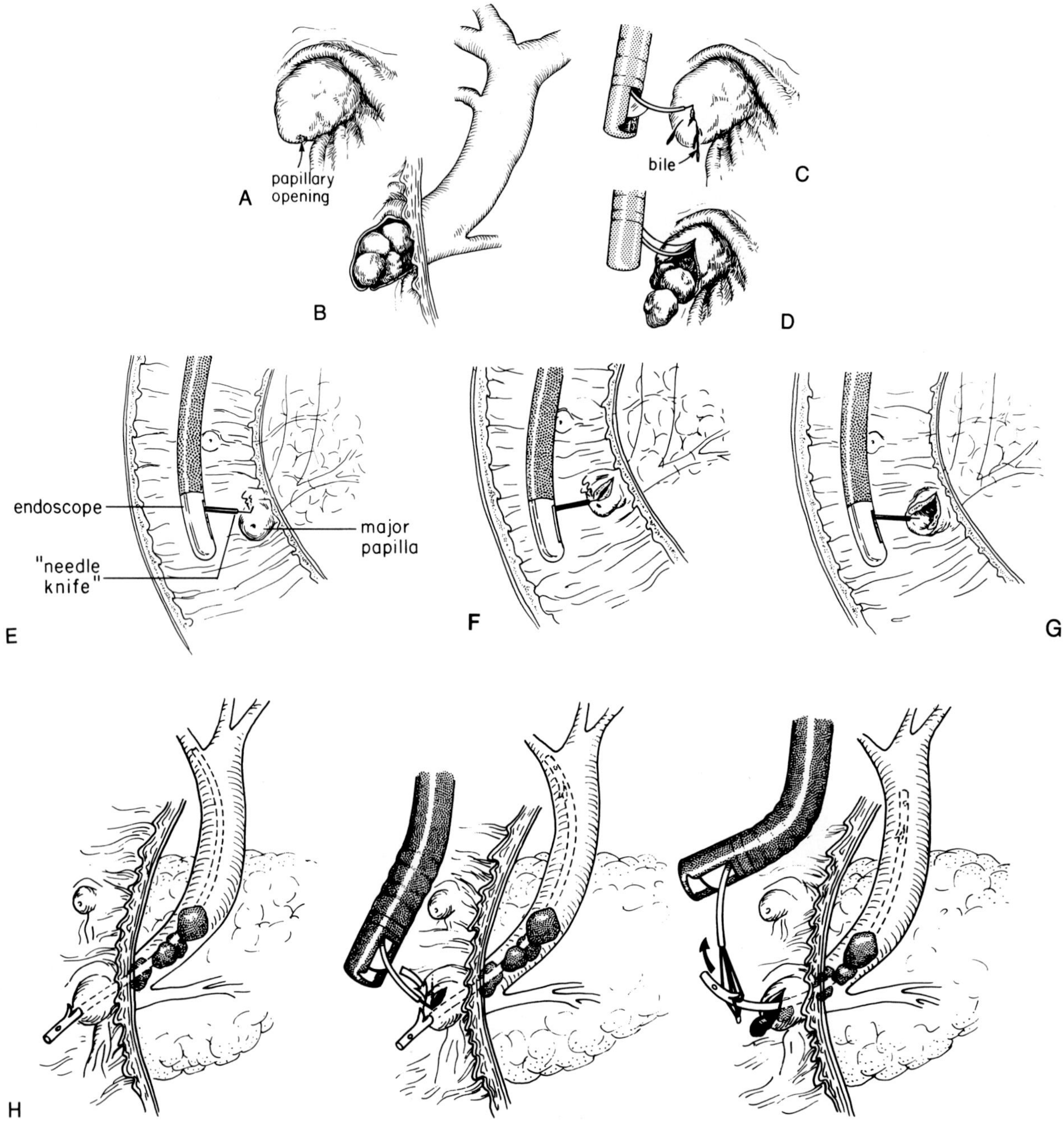

FIG. 10.33. A: A prominent, bulging papilla. The orifice is located beneath the bulge and is technically difficult to cannulate. **B:** The cause for papillary bulging. In this picture, the roof of the papilla has been removed by the artist to demonstrate obstructing stones. **C:** The needle knife being inserted into the bulging papilla, creating a fistula through which bile will flow. **D:** The fistula is entered with a sphincterotome, and the sphincterotomy is completed. Some stones are seen passing spontaneously after enlargement of the sphincterotomy. **E:** De novo needle-knife incision of major papilla is begun at apex with sweeps downward toward the papilla. **F:** The papilla is opening. **G:** A complete incision is accomplished. **H: Left:** A prosthesis has been placed into the papilla. **Middle:** A needle knife is used to open the papilla, using the stent as a guide. **Right:** After the needle-knife sphincterotomy, the stent is removed, and the stones can be removed actively or be allowed to pass spontaneously. I use this technique in patients in whom stents were placed at presentation with cholangitis. After the patient is stabilized, sphincterotomy can be performed later utilizing the stent as a guide. (E, F, G, H: From reference 21, with permission.)

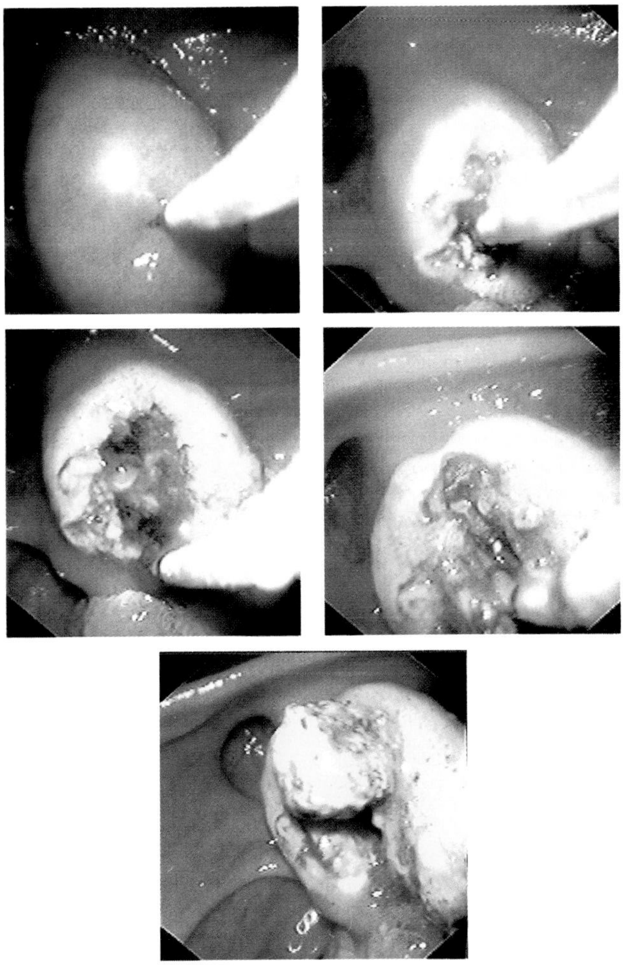

FIG. 10.34. Upper left: A sequence of videoimages illustrating the stepwise performance of a sphincterotomy on a bulging, cystlike bile duct. The needle knife is placed into position before cautery current is applied. **Upper right:** The performance of the fistulotomy using the needle knife. **Middle left:** The bile duct has been opened, and bile streams from the opening. **Middle right:** A standard sphincterotome is placed into the fistula, and the incision is extended to the upper sphincter. **Bottom:** After the sphincterotomy, a stone exits the opening, having passed spontaneously.

A

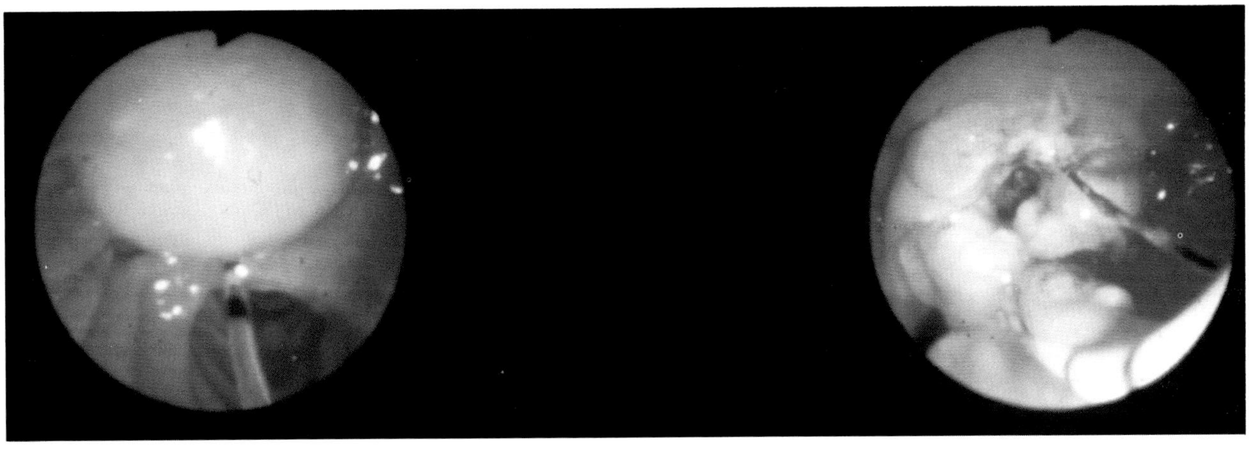

FIG. 10.35. A: Left: A choledochocele with its characteristic cystlike protrusion. **Right:** The papillary orifice was identified and cannulated with a catheter. A sphincterotome was subsequently inserted, and a sphincterotomy performed.

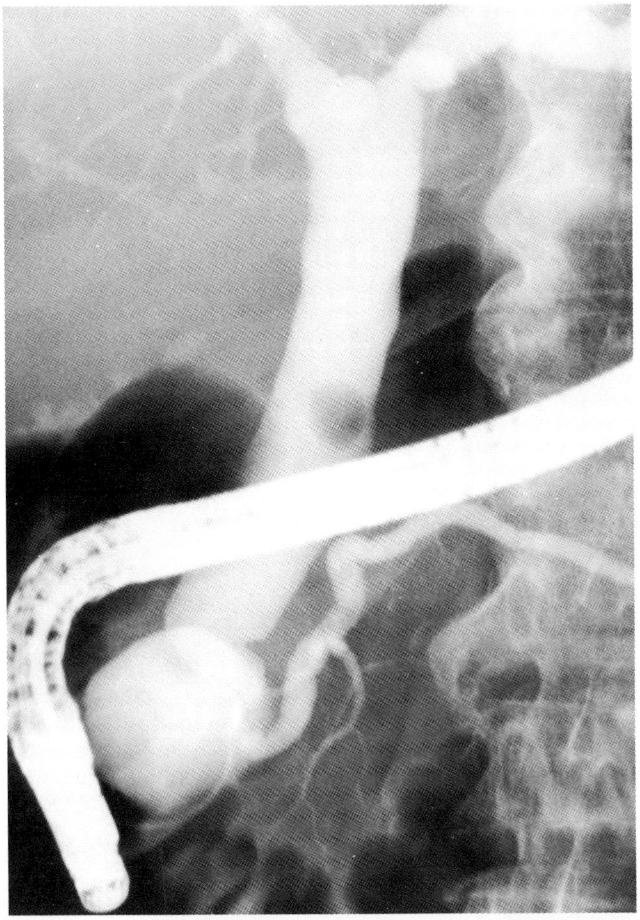

B

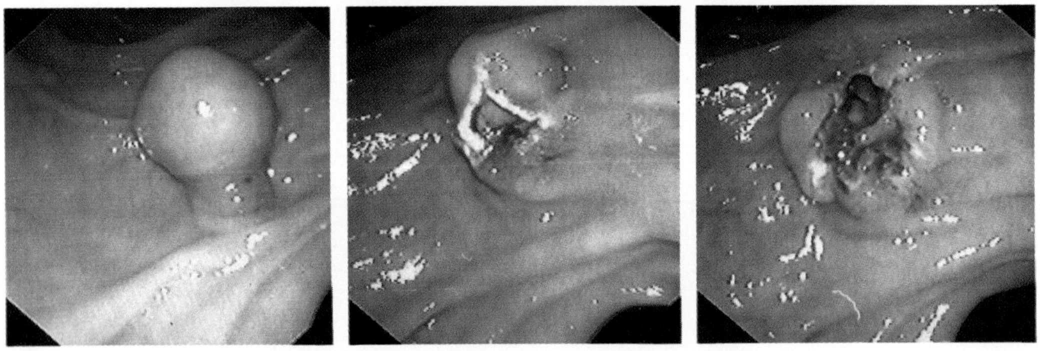

C

FIG. 10.35. (*Continued*). **B:** A cystlike protrusion at the distal end of the common bile duct, affecting the bile duct (dilated with a stone) and pancreatic duct (dilated). **C: Left:** A choledochocele of the distal common bile duct. **Middle:** The papillary orifice could not be cannulated, and a needle knife was used to unroof the papilla and expose the cyst membrane seen inside the incisional opening. **Right:** The membrane was penetrated with the needle knife, and a sphincterotome was used to open the papilla completely.

in their series were performed in patients with malignancy, when the risk of pancreatitis is lower. In my recently reported series, the procedure was performed in both benign and malignant disease, in patients who had protruberant papillae and in patients with normal-appearing papillae. We advocate the prudent use of needle-knife sphincterotomy, even as a diagnostic tool, when other alternatives have failed and when cholangiography is essential to patient management. Figures 10.34 and 10.35 demonstrate the use of the needle knife in the treatment of choledochoceles or cystlike structures of the intramural portion of the bile duct. These structures can be opened not only with a needle knife but also with other types of special or standard sphincterotomes (43–45).

Although other experts in the field disclaim the use

of precut for diagnosis, most experienced endoscopists, by necessity, utilize the procedure for that purpose when other alternatives have been exhausted and surgery is the only remaining alternative. We all agree that precut sphincterotomy may increase risks and morbidity and do not advocate its use by inexperienced endoscopists. It is better to refer the more difficult cases to experts. If the patient refuses referral and surgery, one must obtain an informed consent to perform precut or needle-knife sphincterotomy, ensuring that all risks and alternatives have been carefully explained but agreeing to perform the procedure only if the primary care physician and surgeon concur with that approach. As a matter of fact, all therapeutic procedures should be performed under these conditions, incorporating a team approach and agreement among the team members to proceed.

SPHINCTEROTOMY OF THE PANCREATIC DUCT SPHINCTER

The performance of a sphincterotomy of the pancreatic sphincter can be riskier than one performed on the bile duct sphincter, principally because of the differences in anatomy. This is due to the fact that the pancreatic duct enters the duodenum in a more perpendicular plane, restricting the length of the incision that can be safely made. The bile duct enters more parallel to the duodenal wall, providing a longer intramural segment and permitting a longer incision that transects the entire sphincter mechanism.

On the other hand, sphincterotomy of the pancreatic duct is restricted, and I rarely use a standard sphincterotome in the pancreas unless I confirm a long intramural segment that will minimize the risk of per-

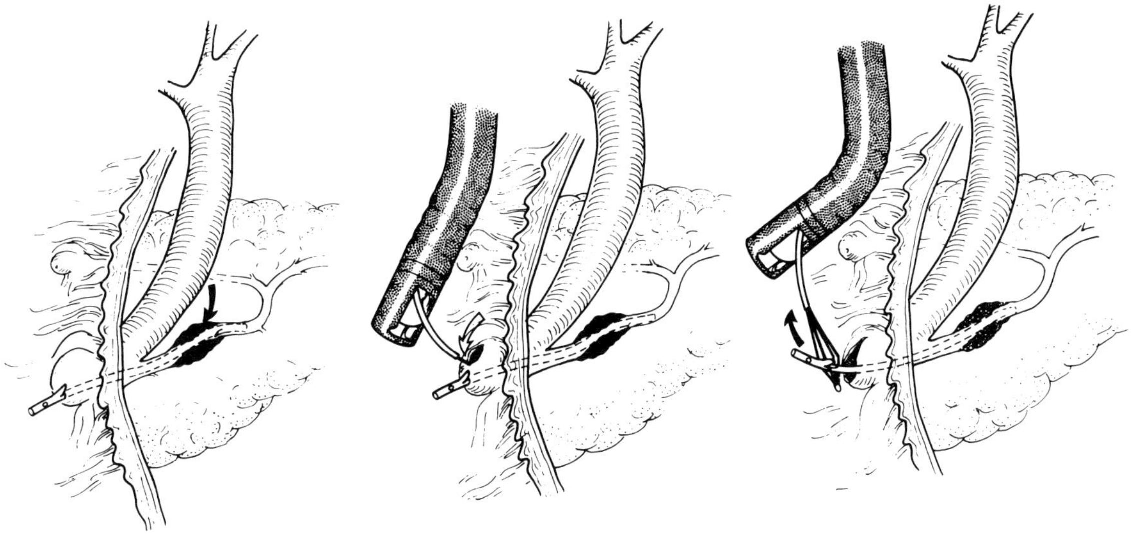

A

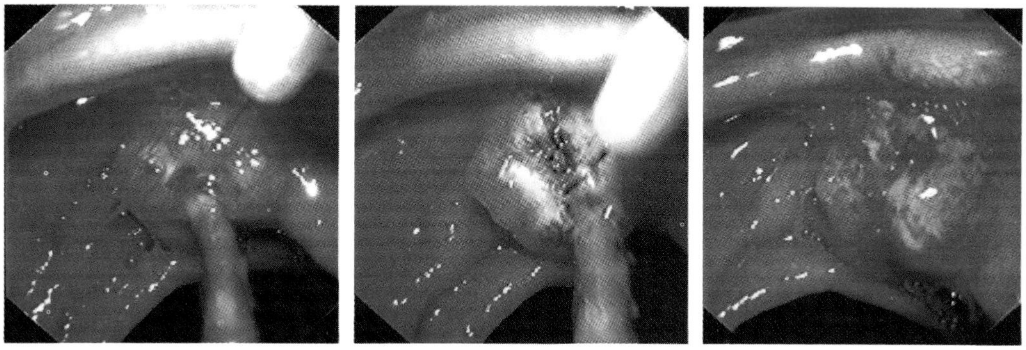

B

FIG. 10.36. A: Left: The insertion of a prosthesis into the main pancreatic duct. A stricture is evident (*arrow*) in the duct. **Middle:** A sphincterotomy of the pancreatic duct sphincter is performed using carefully controlled sweeps with the needle knife. **Right:** The stent provides protection to the bowel wall for a prescribed period of time while the sphincterotomy heals over the stent and is then removed using a basket (as shown) or a snare. **B:** The technique for performing a safe sphincterotomy of the pancreatic duct using an indwelling stent as a guide. **Left:** The stent is in position in the pancreatic duct. **Middle:** The needle knife is advanced to the papillary orifice, pressure applied by the needle to the mucosa, and cautery current applied. **Right:** The completion of a pancreatic sphincterotomy.

foration. By comparison to the descriptions of techniques for performing sphincterotomy of the bile duct sphincter, little has been written or reported on the technique of performing sphincterotomy on the pancreatic sphincter (45–51).

In order to perform a sphincterotomy of the pancreatic sphincter safely, I have incorporated the insertion of a prosthesis, performing the incision over a prosthesis using a needle knife (24). This is similar to the method I use for sphincterotomy in Billroth II and periampullary diverticula situations. As shown in the accompanying illustrations, a prosthesis is placed prior to the sphincterotomy, and the sphincterotomy is completed over the prosthesis, which protects the duodenal wall (Fig. 10.36). After completing the sphincterotomy, I leave the prosthesis in place for several days to weeks in order to minimize the occurrence of pancreatitis, which can ensue if the prosthesis is removed and edema develops.

SEPTOTOMY

Septotomy, incising the septum between the bile duct and the pancreatic duct, can be performed in a similar manner, especially if a bile duct sphincterotomy has been previously performed. It is thought that pancreatitis occurs or recurs in patients who have undergone bile duct sphincterotomy because of the coexistence of a hypertensive pancreatic sphincter (52). In this situation, the bile duct sphincterotomy is reassessed, fibrosis or narrowing of the pancreatic sphincter is confirmed, a stent is placed into the pancreatic duct, and the sphincterotomy is performed (Fig. 10.37).

The safety of this procedure is ensured because the incision is controlled and the duodenal wall is protected by the stent. With this technique, only two cases of mild pancreatitis have occurred in 33 patients (6.1%), and the patients were discharged after a mean hospital stay of only 2 days.

A

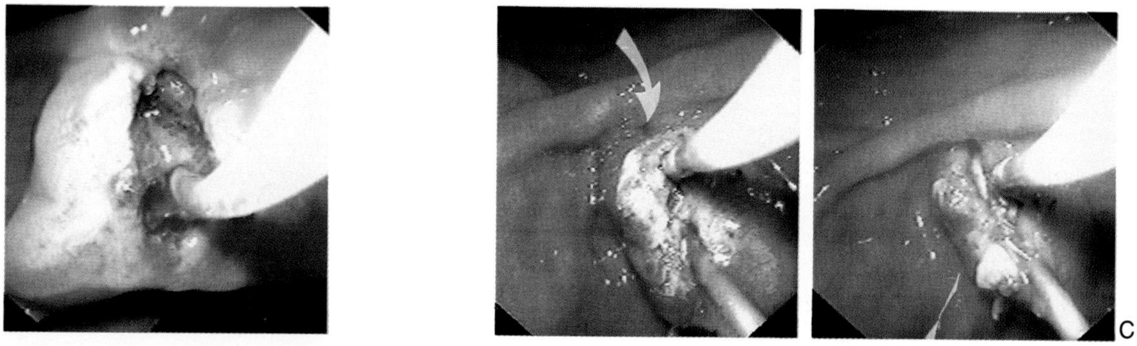

C

B

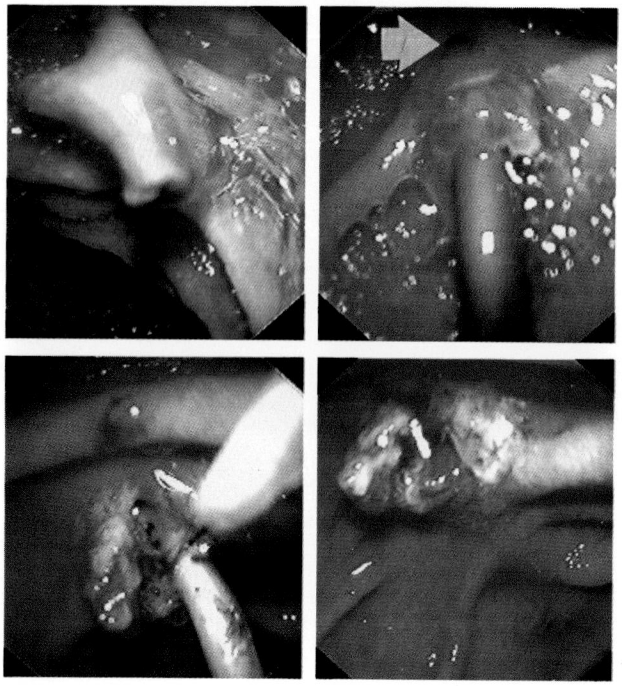

FIG. 10.37. A: The open papilla after a bile duct sphincterotomy. The cannula is visible in the stenotic pancreatic orifice. A septotomy and sphincterotomy of the pancreatic duct sphincter would incise all the tissue present from the catheter to the apex of the bile duct sphincterotomy. **B: Upper left:** An occluded pancreatic stent, which was placed to treat recurrent symptoms of pancreatitis despite a previous biliary sphincterotomy. The patient's symptoms were relieved after stent placement but returned subsequent to stent occlusion. **Upper right:** A close-up view of the papilla. The bile duct sphincterotomy is seen cephalad to the stent (*arrow*). **Lower left:** The needle knife is being used to open the pancreatic sphincter. A septotomy was ultimately performed and incised the septum between the bile duct and the pancreatic duct. **Lower right:** The completed septotomy. **C: Left:** A pancreatic stent is in place while a septotomy of both ducts (bile and pancreas) is carried out with a needle knife. The small bile duct sphincterotomy is seen cephalad (superior) to the incision (*arrow*). **Right:** The completed septotomy exposes the intramural portion of the stent. The incision extended through the bile duct sphincterotomy.

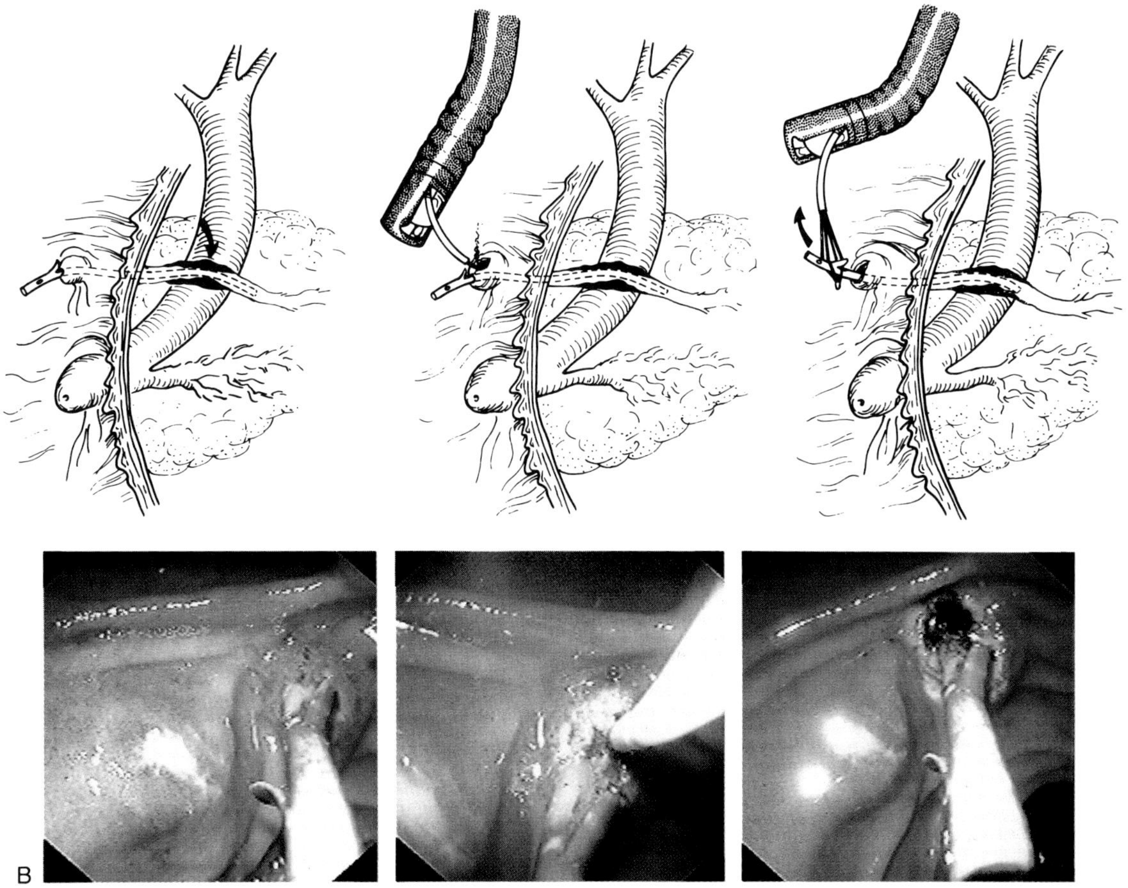

A

B

FIG. 10.38. A: Left: The presence of a prosthesis in the dorsal duct of pancreas divisum. A stricture (*arrow*) is evident in the dorsal duct. **Middle:** A needle-knife sphincterotome is being used to perform a sphincterotomy of the minor papilla. **Right:** After the sphincterotomy of the minor papilla, the prosthesis is removed using a basket. **B:** The technique of performing a catheter-guided sphincterotomy in pancreas divisum using the needle knife. **Left:** A prosthesis is visible exiting from the minor papilla, and the needle knife is poised and positioned to make the incision. **Middle:** The technique of performing the sphincterotomy over the prosthesis using the needle knife. **Right:** The completed sphincterotomy.

Even if a stone is present in the pancreatic duct, I usually place a prosthesis, perform a sphincterotomy, remove the prosthesis, remove the stone, and replace a prosthesis. This approach, though somewhat cumbersome, results in a low morbidity rate.

THE APPROACH TO SPHINCTEROTOMY OF THE MINOR PAPILLA—PANCREAS DIVISUM

Sphincterotomy of the minor papilla is all but impossible to perform because of the miniscule size of the minor papilla and the degree of difficulty in selectively cannulating this structure. It is rare to be able to place a sphincterotome into the minor papilla without having previously performed a precut sphincterotomy or placing a guidewire and inserting a wire-guided sphincterotome. The dorsal pancreatic duct, like the ventral pancreatic duct, presents in a perpendicular plane, allowing for possible perforation, so I advise using the prosthesis-guided system as previously described (24) (Figs. 10.38, 10.39). Again, morbidity is reduced by leaving the prosthesis in place for an extended period after performing the sphincterotomy, and it can be removed at any time on an outpatient basis.

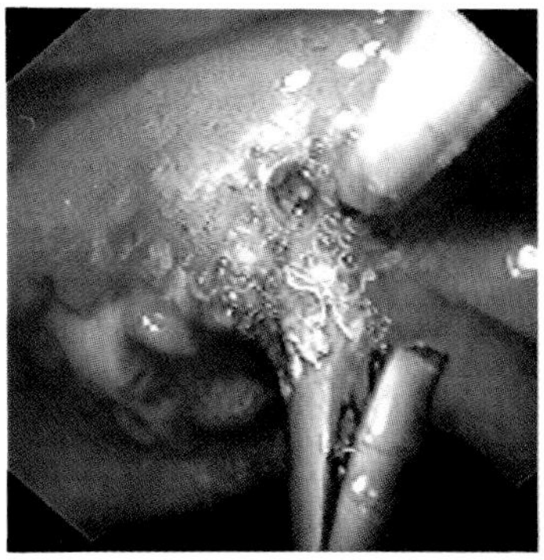

FIG. 10.39. The use of the needle knife in performing a stent-guided sphincterotomy of the minor papilla. Note the granulation tissue and edema surrounding the stent, which was an unusual reaction to the stent in this patient.

Often, one can only place a 5 French stent on initial evaluation and treatment of patients with pancreas divisum. I usually wait to determine if decompression of the dorsal pancreatic duct in pancreas divisum is effective before performing a sphincterotomy. When symptoms recur with stent occlusion, the needle knife can be used to enlarge the sphincter opening, the small prosthesis can be removed, and a larger prosthesis can be placed. When the larger prosthesis occludes, and symptoms recur (usually within 4 to 6 months), the prosthesis can be removed. The results of an endoscopic sphincterotomy can then be fully appreciated, evaluated, and analyzed. Results of endotherapy for pancreas divisum are presented in Chapter 12.

SPHINCTEROTOMY AND SPONTANEOUS OR ACQUIRED PERIAMPULLARY FISTULAE

Occasionally, when examining the papilla, the endoscopist may appreciate a second opening on the superior aspect of the papillary mound (53–56). These are fistulae, and they generally either result from surgical probing during common bile duct exploration or develop spontaneously from stone erosion or, rarely, tumor. A surgical probe or dilator, when passed into a choledochotomy incision and down the distal bile duct to the sphincter, may penetrate the duodenal wall. The surgeon, during palpation, appreciates free passage of the probe into the duodenum and assumes that the probe or dilator passed through the sphincter. However, because of anatomic variations of the papilla, such as a long intramural segment or an angulated distal bile duct, the probe may pass straight through the least resistant portion of the papilla, usually the intramural portion, and not through the sphincter. A spontaneous fistula can occur, which is usually of no consequence. Occasionally, however, stone material or gastrointestinal contents may accumulate, simulating a sump syndrome. In this situation a sphincterotomy, either from the papillary orifice or the fistula, will permit spontaneous passage of the material, relieving the obstruction (Fig. 10.40). Another type of therapy for this situation is shown in the artist's drawing (Fig. 10.41B). After a stent is placed through the papillary orifice, a needle knife is used to open the fistula toward the sphincter, completing the sphincterotomy. The stent and stones are then removed.

A periampullary fistula may form spontaneously as a result of stone erosion through the intramural portion of the papilla. If the stone or stones impact in the ampulla, the wall of the papilla may erode because of pressure, ischemia, and necrosis, resulting in the formation of a fistula. Recurrent fever, chills, intermittent jaundice, and biochemical evidence of cholestasis should alert the physician to suspect the diganosis of stone disease, and he or she should request an ERCP to confirm the diagnosis. A sphincterotomy will rectify this problem by allowing the stones or sludge to pass or the material to be extracted by a balloon or basket.

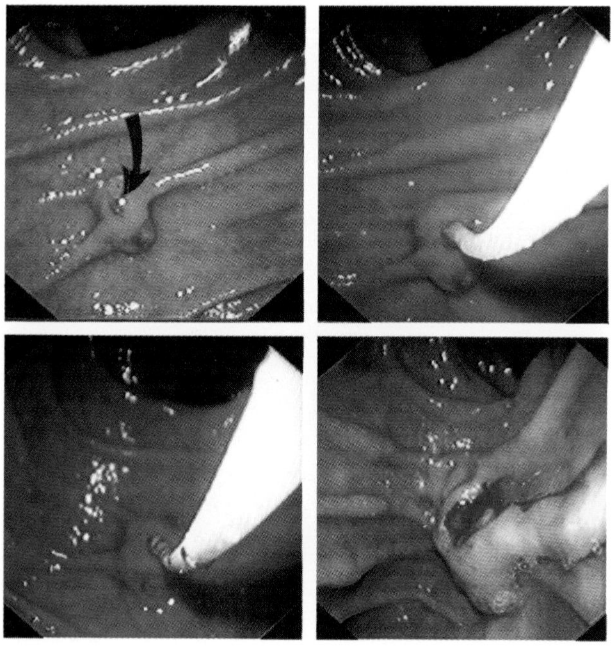

FIG. 10.40. Upper left: A videoendoscopic image of a normal-appearing papilla. Close inspection of the papilla reveals a second opening more proximal to the papillary orifice (*arrow*). In general, the opening to the fistula is epithelialized and has an appearance similar to the papillary orifice. Easy access to the bile duct in this situation is the clue that the opening is a fistula, especially when attempts to opacify the pancreatic duct fail. **Upper right:** A cannula is passed into the fistula. Note the papillary orifice inferior to the fistulous communication. **Lower left:** A sphincterotome is placed into the fistula in preparation for a sphincterotomy. **Lower right:** The appearance of the papilla is appreciated after the sphincterotomy. Note that the papillary orifice is present and intact.

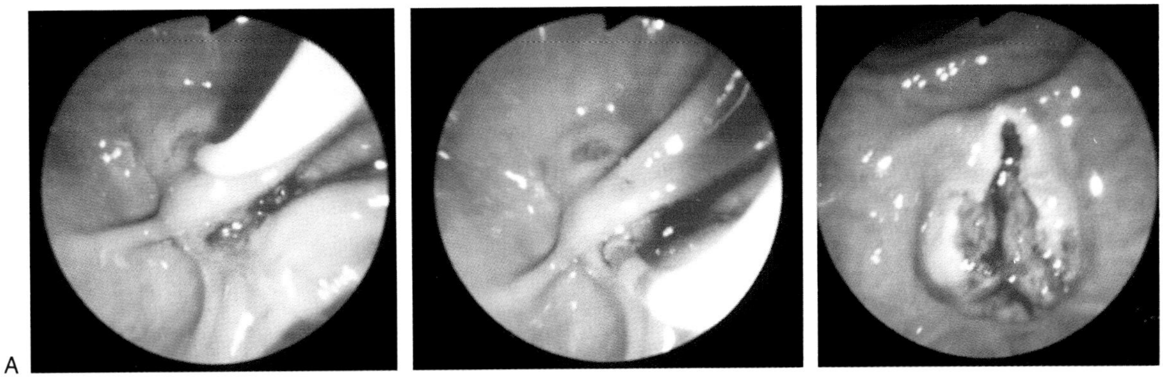

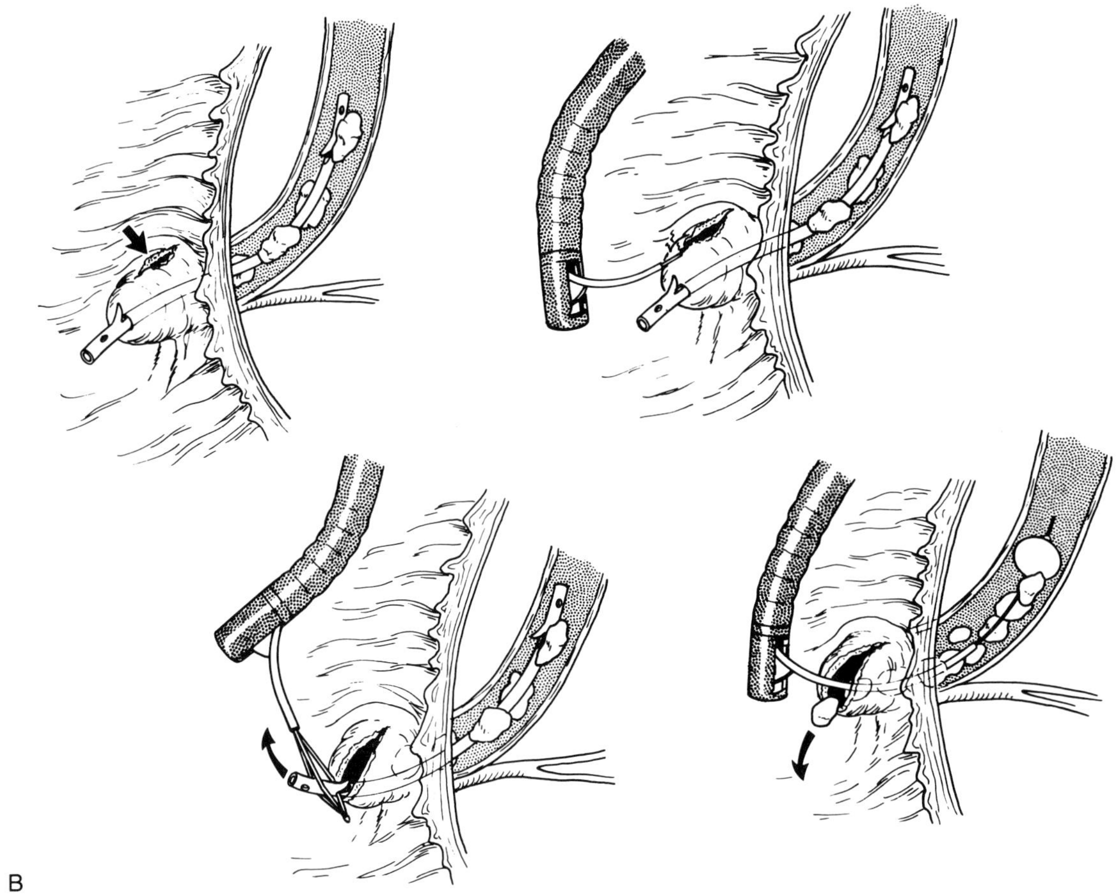

FIG. 10.41. Left: An ampulla with a second opening appearing superior to the papillary orifice, which is an acquired fistula. **Middle:** Cannulation of the papilla. **Right:** Completion of sphincterotomy through the fistula. **B: Upper left:** A spontaneous fistula (*arrow*) that resulted from stone erosion. Stones are seen in the bile duct. A stent has been placed through the papilla into the bile duct to prevent cholangitis. **Upper right:** A needle knife is being used to open or extend the fistula, completing the sphincterotomy. **Lower left:** A stent is being removed with a basket. **Lower right:** The stones are being removed with an occlusion balloon.

SUMP SYNDROME: MANAGEMENT WITH SPHINCTEROTOMY OR STONE—FOREIGN BODY EXTRACTION

The sump syndrome is a clinical syndrome that may develop after surgical formation of a biliary-enteric anastomosis, such as choledochoduodenostomy or choledochojejunostomy (57,58). When the biliary-enteric anastamosis is fashioned, the surgeon attempts to form an enterostomy stoma as large as 2.5 cm, which is certainly adequate enough for most stones to pass spontaneously. Often, after surgery, the surgeon will indicate that a stone was palpated in the distal common bile duct, but it could either not be removed or was not removed, so a choledochoduodenostomy was formed for drainage. Most patients do well following this type of surgery, and few present with recurrent cholestasis, cholangitis, pancreatitis, or retained stones. However, under certain conditions such as stenosis of the enterostomy stoma in combination with possible dysfunction of the sphincter of Oddi, cholestasis, cholangitis, and pancreatitis occur. Biochemical abnormalities are usually present, and air is present in the biliary tree on a flat film of the abdomen. Obstruction of the bile duct secondary to stone material or a phytobezoar should be a consideration included in the differential diagnosis (59).

A patent biliary-enteric anastomosis permits reflux of gastrointestinal contents into the bile duct. With an adequate stoma there should be spontaneous egress of biliary contents through the stoma without obstructive symptoms. However, if the biliary-enteric anastamosis has partially stenosed, egress of biliary contents, especially particulate matter, may not occur, and obstruction to the biliary tree may result. The sump occurs as a result of stone material or gastrointestinal contents accumulating in the dependent portion of the common bile duct, or in that portion of the bile duct to the anastamosis.

Confirming the diagnosis of a sump syndrome is not difficult. Air in the biliary tree may provide the initial clue. Obviously, if the patient is not in shock or septic, the presence of air in the biliary tree corroborates the impression of a biliary-enteric anastamosis (when a patient presents with shock, air in the biliary tree usually connotes an overwhelming infection caused by gas-producing bacteria). Second, at upper endoscopy and specifically ERCP, the enterostomy stoma can be visualized and inspected, and foreign material may be seen through the enterostomy in the bile duct (Fig. 10.42). Injection of contrast into the bile duct opacifies the biliary tree and, in so doing, should identify filling defects in the biliary tree. However, because an enteric-biliary anastomosis exists, air bubbles are present and can be confused for stones or debris. Definition of the biliary tree and confirmation of stones is provided by performing per oral choledochoscopy using a standard or thin-caliber upper endoscope (60) (Fig. 10.43). This technique is performed by inserting the endoscope through the enterostomy into the biliary

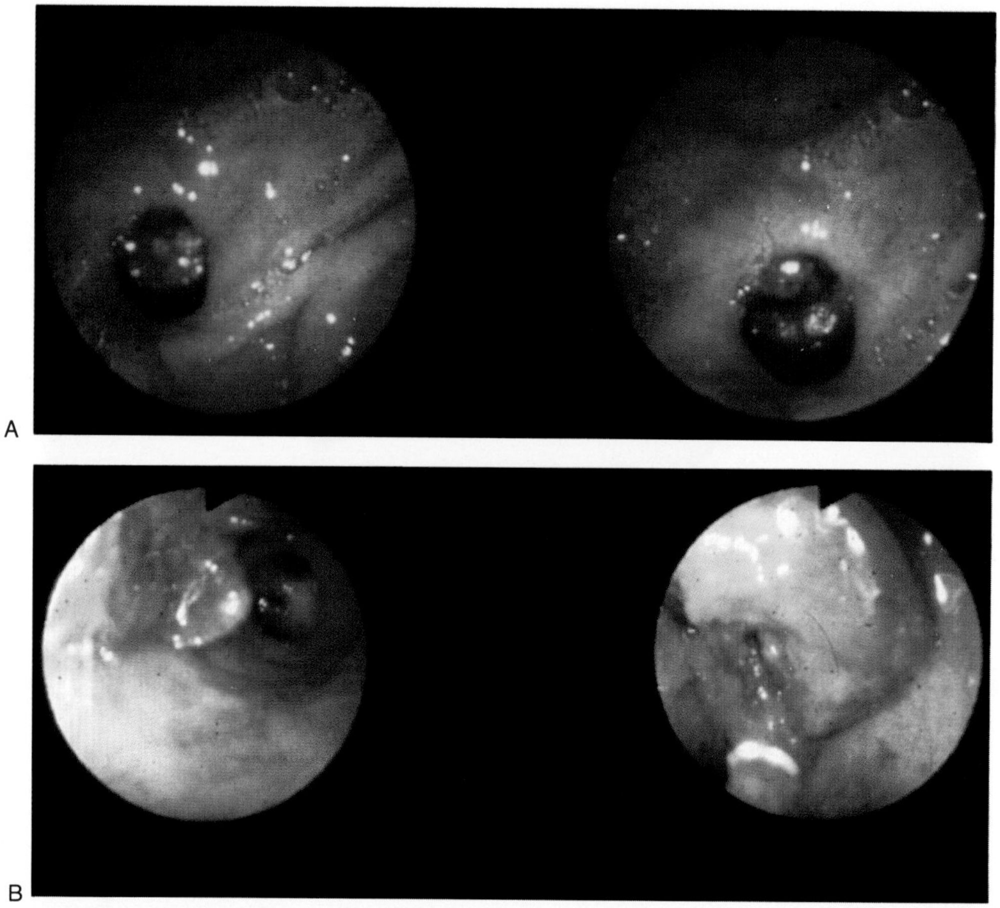

FIG. 10.42. A: Left, right: A partially stenosed choledochoduodenostomy. Foreign material (phytobezoar) is seen on the bile duct side of the anastamosis. (From ref. 59, with permission.) **B: Left:** After advancing a forward-viewing fiberscope into the choledochoduodenostomy, one can appreciate foreign material. **Right:** A phytobezoar being extracted by an accessory.

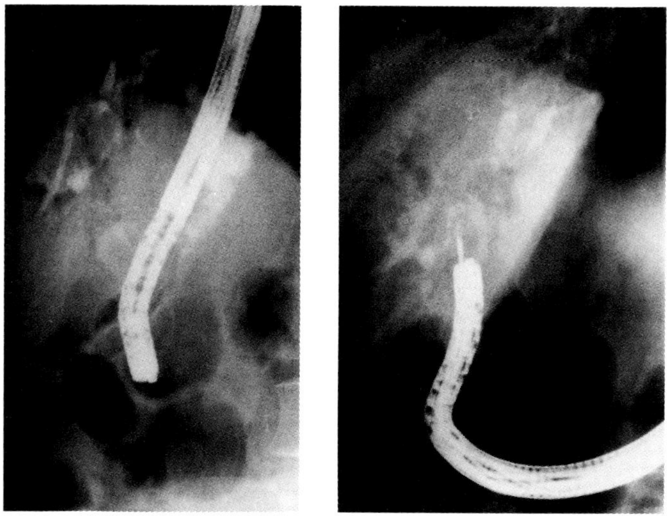

FIG. 10.43. Left: An endoscope being advanced through an enterostomy of a choledochoduodenostomy into the distal common bile duct. **Right:** The endoscope has been removed from the distal bile duct and has been inserted into the proximal bile duct. A foreign body device extends from the tip of the endoscope. (From ref. 59, with permission.)

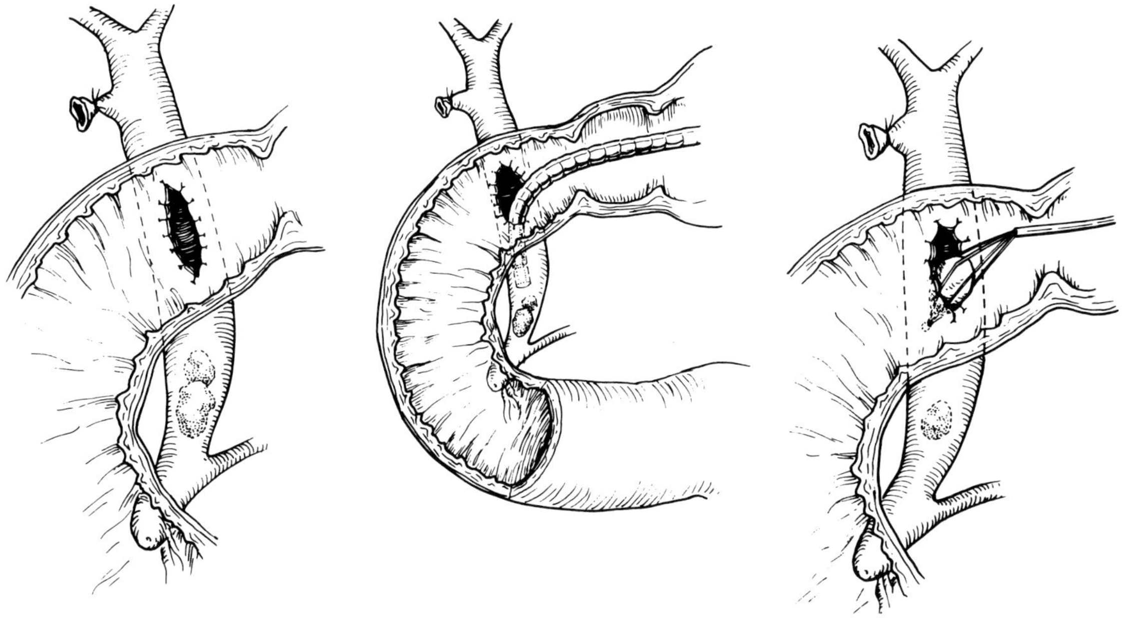

A B C

FIG. 10.44. A: The formation of a choledochoduodenostomy, which is of adequate size, and the presence of stones or filling defects in the distal segment of the bile duct, the sump syndrome. **B:** An endoscope is advanced into the bile duct via the enterostomy for examination of the duct and confirmation of stones. **C:** A basket is passed through the endoscope and into the bile duct, and, under direct vision, a stone is entrapped and removed from the bile duct.

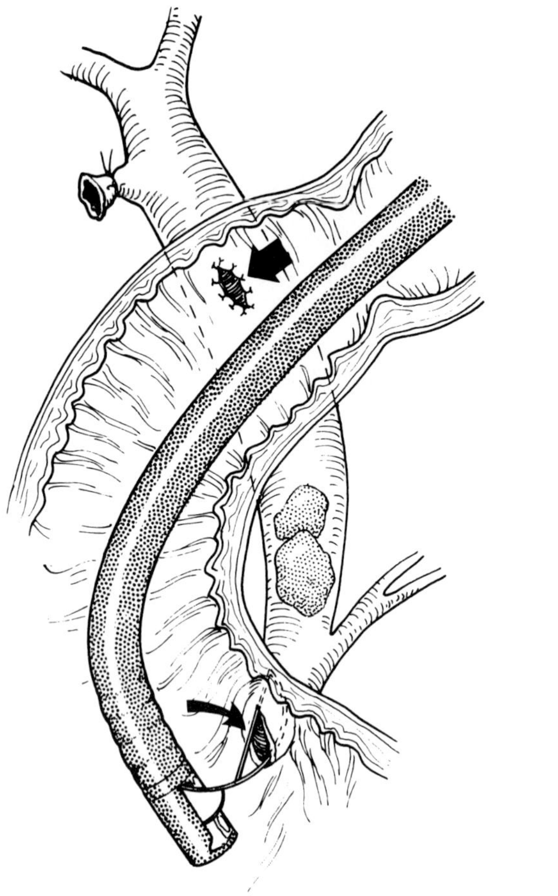

FIG. 10.45. A sump syndrome with stones in the segment of the bile duct distal to the choledochoduodenostomy. The enterostomy has partially stenosed, and the only endoscopic option remaining is sphincterotomy. The sphincterotome has been placed into the sphincter and aligned, and the incision is being carried out.

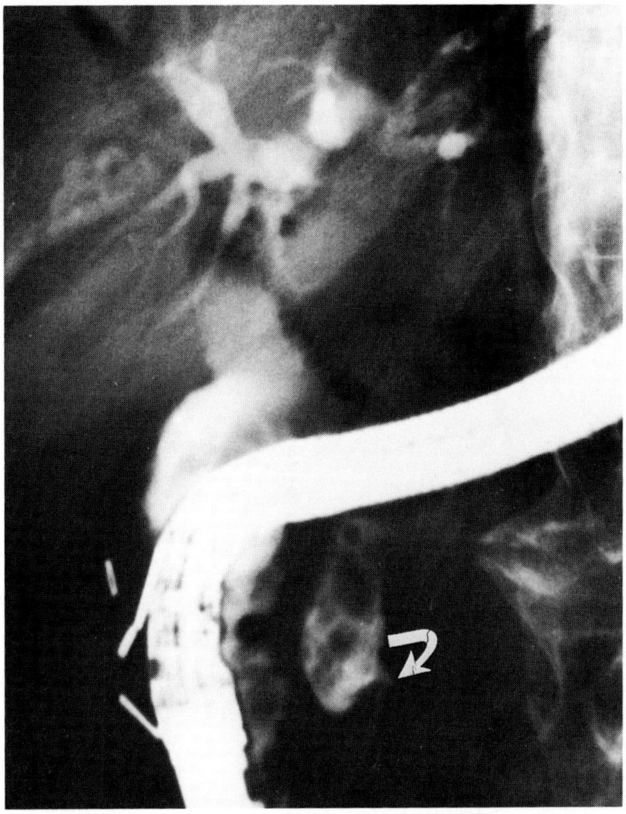

FIG. 10.46. A sump syndrome. Stenosis of the distal common bile duct is visible (*arrow*), and stones are present in the duct. Contrast is visible extravasating into the duodenum through the choledochoduodenostomy into the duodenum, seen above the endoscope.

tree. While the endoscope is in the duct and after a foreign object or stone has been identified, a basket or forceps can be used to remove the object (Figs. 10.44, 10.45). Alternatively, the debris or stones can be removed indirectly by passing a basket from the endoscope through the enterostomy into the duct and removing the debris (61). If the stoma is small, a sphincterotomy, which is more definitive and usually prevents obstruction by debris, is recommended (62–65). I have treated 43 patients presenting with the sump syndrome with sphincterotomy (Figs. 10.46, 10.47; Table 10.3) with excellent results, and I recommend endoscopic management for this condition. I do not recommend that an endoscopist attempt to enlarge the enterostomy stoma using electrocautery techniques because this is fraught with danger (i.e., bleeding and perforation).

TABLE 10.3. *Sump syndrome*

Patients	43
Age range 26–83 years	
Women	23
Men	20
Choledochoduodenostomy	37
Choledochojejunostomy	6
Presenting symptoms	
Cholangitis	19
Cholestasis	17
Pancreatitis	7
Mode of treatment	
Sphincterotomy	39
Extraction	3
Dissolution (bile acids)	1

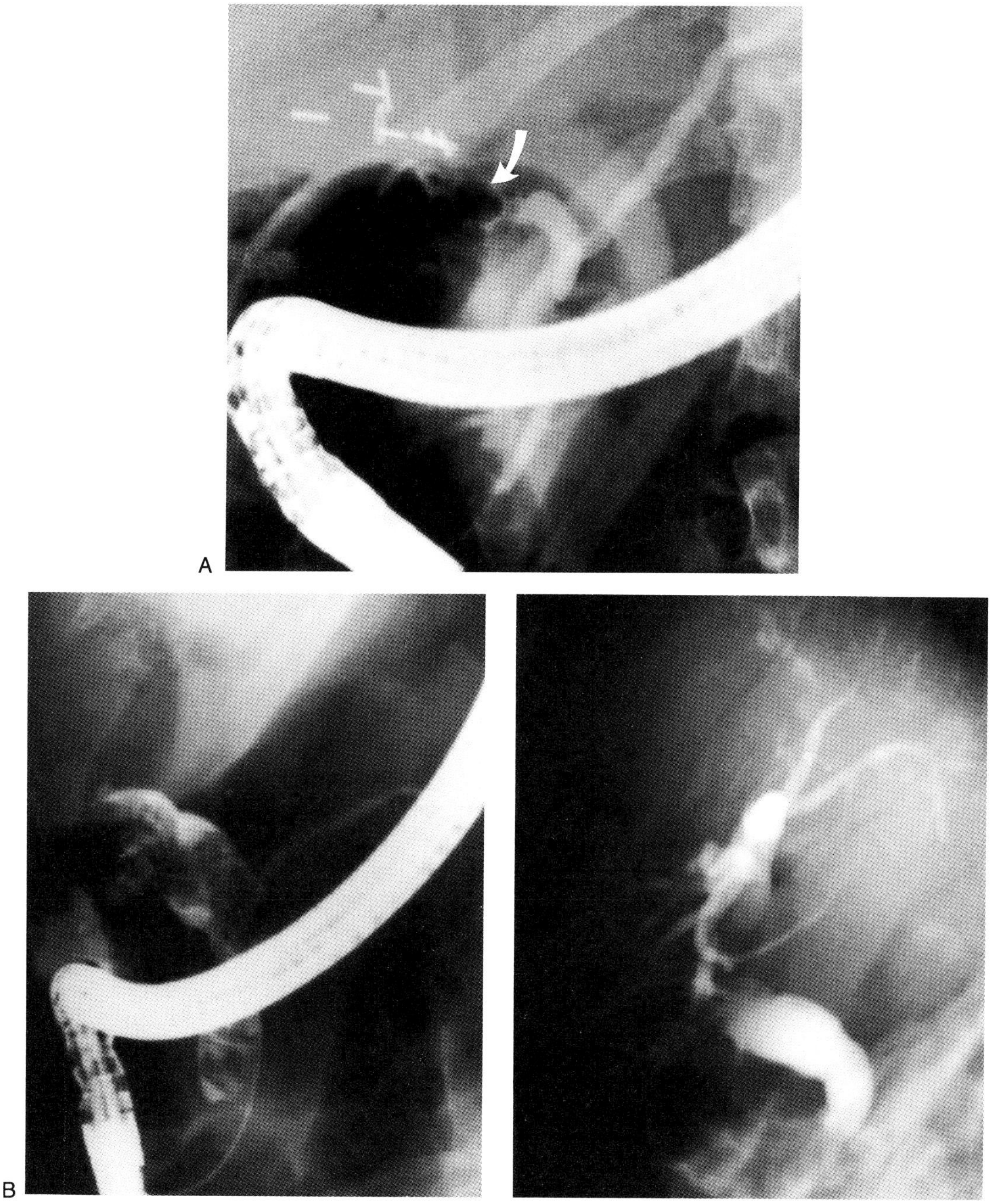

FIG. 10.47. A: Nondilated ducts in this radiograph in a young patient with recurrent pain status post choledochoduodenostomy. Note the lucent defect (*arrow*) occluding the enterostomy, and air is present in the biliary tree. After a sphincterotomy, a balloon catheter was used to dislodge the stone and reestablish continuity of the bile duct. **B: Left:** A cholangiogram obtained in a patient who had undergone a choledochoenterostomy that partially occluded. However, air was present in the proximal biliary tree and stones, and other debris were seen in the distal common bile duct. **Right:** After a sphincterotomy has been performed and the duct has been cleared with a basket and occlusion balloon, this cholangiogram revealed no retained debris.

SPHINCTEROTOMY—GALLBLADDER IN SITU

Controversy still surrounds the concept of performing a sphincterotomy while leaving the gallbladder *in situ* (66–70). Although there is no evidence that leaving the gallbladder *in situ* after sphincterotomy increases the risk of cholecystitis, surgeons continue to proclaim that leaving the source of disease in place *would* increase the incidence of cholecystitis. No data support this claim, and a number of endoscopic studies attest to the safety of sphincterotomy in the presence of an intact gallbladder (71–75). The critical determinants in performing a sphincterotomy are, more specifically, the status of the gallbladder at the time of ERCP and the possible coexistence of cholecystitis. The incidence of cholecystitis following sphincterotomy has been acceptably low, but it has been intimated that its occurrence might be increased when an obstructed cystic duct is demonstrated at the time of ERCP and ES (76). The significance of an obstructed cystic duct requires further study and data analysis, and this finding should be considered when a sphincterotomy is contemplated. Antibiotics should be administered after the endoscopic procedure.

The studies listed in Table 10.4 are open studies, most of which were carried out in a prospective but nonrandomized fashion. For obvious reasons, there are no controlled trials of the performance of sphincterotomy in the presence of an intact gallbladder, but the open, prospective trials are credible. However, at least one randomized trial and one prospective study compared ERCP, sphincterotomy, and clearance of the bile duct followed by cholecystectomy to surgery, cholecystectomy, and surgical common bile duct exploration (77,78). These trials were undertaken to determine if sphincterotomy and bile duct clearance by endoscopy would reduce the complications associated with cholecystectomy and surgical common bile duct exploration. There were problems with randomizing the patient groups in the randomized study because randomization would be difficult in any trial comparing endoscopy with surgery. Patients who appeared to be at greater risk were usually placed into the endoscopic group. As a result, in this trial, more complications occurred in the endoscopic group, but there were no statistical differences in morbidity and mortality between the endoscopic and surgical groups. However, the most important finding in this study showed that the period of hospitalization was shorter in the endoscopic-surgical group than in the pure surgical component. Although this finding was not statistically significant, it is the most significant finding of this randomized trial because reducing hospital stay is critical in today's climate of cost effectiveness. With the

TABLE 10.4. *Endoscopic sphincterotomy—intact gallbladder*

Endoscopic series			
Study	Patients	Follow-up	Cholecystectomy
Cotton	118	2–9 yrs	6 (5.1%)
Escourrou	130	6 mo–5.5 yrs	7 (5.4%)
Davidson	105	1–8 yrs	6 (7.1%)
Siegel	1272	0–11 yrs	108 (8.5%)
Rosseland	66	0–8 yrs	8 (12%)
Tanaka	122	0.5–10 yrs	5 (4.1%)
Martin	70	0–4 yrs	9 (12.86%)

enormous costs of hospitalization, each day saved—which, in the case of cholecystectomy and common bile duct exploration, would be multiplied by more than 100,000 patients annually in the United States—is considerable and would affect the delivery of health care.

For a patient who presents with cholestasis or abnormal liver chemistries and an intact gallbladder, in light of these studies I recommend ERCP, sphincterotomy, and bile duct clearance. If the patient is agreeable and physically capable, a laparoscopic cholecystectomy should be performed shortly thereafter. This combination of procedures promises to be the most cost-effective approach to the management of gallstone disease today. Until laparoscopists develop the technology and can perform an adequate common duct exploration, endoscopic sphincterotomy appears to be the method of choice for clearing the bile duct.

Another significant point, convalescence, is usually not taken into consideration when analyzing the results and follow-up of patients after discharge from hospital. Patients who undergo endoscopic sphincterotomy and an open cholecystectomy tend to return home from the hospital sooner, convalesce more quickly, and return to their usual activities much sooner than those undergoing an open bile duct exploration. This finding will be even more significant when one looks at the data collected from the combined performance of endoscopic sphincterotomy and bile duct clearance followed by laparoscopic cholecystectomy. Data from Reddick and Olsen indicate that patients undergoing laparoscopic colecystectomy (lap chole) alone return to work in a few days (mean 6.5 days), compared to a 30-day convalescence from open cholecystectomy (79). That figure was generated from studies comparing "mini lap," or "bandaid," cholecystectomy to lap chole. The results of the mini lap cholecystectomy were better than those of the standard, open cholecystectomy.

The incidence of cholecystitis following sphincterotomy in patients with gallbladders *in situ,* shown in Table 10.4, is approximately 8% to 9%. The rate for elective cholecystectomy status post sphincterotomy is about the same. Long-term follow-up of patients who have undergone ES with an *in situ* gallbladder may prove critical to the management of patients with gallstone disease. Some investigators in Europe (80) actually have performed sphincterotomy in patients with gallbladder disease but without evidence of bile duct disease (Fig. 10.47). The annual incidence of symptomatic cholecystitis is accepted to be 2% to 4% (81). Long-term follow-up data from our series and from European and Japanese studies support the hypothesis that endoscopic sphincterotomy actually may reduce the annual incidence of cholecystitis (82–89). Sphincterotomy alters the physiology of the gallbladder and bile acid composition and concentration and may contribute to the dissolution of gallstones or the extrusion of smaller stones from the gallbladder (90–94). Despite the presence of enteric bacteria in the bile duct and gallbladder, the incidence of infection is not increased and there is no alteration of bile acids (i.e., dehydroxylation and deconjugation) that would contribute to stone formation (95). Therefore, contrary to the supposition that sphincterotomy may increase the incidence of cholecystitis, sphincterotomy may actually reduce it. Although this may be obsolete because of the advent of laparoscopic cholecystectomy, *endoscopic sphincterotomy may prove to be effective in the treatment of gallbladder disease*. This conclusion is based on the long-term follow-up of patients who have undergone endoscopic sphincterotomy with gallbladders *in situ* and who have done well without evidence of cholecystitis.

Performance of endoscopic sphincterotomy in elderly, high-risk patients with an intact gallbladder has been acceptable and is preferred by many physicians and surgeons as the index therapeutic procedure for such patients presenting with cholestasis, jaundice, and evidence of cholangitis and/or gallstone pancreatitis (96). The usual attitude is to await results of sphincterotomy before considering cholecystectomy. Our group has modified this approach over the years and has not limited the performance of sphincterotomy to patients who are elderly (with *in situ* gallbladders) or at great risk. In fact, we perform the procedure in many young, fit patients without untoward effects. This approach has given us a unique opportunity to accrue long-term follow-up data to determine the efficacy of sphincterotomy and its effect on the intact gallbladder.

My current recommendation to perform ES in elderly as well as young patients with *in situ* gallbladders has been altered only slightly with the advent of laparoscopic cholecystectomy. I recommend the performance of ERCP prior to laparoscopic cholecystectomy in all patients who present with cholestasis, jaundice, or gallstone pancreatitis, regardless of age or risk factors. This recommendation is valid because the current technology for performing laparoscopic cholecystectomy is developing, and common bile duct exploration is arduous and inefficient. For the time being, ERCP and ES excel in this area, and, until the laparoscopic techniques advance into the bile duct, most surgeons prefer the other endoscopic procedure, ES.

ENDOSCOPIC SPHINCTEROTOMY IN THE MANAGEMENT OF CHOLANGITIS

Acute cholangitis and suppurative cholangitis occur commonly as manifestations and complications of stone disease (80%) (97–103) and can occur concomitantly with cholecystitis (up to 10%) (104–106). Ten percent of patients with obstructing bile duct neoplasms (carcinoma of the pancreas or ampulla) or benign obstructive disease such as papillary stenosis present with a clinical picture of cholangitis, but this associated complication occurs more frequently after manipulation of the bile duct (i.e., following percutaneous or endoscopic cholangiography). Prior to the advent of radiologic and endoscopic interventional techniques, the management of this life-threatening condition was surgical; however, the mortality associated with surgery was excessive, as high as 40% (97,102–105). Several reports comparing the decompression modalities—endoscopic, radiologic, and surgical—concluded that the endoscopic approach to this condition was the most efficacious of the three (Table 10.5) (97–125). The highest mortality reported with endoscopic techniques, sphincterotomy, or insertion of stents or nasobiliary tubes is 7.6%. For comparison, the mortalities reported from the radiologic and surgical series, which included their most seriously ill patients, were reportedly as high as 29% and 40%, respectively. Surgical mortality under optimal conditions (in other words, with a stable patient who is normotensive and without other comorbid or intercurrent medical problems) has been reported to be as low as 9%, whereas the lowest mortality reported for the percutaneous technique, under the same conditions, was 5%. In our experience in managing 947 patients with cholangitis, the majority of whom were stable, the overall mortality was low, 0.42% (4 in 947). Although the endoscopic techniques are safe, deaths do occur. In our series, the mortality that occurred among the

TABLE 10.5. *Cholangitis, 30 day mortality: comparison of surgical, radiologic, and endoscopic techniques*

	Surgery	Radiologic	Endoscopic
Welch	40%		
Saharia	14%		
Lygidakis	20%		
Thompson	9%		
Gould		29%	
Kadir		17%	
Pessa		5%	
Kinoshita		14.3%	
Vallon			7.1%
Carr-Locke			4.7%
Leung			4.7%
Gogel			7.6%
Siegel			7.4%[a]

[a] 7.4% ($\frac{2}{27}$ critically ill; two deaths; 2 and 3 weeks; not related to procedure); 1.5% ($\frac{4}{265}$ unstable; includes the 27 critically ill and two deaths); 0.42% ($\frac{4}{947}$ total series, stable and unstable patients)

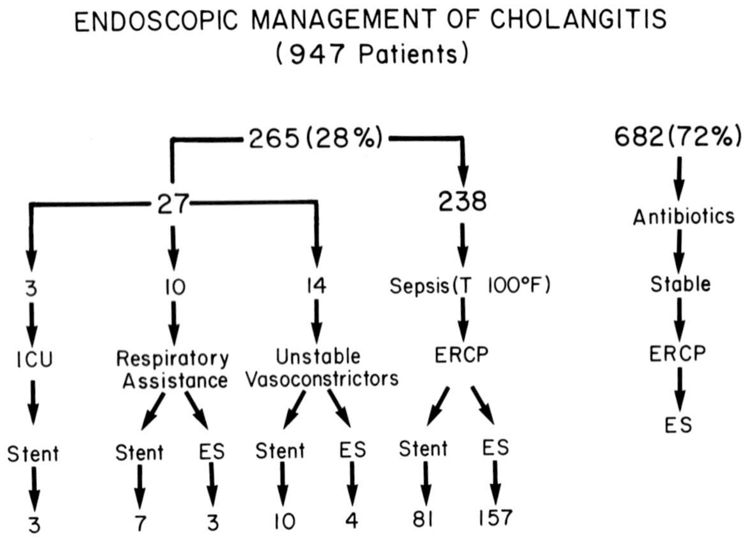

FIG. 10.48. A flow chart identifying the form of presentation of 947 patients with cholangitis and the treatment modalities offered and performed.

critically ill, unstable group was 7.4% (2 in 27), but the combined mortality of the unstable and more stable patients (febrile only) was a respectable 1.5% (4 in 254).

The form of patient presentation and timing of intervention are critical to survival. Suppurative cholangitis, the most serious and morbid presentation occurring in 15% of patients, is associated with Charcot's triad—the clinical combination of abdominal pain, fever, and jaundice—70% of the time (126–128). In our series, Fig. 10.48, all patients with cholangitis fit into one of three distinct stages of illness at presentation. The majority of patients, 682 (72%), were referred to our center after having been stabilized with appropriate fluid and electrolyte replacement and receiving a course of parenteral antibiotic therapy. These patients presented with no fever and were maintained on specific antibiotics (129). As seen from the flowchart (Fig. 10.49), these patients were managed ostensibly with endoscopic sphincterotomy with no mortality and minimal morbidity (Figs. 10.50–10.52). A smaller, less stable group (265 patients) was managed either by

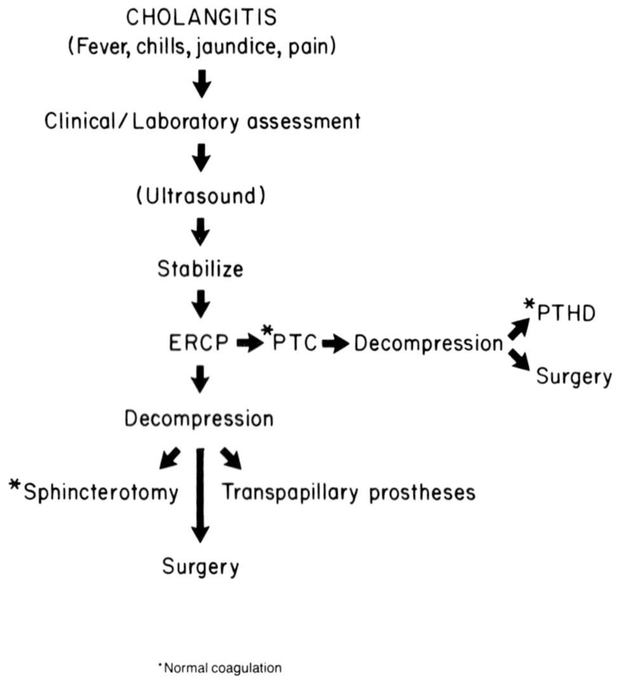

FIG. 10.49. This algorithm describes the author's approach to patients presenting with the clinical syndrome of cholangitis.

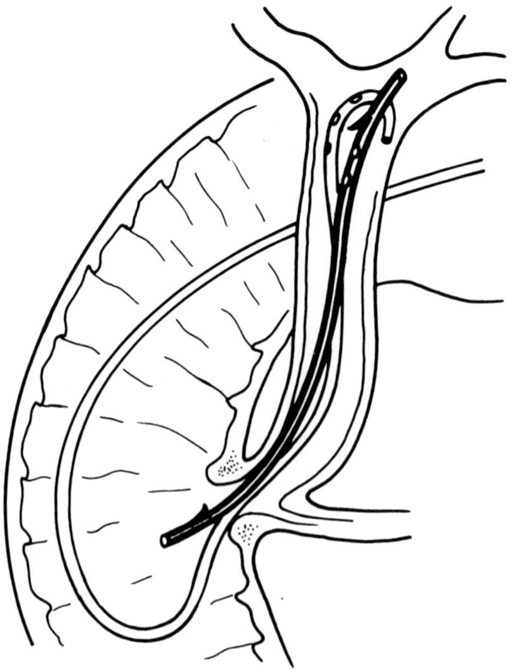

FIG. 10.50. The placement of both a nasobiliary tube and endoprosthesis to manage patients presenting with cholangitis.

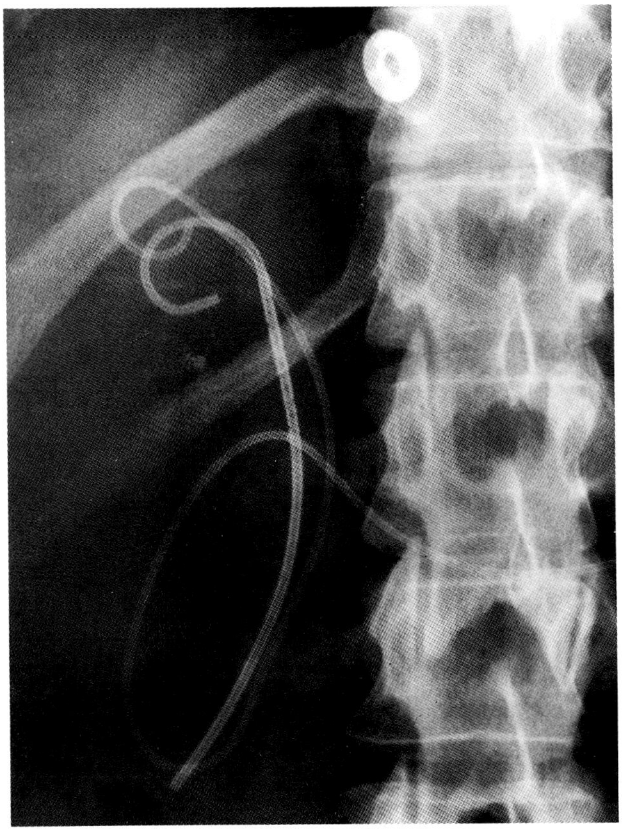

FIG. 10.51. A nasobiliary tube and an endoprosthesis that were placed into the bile duct of a patient presenting with cholangitis.

insertion of endoprostheses into the bile duct or sphincterotomy. This latter group exhibited fever exceeding 100°F and required intravenous antibiotics. The decision to perform a sphincterotomy was made at the time of the procedure and was critical because of the possibility of associated complications. If these patients were too ill to undergo surgery initially, the decision to perform sphincterotomy was made judiciously at endoscopy, because a serious complication might necessitate emergency surgery. When in doubt, or if the procedure needed to be performed expeditiously, a prosthesis was inserted as a temporizing measure (Figs. 10.53, 10.54). Twenty-seven (27) patients were critically ill and required supportive care including vasopressors; ten were on ventilatory assistance, and three who were too unstable to be moved were treated in the intensive care unit, without fluoroscopic control. In this group of three, the endoscope cart was brought to the bedside in the ICU, endoscopy was performed, the papilla was cannulated with the catheter, and bile or pus was aspirated to confirm selective cannulation of the bile duct. After confirmation of the location of the catheter (visible bile or pus or aspiration), a guidewire and prosthesis were inserted blindly. The flowchart stratifies the modes of presentation and treatment of this large series of patients.

Etiology

Cholangitis is most commonly caused by obstruction to the biliary tree, usually secondary to stone disease and intercurrent infection. Because of obstruction of the bile duct, the resultant increased pressure within the hepaticobiliary tree, increased intrabiliary pressure producing hepaticovenous reflux of bacteria, facilitates entry of bacteria into the systemic circulation, accounting for sepsis and its multivariate manifestations (130–141). Both the surgical and the radiologic experiences in managing patients with acute cholangitis have been associated with severe complications and resultant mortality. Although the endoscopic experience has been associated with fewer fatal complications, the mortality is significant. Most investigators agree that if endoscopic facilities and expertise are available when a patient presents with cholangitis, this approach is preferable to surgery and interventional radiologic procedures. Ideally, the patient should be stabilized or made as stable as possible before undertaking the endoscopic procedure. The procedure can be performed on patients who have undergone endotracheal intubation and are on ventilatory assistance. Although moving the patient and managing this extra equipment is rather cumbersome, endoscopy can be

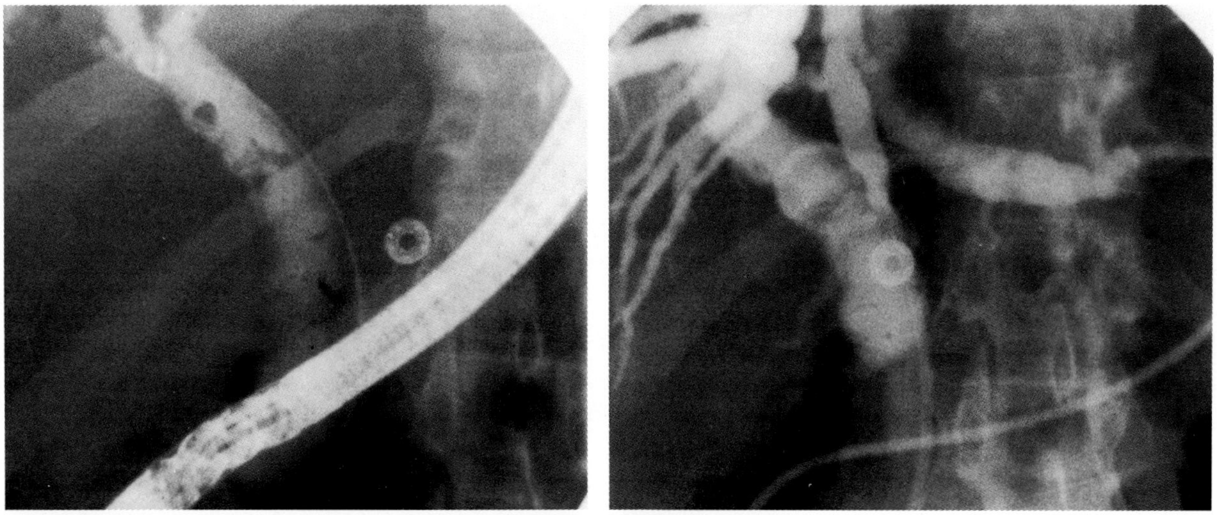

A

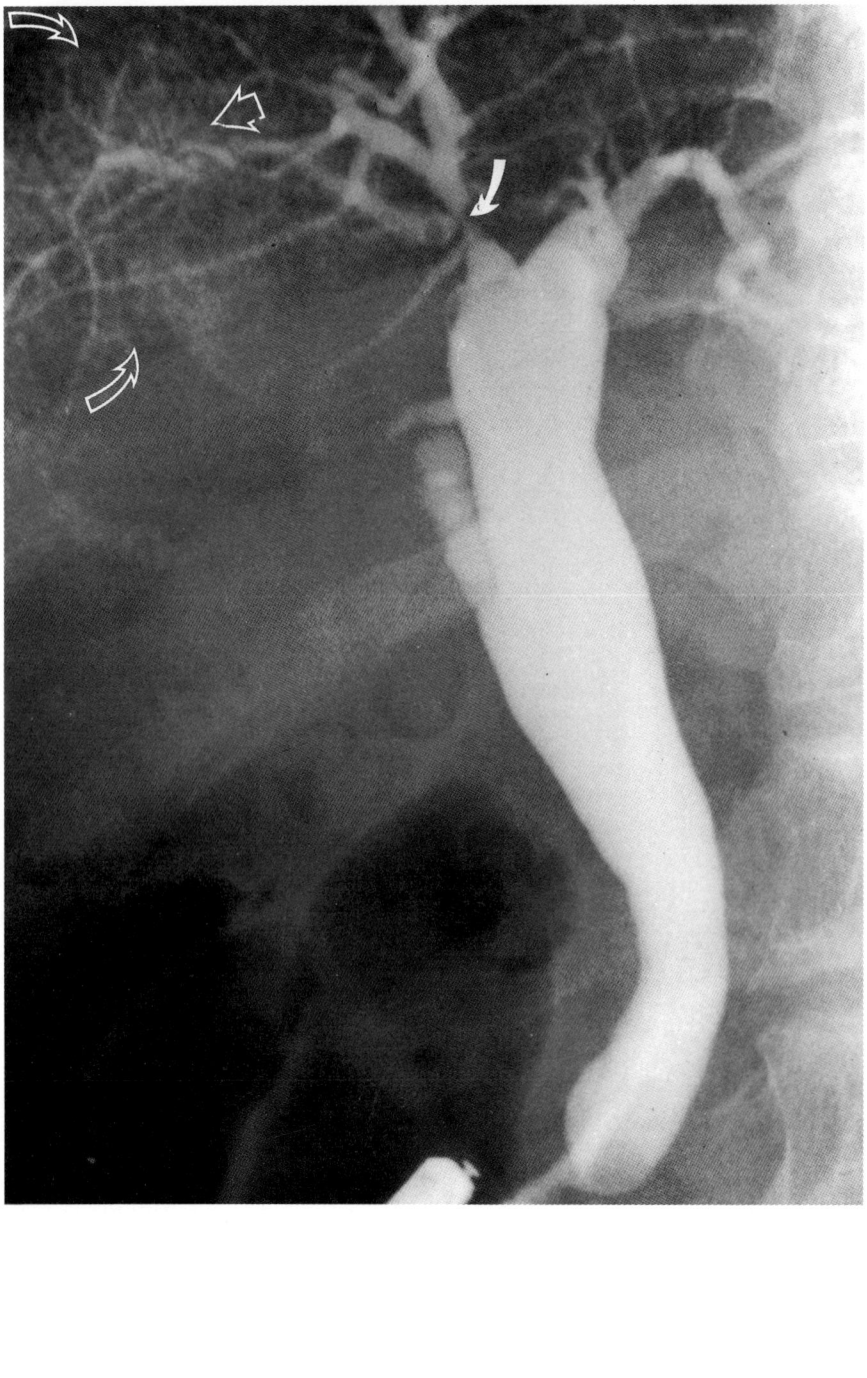

B

FIG. 10.52. A: Left: A cholangiogram obtained in a patient presenting with cholangitis. Stones are seen floating in the bile duct. **Right:** A nasobiliary tube has been placed into the patient's bile duct. After performance of a sphincterotomy and irrigation of the tube, the stones have passed, and the patient's clinical condition has improved. **B:** A radiograph obtained in a patient with a Bilroth II gastrectomy that demonstrates two significant findings. The first is papillary stenosis with a dilated bile duct. The second is a stricture of the right hepatic duct (*arrow*) and evidence of hepatic abcesses in the right lobe (*open arrows*).

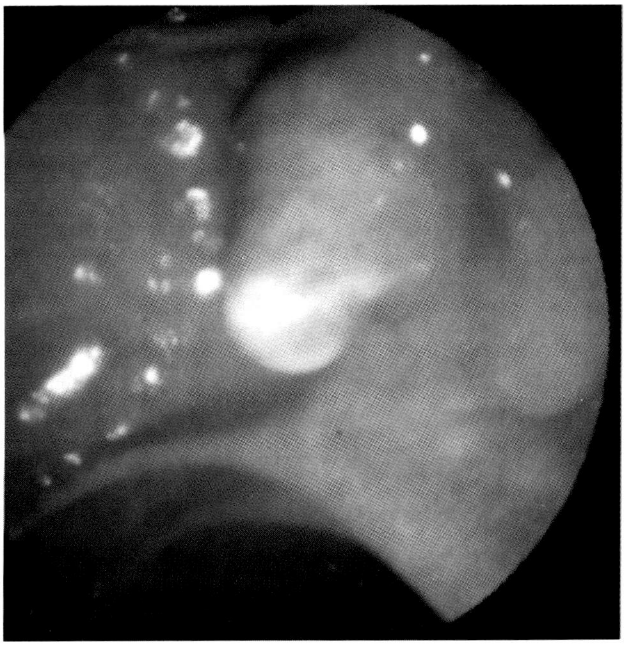

FIG. 10.53. An endoscopic picture of a prominent papilla with pus exuding from its orifice. The patient presented with cholangitis.

successfully performed in the procedure room, which is equipped with a fluoroscope and spot film device. Our success is due in great measure to our close working relationship with our anesthesiologists, who are willing to stand by during these high-risk procedures. No immediate death has occurred in this large group

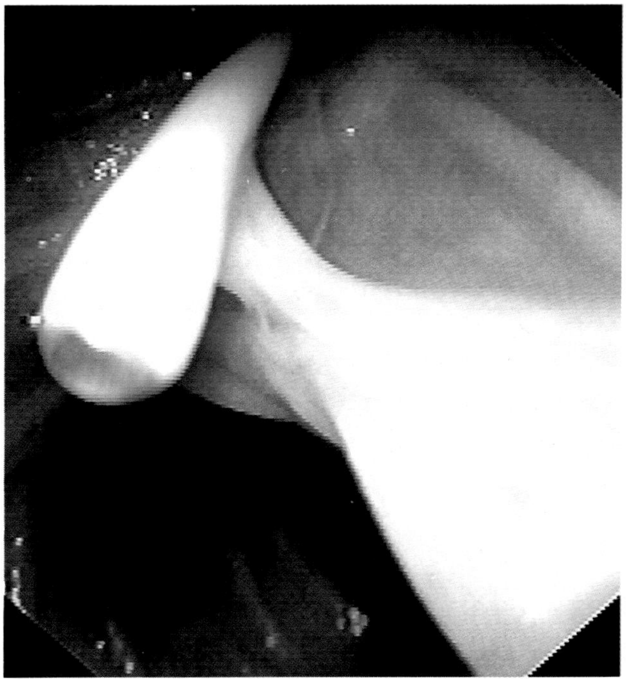

FIG. 10.54. Pus (purulent material) exuding from the side flap hole of a prosthesis placed into a patient with cholangitis.

of patients. The four deaths in the entire series occurred within 10 to 21 days after performing ERCP, but only one was procedure related.

Suppurative cholangitis is a life-threatening disease that may be successfully managed by endoscopic techniques. All endoscopists are encouraged to hone their skills precisely in order to perform a sphincterotomy expeditiously and to insert prostheses in an emergency setting despite the presence of sepsis or shock. The risks of the procedure should be carefully explained to the patient or the patient's family or survivors. Serious complications do occur with endoscopy because of associated multiorgan failure, a critical point that cannot be overemphasized. Appropriate consultations and ancillary support will enhance patient survival. From our experience and that of others, the procedure can be a life-saving one, and the minimal risks certainly justify the results.

Figure 10.49 is presented to assist the primary care physician, gastroenterologist, and surgeon in providing an expeditious evaluation of patients presenting with sepsis secondary to cholangitis. The most readily available scanning procedure, the sonogram, is portable, provides valuable information, and is not invasive, but it is not specific. It is valuable in demonstrating a dilated biliary tree. HIDA scans and scintigraphy are usually not helpful, especially when the patient is deeply jaundiced (142–145). Other important ancillary studies, blood chemistries, and blood counts are quickly obtained, and the patient may be stabilized by the administration of fluids, electrolytes, vasopressors if necessary, and antibiotics. Once the diagnosis is confirmed, if the patient's condition is unstable or deteriorating, an ERCP may be scheduled and arranged urgently. Obviously, the advantage of performing ERCP or percutaneous cholangiography is the additional capability of providing therapy with the diagnostic component (107–117). If the patient can be stabilized, the procedure should be postponed or rescheduled as an elective one. The latter option is preferable, especially if stones are to be removed or lithotripsy carried out, techniques that prolong the index procedure. One is always secure in accepting the option of placing a prosthesis and leaving it in the bile duct indefinitely until the patient becomes stable enough for endoscopy. At that time one can carry out definitive therapy.

SPHINCTEROTOMY IN THE MANAGEMENT OF GALLSTONE PANCREATITIS (See Chapter 9)

Sphincterotomy—Results and Complications (Tables 10.6, 10.7, 10.8)

ES is the only endoscopic procedure with predictable morbidity and mortality. Fortunately, the complica-

TABLE 10.6. *Endoscopic sphincterotomy—experience in 5,370 procedures*

	Attempted	Performed	% Success
Common duct stones	4,159	4,088	98.3
Tumors	590	543	92.0
Papillary stenosis	621	597	96.1
Total	5,370	5,228	97.4
Intact gall bladder		1,516 (28% of total)	
Age range		17–101 years	
Mean age		68.3	
Patients over 65		3,651 (68%)	
History of cholangitis		1,452 (30%, stones plus stenosis)	
Mean hospital stay		4.1 days	

tions associated with the performance of sphincterotomy have remained constant or even low, despite the relatively universal performance of this procedure. As experience has accumulated, the rate of success for the performance of sphincterotomy has increased, and complications have declined. The rate of success has increased because of the experience of the endoscopists as well as the availability of accessories such as the wire-guided sphincterotome and the needle knife. Experienced endoscopists employ all the accessories in the performance of sphincterotomy and invoke many options to complete the procedure successfully. They may have to repeat the procedure more than once to succeed. Because most endoscopists and patients are willing to undergo the procedure a second time and occasionally a third rather than face surgery, endoscopists have had additional opportunities to complete the procedure, thus improving success rates. As long as there is not an increased risk to performing the procedure a second or third time and the endoscopist is willing to accept a more global fee instead of a fee for each procedure, this approach to difficult cannulation and sphincterotomy will help to reduce overwhelming costs to the health care delivery system and reinforces the message of cost containment.

Complications do occur following the performance of ERCP and ES, and the endoscopist should be able to recognize and manage these. All references to

TABLE 10.7. *Complications of endoscopic sphincterotomy (N = 5,370)*

Bleeding	94	5.2% (Bleeding, Cholangitis, Pancreatitis, Perforation combined)
Cholangitis	53	
Pancreatitis	103	
Perforation, pain	21	
Emergency surgery	15	0.28%
Deaths	5	0.09%
Transfusion	35	0.7%

TABLE 10.8. *Complications of ES in 5,370 cases (N = 271, 5.2%)*

Complication	Number of patients	%
Bleeding	94	1.75
Cholangitis (infection)	53	0.99
Pancreatitis	103	1.92
Perforation	21	0.39
Emergency surgery	15	0.28
Transfusion	35	0.68
Deaths	5	0.093
Total	271	5.2%

ERCP and ES clearly describe the frequency and occurrence of bleeding, pancreatitis, perforation, and infection (135–169), which are expected despite appropriate preparation and performance of the procedure. As one reads the original and subsequent reports of these procedures, one can appreciate the fact that despite the universal performance of procedures, which were originally performed by a handful of experts, the morbidity and mortality associated with ES have remained level, a clear indication of the preparation, training, and awareness of the endoscopists.

The following are summaries of the most frequent complications, with special sections for proper preparation for, avoidance of, and management of these complications. Appropriate tables are available to familiarize the endoscopist with these potential risks and to outline diagnostic and treatment plans. Although the tables are simplistic, even the experienced endoscopist will benefit from them.

PREVENTION AND MANAGEMENT OF COMPLICATIONS OF SPHINCTEROTOMY

Equipment Check (Table 10.9)

Before performing any endoscopic procedure, especially therapeutic, the endoscopist should ensure that the equipment is functioning and in good working order. It is routine to check the endoscope, light source, suction, accessories, and the electrocoagulation generator. If everything checks satisfactorily, one can initiate the procedure, having been assured that the hardware is functioning.

TABLE 10.9. *Prevention of Complications*

Equipment check
Endoscope and light source
Sphincterotomes
Handles and contact points
Active cord
Electrocautery generator
Pretest equipment

TABLE 10.10. *Prevention of complications, bleeding*

Complete history to rule out bleeding diathesis.
Stop medications that affect coagulation. Allow enough time for coagulation factors to return to normal range and for platelets to regain function.
Type and screen 2 units of RBCs.
Keep sclerotherapy needle available and epinephrine-saline 1:3,000 drawn up.
Keep balloon catheters for tamponade.
Have a surgeon available.
Keep optional items for standby
Laser
Bicap or heater probe

Bleeding (Tables 10.10, 10.11)

Bleeding is the most common complication of sphincterotomy, but it can be controlled in the majority of cases. Preparation is crucial in preventing serious complications associated with bleeding. First a careful history must be obtained to ascertain the patient's tendency to bleed and to elicit a prior history of bleeding diatheses. Coagulation factor deficiencies will be known to the patient, and replacement of these factors before the procedure will avoid complications. Serious bleeding usually occurs when the incision is extended to the apex of the intramural segment, which is in close proximity to the horizontal duodenal fold. In general, venous bleeding will stop spontaneously, but arteriolar bleeding may persist. Most bleeding stops spontaneously, but blood replacement may be necessary if bleeding is substantial, is continuous, and exceeds 4 units. In my experience, moderate bleeding will cease during the manipulation phase of the procedure and will not require further attention or care. If the endoscopic field is obscured by blood, this usually connotes more serious or heavy bleeding that will require attention. Fastidious follow-up by the endoscopist will usually help to avoid catastrophe.

TABLE 10.11. *Management of bleeding*

Assess degree of bleeding
Venous—will stop spontaneously
Arteriole—may continue, usually slows, stops
Balloon tamponade
Epinephrine 1:3,000 injections
Clinical assessment
Vital signs q 30 min
CBC q2h–3h
N-G tube if patient nauseated or vomiting
N-G tube return bloody
X-match blood
Transfusions if H/H drop below 10/30
If diaphoretic
Increase fluid replacement
Increase blood transfusions
Unstable, vomiting blood, and passing "currant jelly" stools
Increase transfusions
Vasopressors if necessary
ICU
Prepare for surgery

It has been my policy to inject the sphincterotomy site if bleeding persists during or after the manipulation sequence of the procedure. Bleeding usually stops while a basket or balloon catheter is passed to retrieve stones and does not recur, even after the trauma of removing the stone. If bleeding continues, I inject the site with 3 cc of 1:3,000 epinephrine using a sclerotherapy needle (Microvasive or Olympus Corporation) (Figs. 10.55, 10.56). Since the incorporation of sclerotherapy into my postsphincterotomy routine, most bleeds have stopped, and transfusion requirements have decreased. Obviously, if heavy bleeding continues, more aggressive action should be instituted. I have had only one patient who required immediate surgery 3 hours after sphincterotomy. This patient had a Billroth II gastrectomy and aortic insufficiency with a wide pulse pressure. I was unable to inject epinephrine into the sphincterotomy site because blood obscured the field and the endoscope slipped out of the afferent limb and could not be replaced. The patient vomited a large amount of fresh blood and clots, became diaphoretic and unstable, and went to surgery within 3

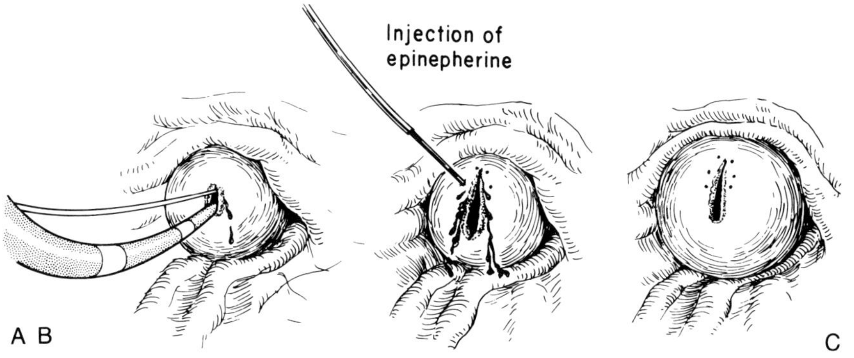

FIG. 10.55. A: This artist's illustration shows a sphincterotomy being performed. Blood droplets are seen. **B:** After completing the sphincterotomy, bleeding persists. The artist demonstrates the injection technique using an endoscopic sclerotherapy needle containing epinephrine 1:3000. **C:** The papilla has swollen because of the intramural injections around the sphincterotomy incision. This is the mechanism for stopping the bleeding.

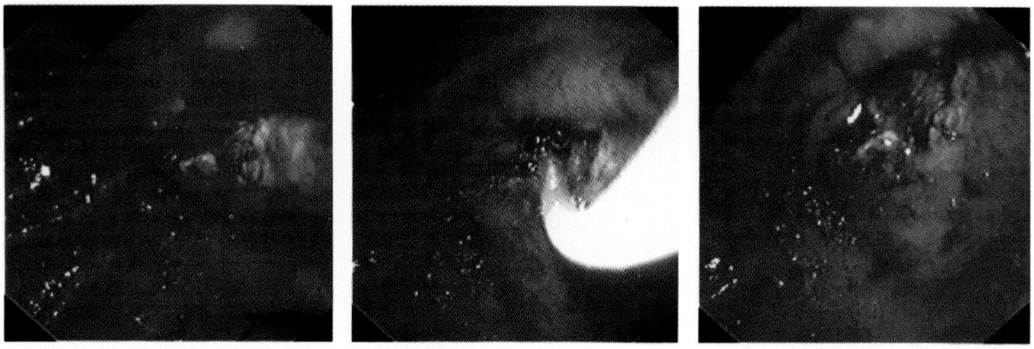

FIG. 10.56. Left: Persistent bleeding from a sphincterotomy. **Middle:** Epinephrine injections are being made into the wall and apex of the incision. The bleeding has stopped. **Right:** No bleeding is seen. Note the edematous sphincterotomy orifice created by the submucosal injections.

hours. This scenario is fortunately rare, and even rarer is death owing to exsanguination. Remember, bleeding can occur within the first 48 hours and up to 7 to 10 days after the procedure when the clot has sloughed. Patients should understand the potential complications and be alerted to symptoms and their chronology, and they should know to call the endoscopist at any time.

Pancreatitis (Tables 10.12, 10.13)

Pancreatitis occurs as frequently as bleeding following sphincterotomy, which is estimated to occur in 2 to 3% of cases. Unlike bleeding and infection, one can do little to prevent its occurrence. It has been my impression that patients with subclinical pancreatitis are more likely to develop severe complications, including phlegmon formation. Because of the large volume of ERCPs performed at my institutions I can predict that two serious cases of pancreatitis with phlegmon will develop annually. This occurrence is not overwhelming when compared to the number of procedures performed annually, but the problem is enigmatic and difficult to manage. Because hospitalization and treatment of severe pancreatitis is long-term and difficult to manage independently, I have, by necessity, utilized a team approach. The team is composed of an intensivist, a nutritionist-physician, an infectious disease specialist, and a surgeon. The intensivist manages the fluid and electrolyte, balance, cardiac, and pulmonary problems; the nutritionist oversees the total parenteral nutrition, and the infectious disease person manages intercurrent infections. The surgeon, justifiably, coordinates the team with me.

TABLE 10.12. *Prevention of complications*

Pancreatitis
Take history of recurrent disease.
Check for recent pancreatitis.
Avoid prolonged procedure.
Check volume of contrast injected.

The first death in my series associated with pancreatitis was complicated by respiratory failure (ARDS) and voluntary extubation, but the remainder of these seriously ill patients have survived. Only one patient underwent surgery after failure of percutaneous drainage to evacuate necrotic debris, and none were treated with peritoneal dialysis after the first fatality. Long-term hospitalization is necessary for the seriously ill until the phlegmon has resolved and the necrotic debris has absorbed. The mean hospitalization for the seriously ill patients was 22 days, with a range of 11 to 75 days. The mean hospitalization for uncomplicated, edematous pancreatitis is 4.1 days, and the range of stay for the less severe problems is 2 to 17 days.

A low-grade fever usually accompanies inflammation of pancreatitis. If there is no evidence of infection (i.e., negative blood, urine, and sputum cultures and negative chest x-rays), antibiotics may be superfluous and may contribute to intercurrent problems such as pseudomembranous colitis and sensitivity reactions.

TABLE 10.13. *Management of pancreatitis*

NPO
NG tube if patient nauseated, abdomen distended
IV infusions: replace volume and electrolytes
Serial serum amylase levels if patient manifests clinical symptoms
Ultrasound—CT scan every 48–96 hours if no clinical improvement
CT scan every 10–14 days to follow progression or regression of phlegmon and intraperitoneal—retroperitoneal collections.
Serial CBCs, electrolytes, and calcium levels: replace or replenish electrolytes and calcium as needed
Transfusion if H/H <10/30
Assess pulmonary function if clinically appropriate
Chest radiographs
Respiratory therapy for atelectasis and improvement of tidal volume
Antibiotics if temperature >101°F and WBCs >14,000 with left shift
Total parenteral nutrition if albumin/protein and other essential parameters down and patient not eating

Even when a phlegmon is present and the white blood cell count remains normal or slightly elevated with only a few bands, antibiotics may not be helpful. Close observation is the watchword and has been most effective in my series. If intraperitoneal or retoperitoneal collections develop, percutaneous drainage may be accomplished. If appropriate stains and cultures of this necrotic material are positive, specific antibiotics should be administered, and more definitive surgical drainage procedures should be planned if the material continues to accumulate and is unresponsive to specific antibiotics and percutaneous drainage. Often in such patients, shotgun antibiotic therapy is associated with intercurrent problems including overgrowth of *Candida albicans* and *Clostridium difficile*, so the physician and his or her team should be prepared to manage these problems.

If checked after ERCP and ES, the serum amylase may be abnormal in 20 to 30% of patients (chemical pancreatitis). It is my rule not to order amylase levels routinely after these procedures; if a clinical syndrome develops and the accompanying symptoms are compatible with clinical pancreatitis, I request serial amylase levels to correlate these findings. Often, in both complicated and uncomplicated cases, the serum amylase will be elevated, but, within 2 to 6 days (mean 4 days), the amylase will return to normal. The amylase level cannot be used as a prognostic sign because it usually returns to normal despite subsequent development of more serious complications such as the formation of a phlegmon or pseudocysts. The only positive prognostic sign is the patient's clinical improvement as manifested by a decrease in pain, return of bowel sounds, passage of flatus and stool, a return of appetite, and a feeling of well being. The best course of treatment for these patients is aggressive support with as little intervention as possible.

Why do patients develop pancreatitis secondary to ERCP and ES? As previously mentioned, most patients have a predisposition to this problem, the so-called subclinical form (Chapter 9) and have experienced symptoms referable to pancreatitis prior to ERCP. These symptoms become fulminant after (A) injection of contrast—volume, pressure, or both; (B) persistent palpation and probing of the papilla without successful cannulation, injection, or opacification; (C) manipulation with an accessory, that is, a guidewire or sphincterotome; and (D) edema secondary to cautery application. Prevention is therefore unfeasible, especially because the radiographic study or attempted study is indicated. Care and caution are advised, but, despite this cautious approach, if pancreatitis ensues, the endoscopist is not to blame and no departure from the standards of practice can be established (unless there was a departure from the procedure explained during the informed consent).

Precut sphincterotomy or needle-knife precut fistulotomy may increase the incidence of pancreatitis, but even this assumption is mostly conjectural since there are only a few anecdotal reports to support this inference. If the patient and/or relatives have been fully informed of the potential complications and alternatives, the endoscopist proceeds cautiously with the knowledge that the patient has been fully informed. Of course, only experienced endoscopists should undertake procedures that are considered difficult and are associated with increased risks.

The management of pancreatitis is not universal and differs among individuals. As long as one advises bowel rest and institutes active therapy (i.e., replacement of the intravascular volume and electrolytes and management of metabolic imbalances that develop), the treatment is considered adequate and within the accepted standards of practice. If abdominal distention worsens and associated nausea and regurgitation occur, a nasogastric tube can be placed to provide relief of these symptoms.

Fortunately, most patients who suffer post-ERCP or post-ES pancreatitis recover completely, but many endure pain during this recovery. Some patients, unfortunately, require surgery, which may be difficult and may not have gratifying results with the exception of evacuating necrotic debris. Our team defers surgery if possible, acquiescing to nature while supporting the patient through the long and depressing hospitalization.

Perforation (Tables 10.14, 10.15)

Retroperitoneal perforation has been reported to occur in 2% of patients who have undergone ES. This figure is even lower today because of the shortened sphincterotome wire, which restricts the length of the incision. As indicated in Table 10.12, perforation can be and has been reduced by performing a limited, controlled incision. If one routinely uses a sphincterotome with a 20 mm to 25 mm wire and inserts only one-half of this wire, perforation will be infrequent. Obviously, despite the availability of improved accessories and

TABLE 10.14. *Prevention of complications*

Perforation
Replace short length of sphincterotome wire into sphincter (prevents perforation if "zipper cut" occurs).
Apply cautery in short bursts.
Stop cautery when dessication seen; proceed slowly in short increments.
Be in control.

TABLE 10.15. *Management of complications*

Perforation
NPO
Nasobiliary tube, if possible to insert
Nasogastric tube for abdominal distention
Intravenous fluids and broad spectrum antibiotic coverage
Parenteral analgesics
Flat and upright x-rays of abdomen in first 24–48 hrs
Gastrographin (TM) through NG tube to assess leak
Supportive-anticipatory care
Abdominal ultrasound/CT abdomen 48–96 hours if other studies equivocal Serial CT exams if intraperitoneal collections present
Surgical standby
If severe, prolonged, consider TPN
CT-guided drainage if localized

increasing experience with sphincterotomy, it is possible to eliminate this complication completely, especially in the patient whose distal bile duct is contained in a very short intramural segment of the duodenum. Also, making a controlled incision in short increments minimizes complications, but even this is not always possible. In some patients, there is resistence at the papilla that defies cutting. Until this impedence is overcome, no visible cutting takes place; only desiccation and smoke are seen. Suddenly a zipper cut occurs as the cautery current transects this area of resistence and easily cuts through the softer, less fibrotic sphincter area. If a short length of wire is positioned in the papilla when this rapid cutting occurs, a perforation is avoided (although bleeding may still occur).

It is difficult to recognize a perforation endoscopically, because it is rare to visualize the retroperitoneum. Contrast usually extravasates into the retroperitoneum when a post-ES cholangiogram is obtained (Fig. 10.57), or one may be able to appreciate air in the retroperitoneum, as illustrated in Fig. 10.58. The psoas margins are obscured, and the kidney may be readily visible or outlined by air. Subdiaphragmatic air is rare because the peritoneum has not been breached, but this finding may accompany a retroperitoneal leak because air may track anywhere in the abdominal cavity. Two patients in my series developed subcutaneous emphysema extending up the back, neck, and face without developing a frank perforation! In order to prove a leak, the patient must ingest Gastrographin (TM) or any type of water-soluble contrast material or have contrast injected in the nasogastric tube.

If a retroperitoneal leak is suspected or proved, further leakage can be minimized by inserting a nasobiliary tube, if possible, and a nasogastric (NG) tube. If a nasobiliary tube cannot be inserted, I recommend placing an NG tube when this complication (retroperitoneal perforation) is appreciated or recognized. The patient will not take oral nourishment, so appropriate intravenous infusions should be given. The patient may experience pain and will require analgesics for a short period of time. Broad-spectrum antibiotics to cover aerobes, anaerobes, enterococci, and bacteroides are recommended until specific cultures are obtained.

A retroperitoneal leak has usually been associated with few, if any, sequelae, but all of us have had at least one patient (two in my series) who developed multiple complications ranging from diffuse loculated collections that required percutaneous and subsequent surgical drainage to respiratory distress requiring endotrachael intubation. Fortunately, I have not experienced a death in this group of patients who recovered and returned to normal activity. Their hospitalizations ranged from 8 days to 45 days, with a mean of 17 days. The distinction between air and liquid extravasation into the retroperitonium is a critical determinant for early recovery (air) or a more complicated course (contaminated liquid). Air, which is usually not contaminated, may leak into the retroperitoneum after a small sphincterotomy because of the high pressures and volume of air delivered into the duodenum through the

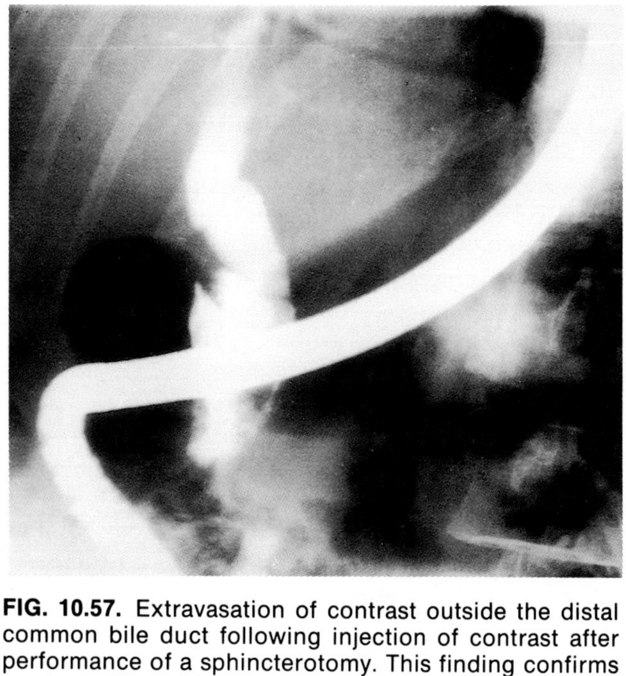

FIG. 10.57. Extravasation of contrast outside the distal common bile duct following injection of contrast after performance of a sphincterotomy. This finding confirms a retroperitoneal leak.

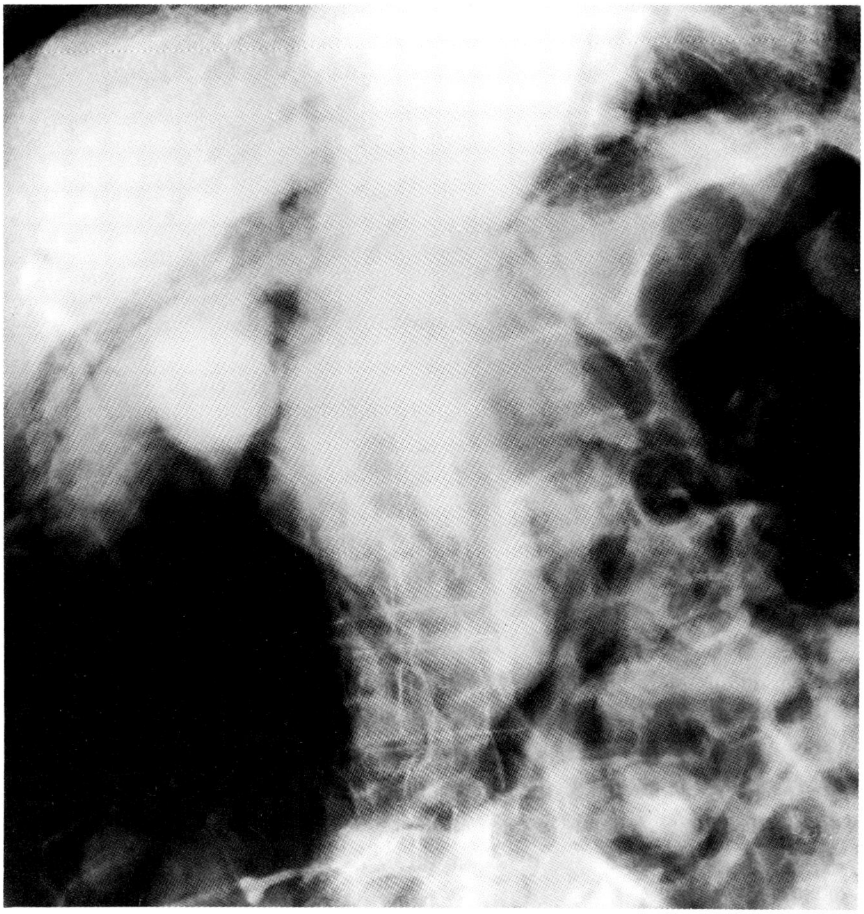

FIG. 10.58. A radiograph of a patient taken after performance of a sphincterotomy, demonstrating diffuse retroperitoneal air obliterating the psoas margins and outlining the inferior margin of the liver.

endoscope. When this occurs, the patient recovers quickly without complications because the leak seals rapidly and does not form a fistula through which fluid may continue to flow. Because the patient is fasting, little fluid is present in the duodenum, and fluid leakage is unlikely because a small perforation will heal rapidly. With a larger perforation, however, fluid may leak, especially if the patient does not remain NPO.

Prevention of perforation is not always possible, but a carefully controlled sphincterotomy will reduce its frequency or occurrence. The second best option is early recognition and aggressive treatment. It is not necessary to perform a Gastrographin study if the flat and upright x-rays corroborate the clinical impression and the patient shows signs of improvement. If the patient's condition deteriorates rapidly, a contrast study may be helpful to confirm persistence of the leak or spontaneous closure of the tract or to determine if early radiologic or surgical intervention will be necessary.

Infection (Cholangitis) (Tables 10.16, 10.17)

Cholangitis occurs infrequently after sphincterotomy and then usually because of retained stones or inadequate drainage. The term *cholangitis* has been inappropriately used to describe an infection that may occur following ERCP or ES. Cholangitis, as described by Charcot and others (126–128), is associated with

TABLE 10.16. *Prevention of complications*

Infection
After performing sphincterotomy, empty bile duct of stones or place prosthesis for stone disease or strictures.
If anticipated (recent history infection, or obstructed duct), give prophylactic antibiotics Recommended antibiotics: cephalosporins, aminoglycosides, metronidazole

TABLE 10.17. *Management of infection*

Blood cultures when temperature >101°F (38.5°C)
If single antibiotic ineffective: ampicillin, gentamicin
If double antibiotics ineffective: ampicillin, gentamicin, clindamycin
Infectious disease consult and monitor

fever, shaking chills, and pain, which is not always the scenario following ERCP or ES. Frequently a patient presenting with bile duct stones has previously been treated with antibiotics because of infection. The patient may have presented on the most recent occasion without signs of infection or clinical evidence of cholangitis. Often fever or infection follow ERCP and manipulation of the biliary tree in patients presenting with a recent history of infection. Preventing infection or cholangitis during or subsequent to ERCP requires prophylactic antibiotics and continuation of these drugs after the procedure. The most important factor influencing subsequent infection is establishing drainage of the bile duct, either clearing the duct after sphincterotomy or placing a prosthesis or nasobiliary catheter. If the bile duct drains freely following manipulation, infection is less likely to occur.

It has been my policy to follow each patient carefully after biliary tract manipulation, to continue parenteral antibiotics during hospitalization, and to continue antibiotics by mouth after discharge. I also make every attempt to establish drainage before completing the endoscopic procedure. If it is not possible to place an endoscopic drain, I request percutaneous drainage. These principles help to minimize complications. Establishing drainage for a bifurcation tumor is, of course, different and often requires a multidisciplinary approach (Chapter 12).

In general, infections of the biliary tree following ERCP are usually not as disconcerting as are bleeding, perforation, and pancreatitis because infections can be controlled by antibiotics and drainage. Nevertheless, management of infections is no less aggressive because the problem was not anticipated; it is our desire to regain control as soon as possible. Frequent blood cultures and consultations with infectious disease consultants may be necessary in order for the patient to recover completely.

POSTSPHINCTEROTOMY HEALING

In my experience, if an adequate sphincterotomy has been performed, it should be comparable to a surgical sphincteroplasty (170). The sphincterotomy should remain patent and nearly the same size as originally formed in 80 to 90% of cases (Table 10.18; Fig. 10.59), and it may become smaller but functional in perhaps 5% of patients. Fewer than 5% of sphincterotomies close and require extension. Despite earlier reports of presumed bleeding when extending a sphincterotomy, I have extended 40 sphincterotomies, and none have bled.

TABLE 10.18. *Follow-up of sphincterotomy*

Sphincterotomy success	98%
Sphincterotomy stoma size same on follow-up	80%
Narrowing of sphincterotomy	12%
Stenosis of sphincterotomy	8%

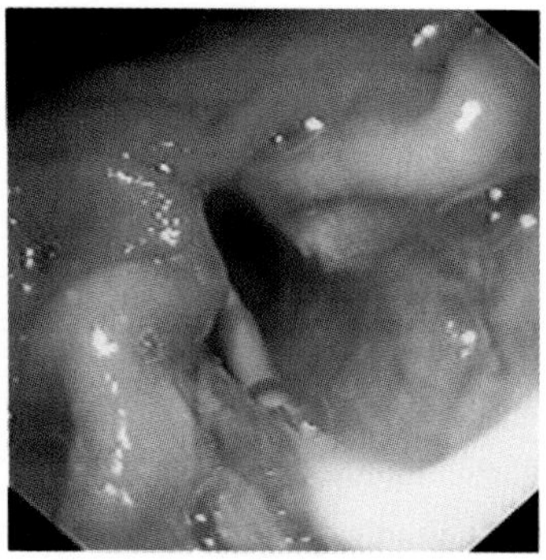

FIG 10.59. A wide-open sphincterotomy and a balloon catheter inserted. This picture was taken 2 months after sphincterotomy, and this wide opening should remain the same on repeat examination for years.

An easy method to test the patency of a sphincterotomy without repeating an ERCP in a patient with recurrent biliary symptoms or nonspecific upper gastrointestinal complaints is to perform an upper GI series. If the sphincterotomy is patent and the patient is positioned for reflux, barium will enter and opacify the biliary tree (Fig. 10.60). If the patient's symptoms persist, I recommend a repeat ERCP and possible manometric studies; however, emphasis should be placed on obtaining a pancreatogram to rule out the presence

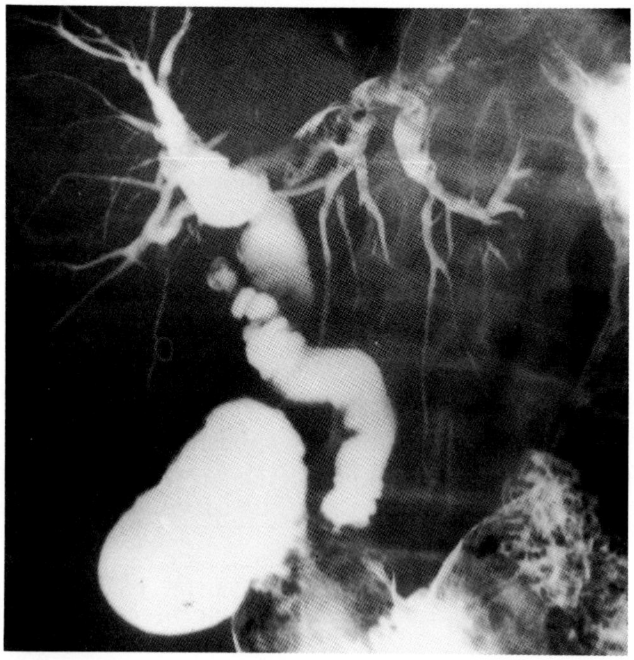

FIG. 10.60. Barium easily refluxing into the biliary tree during an upper GI series examination. This reflux should occur after an adequate sphincterotomy, obviating the need for repeat intubation if recurrent symptoms are obscure.

of hypertensive pancreatic sphincter, pancreatitis, and pancreas divisum, additional causes for the postcholecystectomy syndrome.

SUMMARY

Endoscopic sphincterotomy is the only endoscopic procedure that has predictable morbidity and mortality. Endoscopists performing this procedure should be aware of the potential complications and must be prepared to handle any of these situations. A surgeon should be aware of the procedure so that in the event of a complication, there is no unnecessary delay in performance of surgery. Adherence to these recommendations will avoid misadventure and will permit the continued performance of this valuable procedure.

More endoscopists perform sphincterotomy now than when the procedure was originally introduced. Despite the increased utilization of the procedure, the morbidity and mortality rates have stabilized and remain acceptable. The overall morbidity has not exceeded 8% to 10%, and mortality remains about 1% worldwide (1–11, 146–169). Tables 10.6, 10.7, and 10.8 summarize my own personal experience with sphincterotomy and the complications incurred with this procedure. Emergency surgical intervention has also remained at acceptable levels, with only approximately 1% of patients who undergo endoscopic sphincterotomy requiring surgical intervention.

REFERENCES

1. Kawai K, Akasaka Y, Murakami K, et al. Endoscopic sphincterotomy of the ampulla of Vater. *Gastrointest Endosc* 1974;20:148–51.
2. Classen M, Demling. Endoskopische Spinkterotomie der Papilla Vateri um Steinextrakation aus dem Ductus Choledochus. *Dtsch Med Wochenschr* 1974;99:496–7.
3. Koch H. Endoscopic papillotomy. *Endoscopy* 1975;7:89.
4. Zimmon DS, Falkenstein DB, Kessler RE. Endoscopic papillotomy for choledocholithiasis. *N Engl J Med* 1975;293:1181.
5. Classen M, Safrany L. Endoscopic papillotomy and removal of gallstones. *Br Med J* 1975;4:371–4.
6. Safrany L. Duodenoscopic sphincterotomy and gall stone removal. *Gastroenterology* 1977;72:338–43.
7. Geenen JE, Hogan J, Shaffer RD, et al. Endoscopic electrosurgical papillotomy and manometry in biliary tract disease. *JAMA* 1977;237:2075–8.
8. Cotton PB. Progress report, ERCP. *Gut* 1977;18:316–41.
9. Siegel JH. ERCP update: diagnostic and therapeutic applications. *Gastrointest Radiol* 1978;3:311–8.
10. Siegel JH. Endoscopic management of choledocholithiasis and papillary stenosis. *Surg Gynecol Obstet* 1979;148:747–52.
11. Siegel JH. Endoscopy and papillotomy in diseases of the biliary tract and pancreas. *J Clin Gastroenterol* 1980;2:337–47.
12. Riemann JF, Demling L. Lithotripsy of bile duct stones. *Endoscopy* 1983;15:191.
13. Siegel JH, Ben-Zvi JS, Pullano W. Mechanical lithotripsy of common duct stones. *Gastrointest Endosc* 1990;36:351–6.
14. Siegel JH, Pullano WH. Lithotripsy—to crush or explode? State of the art. *Gastrointest Endosc* 1986;15:191 (abst).
15. Siegel JH, Pullano W. Two new methods for selective bile duct cannulation and sphincterotomy. *Gastrointest Endosc* 1987;33:438–40.
16. Tucker RD, Silvis SE. Induced current on the guide wire during sphincterotomy. *Gastrointest Endosc* 1989;35:45–7.
17. Cass OW. Modify technique for wire-guided papillotomy. *Gastrointest Endosc* 1990;30:537–9.
18. Geenen JE, Vennes JA, Silvis SE. Resume of a seminar on endoscopic retrograde sphincterotomy (ERS). *Gastrointest Endosc* 1981;27:31–8.
19. Siegel JH. Precut papillotomy: a method to improve success of ERCP and papillotomy. *Endoscopy* 1980;12:130–3.
20. Booth FV, Doerr RJ, Khalafi RS, Luchette FA, Flint LM Jr. Surgical management of complications of endoscopic sphinterotomy with precut papillotomy. *Am J Surg* 1990;159:132–5.
21. Siegel JH, Ben Zvi JS, Pullano W. The needle knife: a valuable tool in diagnostic and therapeutic ERCP. *Gastrointest Endosc* 1989;35:499–503.
22. Cotton PB. Precut papillotomy—a risky technique for experts only. *Gastrointest Endosc* 1989;35:578–9.
23. Vaira D, Dowsett JF, Hatfield ARW, et al. Is duodenal diverticulum a risk factor for sphincterotomy? *Gut* 1989;30:939–42.
24. Veerappan A, Kothur R, Patel N, et al. A safer technique for performing endoscopic sphincterotomy (ES) in high risk situations: Bilroth II (BII), periampullary diverticula (PAD), Wirsung sphincter (WS) and Santorini sphincter (SS). *Am J Gastroenterol* 1990;85:1259 (abst).
25. Shorvon PJ, Cotton PB, Mason RR, Siegel JH, Hatfield ARW. Percutaneous transhepatic assistance for duodenoscopic sphincterotomy. *Gut* 1985;26:1373–6.
26. Siegel JH, Yatto RP. ERCP and endoscopic papillotomy in patients with a Bilroth II gastrectomy: report of method. *Gastrointest Endosc* 1983;29:116–8.
27. Safrany L, Neuhaus B, Portocarrero G, et al. Endoscopic sphincterotomy in patients with Bilroth II gastrectomy. *Endoscopy* 1980:12:16–22.
28. Rosseland AR, Osnes M, Kruse A. Endoscopic sphincterotomy (EST) in patients with Bilroth II gastrectomy. *Endoscopy* 1981;13:19–24.
29. Thon HJ, Loffler A, Buess G, et al. Is ERCP a reasonable diagnostic method for excluding pancreatic and hepaticobiliary disease in patients with a Bilroth II resection? *Endoscopy* 1983;15:93–5.
30. Forbes A, Cotton PB. ERCP and sphincterotomy after Bilroth II gastrectomy. *Gut* 1984;25:971–4.
31. Nordhock I, Airo I. Endoscopic retrograde cholangiopancreatography (ERCP) and sphincterotomy after BII resection. *Ann Chir Gynaecol* 1988;77:64–9.
32. Osnes M, Rosseland AR, Aabakken L. Endoscopic retrograde cholangiopancreatography and endoscopic papillotomy in patients with a previous Bilroth-II resection. *Gut* 1986;27:1193–8.
33. Ricci E, Bertoni G, Congliaro R, et al. Endoscopic sphincterotomy in Bilroth II patients: an improved method using a diathermic needle as a sphincterotome and a nasobiliary drain as a guide. *Gastrointest Endosc* 1989;35:47–50.
34. Robertson DAF, Ayres R, Hacking CN, et al. Experience with a combined percutaneous and endoscopic approach to stent insertion in malignant obstructive jaundice. *Lancet* 1987;2:1449–52.
35. Osnes M, Kahrs T. Endoscopic choledochoduodenostomy for choledocholithiasis through choledochoduodenal fistula. *Endoscopy* 1977;9:162–5.
36. Osnes M. Endoscopic choledochoduodenostomy for common bile duct obstructions. *Lancet* 1979;1:1059–60.
37. Shapira L, Khawaja FI. Endoscopic fistulosphincterotomy: an alternative method of sphincterotomy using a new sphincterotome. *Endoscopy* 1982;14:58–60.
38. Caletti GC, Vercucchi G, Bolondi L, Labo G. Diathermy ERCP—an alternative method for endoscopic retrograde cholangiopancreatography in jaundiced patients. *Gastrointest Endosc* 1980;26:13–15.
39. Kozarek RA, Sanowski RA. Endoscopic choledochoduodenostomy. *Gastrointest Endosc* 1983;29:119–21.

40. Huibregtse K, Katon RM, Tytgat GNJ. Precut papillotomy via fine-needle papillotome: a safe and effective technique. *Gastrointest Endosc* 1986;32:403–5.
41. Leung JWC, Banez VP, Chung SCS. Precut (needle knife) papillotomy for impacted common bile stone at the ampulla. *Am J Gastroenterol* 1990;85:991–3.
42. Sloof M, Baker R, Lavelle MI, et al. What is involved in endoscopic sphincterotomy for gallstones? *Br J Surg* 1980;67:18–21.
43. Siegel JH, Harding GT, Chateau F. Endoscopic incision of choledochal cysts (choledochocele). *Endoscopy* 1981;13:200–2.
44. Venu RP, Geenen JE, Hogan WJ, et al. Role of endoscopic retrograde cholangiopancreatography in the diagnosis and treatment of choledochocele. *Gastroenterology* 1984;87:1144.
45. Gerritsen JJ, Janssens AR, Kroon HM. Choledochocele: treatment by endoscopic sphincterotomy. *Br J Surg* 1988;75:495–6.
46. Siegel JH, Yatto RP. Endoscopic management of chronic pancreatitis. *Gastrointest Endosc* 1981;27:240.
47. Huibregtse K, Schneider B, Vrij AA, Tytgat GNJ. Endoscopic pancreatic drainage in chronic pancreatitis. *Gastrointest Endosc* 1988;34:9–15.
48. Soehendra N, Grimm H, Schreiber H. Endoscopic transpapillary drainage of the pancreatic duct in chronic pancreatitis. *Dtsch Med Wochenschr* 1986;111:727–31.
49. McCarthy J, Geenen JE, Hogan WJ. Preliminary experience with endoscopic stent placement in benign diseases. *Gastrointest Endosc* 1988;34:16–8.
50. Geenen JE. ASGE distinguished lecture—endoscopic therapy of pancreatic disease: a new horizon. *Gastrointest Endosc* 1988;34:386–9.
51. Ponsky JL, Duppler DW. Sphincterotomy and removal of pancreatic duct stones. *Am Surg* 1987;53:613–6.
52. Guelrud M, Siegel JH. Hypertensive pancreatic duct sphincter as cause of recurrent pancreatitis: successful treatment with hydrostatic balloon dilatation. *Dig Dis Sci* 1984;29:225–31.
53. Siegel JH. The double papilla of Vater. *Gastrointest Endosc* 1986;32:119 (letter).
54. Hunt DR, Blumgart LH. Iatrogenic choledochoduodenal fistula: an unsuspected cause of post-cholecystectomy symptoms. *Br J Surg* 1980;67:10–3.
55. Tanaka M, Ikeda S. Parapapillary choledochoduodenal fistula: an analysis of 83 consecutive patients diagnosed at ERCP. *Gastrointest Endosc* 1983;29:89–93.
56. Martin DF, Tweedle DE. The etiology and significance of distal choledochoduodenal fistula. *Br J Surg* 1984;71:632–4.
57. Engelberg M, Avraham I, Redman S, et al. Choledochoduodenostomy. A useful procedure in the management of benign disorders of the biliary tract. A review of 53 cases. *Am Surg* 1976;183:476.
58. Akiyama H, Ikezawa H, Kawega S, et al. Unexpected problems of external choledochoduodenostomy. *Am J Surg* 1980;140:660.
59. Siegel JH. Biliary bezoar: the sump syndrome and choledochenterostomy. *Endoscopy* 1983;14:238–40.
60. Siegel JH. Peroral choledochoscopy in the sump syndrome: use of a thin caliber endoscope to negotiate a choledochoduodenostomy. *Gastrointest Endosc* 1982;28:192–3.
61. Barkin MS, Silvis S, Greenwald R. Endoscopic therapy of the "sump" syndrome. *Dig Dis Sci* 1980;25:597.
62. Siegel JH. Duodenoscopic sphincterotomy in the treatment of the sump syndrome. *Dig Dis Sci* 1981;26:922.
63. Marbet UA, Stalder GA, Faust H. Harder F, Gyr K. Endoscopic sphincterotomy and surgical approaches in the treatment of the "sump syndrome." *Gut* 1987;28:142–5.
64. Miros M, Kerlin P, Strong R, Hartley L, Dickey D. Post-choledochoenterostomy "sump syndrome." *Aust N Z J Surg* 1990;60:109–12.
65. Polydorou A, Dowsett JF, Vaira D, Salmon PR, Cotton PB, Russell RC. Endoscopy therapy of the sump syndrome. *Endoscopy* 1989;21:126–30.
66. Dresemann G, Kautz G, Bunte H. Long-term results of endoscopic sphincterotomy in patients with gallbladder in situ. *Dtsch Med Wochenschr* 1988;113:500–5.
67. Olaison G, Kald B, Karlqvist PA, Lindstrom E, Anderberg B. Endoscopic removal of common bile duct stones without subsequent cholecystectomy. *Acta Chir Scand* 1987;153:541–3.
68. Hansell DT, Miller MA, Murray WR, Gray GR, Gillespie G. Endoscopic sphincterotomy for bile duct stones in patients with intact gallbladders. *Br J Surg* 1989;76:856–8.
69. Way LW. Trends in the treatment of gallstone disease: putting the options into context. *Am J Surg* 1989;158:251–3.
70. Siegel JH, Safrany L, Ben-Zvi JS, et al. The significance of duodenoscopic sphincterotomy in patients with gallbladder in situ: report of a series of 1272 patients. *Am J Gastroenterol* 1988;83:1255–8.
71. Neoptolemos JP, Carr-Locke DL, Fraser I, Fossard DP. The management of common bile duct calculi by endoscopic sphincterotomy in patients with gallbladders in situ. *Br J Surg* 1984;71:69–71.
72. Hansell DT, Millar MA, Murray WR, Gray GR, Gillespie G. Endoscopic sphincterotomy for bile duct stones in patients with intact gallbladders.
73. Cotton PB. Endoscopic management of bile duct stones (apples and oranges). *Gut* 1984;25:587–97.
74. Neoptolemos JP, Shaw DE, Carr-Locke DL. A multivariate analysis of preoperative risk factors in patients with common bile duct stones. Implications for treatment. *Ann Surg* 1989;209:157–61.
75. Jacobson IM. Endoscopic sphincterotomy in patients with intact gallbladders. In: Jacobson IM, ed. *ERCP: diagnostic and therapeutic applications*. New York: Elsevier, 1989;127–38.
76. Worthley CS, Toouli J. Gallbladder (GB) nonfilling contraindicates leaving the GB in situ after endoscopic sphincterotomy (ES). *Gastrointest Endosc* 1987;33:160 (abst).
77. Neoptolemos JP, Carr-Locke DL, Fossard DP. Prospective randomized study of preoperative endoscopic sphincterotomy versus surgery alone for common bile duct stones. *Br J Surg* 1987;294:470–4.
78. Van Stiegmann G, Pearlman NW, Goff JS, Sun JH, Norton LW. Endoscopic cholangiography and stone removal prior to cholecystectomy. *Arch Surg* 1989;124:787–90.
79. Reddick EJ, Olsen DO. Laparoscopic cholecystectomy. *Surg Endosc* 1989;3:131–3.
80. Halver B. Endoscopic symptomatic treatment of gallbladder stones. *Scand J Gastroenterol* 1986;21(suppl 120):32.
81. Gracie WA, Ransahoff DF. Natural history of silent gallstones: the innocent gallstone is not a myth. *N Engl J Med* 1982;307:798.
82. Seifert E. Endoscopic papillotomy and removal of gallstones. *Am J Gastroenterol* 1978;69:154–9.
83. Siegel JH, Pullano WE, Safrany L, et al. Does endoscopic sphincterotomy reduce the annual incidence of cholecystitis in patients with intact gallbladder? An analysis of long-term results in 1555 patients. *Gastrointest Endosc* 1988;34:192 (abst).
84. Martin DE, Tweedle DE. Endoscopic management of common duct stones without cholecystectomy. *Br J Surg* 1987;74:209–11.
85. Davidson BR, Neoptolemos JP, Carr-Locke DL. Endoscopic sphincterotomy for common bile duct calculi patients with gallbladder in situ considered unfit for surgery. *Gut* 1988;29:114–20.
86. Lamont DD, Passi RB. Fate of the gallbladder with cholelithiasis after endoscopic sphincterotomy for choledocholithiasis. *Can J Surg* 1989;32:15–8.
87. Heinerman PM, Boeckl O, Pimpl W. Selective ERCP and preoperative stone removal in bile duct surgery. *Ann Surg* 1989;209:267–72.
88. Ingoldby CJ, el-Saadi J, Hall R, Denyer ME. Late results of endoscopic sphincterotomy for bile duct stones in elderly patients with gallbladders in situ. *Gut* 1989;30:1129–31.
89. Tanaka M, Ikeda S, Yoshimoto H, Matsumoto S. The long term fate of the gallbladder after endoscopic sphincterotomy. Complete followup study of 122 patients. *Am J Surg* 1987;154:505–9.
90. Cohn MS, Schwartz SI, Faloon WW, Adams JT. Effect of sphincteroplasty on gallbladder function and bile composition. *Ann Surg* 1979;189:317–21.

91. Sauerbruch T, Stellaard F, Paumgartner G. Effect of endoscopic sphincterotomy on bile acid pool size and bile lipid composition in man. *Digestion* 1983;27:87–92.
92. Stellaard F, Sauerbruch T, Brunholzl C, et al. Bile acid pattern and cholesterol saturation of bile after cholecystectomy and endoscopic sphincterotomy. *Digestion* 1983;26:153–8.
93. Hutton SW, Sievert CE Jr, Vennes JA, Duane WC. The effect of sphincterotomy on gallstone formation in the prairie dog. *Gastroenterology* 1981;81:663–7.
94. Hutton SW, Sievert CE Jr, Vennes JA, Shafer RB, Duane WC. Spontaneous passage of glass beads from the canine gallbladder: facilitation by sphincterotomy. *Gastroenterology* 1988; 94:1031–35.
95. Gregg JA, DeGirolami P, Carr-Locke DL. Effects of sphincteroplasty and endoscopic sphincterotomy on the bacteriologic characteristics of the common bile duct. *Am J Surg* 1985;149:668–71.
96. Siegel JH. Endoscopic sphincterotomy: when is it appropriate? In: Barkin JS, Rogers AI, eds. *Difficult decisions in digestive diseases.* Boca Raton: Year Book Medical Publishers, 1989:551–7.
97. Thompson JE, Thompkins RK, Longmire WP. Factors in management of acute cholangitis. *Ann Surg* 1982;195:137–45.
98. Saharia PC, Cameron JL. Clinical management of acute cholangitis. *Surg Gynecol Obstet* 1976;142:369–72.
99. Saik RP, Greenburg AG, Farris JM, et al. Spectrum of cholangitis. *Am J Surg* 1975;130:143–50.
100. Hinchey EJ, Couper CE. Acute obstructive suppurative cholangitis. *Am J Surg* 1969;117:62.
101. Cole WN. Suppurative cholangitis. *Surg Clin North Am* 1947;27:23–6.
102. Welch JP, Donaldson GA. The urgency of diagnosis and surgical treatment of acute suppurative cholangitis. *Am J Surg* 1976;131:527.
103. O'Connor MJ, Schwartz ML, McQuarrie DG, et al. Acute bacterial cholangitis; an analysis of clinical manifestations. *Arch Surg* 1982;117:437.
104. Dow RW, Lindenauer SM. Acute obstructive suppurative cholangitis. *Ann Surg* 1969;169:272.
105. Glenn F, Moody FG. Acute obstructive suppurative cholangitis. *Surg Gynecol Obstet* 1961;113:265.
106. Pitkin H, Beal JM. Choledocholithiasis associated with acute cholecystitis. *Arch Surg* 1979;114:887.
107. Gogel HK, Runyon BA, Volpicelli NA, Palmer RC. Acute suppurative obstructive cholangitis due to stones: treatment by urgent endoscopic sphincterotomy. *Gastrointest Endosc* 1987;33:210–3.
108. Siegel JH, Ramsey WH, Pullano W. Endoscopic management of 947 patients with cholangitis: proven safety and efficacy. *Gastrointest Endosc* 1986;32:154 (abst).
109. Leese T, Neoptolemos JP, Baker AR, et al. Management of acute cholangitis and the impact of endoscopic sphincterotomy. *Br J Surg* 1986;73:988–92.
110. Leung JWC, Chung SCS, Sung JJY, et al. Urgent endoscopic drainage for acute suppurative cholangitis. *Lancet* 1989;1307–9.
111. Choi TK, Wong J. Endoscopic retrograde cholangiopancreatography and endoscopic papillotomy in recurrent pyogenic cholangitis. *Clin Gastroenterol* 1986;151:393–415.
112. Chau EM, Leong LL, Chan FL. Recurrent pyogenic cholangitis: ultrasound evaluation compared with endoscopic retrograde cholangiopancreatography. *Clin Radiol* 1987;38:79–85.
113. Fritsch WP. Therapy of bacterial cholangitis. *Dtsch Med Wochenschr* 1986;111:304–6.
114. Neoptolemos JP, Carr-Locke DL, Lesse T, James D. Acute cholangitis in association with acute pancreatitis: incidence, clinical features and outcome in relation to ERCP and endoscopic sphincterotomy. *Br J Surg* 1987;1103–6.
115. Kiil J, Kruse A, Rokkjaer M. Large bile duct stones treated by endoscopic biliary drainage. *Surgery* 1989;105:51–6.
116. Kopiela T, Karcz D, Marecik J. Endoscopic sphincterotomy as a therapeutic measure in cholangitis and as prophylaxis against recurrent biliary tract stones. *Endoscopy* 1987;19:14–6.
117. Vennes JA. Management of calculi in the common duct. *Semin Liver Dis* 1983;3:162–71.
118. Dodd GD. Percutaneous transhepatic cholangiography. *Surg Clin North Am* 1967;47:1095–1106.
119. Molnar W, Stockhum AE. Relief of obstructive jaundice through percutaneous transhepatic catheter: a new therapeutic method. *Am J Radiol* 1974:122:356–67.
120. Joseph PK, Bizer LS, Sprayraegen SS, et al. Percutaneous transhepatic biliary drainage: results and complications in 81 patients. *JAMA* 1986;255:2763–7.
121. Smith RC, Pooley M, George CR, et al. Preoperative percutaneous transhepatic internal drainage in obstructive jaundice: a randomized, controlled trial examining renal function. *Surgery* 1985;97:641–7.
122. McPherson GA, Benjamin IS, Hodgson HJ, et al. Preoperative percutaneous biliary drainage: the results of a controlled trial. *Br J Surg* 1984;71:371–5.
123. Audiosio A, Bozzetti F, Severini A, et al. The occurrence of cholangitis after percutaneous drainage: evaluation of some risk factors. *Surgery* 1988;103:507–12.
124. Gould RJ, Vogelzang RL, Niemann HL, et al. Percutaneous biliary drainage as an initial therapy in sepsis of the biliary tract. *Surg Gynecol Obstet* 1985;160:523–7.
125. Kadir S, Baassiri A, Barth KH, et al. Percutaneous biliary drainage in the management of biliary sepsis. *Am J Roentgenol* 1982;138:25–9.
126. Charcot JM. Lecon sur les Maladies du Foie des Voies Filiares et des Reins. Paris: Faculte de Medecine de Paris, 1877.
127. Reynolds BM, Dargan EL. Acute obstructive cholangitis: a distinct clinical syndrome. *Ann Surg* 1959;150:299.
128. Boey JH, Way LW. Acute cholangitis. *Ann Surg* 1980;191:264.
129. Keighely MRB, Drysdale RB, Quoraishi AH, et al. Antibiotic treatment of biliary sepsis. *Surg Clin North Am* 1975;55:1379.
130. Lygidakis N. Incidence of bile infection in patients with choledocholithiasis. *Am J Gastroenterol* 1982;77:12.
131. Rogers L. Biliary abscess of the liver with operation. *Br Med J* 1903;2:706–7.
132. Neoptolemos JP, Macpherson DS, Holm J, et al. Pyogenic liver abscess: a study of forty-four cases in two centres. *Acta Chir Scand* 1982;148:415–21.
133. Lygidakis NJ, Brummelkamp WH. The significance of intrabiliary pressure in acute cholangitis. *Surg Gynecol Obstet* 1985;161:465–9.
134. Kinoshita H, Hitohashi K, Igawa S, et al. Cholangitis. *World J Surg* 1984;8:963–9.
135. Edlung YA, Mollstedt BO, Ouchterlony O. Bacteriological investigation of the biliary system and liver in biliary tract disease correlated to clinical data and microstructure of the gallbladder and liver. *Acta Chir Scand* 1959;116:461–76.
136. Huang T, Bass JAB, Williams RD, et al. The significance of biliary pressure in cholangitis. *Arch Surg* 1969;89:629–32.
137. Finegold SM. Anaerobes in biliary tract infections. *Arch Intern Med* 1979;139:1338.
138. Hinshaw DB. Acute obstructive suppurative cholangitis. *Surg Clin North Am* 1973;53:1089.
139. Bourgault AM, England DM, Rosenblatt FE. Clinical characteristics of anaerobic bactibilia. *Arch Intern Med* 1979;139:1346.
140. Shimada K, Inamatsu T, Yamashiro M. Anaerobic bacteria in biliary disease of elderly patients. *J Infect Dis* 1977;135:850.
141. Schotton WE, Desprez JD, Holden WA. A bacteriological study of portal vein blood in man. *Arch Surg* 1955;71:404–9.
142. Taylor KJW, Rosenfield AT, Spiro HM. Diagnostic accuracy of gray scale ultrasonography for the jaundiced patient. *Arch Intern Med* 1979;139:60–3.
143. Einstein DM, Lapin SA, Ralls PW, et al. The insensitivity of sonography in the detection of choledocholithiasis. *Am J Roentgenol* 1984;143:725–8.
144. Kaplun L, Weisman HS, Rosenblatt RR, et al. The early diagnosis of common bile duct obstruction using cholescintigraphy. *JAMA* 1985;254(17):2431.
145. Miller DR, Egbert RM, Braunstein P. Comparison of ultrasound and hepaticobiliary imaging in the early detection of acute total common bile duct obstruction. *Arch Surg* 1984;119:1233–7.

146. Nebel OT, et al. Complications associated with endoscopic retrograde cholangiopancreatography. Results of the 1974 A/S G/E survey. *Gastrointest Endosc* 1975;22:34.
147. Zimmon DS, Falkenstein DB, Riccobono C, Aaron B. Complications of endoscopic retrograde cholangiopancreatography (ERCP). Analysis of 300 consecutive cases. *Gastroenterology* 1975;69:303.
148. Bilbao MK, Dotter CT, Lee TG, Katon RM. Complications of endoscopic retrograde cholangiopancreatography (ERCP). A study of 10,000 cases. *Gastroenterology* 1976;70:314.
149. Cotton PB. ERCP. *Gut* 1977;18:316.
150. Kawai K, Akasaka Y, Murakami K, et al. Endoscopic sphincterotomy of the ampulla of vater. *Gastrointest Endosc* 1974;20:148–51.
151. Classen M, Demling L. Endoskopische sphincterotomie der papilla vateri und steinextraktion aus ductus choledochus. *Dtsch Med Wochenschr* 1974;99:496–7.
152. Cotton PB, Vallon AG, British experience with duodenoscopic sphincterotomy for removal of bile duct stones. *Br J Surg* 1981;68:373–5.
153. Escourro J, Cordova JA, Lazorthes F, et al. Early and late complications after sphincterotomy for biliary lithiasis with and without gallbladder in situ. *Gut* 1984;25:598–602.
154. Winstanley PA, Ellis WR, Hamilton I, et al. Medium term complications of endoscopic biliary sphincterotomy. *Gut* 1985;26:730–3.
155. Silvis SE, Vennes JA. *Endoscopic retrograde sphincterotomy.* In: Silvis SE, ed. Therapeutic gastrointestinal endoscopy. 2nd ed. New York: Igaku-Shoin, 1990;225–81.
156. Ossenberg FW, Classen M. *Papilla Vateri-Gallenwege-Pankreas. Themen der Medizen 2.* Nurnberg: Wander Pharma, 1980;34.
157. Geenen JE, Vennes JA, Silvis SE. Resume of a seminar on endoscopic sphincterotomy. *Gastrointest Endosc* 1981;27:31–8.
158. Leese T, Neoptolemos JP, Carr-Locke DL. Successes, failures, early complications and their management following endoscopic sphincterotomy: results in 394 consecutive patients from a single centre. *Br J Surg* 1985;72:215–9.
159. Dunham F, Burgeois N, Gelin M, Jeanmart J, Toussaint J, Cremer M. Retroperitoneal perforations following endoscopic sphincterotomy, clinical course and management. *Endoscopy* 1982;14:92–6.
160. Silvis SE, Vennes JA. *Endoscopic retrograde sphincterotomy.* In: Silvis SE, ed. Therapeutic gastrointestinal endoscopy. New York: Igaku-Shoin, 1989;198–240.
161. Freidman CJ, Leavell BS Jr, Adams K. A new complication of endoscopic papillotomy. *Gastrointest Endosc* 1983;29:62.
162. Neihaus B, Safrany L. Complications of endoscopic sphincterotomy and their treatment. *Endoscopy* 1981;13:197–9.
163. Halter F, Bangerter U, Gigon JP, Pusterla C. Gallsteone ileus after endoscopic sphincterotomy. *Endoscopy* 1981;13:88–9.
164. McLBooth FV, Doerr RJ, Khalafi RS, et al. Surgical management of complications of endoscopic sphincterotomy with precut papillotomy. *Am J Surg* 1990;159:132–6.
165. Sivak MV. Endoscopic management of bile duct stones. *Am J Surg* 1989;158:228–40.
166. Vaira D, D'Anna L, Ainley C, et al. Endoscopic sphincterotomy in 1000 consecutive patients. *Lancet* 1989;2:431–4.
167. Ostroff JV, Shapiro HA. Complications of endoscopic sphincterotomy. In: Jacobson IM, ed. *ERCP, diagnostic and therapeutic applications.* New York: Elsevier, 1989;61–73.
168. Kuhlman JE, Fishman EK, Milligan FD, Siegelman SS. Complications of endoscopic retrograde sphincterotomy: computed tomographic evaluation. *Gastrointest Radiol* 1989;14:127–32.
169. Siegel JH, Veerappan A. Complications of endoscopic sphincterotomy. In: Kozarek RA, ed. *Clinics of gastrointest endoscopy.* New York: WB Saunders, 1991.
170. Siegel JH. Endoscopic papillotomy: sphincterotomy or sphincteroplasty. *Am J Gastroenterol* 1979;72:511–6.

CHAPTER 11

Stone Extraction, Lithotripsy, Stents and Stones

OCCLUSION BALLOONS

The concept of using an occlusion balloon to extract common bile duct stones is a technique familiar to surgeons who have been performing common duct exploration at the operating table. In the course of performing a choledochotomy and exploring the common bile duct with instruments and accessories, the surgeon typically uses a Fogarty balloon catheter to extract stones from the bile duct and biliary tree (1–4). The balloon catheter is inserted through the choledochotomy into the distal common bile duct, inflated, and withdrawn back through the choledochotomy, carrying stones and stone particles with it. The intrahepatic biliary tree and common hepatic duct are manipulated in a similar fashion to remove stones from these areas.

With the advent of endoscopic sphincterotomy and the incorporation of more aggressive techniques for removing stones (5–16), the safest and most frequently used of these techniques for stone extraction is the occlusion balloon (Fig. 11.1). The double-lumen balloon catheter contains a latex balloon on its tip, which, when deflated, is flat on the catheter, does not occupy additional space in the endoscope channel, and is true to its French size. This characteristic is peculiar to latex because after stretching, it returns to its prestretch position when the dilating medium, air or liquid, is removed from its inflation channel. The smaller 5Fr catheters containing balloons were initially available by necessity because the earlier model endoscopes had biopsy channels of 2.0 mm or 2.2 mm, smaller than the current models, and could accommodate only these small catheters. These catheters fit through the channel of the endoscope and can be manipulated and inserted through the sphincterotomy and into the bile duct in a manner similar to the technique of cannulation. The endoscopic technique was adapted to the technique employed by the surgeon: insertion of the balloon catheter beyond the stone, inflation of the balloon, and gentle withdrawal of the balloon toward the sphincterotomy to extract the stone (Fig. 11.2). The smaller catheters contain a balloon that can be distended to 1 cc or 1.2 cc, which is sufficient for extraction of a stone in a nondilated duct but inadequate for exploration of a dilated biliary tree. In the latter situation, the dilated bile duct is too large, and the balloon cannot or does not occlude the lumen. The stones easily slip by the smaller balloon remaining in the duct rather than being withdrawn to the sphincterotomy for extraction.

With the introduction of large-channel endoscopes, larger balloon catheters became available. These larger catheters provide not only the additional occlu-

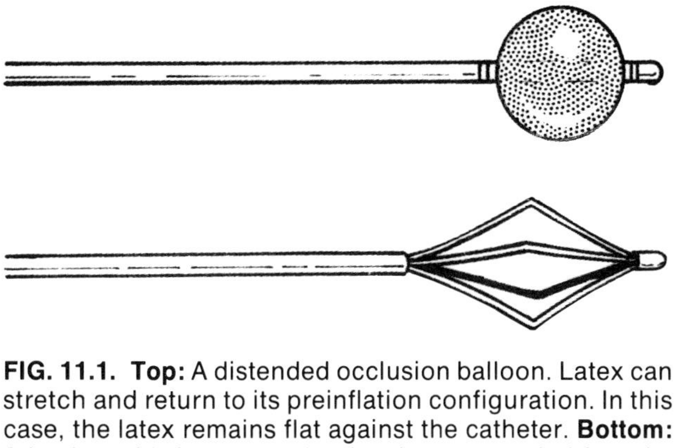

FIG. 11.1. Top: A distended occlusion balloon. Latex can stretch and return to its preinflation configuration. In this case, the latex remains flat against the catheter. **Bottom:** A basket with four arms that has been extended from its sheath. I prefer this configuration, and my preference for material includes a soft, braided-wire construction. The curved Dormia type of baskets that contain a monofilament wire are too rigid and are generally not good for endoscopic use. Baskets are available in different sizes extending out as much as 6 cm. In general, a 2 cm by 4 cm basket will capture most large stones and a 2 cm by 2 cm or 2 cm by 3 cm can be used frequently for small and medium-sized stones.

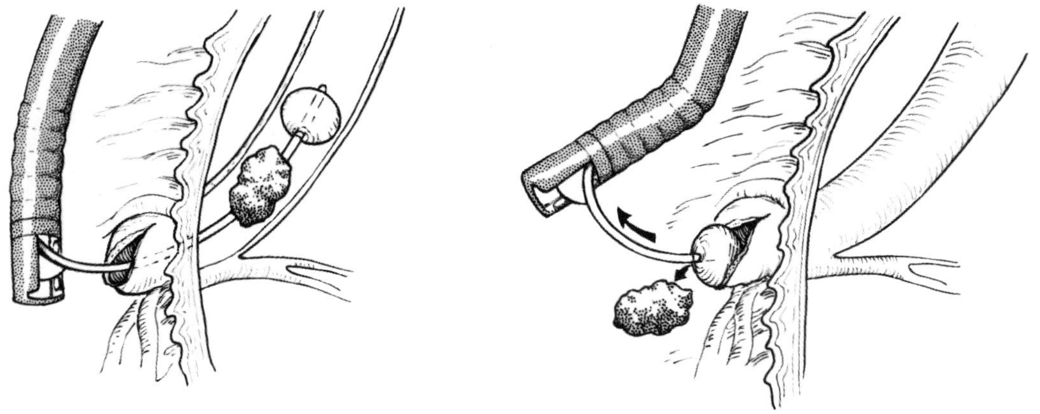

FIG. 11.2. Left: The technique of removing a stone from the common bile duct using an occlusion balloon catheter. A stone is visible in the common bile duct, and the balloon catheter has been advanced above the stone and inflated in preparation to pull the stone out of the duct. **Right:** The balloon has been pulled toward the sphincterotomy with the stone preceding it. As the endoscope is extended and deflected away from the sphincterotomy and tension is maintained on the balloon, the stone and balloon are delivered into the duodenum.

sion size but also the advantage of passing the catheter over a 0.035″ guidewire for selective insertion into the intrahepatic tree or for access into the bile duct when cannulation is difficult or when the balloon catheter, because of its curved configuration, enters the cystic duct instead of the bile duct. The guidewire is helpful for repeat cannulations as well. The larger balloon can be distended to approximately 1.5 cc or cm to 2 cc or cm, which is large enough to occlude the majority of dilated bile ducts. Still, a markedly dilated bile duct may prohibit total occlusion, and other accessories may be necessary to capture the stone.

Removing medium to large stones through a sphincterotomy using a balloon requires manipulation with gentle traction: slowly pulling the stone through the sphincterotomy. If the endoscopist pulls with greater tension and the stone rapidly exits the sphincterotomy, the balloon will slip through the sphincterotomy too rapidly and rupture as it is pulled into the biopsy channel of the endoscope by making contact with the metal edge of the elevator. Therefore, the technique of extracting any stone, but especially medium to large ones, is to pull gently downward on the catheter while deflecting the distal tip of the endoscope. This motion applies extra tension in the appropriate axis and avoids rupturing the balloon. Once again, applying gentle traction to the balloon catheter while deflecting or extending the tip of the endoscope downward provides extra tension on the balloon in the proper axis or orientation (Fig. 11.2) Using the endoscope for the terminal force rather than pulling on the balloon prevents its rupture.

Because of the fragile nature of the balloon's composition and construction (i.e., latex with cement seals), it is not very resistant to force and can be easily damaged or punctured. Even the best of the balloon catheters may begin to leak after applying prolonged traction to a stone.

To strengthen the latex balloon and provide longer life, the balloon may be cooled prior to use to toughen the skin. Also, using cool water or saline to inflate the balloon instead of air strengthens the latex skin and extends its useful life.

In the ideal situation for balloon extraction, one or several small stones, smaller than 0.5 cm, remain in a nondilated bile duct. When the balloon is placed above the stones and inflated, it will fill the lumen of the bile duct; in other words, the balloon should touch the bile duct walls, occluding the lumen, in order to achieve successful extraction. Figures 11.3 through 11.8 are illustrative examples of the use of an occlusion balloon for extraction of multiple stones, large stones, and foreign bodies. Large stones require more skill and experience, and may be best extracted using a basket. The next section describes basket extraction techniques employed by the author for medium to large common bile duct stones.

Text continues on page 232.

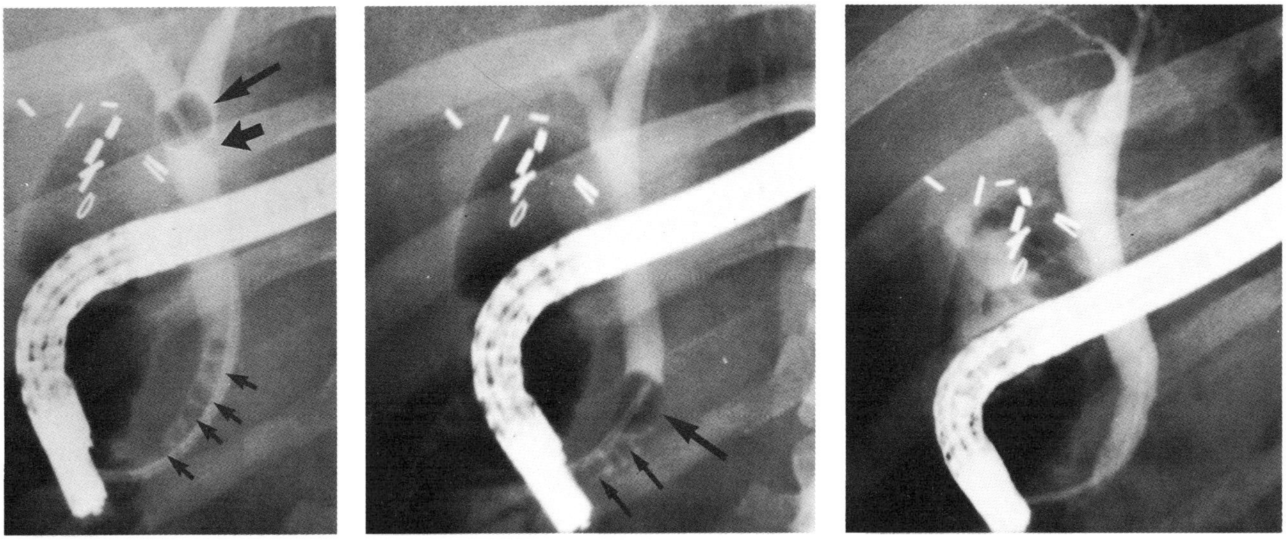

A

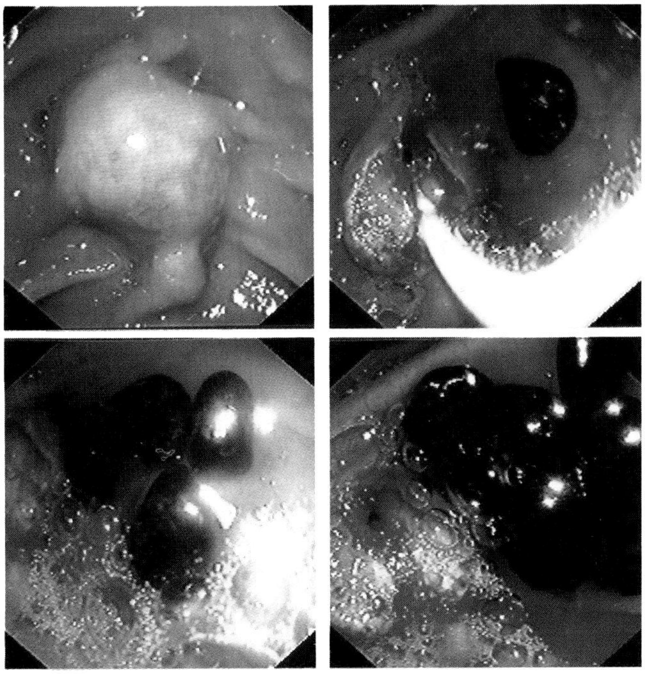

B

FIG. 11.3. A: Left: An ERCP cholangiogram demonstrating a column of common bile duct stones in the distal duct (*small arrows*). The occlusion balloon is inflated at the bile duct bifurcation (*large arrow*). Note the presence of another small stone near the balloon (*short arrow*). **Middle:** The balloon has been withdrawn to the distal common bile duct (*large arrow*). Several stones remain in duct (*small arrow*). **Right:** A cholangiogram taken after stone extraction shows a bile duct free of stones. **B: Upper left:** A videoendoscopic view of a bulging and prominent ampulla. **Upper right:** A sphincterotomy has been completed and a balloon catheter is being advanced into the bile duct. One pigmented stone has been extracted and is located to the right of the balloon catheter. **Lower left:** Several pigmented stones are visible in the duodenum. **Lower right:** More stones have been extracted into the duodenum.

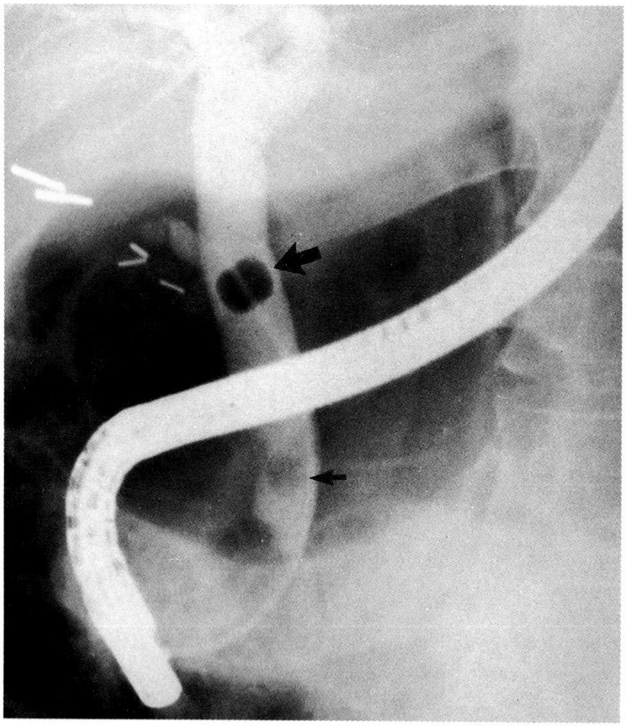

A

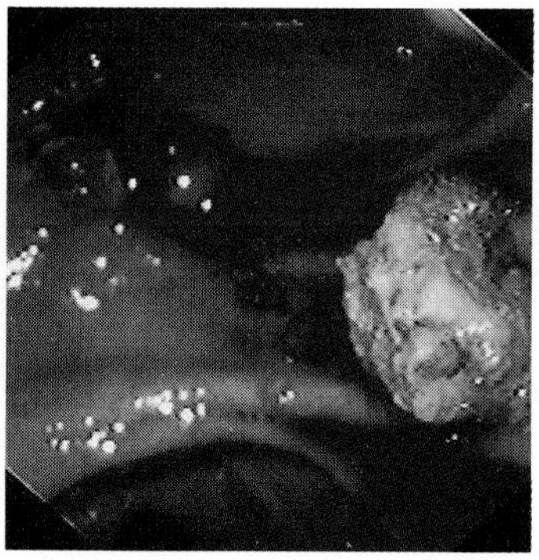

B

FIG. 11.4. A: A medium-sized stone in the distal common bile duct (*small arrow*) and a balloon catheter in the proximal duct (*large arrow*). **B:** A medium-sized cholesterol stone that was extracted through the sphincterotomy using a balloon catheter.

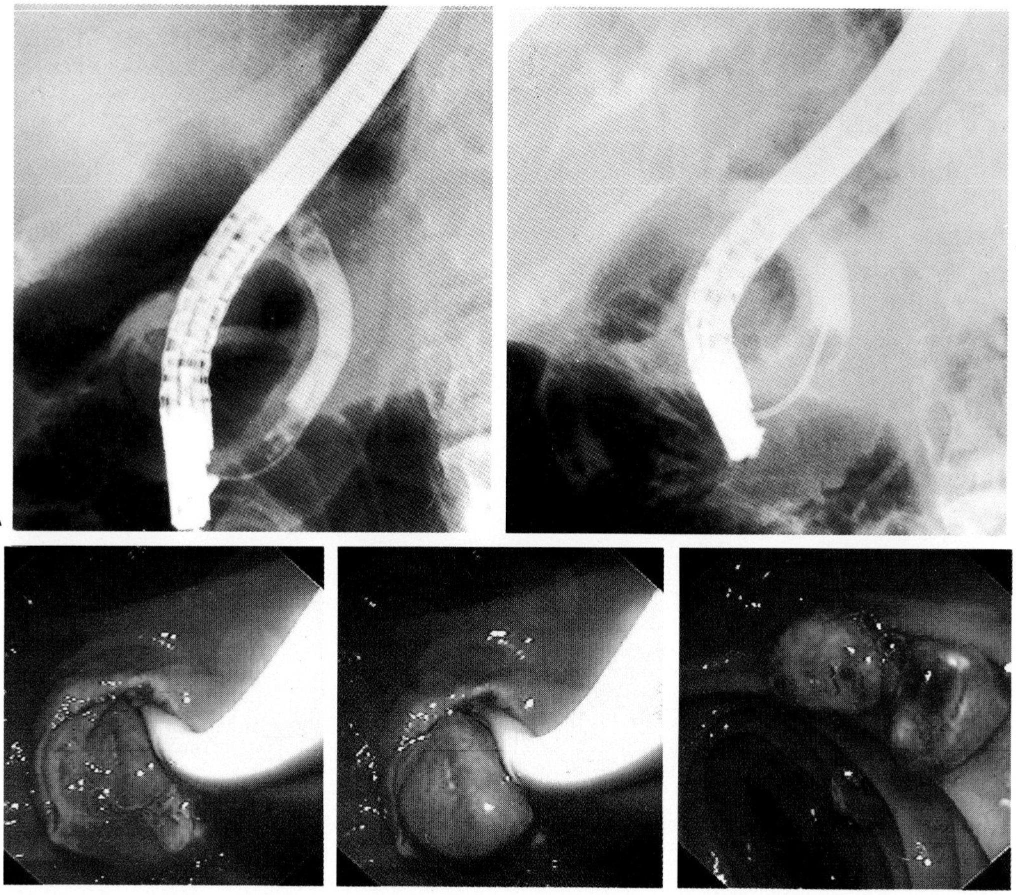

A

B

FIG. 11.5. A: Left: A cholangiogram showing several stones in the common hepatic duct and distal common bile duct. **Right:** After exploration of the common bile duct with a balloon catheter, a follow-up cholangiogram reveals no evidence of stones. **B: Left:** After a sphincterotomy, a balloon catheter is introduced into the bile duct, inflated, and withdrawn to the sphincterotomy. A stone can be seen at the sphincterotomy opening. **Middle:** A large stone is being extracted into the duodenum. **Right:** At least three medium-sized stones are visible in the duodenum after extraction.

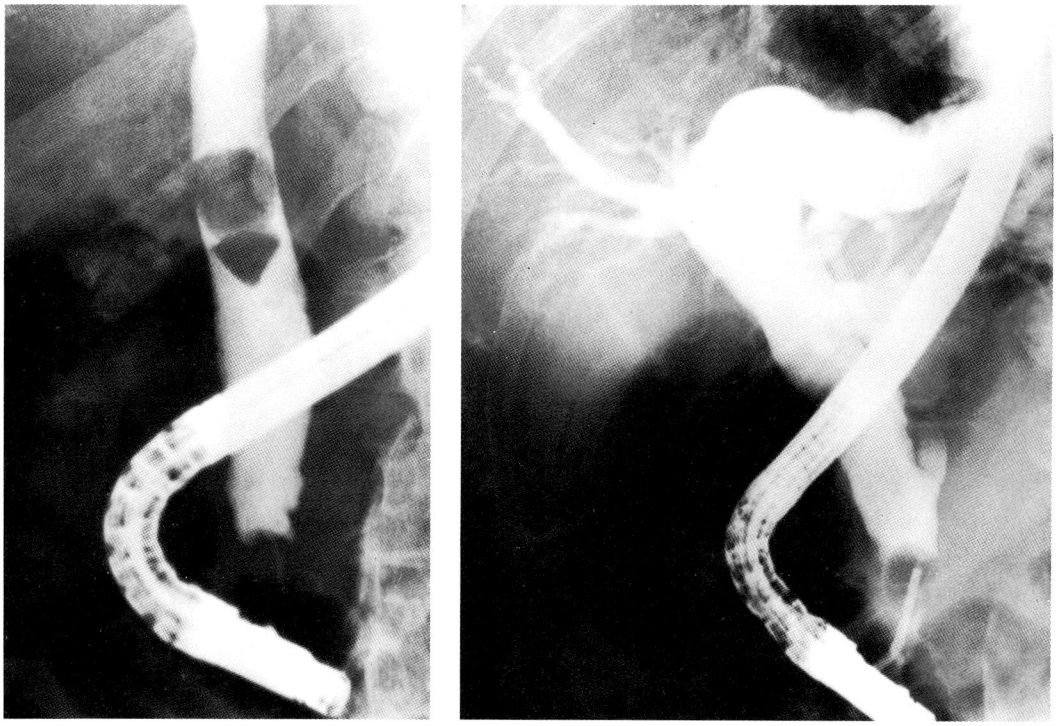

FIG. 11.6. **Left:** Two large stones of odd shape. **Right:** The duct is free of stones after balloon extraction. The balloon is shown inflated in the distal common bile duct. To check for other stones, I recommend placing an inflated balloon at the bifurcation and, while withdrawing the balloon, injecting contrast to ensure that all stones have been removed.

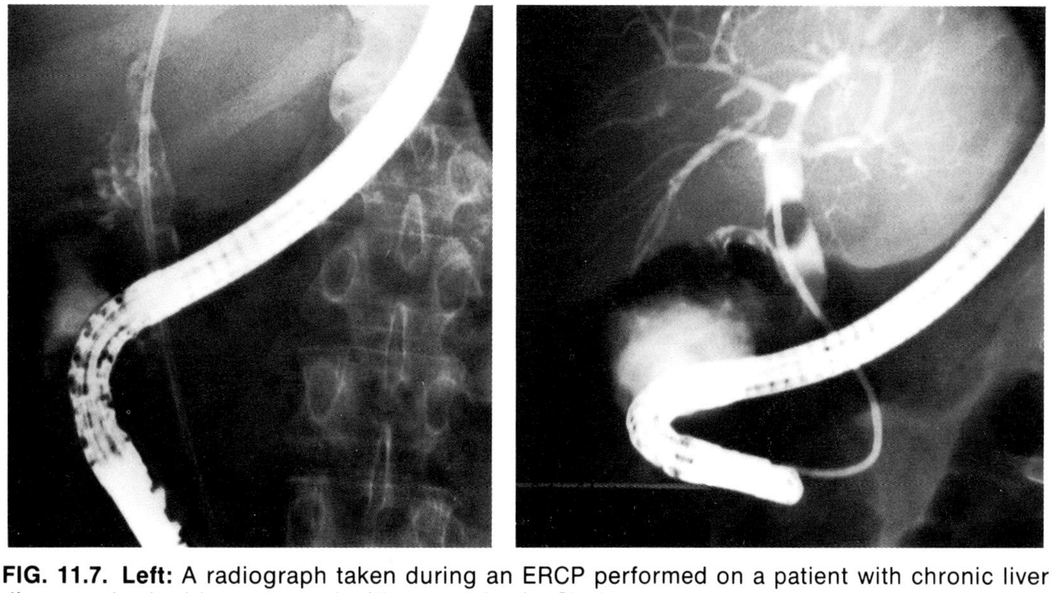

FIG. 11.7. **Left:** A radiograph taken during an ERCP performed on a patient with chronic liver disease who had been treated with a prosthesis. Sludge or stone material has formed around the stent, and the bile duct is filled with lucencies that are visible around the stent. This was sludgelike material that was cleared from the duct with a balloon catheter. **Right:** The postevacuation cholangiogram on the same patient, showing the balloon inflated in the duct and contrast injected through the catheter. Note the attenuated intrahepatic ducts consistent with intrahepatic disease and the normal extrahepatic duct with no evidence of stones or sludge.

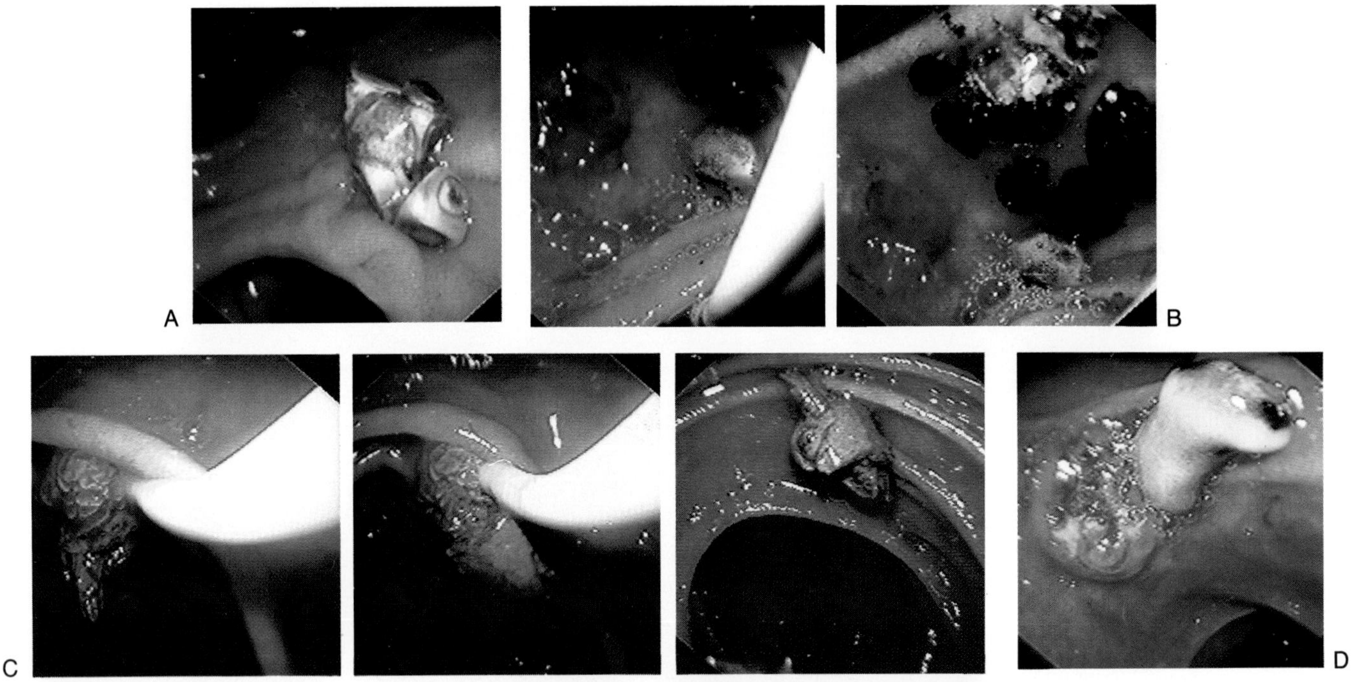

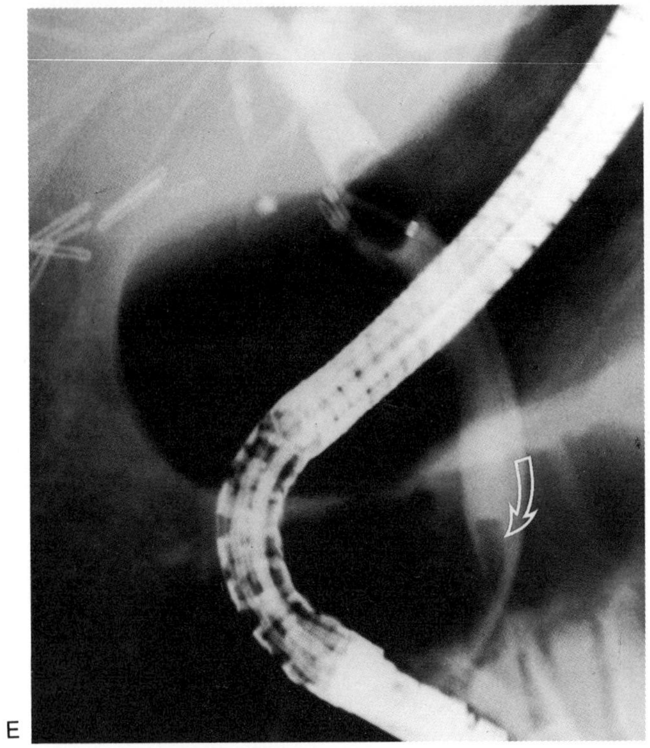

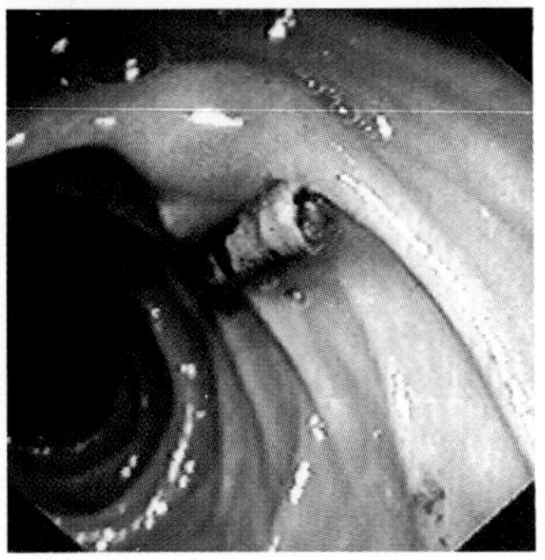

FIG. 11.8. A: Several stones of mixed type that have coalesced to appear as one object. The mixed composition of the stones is appreciated by their different colorations. **B: Left:** Several stones have been extracted through the sphincterotomy, which may be seen to the left of the stones. Note the mixed stones that were extracted. **Right:** More stones have been extracted and confirm the mixed composition, cholesterol and pigmented. **C: Left:**Part of a stent left in this patient's bile duct had fractured and was identified on appropriate radiographs. This videoimage shows the white balloon catheter inserted into the sphincterotomy and the stent being extracted. **Middle:** Stone material exiting from the sphincterotomy. **Right:** The retained stent fragment served as a nidus for stone formation. **D:** An odd-shaped stone that was extracted with a balloon catheter. **E: Left:** A cholangiogram taken in a patient who experienced recurrent pain after cholecystectomy. An operative cholangiogram at cholecystectomy was negative. A linear defect is evident in the distal common duct (*arrow*). A balloon catheter is inflated in the proximal duct. **Right:** A fractured portion of the catheter used for cholangiography, which apparently went undetected after surgery.

Text continued from page 228.

BASKET EXTRACTION

Soon after endoscopic sphincterotomy was developed, baskets, if available, were employed very successfully for the removal of medium to large stones. Endoscopists did not usually actively attempt to remove stones with baskets or balloons but, rather, permitted the stones to pass spontaneously, as they often did if a generous sphincterotomy were performed (7,8,15,17–20). The earlier model baskets were made of monofi-

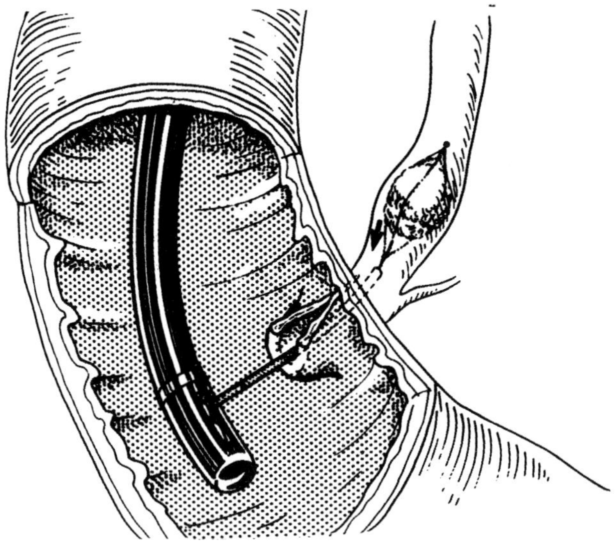

FIG. 11.9. A stone that has been captured in a basket. Once it is trapped, the stone is pulled down to the sphincterotomy for extraction.

lament wire, which was inflexible and stiff, and were configured with either straight arms or curved arms similar to the urologist's Dormia basket. The earlier baskets did not have a sustained "memory" and soon lost the capability of opening large enough to entrap a stone; most experts agree that the retained stone rate after sphincterotomy remains at approximately 8%. However, despite these shortcomings, most of us working in the field in those days managed very successfully using these different types of baskets.

The early endoscope channels were only 2.0 mm or 2.2 mm in diameter, which required 5Fr accessories, including not only the sphincterotomes and balloons but also the baskets. The hardware therefore was restrictive, and the utility of the basket was not as effective as desired. Since the introduction of larger-channel endoscopes, 6Fr and 7Fr catheters containing baskets of different configuration, construction, and size are available and are frequently used (Fig. 11.1).

I prefer basket extraction for stones measuring 1 cm or larger because of the ease in entrapping and extracting the entire stone for retrieval. The basket extraction technique is carried out as follows: The basket catheter is introduced through the sphincterotomy (in almost all cases a sphincterotomy should be performed prior to the insertion of a basket to facilitate the removal of the stone and basket), and this accessory is advanced alongside or slightly above the stone. The basket is then partially or fully opened (the basket is pushed out of the catheter to open), depending on the size of the stone, and the entire accessory, opened basket and catheter, is moved in a to-and-fro fashion in an attempt to entrap the stone (Figs. 11.9, 11.10). The newer, softer, braided-wire baskets can entrap the stone more easily than the monofilament type in my opinion. Entrapment is confirmed when simultaneous movement of the stone and basket is seen on the fluor-

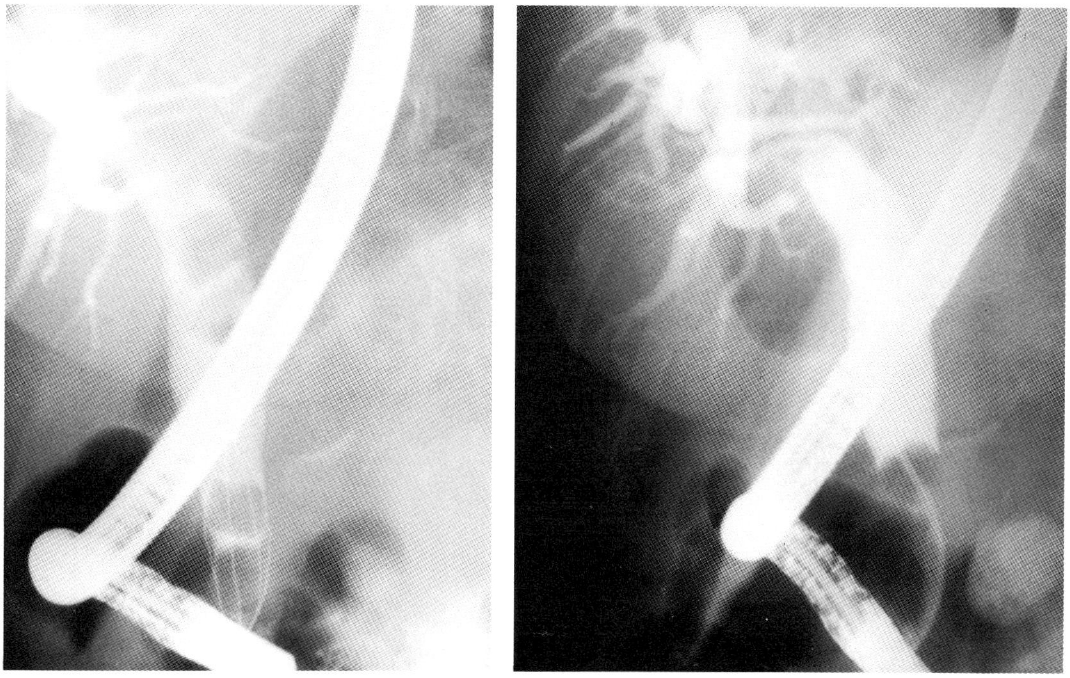

FIG. 11.10. Left: This ERCP radiograph shows several large stones present in the bile duct. The basket has been advanced forward and backward, entrapping two stones. These stones were extracted, the others manipulated. **Right:** An occlusion balloon was then used to ensure that the bile duct was free of stones.

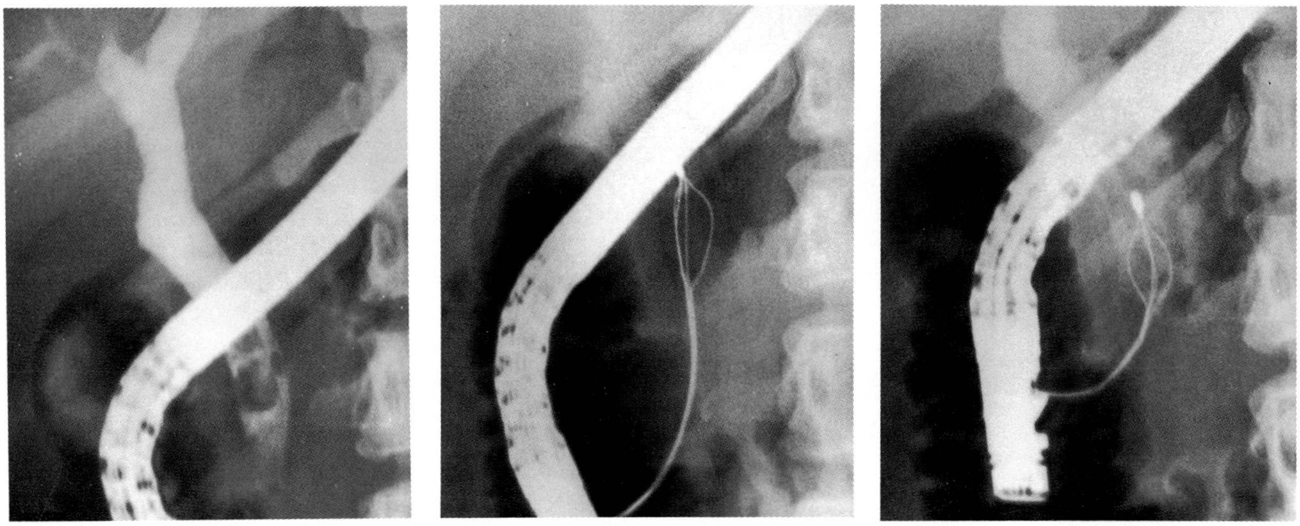

FIG. 11.11. Left: A radiograph showing several stones in the bile duct on cholangiography. **Middle:** The basket has entrapped a stone, but the fourth arm is not completely around the stone. This means the stone may slip from the basket. **Right:** The basket was readjusted to entrap the stone and can be pulled through the sphincterotomy without danger of losing the stone.

oscope screen. Once the stone is entrapped, the basket is gently closed, and the basket and stone are withdrawn to the sphincterotomy (Figs. 11.11–11.21). Again, as in the technique of balloon extraction, gentle traction is applied to the basket, and the distal tip of the endoscope is deflected downward (extended). This action adds an extra force in the correct axis, allowing for successful withdrawal of the basket and the entrapped stone (Fig. 11.22). Figures 11.23 through 11.27 are endoscopic pictures of stones extracted by the basket technique. Endoscopists should not persist in applying continuous traction to the basket catheter if the basket and stone are not visible in the sphincterotomy

Text continues on page 238.

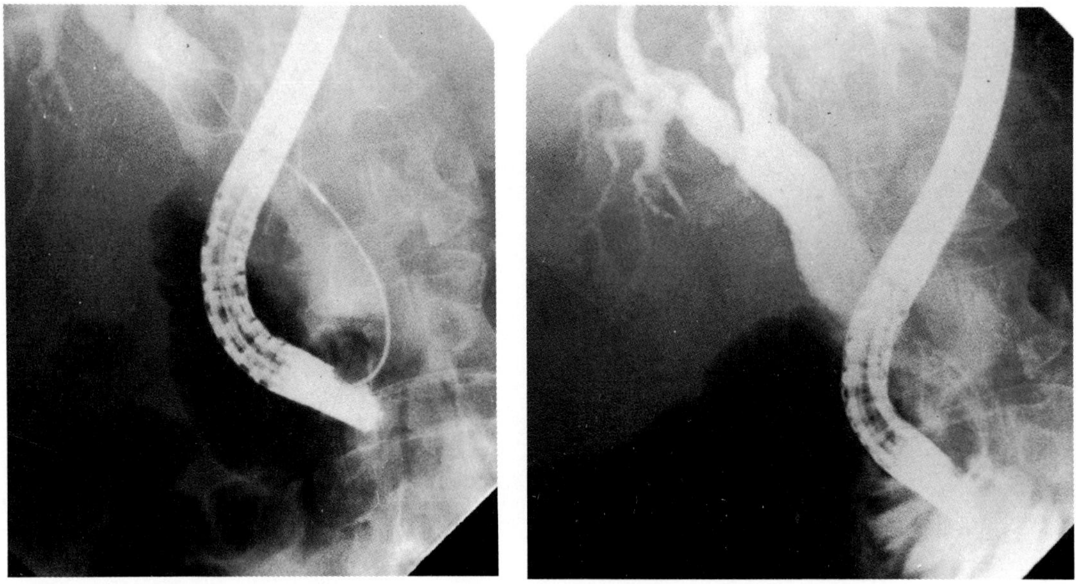

FIG. 11.12. Left: A large stone being entrapped by a basket in the mid bile duct. **Right:** The stone has been removed, as shown on the follow-up cholangiogram.

FIG. 11.15. Left: Several large stones lined up in the bile duct. **Middle:** A basket was used to remove all but one of the stones, and in this radiograph, the last stone has been entrapped. **Right:** The follow-up radiograph demonstrates a bile duct free of stones.

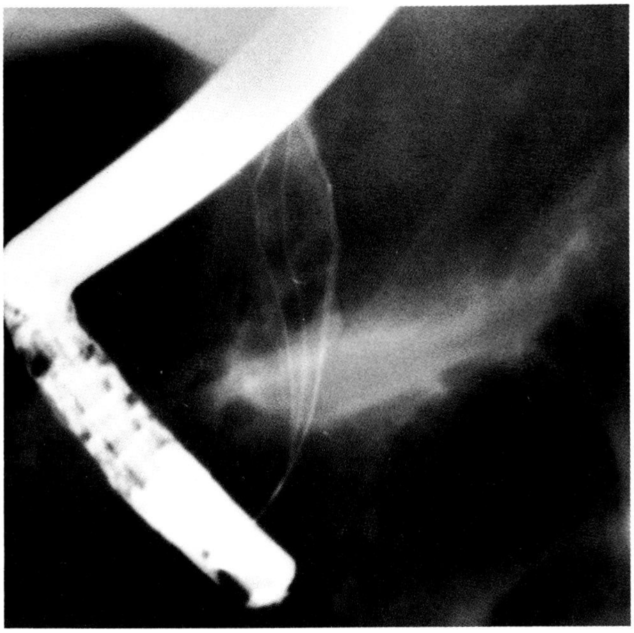

FIG. 11.13. Several small stones are seen entrapped in a single basket. This is unusual because small stones usually slip through the basket cage. However, in this case, the stones coalesced into one and could be removed as a unit. It is not recommended that more than one medium to large stone be entrapped simultaneously: The basket and stones may impact because of the mass.

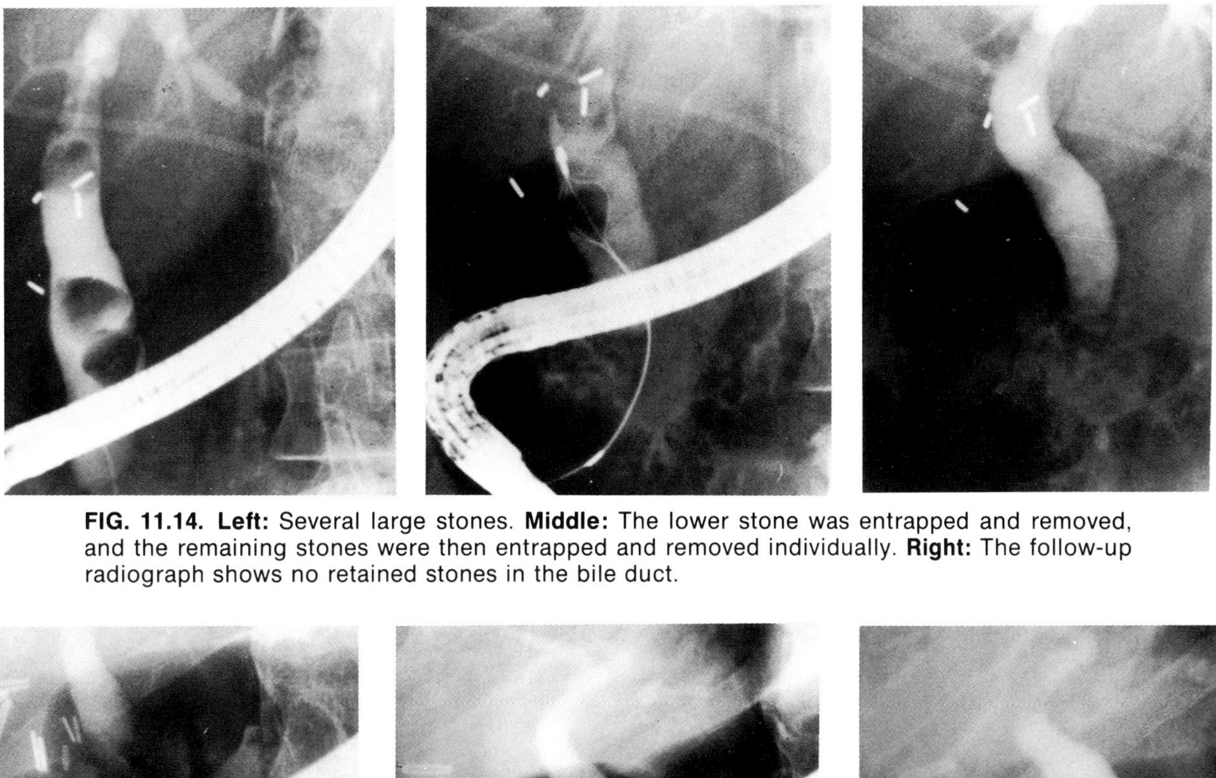

FIG. 11.14. Left: Several large stones. **Middle:** The lower stone was entrapped and removed, and the remaining stones were then entrapped and removed individually. **Right:** The follow-up radiograph shows no retained stones in the bile duct.

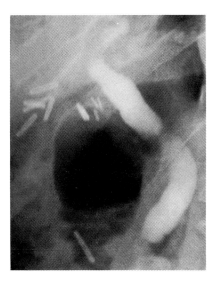

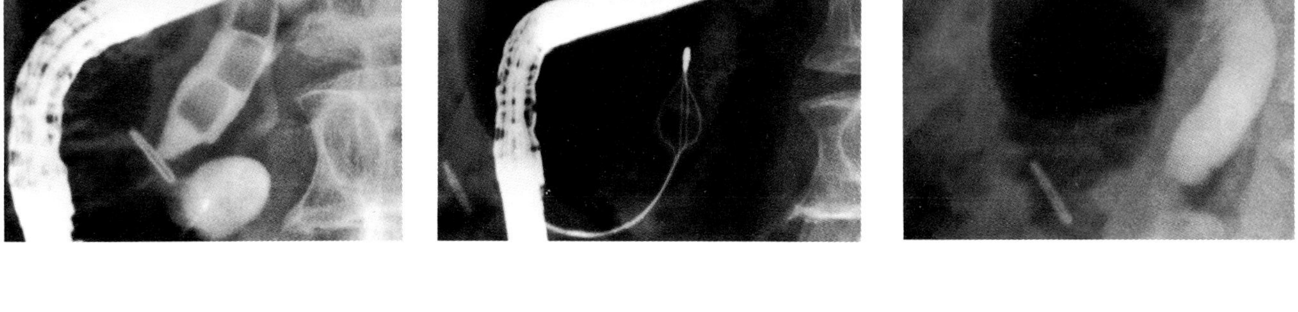

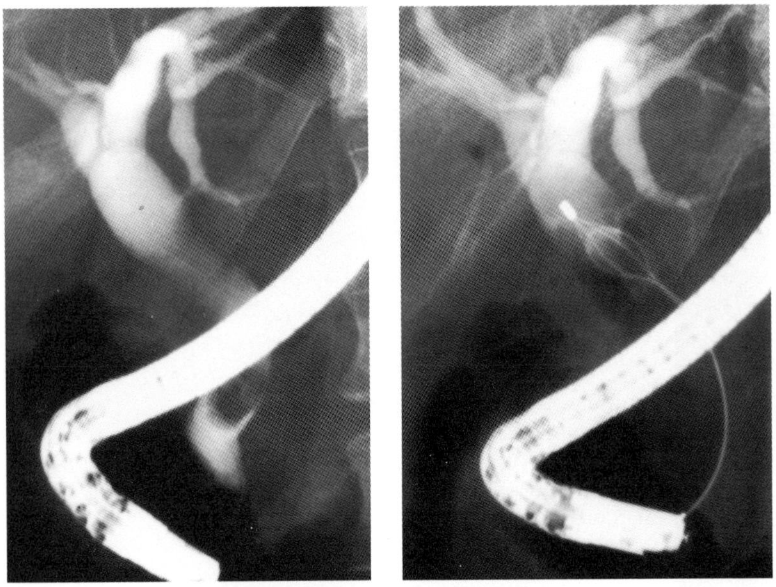

FIG. 11.16. Left: A large stone in the distal common bile duct. Usually a large distal stone or an impacted stone cannot be entrapped with a basket because the arms of the basket may not open large enough in this confined space to entrap the stone. **Right:** The stone was disimpacted and firmly entrapped with the basket.

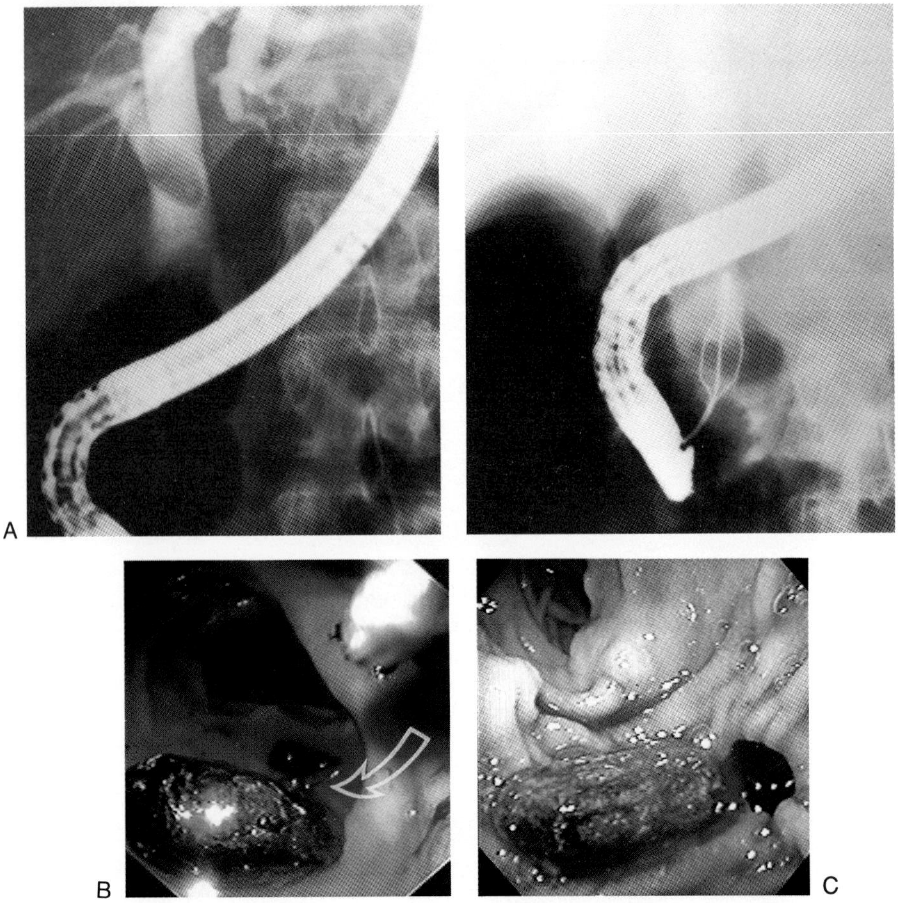

FIG. 11.17. A: Left: This large stone was disimpacted; after forceful disimpaction with a catheter, it floated to the bifurcation of the bile ducts. Fortunately, the stone did not float into either hepatic duct because the basket may not have opened large enough to entrap it. **Right:** The stone was entrapped with the basket and pulled toward the sphincterotomy. **B:** A large, pigmented stone containing prolene suture material (*arrow*), which may have been the nidus for stone formation. **C:** This large stone was extracted with an occlusion balloon. The sphincterotomy is next to a periampullary diverticulum (which is not visible here). Often large stones can be extracted through sphincterotomies formed near a periampullary diverticulum because the sphincter lacks some of the muscle fibers.

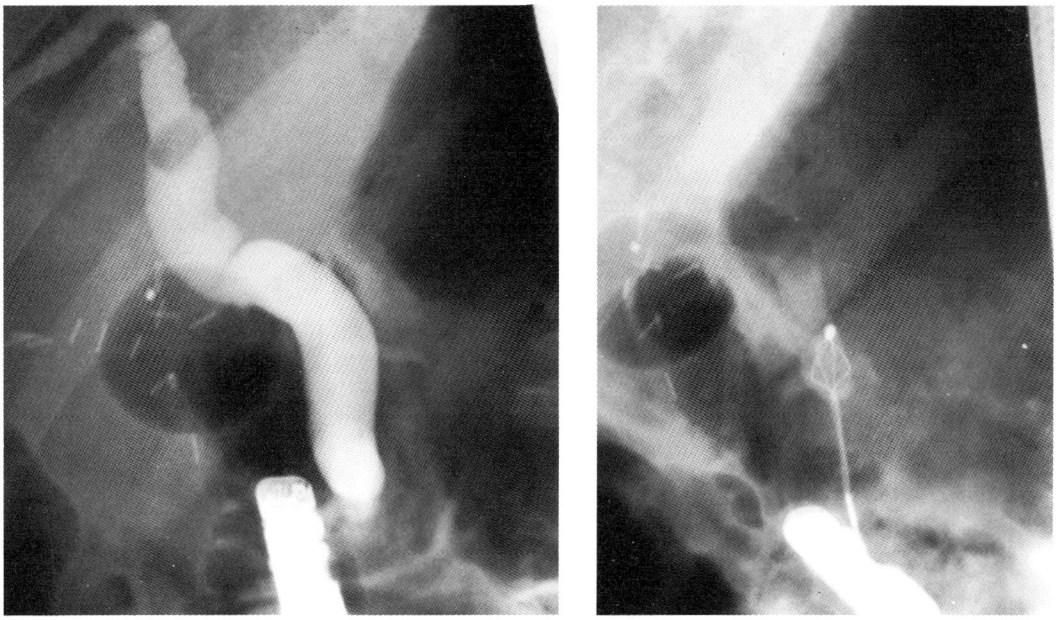

FIG. 11.18. Left: Stones in the bile duct of patients who have undergone a Bilroth II gastric resection may be difficult to entrap because of the position of the endoscope. Looping of the endoscope (which increases friction while decreasing mobility) is a problem encountered when the endoscope is looped and angulated. In this radiograph, a medium-sized stone is visible high in the common hepatic duct. **Right:** A basket has successfully entrapped the stone, and the stone and basket are being pulled down to the sphincterotomy for extraction.

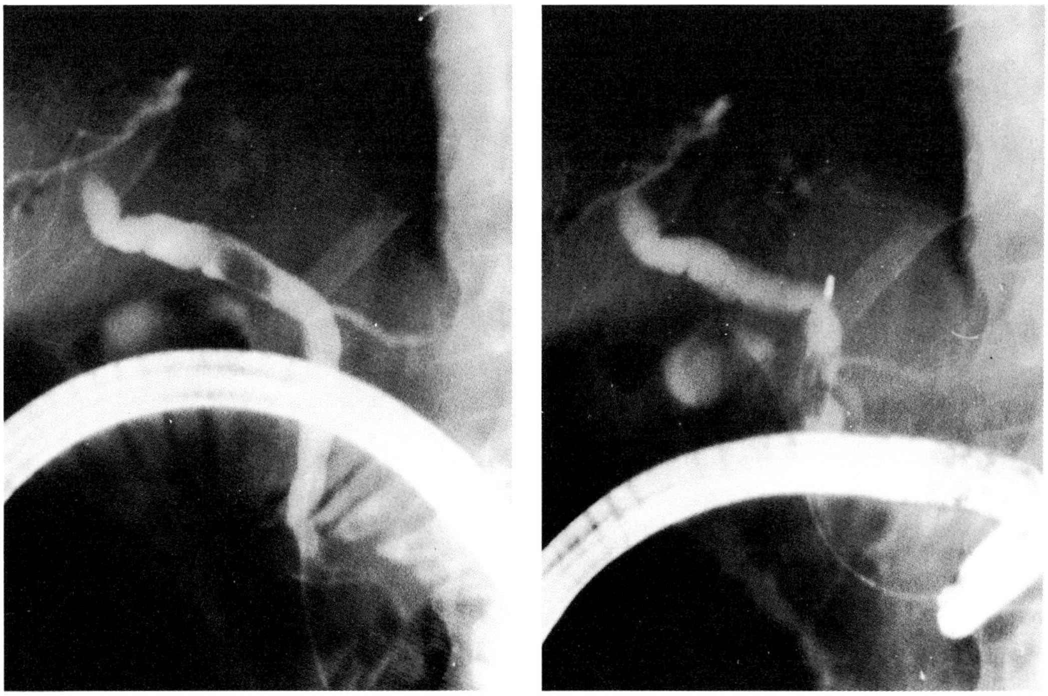

FIG. 11.19. Left: In this case, a long loop was formed by the endoscope when traversing the afferent limb of a patient with a Bilroth II resection. A long, narrow stone is visible in the mid bile duct. **Right:** A basket has been used to entrap the stone to remove it through the sphincterotomy.

Text continued from page 234.
opening (the sphincterotomy incision most likely requires extension). It is not advised that the endoscopist tug with both the basket and endoscope in an upward direction (pulling the endoscope), because this maneuver may tear the sphincterotomy and the bowel wall. Therefore, once again, gentle downward traction with the basket and downward deflection of the distal tip of the endoscope should assist in removing most medium-sized stones that are entrapped in a basket.

If the stone is entrapped in a basket and there is no indication that it can be removed, one must resort to lithotripsy techniques (21). An entrapped basket and stone should not be considered a surgical problem. There are earlier reports of patients undergoing surgery for extraction of an entrapped basket and stone, but mechanical lithotripsy techniques usually make laparotomy unnecessary.

An entrapped basket can occasionally be treated by extending the sphincterotomy to permit easier passage; this requires removing the endoscope over the basket catheter and cable and reintroducing the endoscope into the duodenum. On one occasion, while using cautery to extend the sphincterotomy, I actually touched a basket arm with the cautery device, which shorted the circuit and broke the basket, permitting removal of the entrapped basket from around the stone. I was also once able to capture an entrapped basket and stone using a larger basket (the type utilized for lithotripsy) and to remove it through the sphincterotomy. Figure 11.28 is a radiograph taken after an endoscopic basket was used to entrap a percutaneously placed basket that became impacted on a stone and could not be removed through the T-tube tract. After performing a sphincterotomy, I inserted an endoscopic stone basket and successfully entrapped the percutaneously placed basket containing the stone, allowing removal of the stone, basket, and all the percutaneous hardware.
Text continues on page 243.

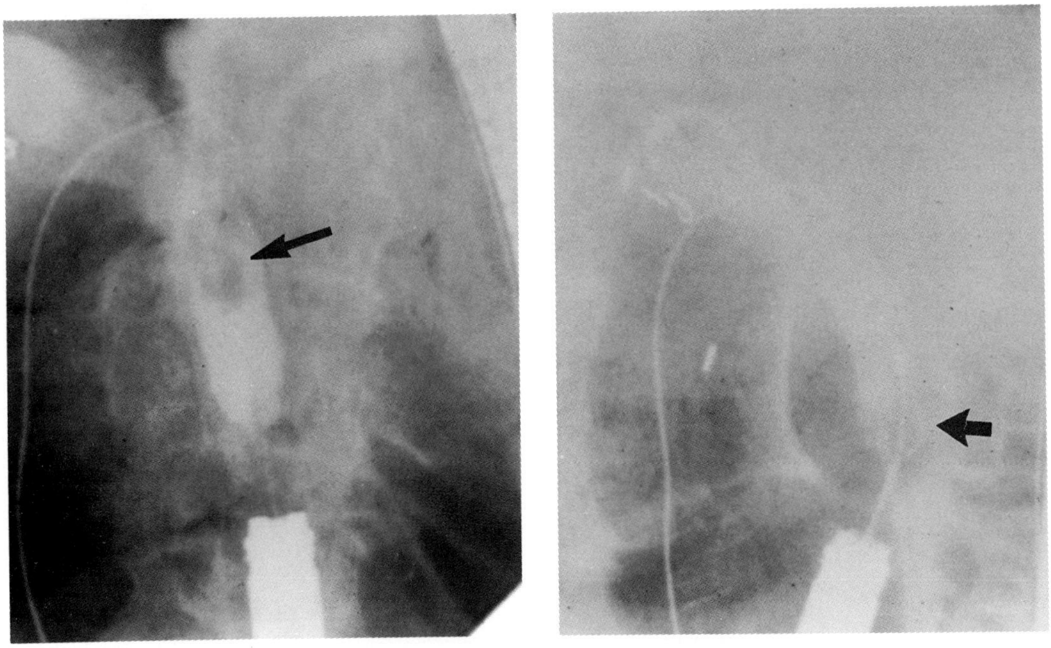

FIG. 11.20. Left: This radiograph demonstrates the use of a colonoscope to traverse a long afferent limb. The papilla could not be reached using the duodenoscope, so a colonoscope was used. Here, a stone may be seen in the bile duct (*arrow*). **Right:** In this underexposed (light) radiograph, the stone can be seen entrapped in a basket (*arrow*), which is contained in the colonoscope.

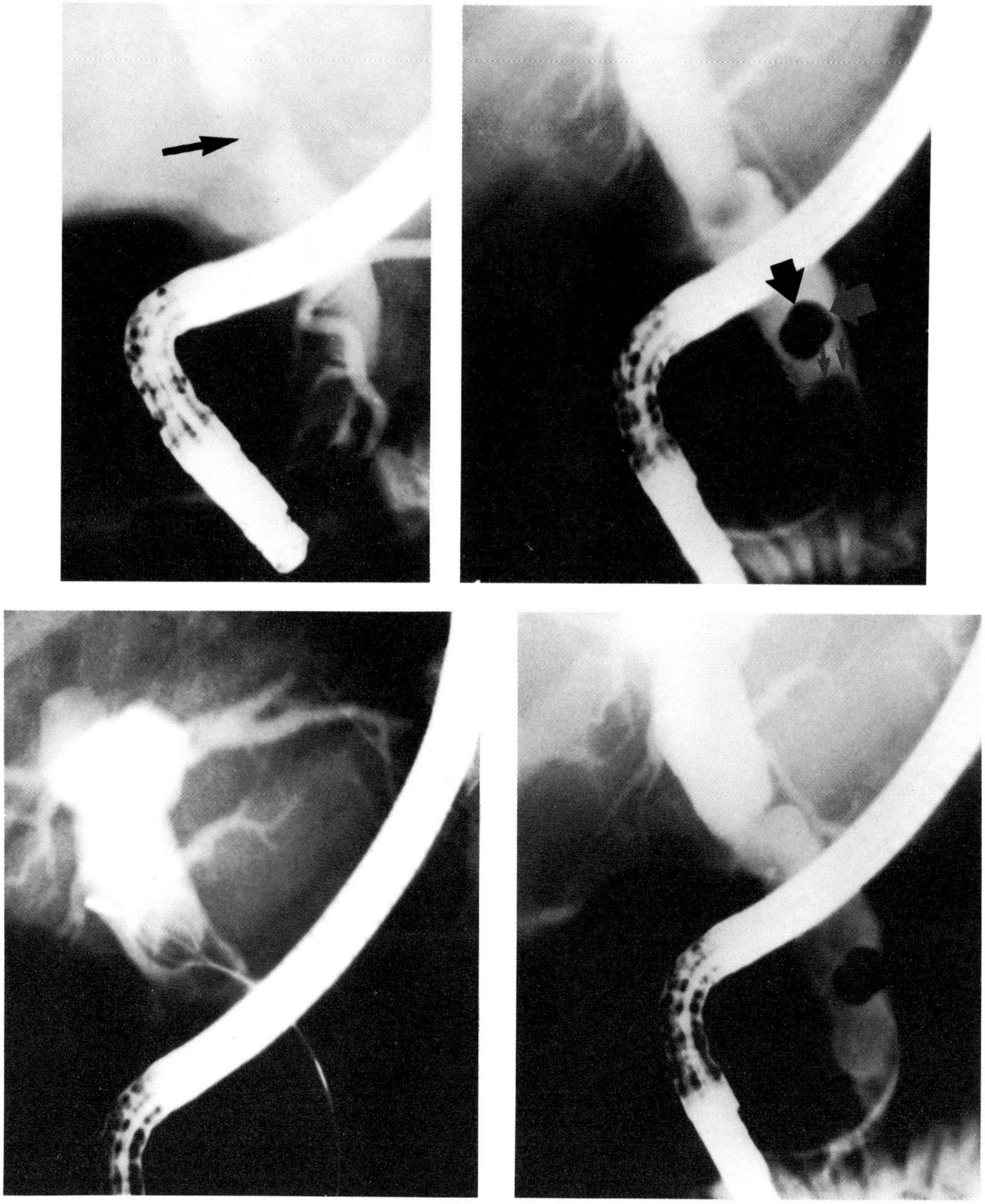

FIG. 11.21. This series of radiographs demonstrates the combined use of occlusion balloons and baskets. **Top Left:** A medium-sized stone in the common hepatic duct (*arrow*). **Top right:** After a balloon is placed and more contrast is injected, a large stone was seen impacted in the distal duct. Note the convex meniscus representing the stone, and, proximal to the stone (*small arrows*), the balloon (*large arrow*). The common hepatic duct stone is still in place. **Bottom left:** The large stone has been entrapped by the basket. **Bottom right:** A balloon was placed into the duct after removal of the large stone to ensure clearance of the duct.

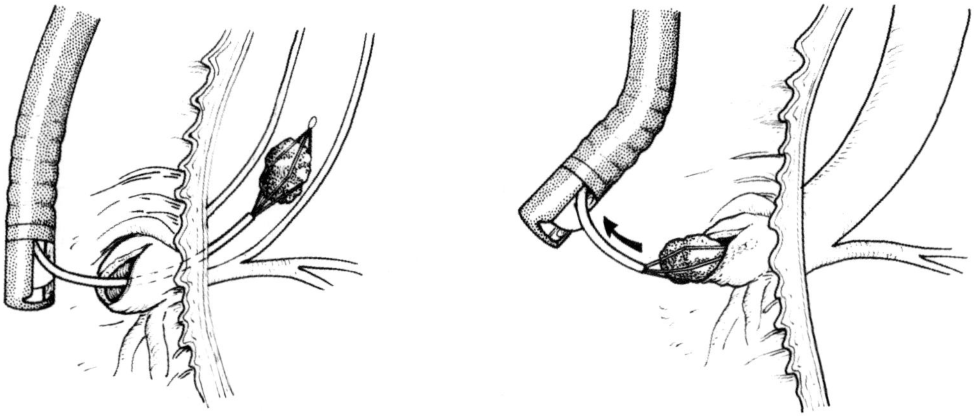

FIG. 11.22. The technique for entrapping a stone in a basket and safely removing it through the sphincterotomy. **Left:** The stone has been entrapped. **Right:** The basket and stone have been withdrawn to the sphincterotomy. In order to remove them from the sphincterotomy, the endoscope is extended downward away from the sphincterotomy, a maneuver that can safely be used to remove a stone and basket through an adequate sphincterotomy.

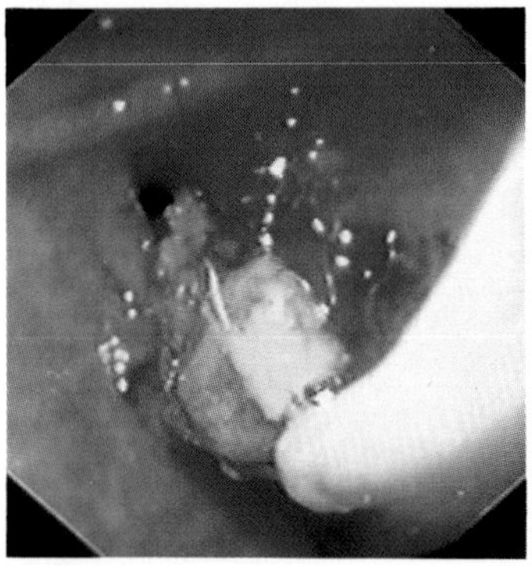

FIG. 11.23. A videoimage of a stone extracted by the basket technique from the bile duct through a sphincterotomy.

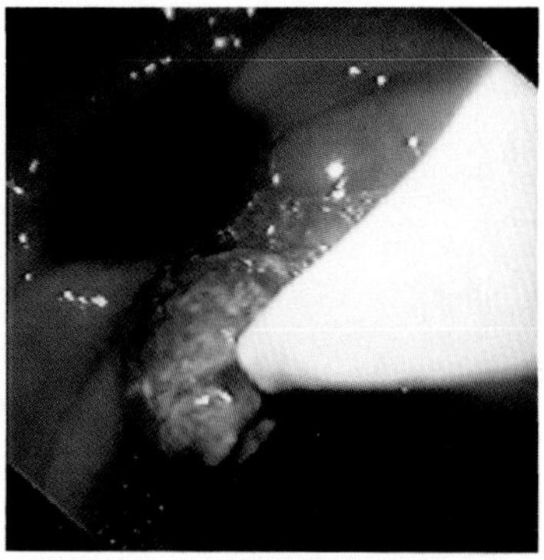

FIG. 11.24. The stone is contained in a basket adjacent to a periampullary diverticulum.

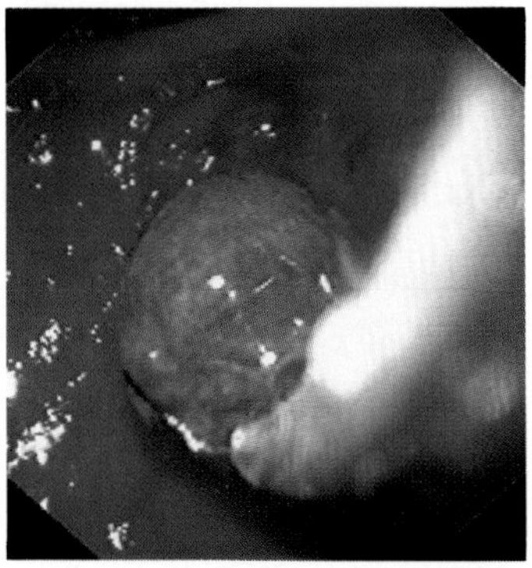

FIG. 11.25. A stone extracted by the basket technique from the bile duct.

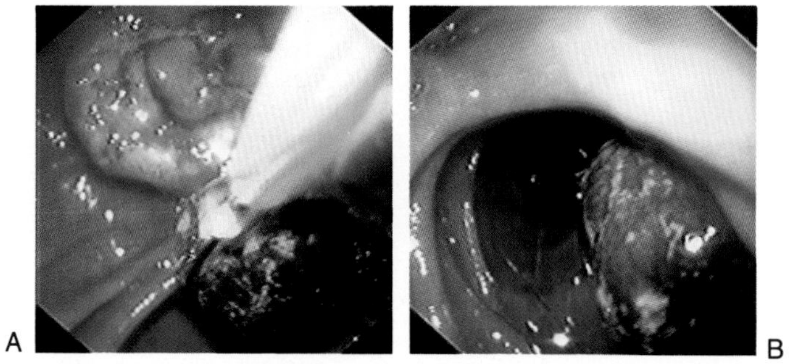

FIG. 11.26. **A:** A stone being removed from the bile duct through a sphincterotomy by the basket technique. **B:** The length of the stone is better appreciated after repositioning it against the duodenal wall.

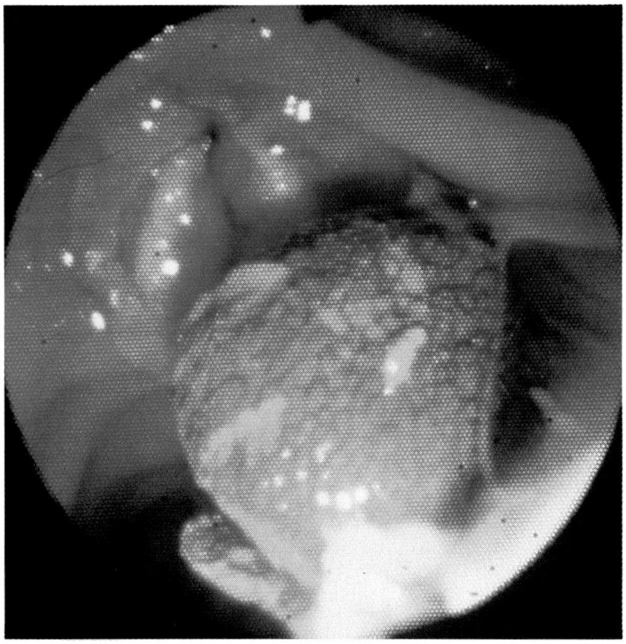
A

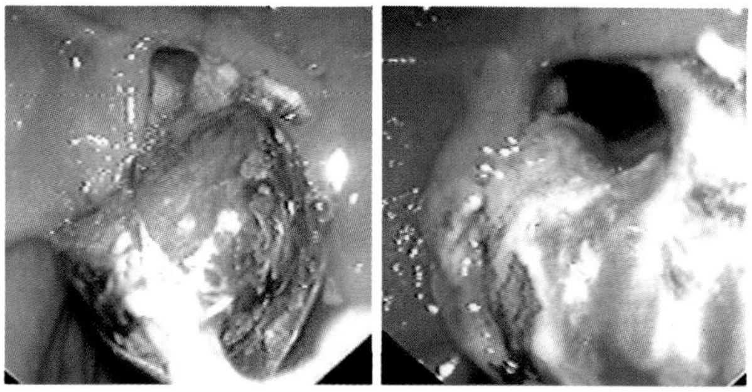
B

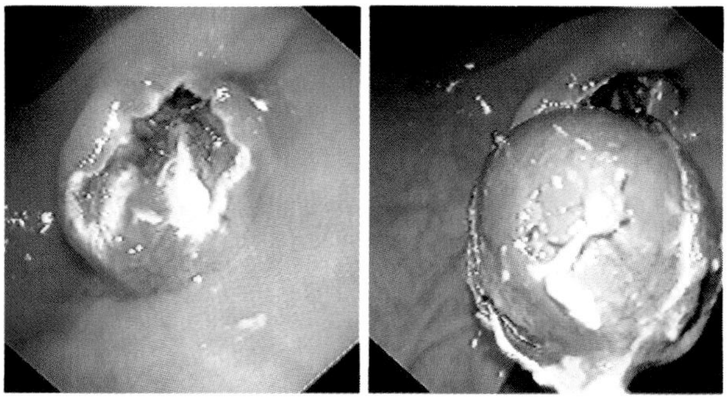
C

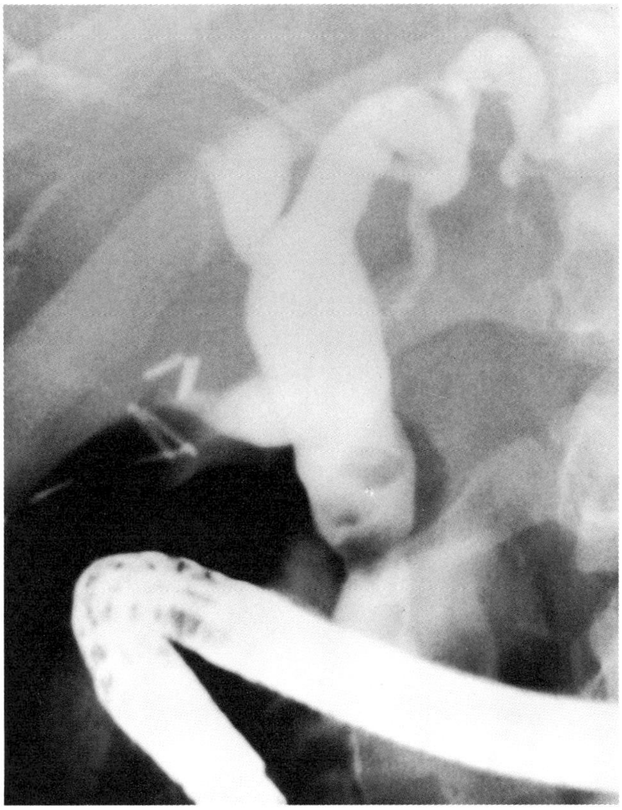
D

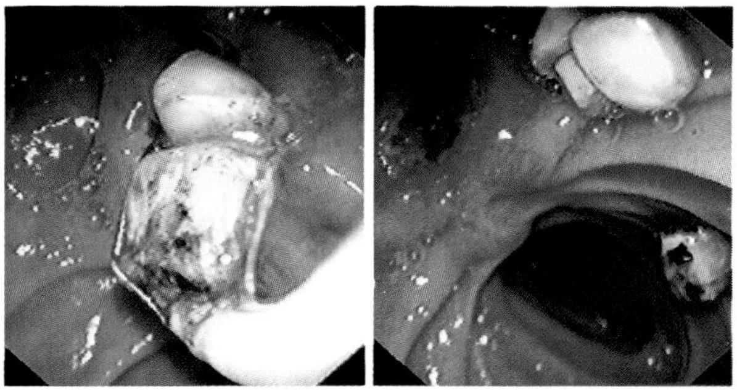
E

FIG. 11.27. A: An endoscopic view of a large stone contained in a basket after removal through the sphincterotomy. The sphincterotomy incision is clearly visible in this picture. **B: Left:** A large stone being extracted from a generous sphincterotomy, which is seen on the right after stone removal. **Right:** The sphincterotomy after removal of the stone. **C: Left:** A generous sphincterotomy has been formed. **Right:** A large stone has been pulled through the sphincterotomy entrapped in a basket. **D:** The cholangiogram shows several stones in the distal common duct. **E: Left:** Several stones are visible in one basket after extraction (same patient as 11.27D). **Right:** The stones have been released from the basket.

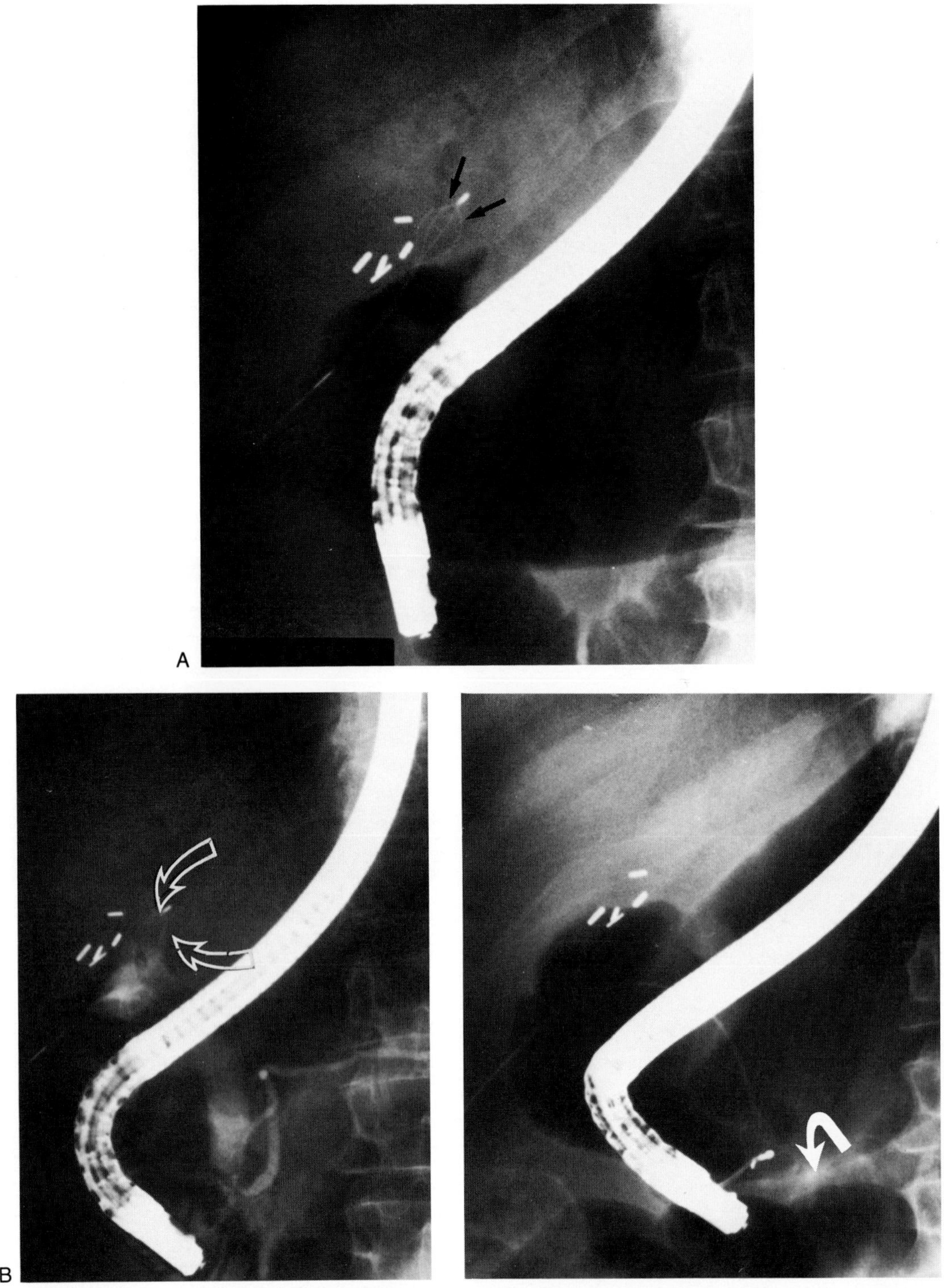

FIG. 11.28. A: A basket containing a stone (*arrows*), which was inserted percutaneously through a mature T-tube tract. The tract, or more specifically, the peritoneal tract, was not mechanically dilated before entrapment, and the stone could not be extracted. Also, the basket containing the stone was entrapped. **B: Left:** After performance of a sphincterotomy, an endoscopic basket was inserted into the bile duct, snaring the tip of the percutaneous basket. **Right:** The percutaneous basket, stone, and wire were pulled through the sphincterotomy into the duodenum.

Text continued from page 238.

REMOVAL OF AN ENTRAPPED BASKET

In order to facilitate removal of an entrapped basket, the handle of the basket may be removed. In most cases, this is accomplished by using a wire cutter to sever the cable. The endoscope is then removed over the Teflon sheath and basket cable; once the basket and cable are freed from the endoscope, it can be reintroduced into the duodenum. If there is room to extend the sphincterotomy, a standard sphincterotome or needle knife can be inserted and the incision extended, which may permit free exit of the basket and stone. Although it is more dangerous to apply electric current, the application of current to one of the arms of the basket may cause the wire to break, thus freeing the basket and stone. The latter technique is not recommended unless the endoscopist is completely familiar with the principles of electrocautery and the patient is totally grounded and not touching metal. Because it is rather simple to apply the lithotripsy coil-spring catheter in this situation, I would recommend this approach rather than cautery, especially if extension of the sphincterotomy still does not permit the removal of the basket and stone.

Dr. M. Osnes of Norway has suggested another method for removing a basket and stone entrapped in the sphincterotomy. He recommends attaching the basket cable to a helmet-pulley apparatus previously used for Sengstaken-Blakemore tubes or an orthopedic pulley system. The basket cable can be attached to a weight, usually 2 lbs. to 5 lbs. (intravenous fluid bags or bottles can also be used for weights and are easy to adjust for the patient's comfort) and suspended from the pulley system. In Osnes's experience, the basket and stone usually erode through the sphincterotomy and are free of the impaction within 24 to 48 hours. Again, since the introduction of the mechanical lithotriptor, the method recommended by Osnes may be redundant if the lithotripsy coil-spring catheter is available.

Despite endoscopists' successful efforts with stone extraction techniques, an estimated 3% to 8% of stones treated endoscopically are retained to pass spontaneously or to be treated by lithotripsy techniques (19–25). Figure 11.29 illustrates a situation that might lead to a retained stone or entrapment of an endoscopic basket containing a stone, but this situation can be remedied by incorporating lithotripsy techniques into our armamentarium.

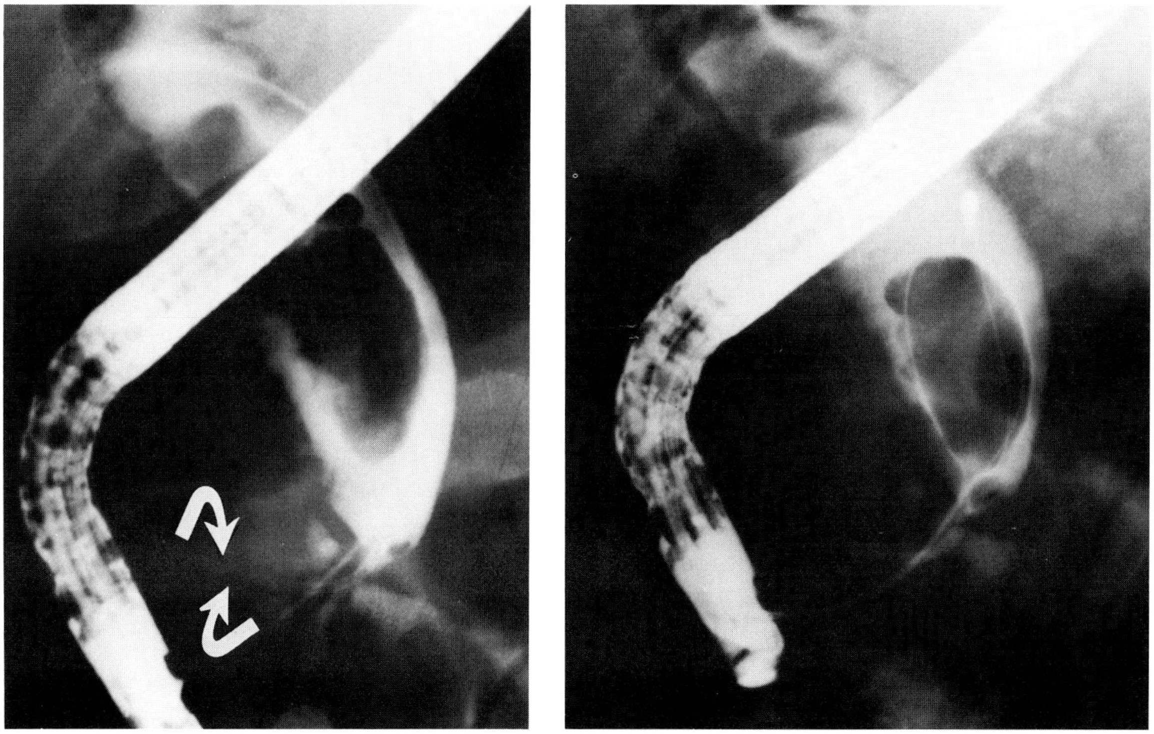

FIG. 11.29. Left: An ERCP demonstrating several stones in the common bile duct, obviously too large for extraction. Note that a prosthesis (*arrows*) had been placed prior to an attempted manipulation of the stones in order to avoid obstruction if entrapment occurred. **Right:** The stone has been entrapped with a large basket in preparation for lithotripsy.

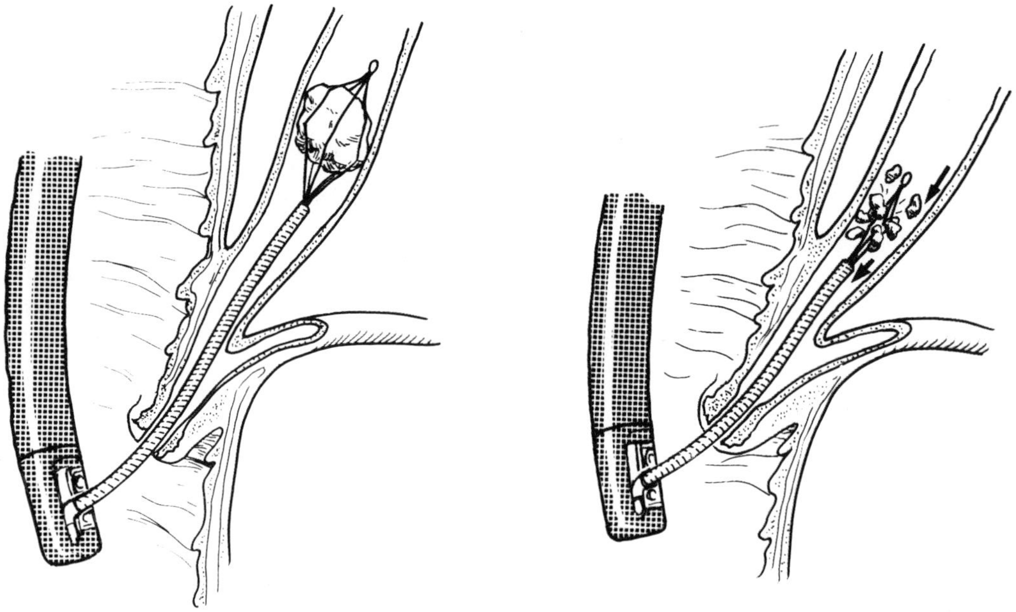

FIG. 11.30. Left: The technique of mechanical lithotripsy using a single-unit device that is advanced intact through the channel of the endoscope. Note that a sphincterotomy has been performed. In this drawing, the stone is entrapped in the basket that comprises the lithotripsy device. **Right:** After entrapment of the stone, the proximal end of the basket cable is attached to a handle, and the handle is turned in the direction that draws the basket into the coil-spring catheter, crushing the stone. (From ref. 21, with permission.)

Mechanical Lithotripsy

Over the course of time, several mechanical lithotripsy systems have been devised and incorporated into our armamentarium (21,26–37). Some models contain a reinforced basket and cable that are self-contained in a coil-spring catheter. This lithotripsy mechanism is advanced through the biopsy channel of a 2.8 mm endoscope, through the sphincterotomy, and into the bile duct (Figs. 11.30–11.35). The coil-spring catheter, which may be too rigid and difficult to manipulate, especially the earlier models, requires more perseverence and effort to cannulate the bile duct selectively. Early failures with this system were common. With any mechanical system, once the stone has been entrapped in the basket, the proximal end of the basket cable is attached to a handle that, when turned, draws the basket and stone toward the coil-spring catheter. The shearing force of the basket drawn into the steel catheter results in fragmentation of the stone (Fig. 11.30).

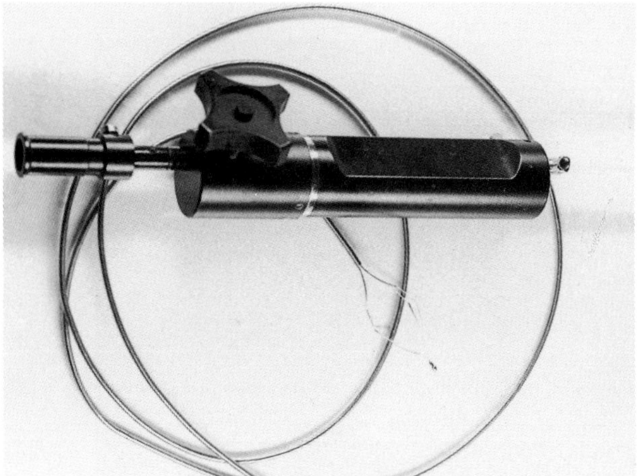

FIG. 11.31. A photograph of a lithotripsy device (Olympus) that contains the basket and coil-spring catheter in a single unit to be used through the 3.2 mm channel duodenoscope.

The earlier devices were more difficult to use because of the stiff coil-spring catheter, but later models were made with more flexible tips. Subsequent models designed for larger-channel endoscopes, usually 3.2 mm (Fig. 11.31), have a more flexible distal tip that is easier to angulate from the duodenoscope into the sphincterotomy. The mechanical crank devices are similar to the earlier models, and the results are as good or better. Because the more flexible coil-spring catheter is easier to insert than earlier models, the endoscopist has a better chance of capturing and crushing a stone.

The disadvantage of a through-the-endoscope mechanical system is the wear that using this system and crushing stones places on the instrument. The advantage is the fact that the patient does not have to undergo multiple intubations because the stone is captured and

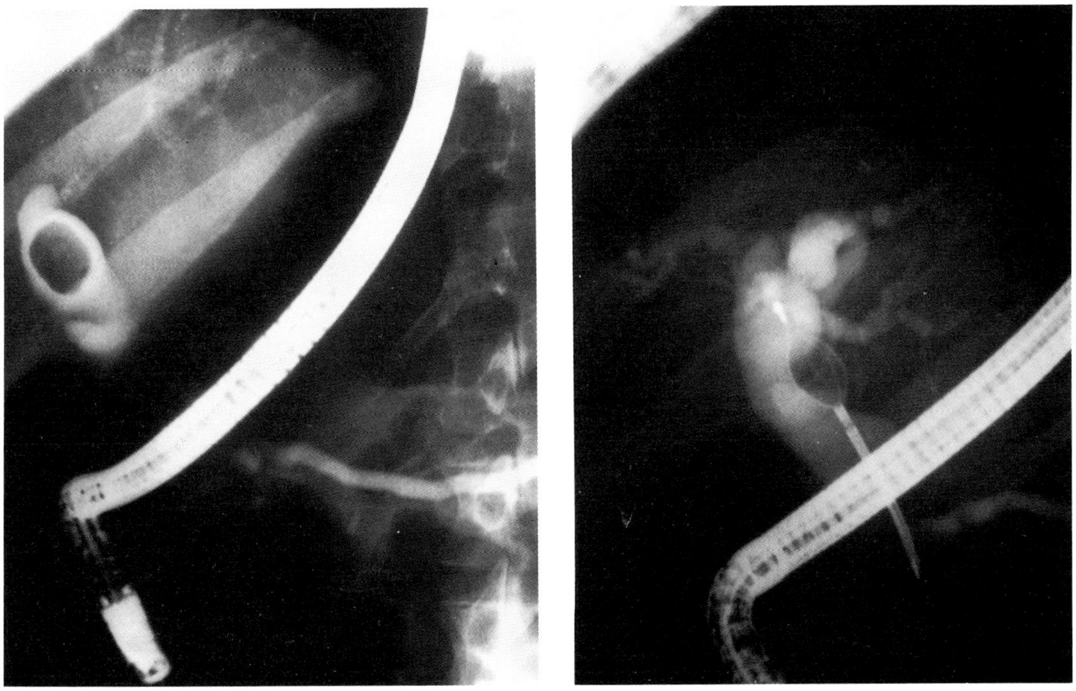

FIG. 11.32. A radiograph demonstrating the effectiveness of the lithotripsy unit that contains the basket within the coil-spring catheter. **Left:** The stones are appreciated in the bile duct. **Right:** The method for cannulating the sphincterotomy with the device and subsequently entrapping the stone.

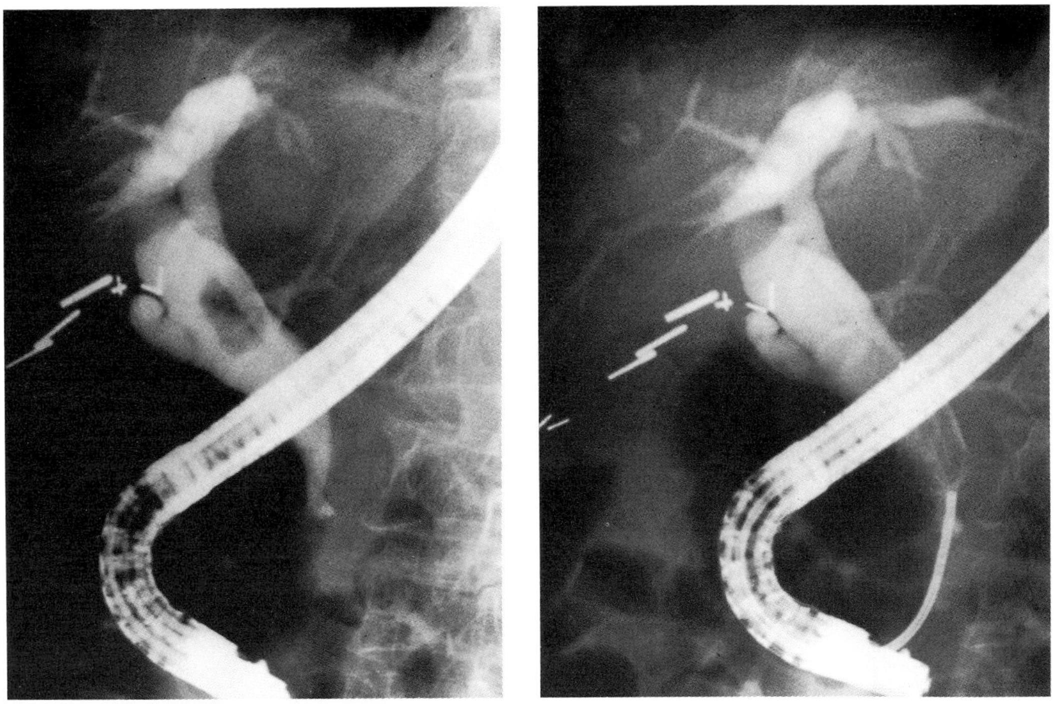

FIG. 11.33. Left: A stone in the bile duct. **Right:** The cannulating and entrapping procedure.

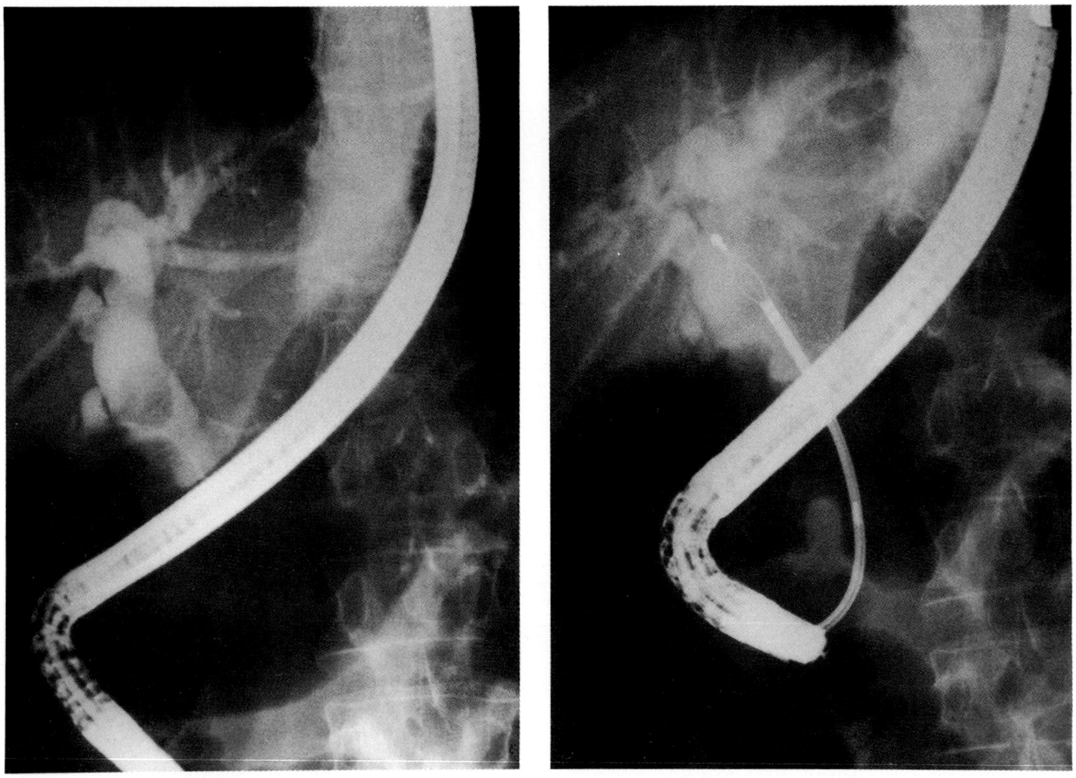

FIG. 11.34. **Left:** Another example of stones in the bile duct. **Right:** The method for cannulating the sphincterotomy and entrapping the stone.

crushed and the duct is rechecked before removing the endoscope. Other lithotripsy devices were introduced to avoid instrument damage, and these devices should make the procedure as accessible and successful. With these devices, the basket, which is a regular stone basket, is advanced through the endoscope and into the bile duct to capture the stone (the usual procedure for stone entrapment). Once the stone is captured and the basket pulled snugly to the sphincterotomy, the handle is removed from the basket by cutting it off with a wire cutter (Wilson-Cook) or by simply unscrewing it (George Percy McGowen). The endoscope then can be removed over the basket catheter and cable, and

Text continues on page 249.

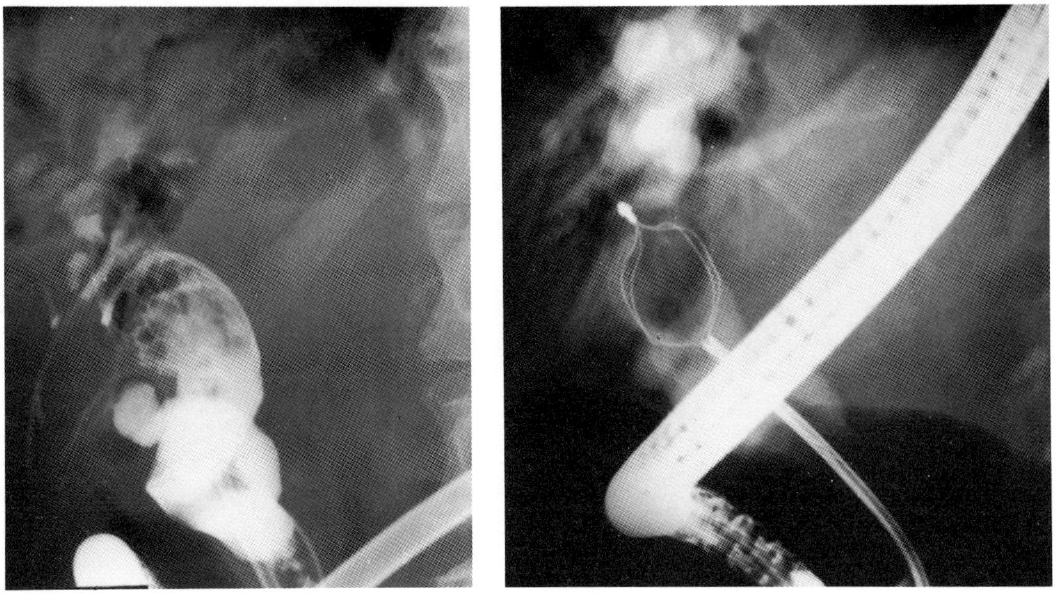

FIG. 11.35. **Left:** Stones in the bile duct. **Right:** The coil-spring catheter and basket.

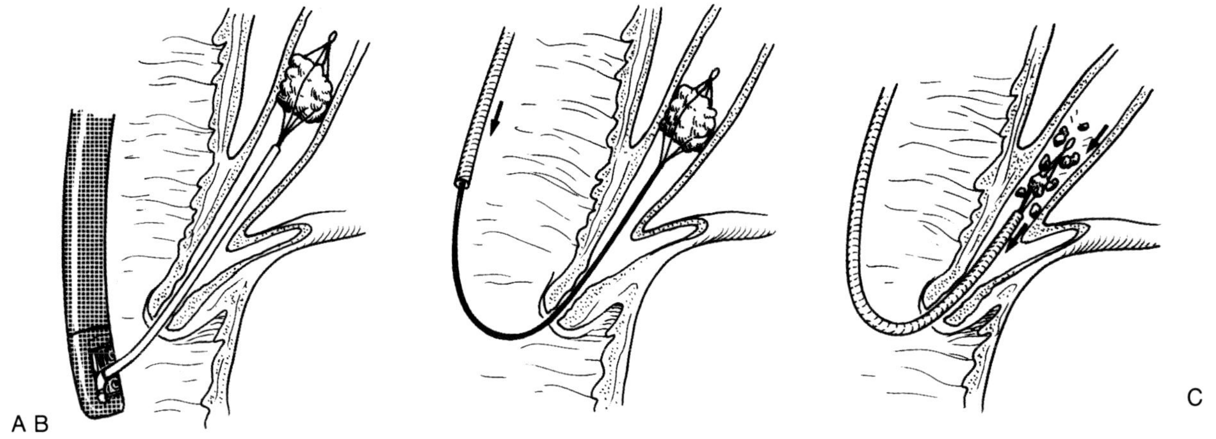

FIG. 11.36. Left: A stone being entrapped by a standard basket, which has been introduced through the endoscope and into the bile duct. **Middle:** The handle of the basket was removed to facilitate removal of the endoscope, and a coil-spring catheter is then advanced over the basket cable to the stone. **Right:** The proximal end of the basket cable has been attached to a crank, which, when turned, draws the stone into the coil-spring catheter, crushing the stone. (From ref. 21, with permission.)

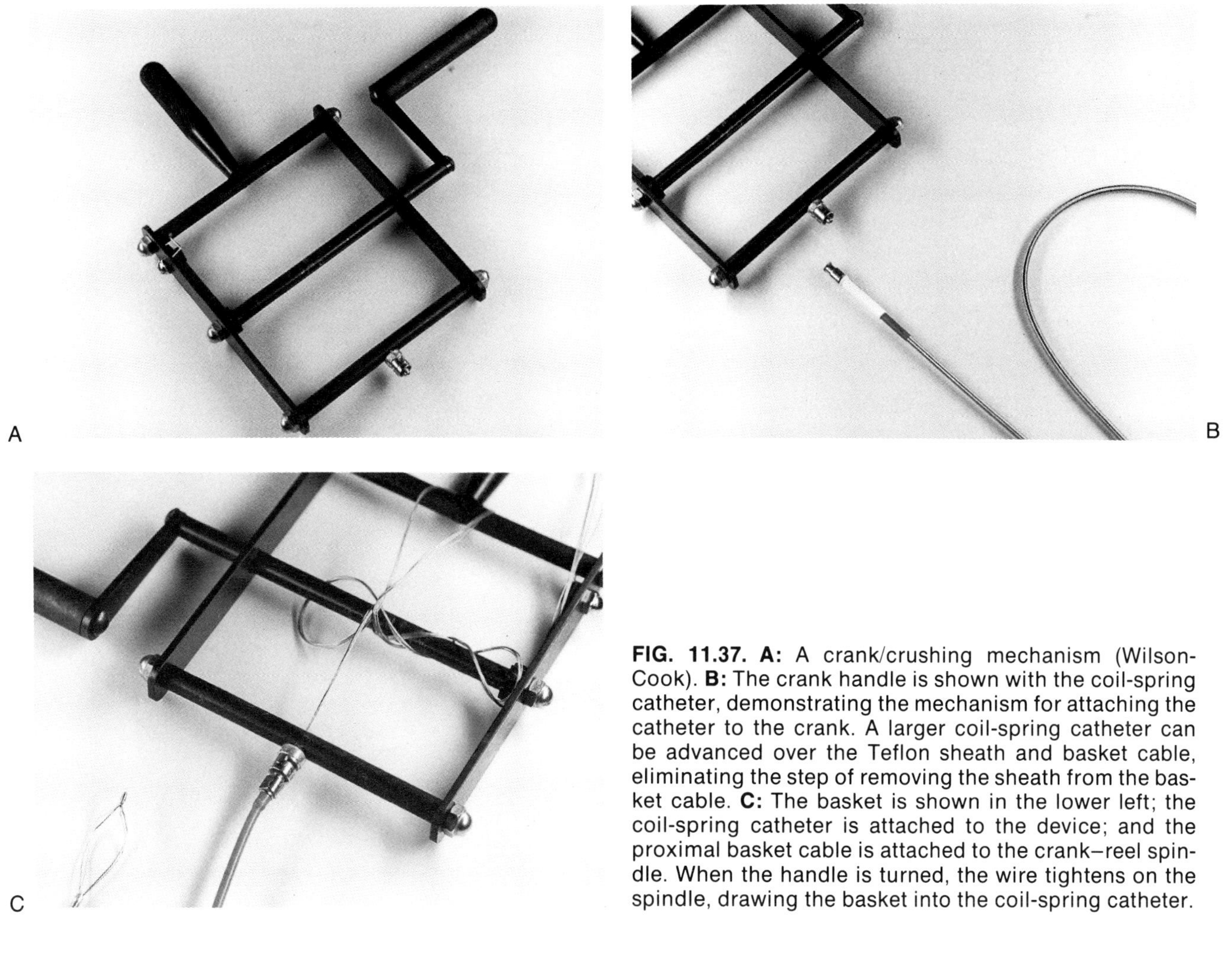

FIG. 11.37. A: A crank/crushing mechanism (Wilson-Cook). **B:** The crank handle is shown with the coil-spring catheter, demonstrating the mechanism for attaching the catheter to the crank. A larger coil-spring catheter can be advanced over the Teflon sheath and basket cable, eliminating the step of removing the sheath from the basket cable. **C:** The basket is shown in the lower left; the coil-spring catheter is attached to the device; and the proximal basket cable is attached to the crank–reel spindle. When the handle is turned, the wire tightens on the spindle, drawing the basket into the coil-spring catheter.

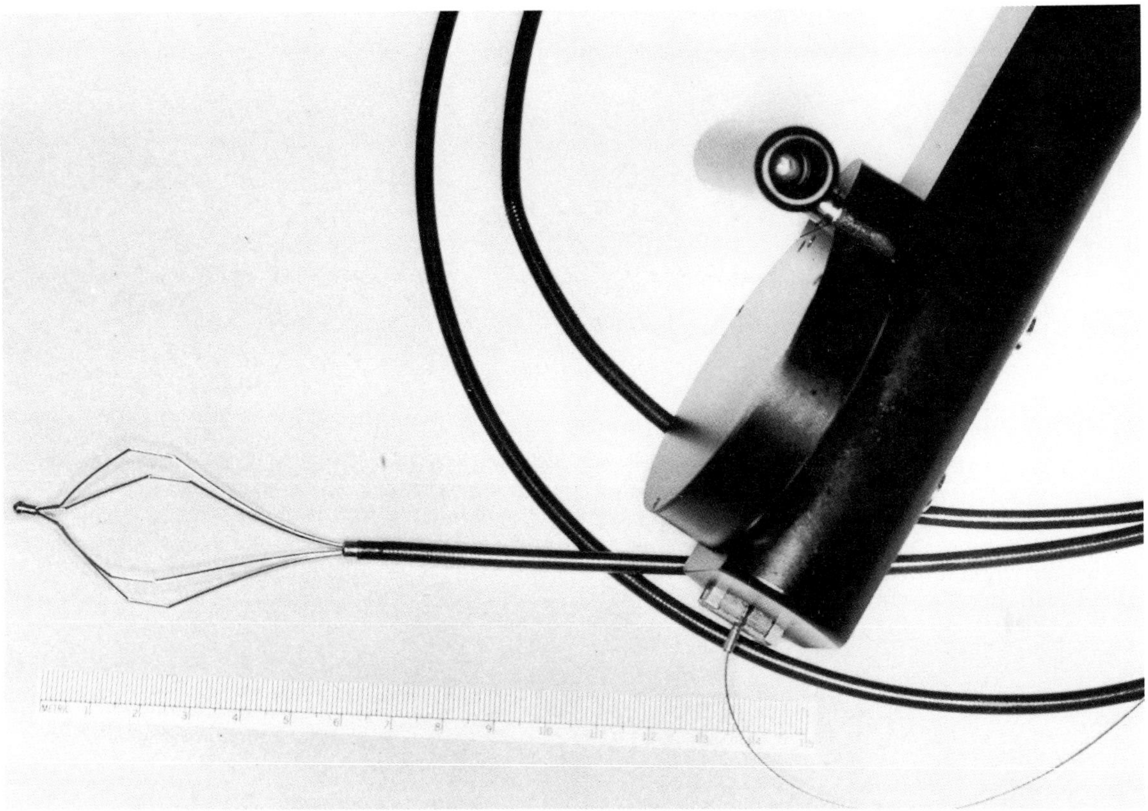

FIG. 11.38. Another type of crank handle, coil-spring catheter and basket used for lithotripsy. With this system (by Olympus) a handle is not attached to the basket cable, thus eliminating the additional step of removing the handle. The basket is contained in a Teflon sheath that remains on the basket cable as the endoscope is removed and as the coil-spring catheter (which has a protective, smooth coating) is advanced over the basket cable and catheter to the basket.

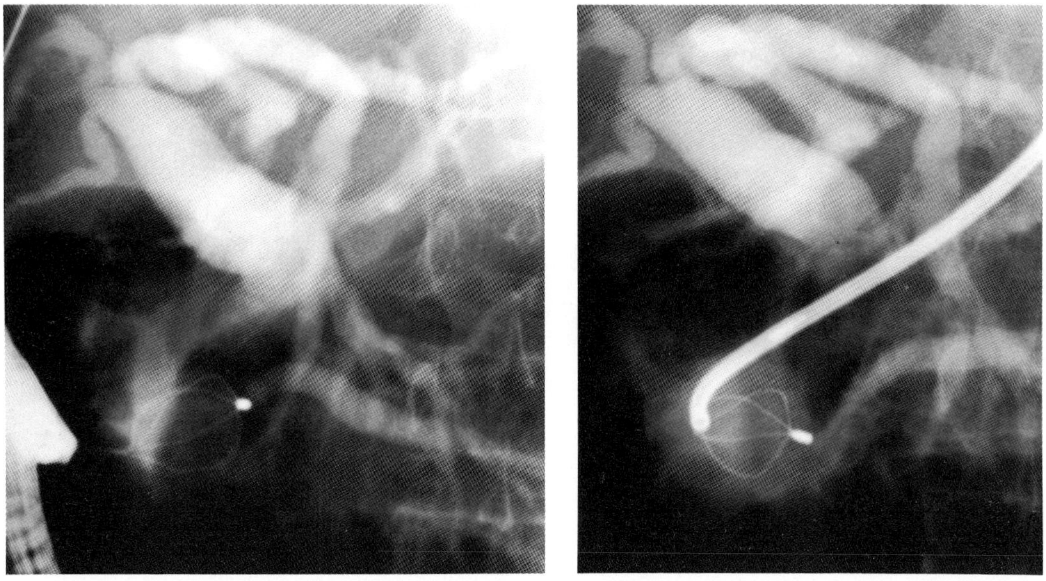

FIG. 11.39. Left: A large stone has been entrapped in a basket and pulled down to the distal common bile duct. **Right:** The endoscope has been removed, and the coil-spring catheter has been advanced to the stone. Next, the proximal end of the basket cable will be attached to a handle and the stone crushed.

Text continued from page 246.
the coil-spring (crushing) catheter may be passed over the catheter and cable down to the sphincterotomy (Fig. 11.36). The proximal cable is attached to a hand crank (Figs. 11.37, 11.38). When the handle is turned, the basket containing the stone is drawn into the coil-spring catheter, and the stone is crushed (Figs. 11.39–11.42).

Another unique lithotripsy system (Olympus Corporation) is a single through-the-endoscope system that utilizes a movable coil-spring catheter into which the Teflon catheter and basket are inserted as one unit. When cannulating the bile duct with this unit, the endoscopist advances the Teflon sheath and basket through the distal end of the endoscope, into the sphincterotomy and bile duct; because the system has a movable coil-spring catheter that remains in the endoscope, cannulation is not more difficult than when using a regular stone retrieval basket. In the bile duct,
Text continues on page 253.

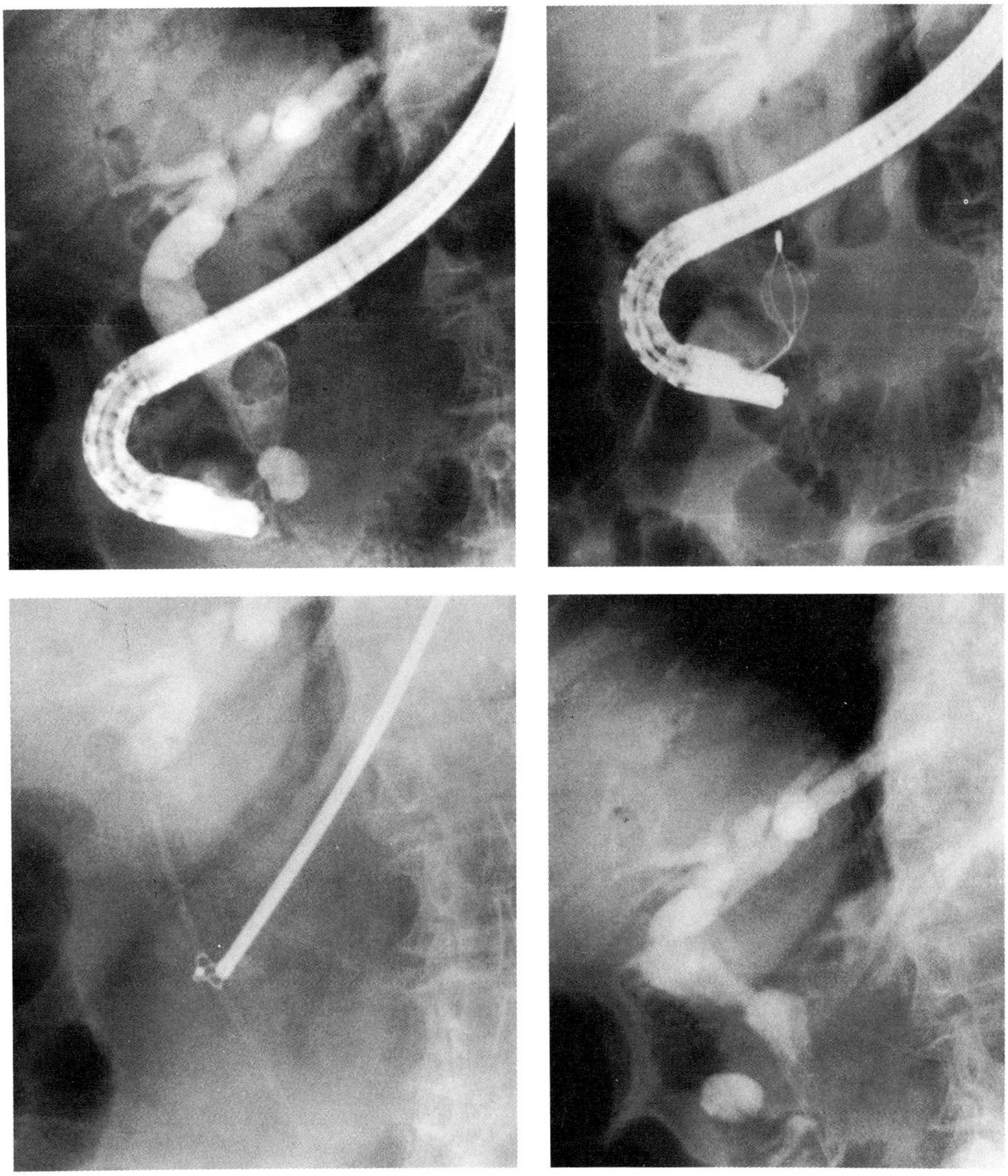

FIG. 11.40. A series of radiographs showing the sequence of mechanical lithotripsy using the separate devices. **Top left:** A cholangiogram that shows a large stone in the common bile duct. **Top right:** The stone has been captured in a basket. **Bottom left:** A prosthesis is visible in the bile duct, which will prevent bile duct obstruction if lithotripsy fails and the stone remains entrapped. Lithotripsy is in progress as noted by the presence of the coil-spring catheter (the endoscope has been removed) and the decrease in diameter of the basket, which is being drawn into the coil-spring catheter. **Bottom right:** A bile duct free of stones.

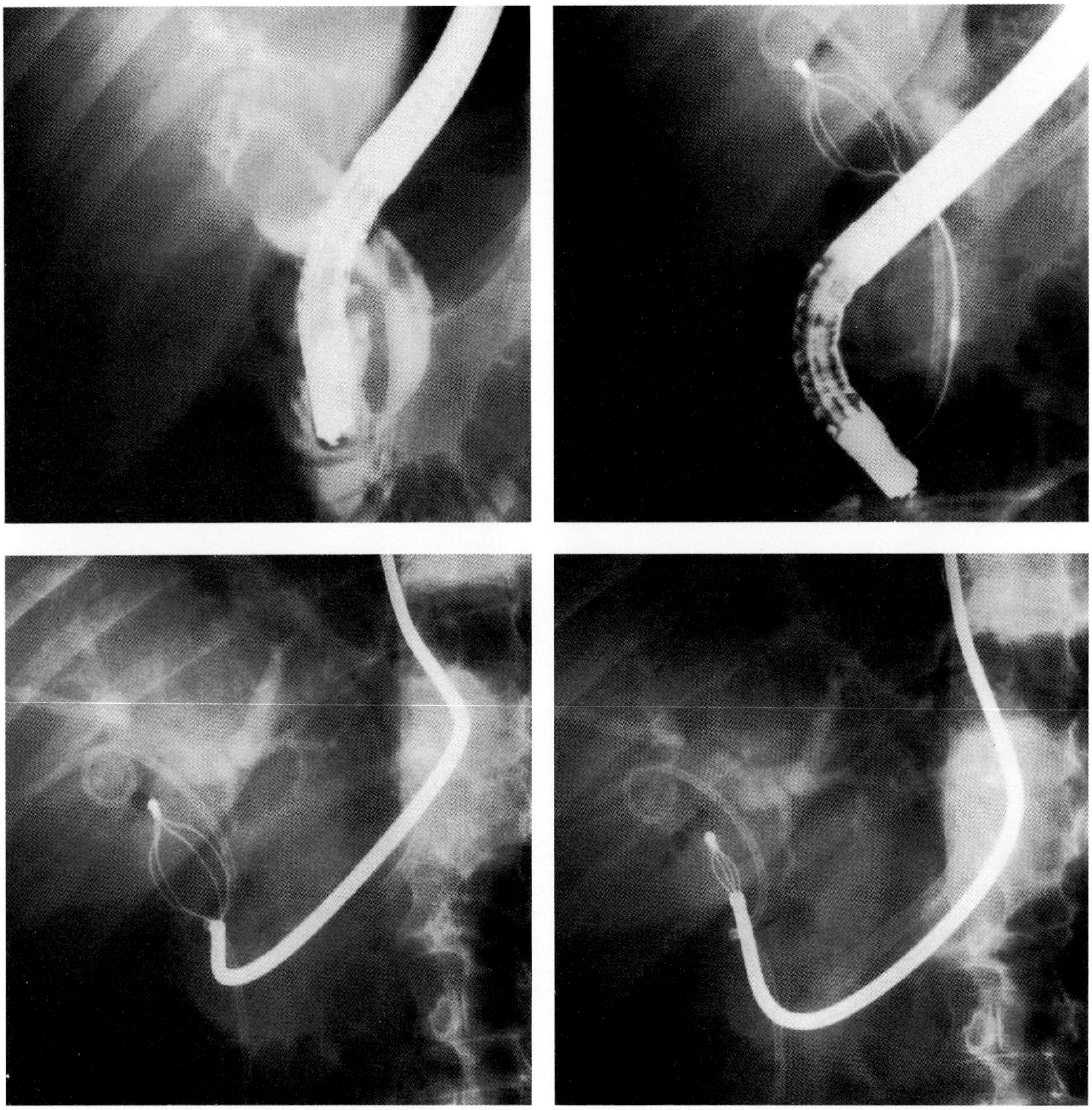

FIG. 11.41. Mechanical lithotripsy of a large stone. **Top left:** The stone is seen on the cholangiogram. **Top right:** The stone has been captured in the basket. **Bottom left:** The endoscope has been removed and the coil-spring catheter has been advanced to the basket. **Bottom right:** Lithotripsy is completed, as evidenced by the decrease in size of the basket as it is drawn into the coil-spring catheter.

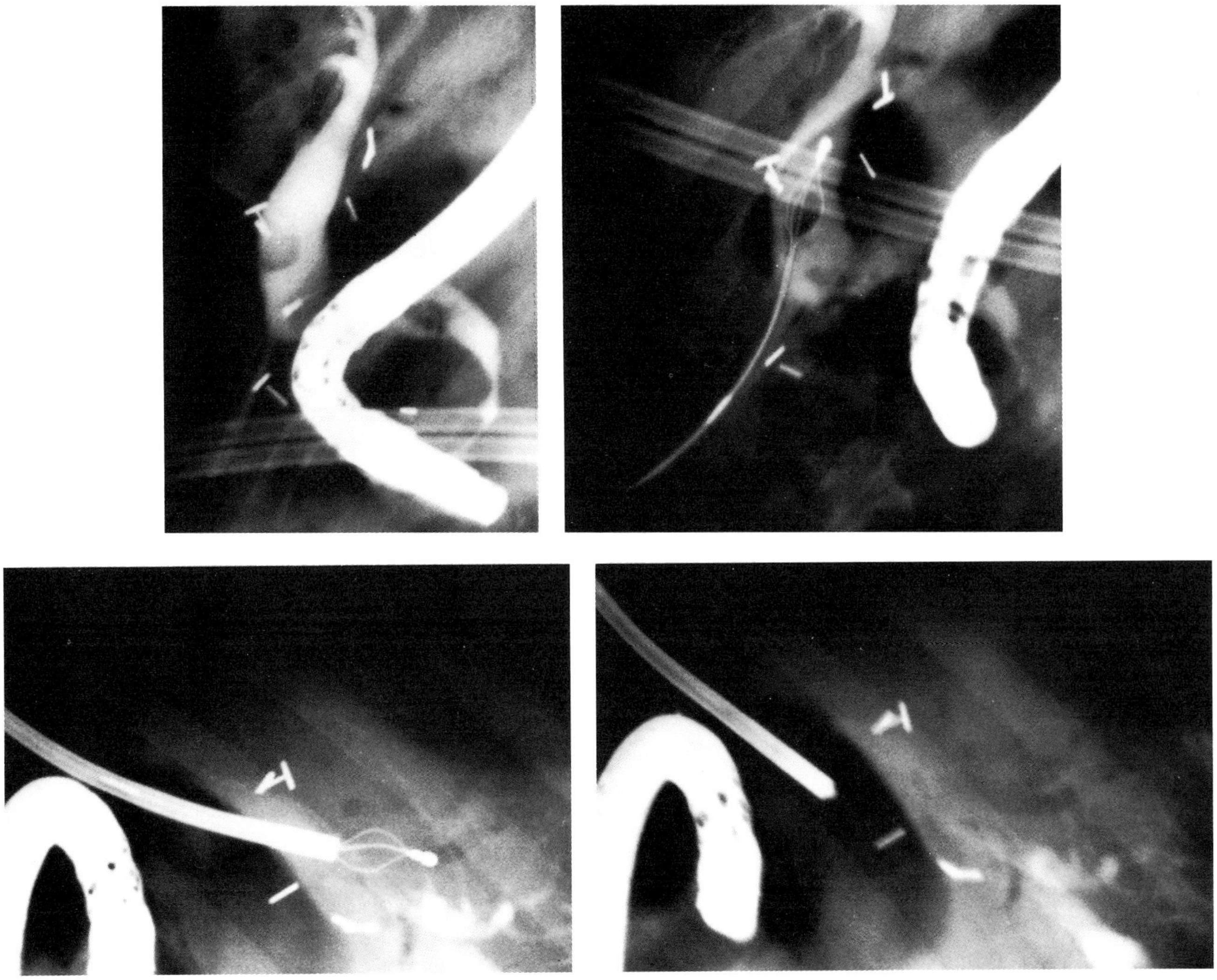

FIG. 11.42. This unique series demonstrates mechanical lithotripsy performed through a percutaneous T-tube tract. **Top left:** A cholangiogram obtained at ERCP demonstrating two medium-sized stones. The endoscopic basket could not negotiate the acute angle of the bile duct to entrap the proximal stone, but the lower stone was captured and removed. **Top right:** The proximal stone was entrapped by a basket, which was passed through the T-tube tract. However, because the peritoneum and tract were not dilated, the stone could not be removed. **Bottom left:** A coil-spring lithotripsy catheter was then advanced over the percutaneous basket cable. **Bottom right:** The stone was crushed after attaching the proximal basket cable to the lithotripsy handle.

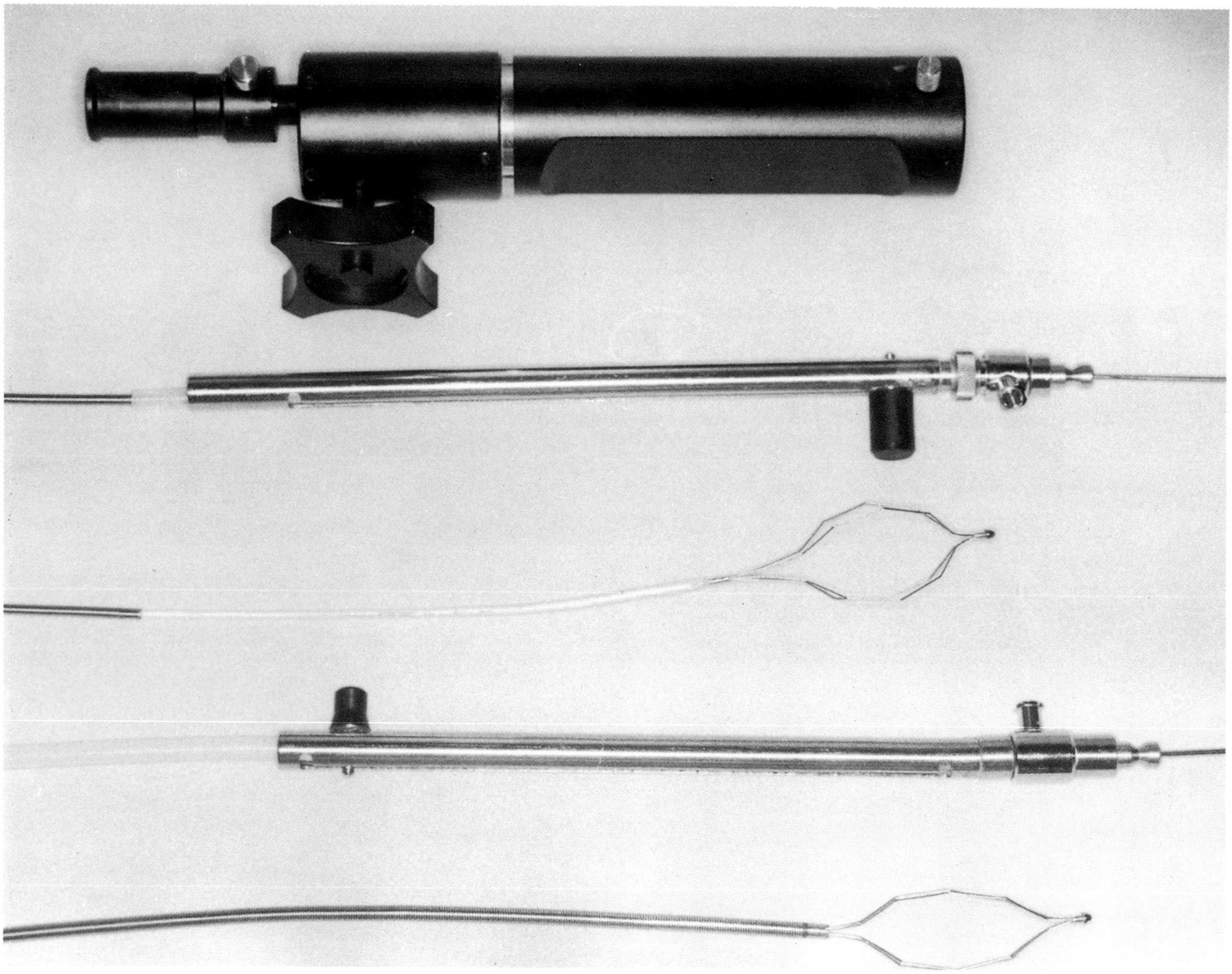

FIG. 11.43. This photograph shows a special lithotripsy handle (Olympus) at the top. The basket and a device (black knob) that moves the coil-spring catheter are on the handle. One basket is extended from the coil-spring catheter and is contained in a Teflon sheath. Note the position of the slide device, which is located near the proximal end of the unit. The other (lower) basket differs from the upper one as the slide device has been pushed down the control unit, advancing the coil-spring catheter to the basket. After a stone is captured in the basket, the proximal end of the basket is inserted into the crank device and the stone crushed. (From ref. 21, with permission.)

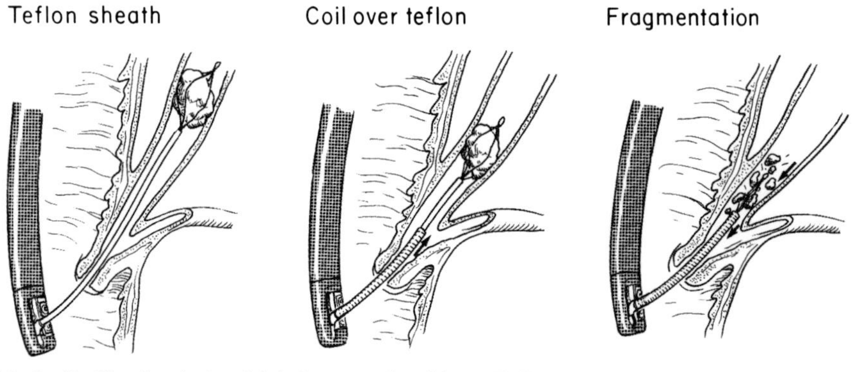

FIG. 11.44. Left: The basket, which is contained in a Teflon sheath, has been inserted into the bile duct, and a stone has been captured. **Middle:** The coil-spring catheter is being advanced over the basket cable toward the stone. **Right:** The stone is crushed after attaching the proximal handle of the basket to the crank device. (From ref. 21, with permission.)

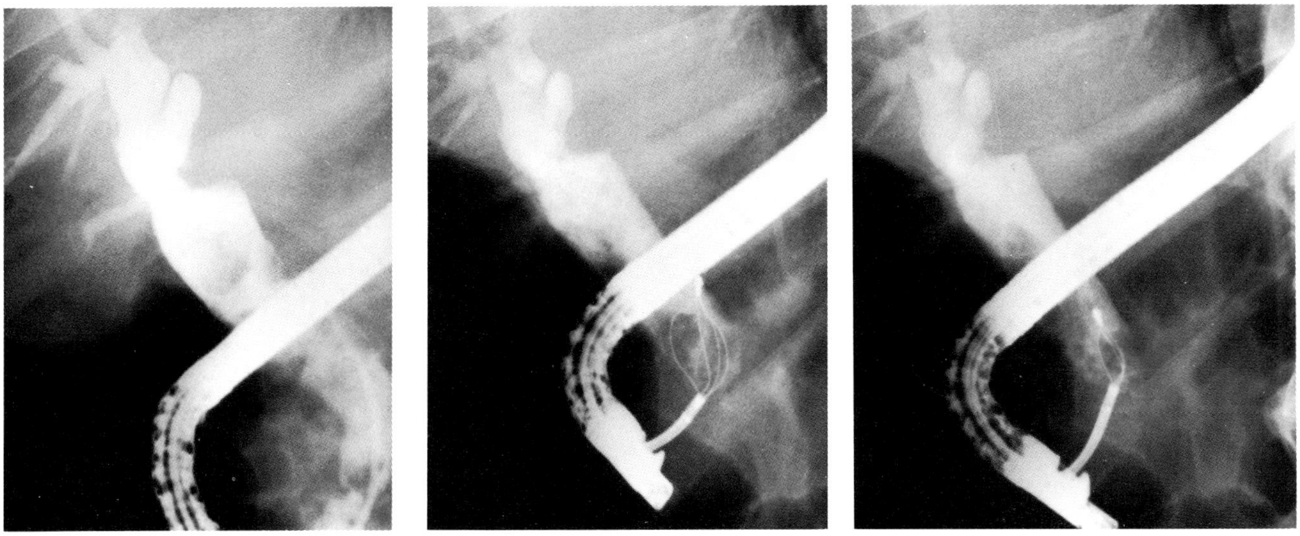

FIG. 11.45. This series of radiographs demonstrates the self-contained Olympus system. **Left:** A large stone is visible in the proximal bile duct. **Middle:** The stone has been captured, and the coil-spring catheter is advanced over the basket cable to the basket in preparation for lithotripsy. **Right:** Lithotripsy is being completed.

Text continued from page 249.
the basket is extended from the Teflon sheath, and the stone is entrapped and drawn toward the sheath. Once the stone has been entrapped in the basket, the proximal handle, which consists of a knob attached to a movable core, is adjusted so that the coil-spring catheter is advanced over the Teflon sheath to the basket by moving or sliding the knob downward on the handle device (Figs. 11.43, 11.44). The proximal end of the basket is then attached to a crank handle, which is turned in a direction that draws the stone and basket toward the coil-spring catheter and results in fragmentation. This one-step system is more efficient and avoids the additional steps of sacrificing the basket handle, withdrawing the instrument, and subsequently advancing the coil-spring catheter–lithotripsy device. This system is available for both 3.2 mm and 4.2 mm duodenoscopes (Figs. 11.45, 11.46). Videoendoscopic pictures, which were taken after mechanical lithotripsy, show stone fragments being removed from the bile duct (Figs. 11.47–11.50).

I have performed mechanical lithotripsy in more than 100 patients who presented with retained stones, using a combination of lithotripsy devices (Table 11.1). Although the procedure had a success rate of 94%, several attempts during separate, selective sessions were necessary using different devices before stone fragmentation was completed. These results reflect earlier work when my associates and I were less experienced and the devices were less functional (Table 11.2). In our more recent experience using the latest model devices, mechanical lithotripsy is accomplished in the majority of patients during the first session. A second procedure may be required in approximately 30% of cases. The procedure is generally safe, and complications with mechanical lithotripsy have been few and not serious (Table 11.3).

Employing the more simple and basic endoscopic extraction techniques for the removal of stones combined with the more complex mechanical lithotripsy techniques for stone fragmentation has been a significant contribution to the field of interventional ERCP. The endoscopist now has several viable options to em-

TABLE 11.1. *Mechanical lithotripsy: demographics*

No. patients	110
Females	71
Males	39
Mean age (yrs)	76
Age range (yrs)	37–99

TABLE 11.2. *Results of mechanical lithotripsy*

No. attempts	110
Initial success	59
Second attempt	35
Third attempt	9
% success	94% (103/110)

TABLE 11.3. *Complications of lithotripsy*

Bleeding	5
Transient fever	13
Transient hyperamylasemia	9
Impacted basket (broken cable)	2
Deaths	0
Surgery	0

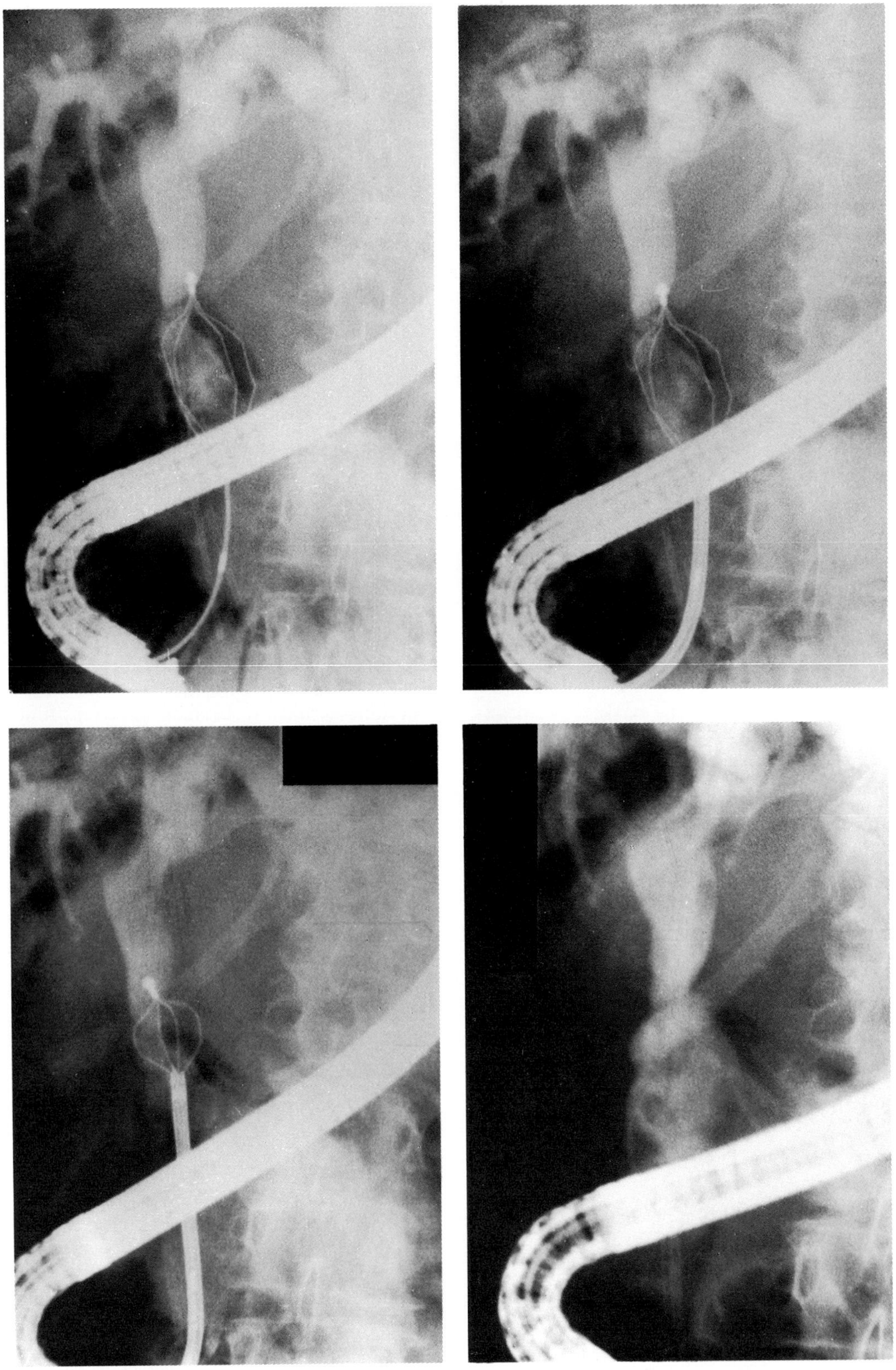

FIG. 11.46. **Top left:** A large stone has been entrapped in a basket. **Top right:** The coil-spring catheter is advanced over the basket cable to the stone and basket. **Bottom left:** The proximal handle has been attached to the basket cable, the crank turned, and the basket drawn into the coil-spring catheter. **Bottom right:** Small stone particles remain in the bile duct.

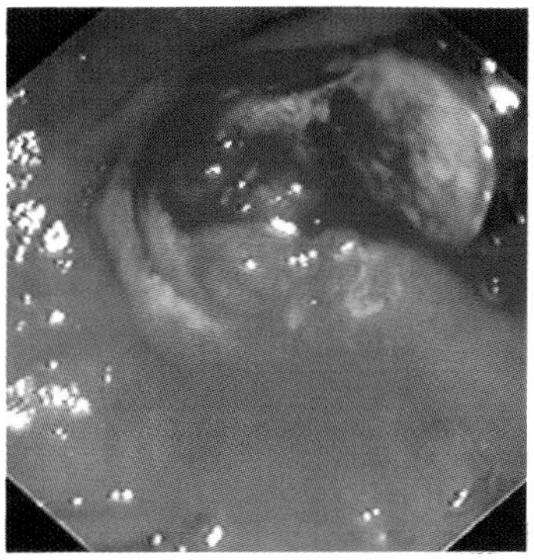

FIG. 11.47. A videoendoscopic image of a stone fragment extracted from the bile duct of a patient who has undergone mechanical lithotripsy. Note the severed or transected margins of the stones, which have been literally cut by the wires of the basket.

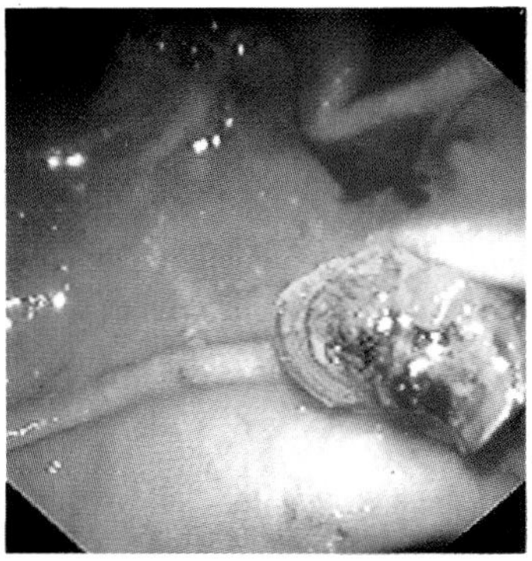

FIG. 11.48. A stone fragment.

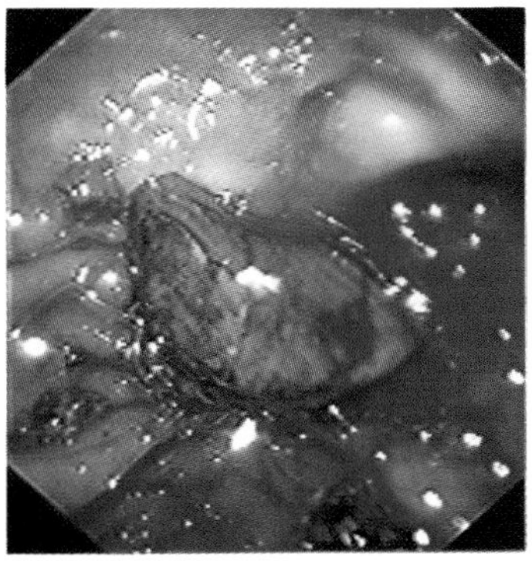

FIG. 11.49. Another stone fragment extracted from the bile duct of a patient who has had mechanical lithotripsy.

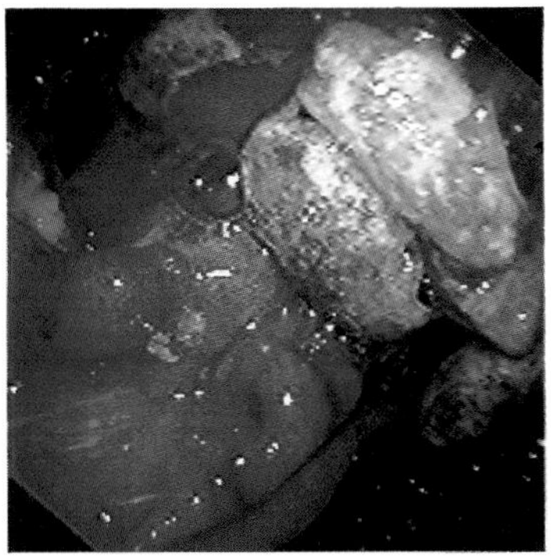

FIG. 11.50. Another example of a stone fragment.

ploy in the management of retained common bile duct stones. He or she may still invoke the simplest option of leaving the stone after sphincterotomy and observing the patient carefully for spontaneous passage of the stone. If the stone cannot be extracted or crushed, the endoscopist can place a prosthesis to prevent stone impaction and cholangitis (see the section on stents and stones in this chapter), which is usually safer than allowing the stone to pass spontaneously, which may result in cholangitis.

Electrohydraulic Lithotripsy

Endoscopists and radiologists again borrowed from another discipline by utilizing a device used previously by urologists for fragmentation of stones, the electrohydraulic lithotriptor (38–45). Urologists have used this device in the treatment of urinary bladder stones with great success. Subsequently, Silvis and coworkers began using this technique on gallstones *in vitro* (46). The results were so impressive that they later implanted gallstones into the bile ducts of dogs and performed electrohydraulic lithotripsy with the generator and probe in these animal models (47). The results were encouraging in the animal model, and Silvis and others embarked on a clinical trial to incorporate this device in the treatment of retained common bile duct stones.

In earlier reports of its clinical use in the United States, electrohydraulic lithotripsy (EHL) was successfully performed in seven patients (46). The manufacturer of the generator (ACMI-Circon) subsequently improved both the generator and the lithotripsy probes to facilitate the procedure and improve the overall efficacy of the devices.

Because of its larger diameter, the original probe had to be placed in a 9Fr balloon catheter (Fig. 11.51) for delivery. This combined accessory was then advanced through a therapeutic endoscope, TJF, which has a 4.2 mm operating channel, through the sphincterotomy, and into the bile duct. In our first trials, the probe and balloon were inserted into the bile duct, the electrohydraulic charge was delivered, and lithotripsy was performed with a modest degree of success. Newer,

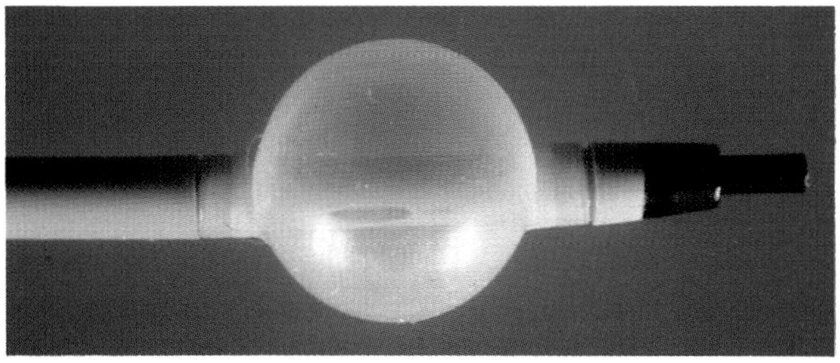

FIG. 11.51. The tip of the electrohydraulic probe contained in a balloon catheter.

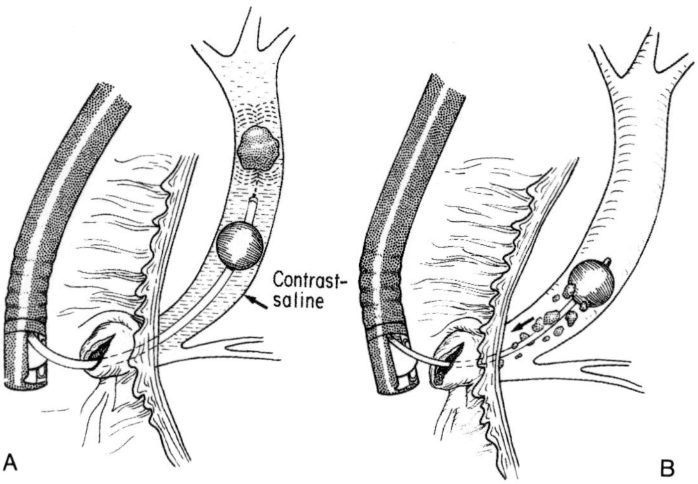

FIG. 11.52. Left: The technique of electrohydraulic lithotripsy using the indirect system of placing the probe, which is contained in a balloon, into the liquid-filled bile duct. **Right:** Under fluoroscopic control, the charge is pulsed toward the stone, fragmenting it. The stone fragments can be removed with the inflated balloon.

smaller probes have subsequently become available. These smaller probes are more efficient and, thus, more powerful, and they have increased our options and methods of delivery. These smaller probes can be placed into a 7Fr balloon, which enables the endoscopist to advance the probe through a standard diagnostic endoscope with either a 2.8 mm or a 3.2 mm channel. With the newer probe, other exciting options are being utilized. The probe can be advanced through a choledochoscope that has been inserted into the bile duct through either a T-tube tract or a percutaneous transhepatic tract (48–50), or it can be advanced through the mother-daughter endoscope system. With the choledochoscope or mother-daughter endoscopes, the procedure is performed under direct visualization, and the stone is fragmented.

The physical effects of electrohydraulic lithotripsy are similar to those of pulsed-dye lasers. The electrohydraulic lithotriptor utilizes a bipolar electrical charge that is discharged through the probe. The bile duct must be filled with an isotonic liquid medium that serves as an interface between the electrical charge and the stone. This mixture usually consists of contract and saline. When the bipolar probe is discharged, the fluid interface immediately adjacent to the stone vaporizes and expands as steam, and when the charge is pulsed, the bombardment of forceful shock waves fragments the stone (Fig. 11.52). We attempted the pro-

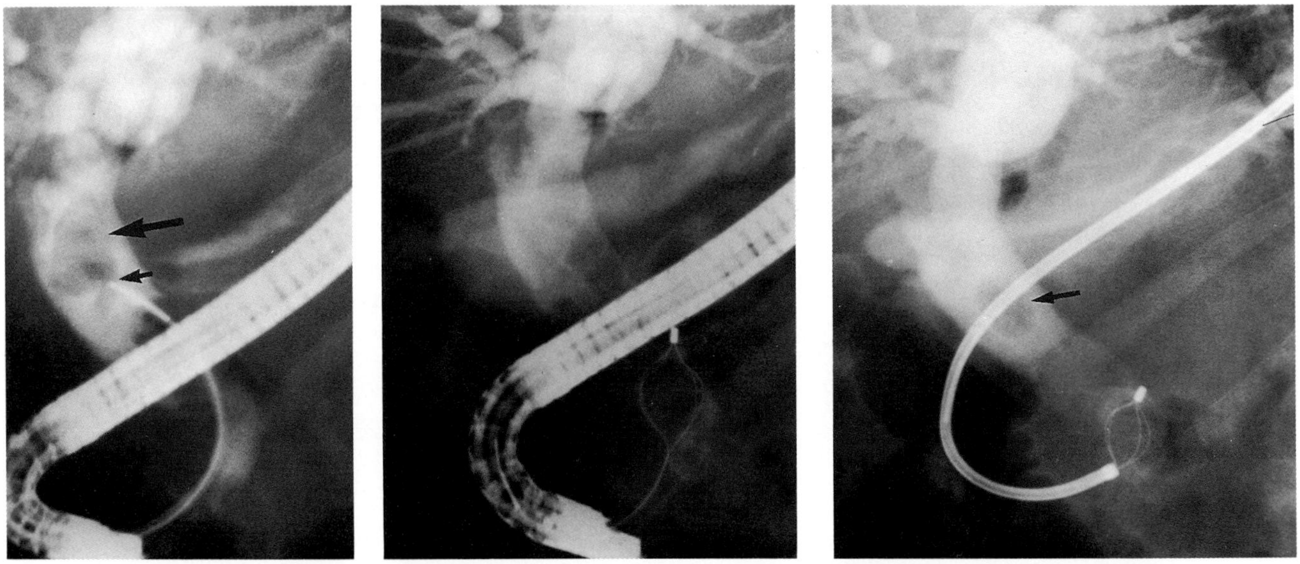

FIG. 11.53. Left: The successful fragmentation of a large stone (*large arrow*) using an electrohydraulic probe (*small arrow*). **Middle:** After the stone was fractured, a basket was used to capture the largest fragment, and this fragment was crushed using a mechanical lithotripter. **Right:** The other fragment (*arrow*) is visible in the bile duct and was removed with a basket.

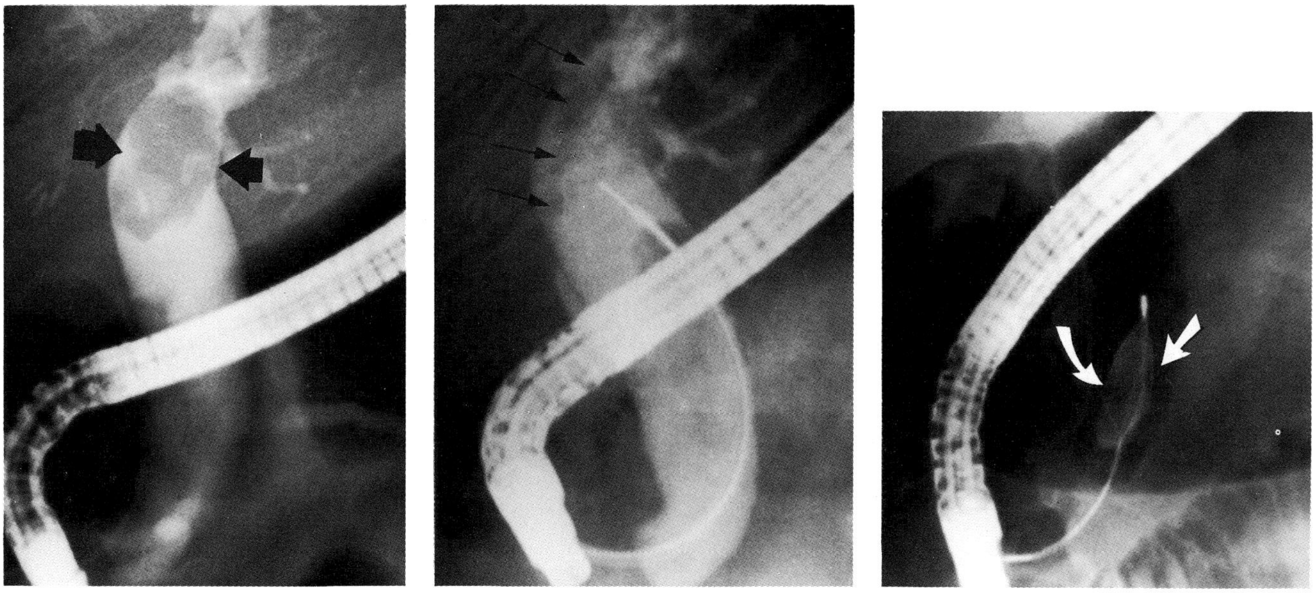

FIG. 11.54. Left: A large stone (*arrows*). **Middle:** The stone was fragmented by electrohydraulic lithotripsy into smaller fragments (*arrows*). **Right:** The largest fragment was removed with a basket (*arrow*). (From ref. 51, with permission.)

cedure in 25 patients and were successful with fragmentation in 20 (80%) (Figs. 11.53–11.61; Table 11.4) (51). The liquid, isotonic interface is essential because the shockwave is actually produced by rapidly expanding steam and not by electrical shock. Placing the probe against the stone without a liquid interface will result only in sparks, and fragmentation will not occur (this caused failure in two patients).

This procedure can be incorporated into the management of patients with retained stones, with or without sphincterotomy. In patients in whom sphincterotomy may not be prudent (Jehovah's Witnesses or

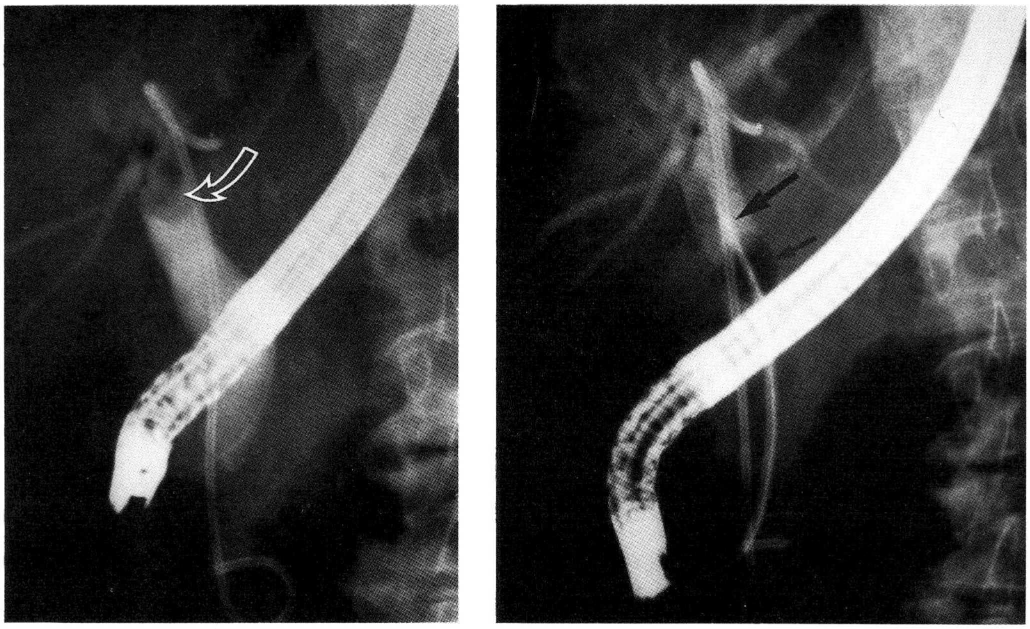

FIG. 11.55. Left: An arrow points to a retained stone located in the common hepatic duct. Note the presence of a prosthesis. **Right:** The stone has been fragmented by the electrohydraulic charge delivered by the probe that was inserted into the duct. The large arrow identifies the probe, and its balloon is identified by a smaller arrow.

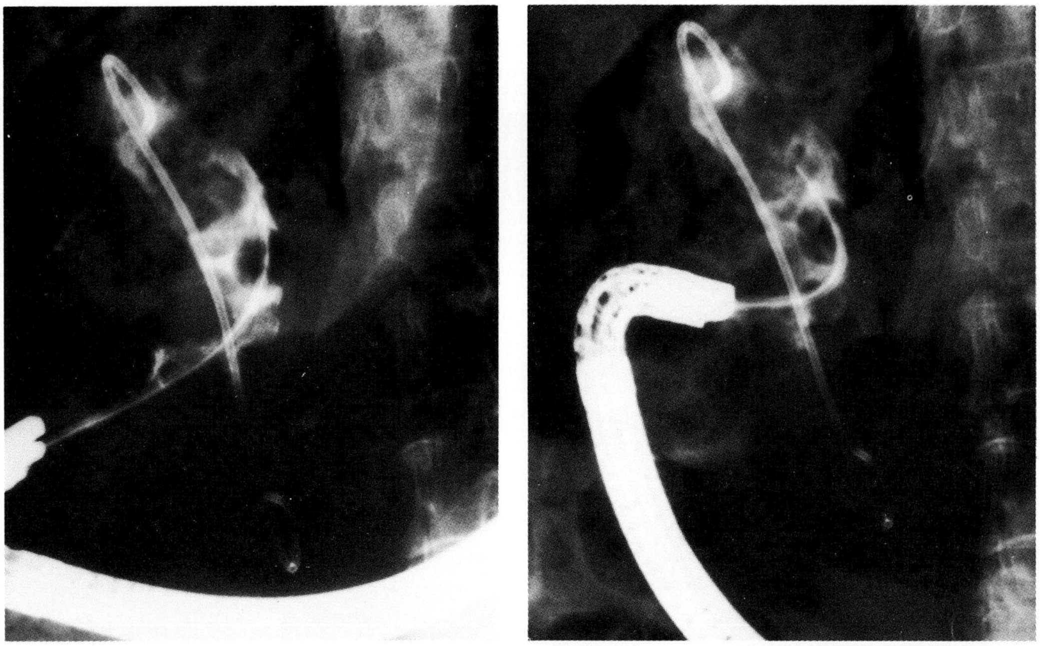

FIG. 11.56. The electrohydraulic lithotripter has been used in patients with a Bilroth II resection as well. **Left:** The probe is placed into a dilated bile duct, which contains a very large stone and a prosthesis. **Right:** The probe is being discharged, and fragmentation of the stone can be appreciated.

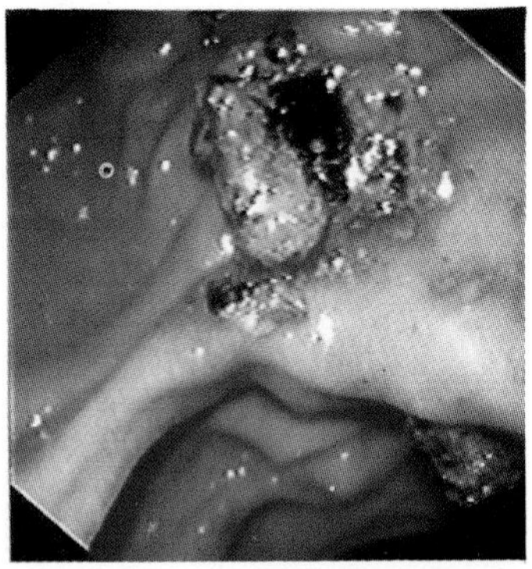

FIG. 11.57. These are videoendoscopic images of stone fragments, small particles, and larger fragments of mixed composition that were extracted from the bile ducts of patients who had undergone endoscopic electrohydraulic lithotripsy.

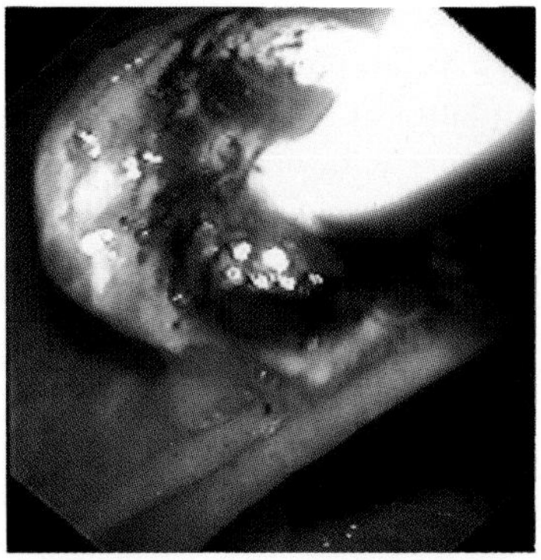

FIG. 11.58. Stone fragments, small particles, and larger fragments of mixed composition.

TABLE 11.4. *Electrohydraulic lithotripsy (EHL)*

Procedure and patients	
Attempted	25
Men	11
Women	14
Successful fragmentation	20 (80%)
Age range	47–79 yrs
Mean age	63.4 yrs

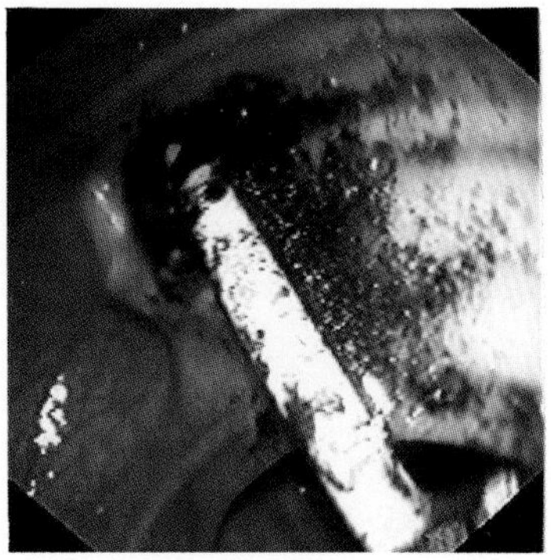

FIG. 11.59. Stone fragments, small particles, and larger fragments of mixed composition.

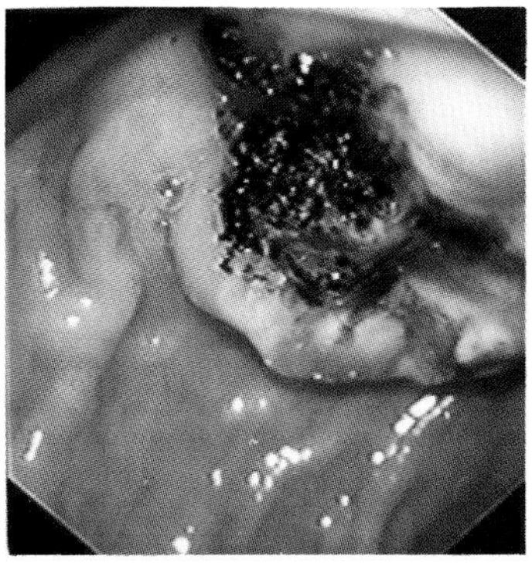

FIG. 11.60. Stone fragments, small particles, and larger fragments of mixed composition.

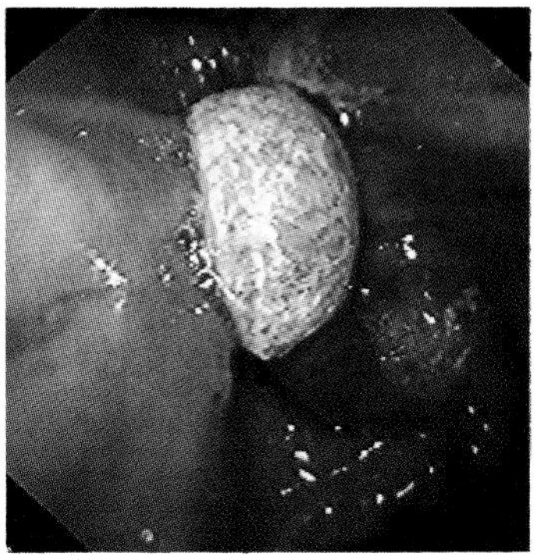

FIG. 11.61. Stone fragments, small particles, and larger fragments of mixed composition.

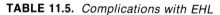

TABLE 11.5. *Complications with EHL*

Transient fever	2
Transient amylase	1
Deaths	0
Surgery	0

patients with bleeding diatheses), dilatation of the sphincter is performed using balloon dilators prior to the insertion of the electrohydraulic probe (Figs. 11.62, 11.63) (51). Small or medium-sized stones can be fragmented with the probe, and the stone fragments can be extracted through the dilated papilla using either a basket or a balloon. The electrohydraulic probe is contained in a balloon catheter, which can serve a dual purpose. During electrohydraulic lithotripsy, the balloon may centralize the probe within the bile duct, avoiding injury to the bile duct walls. After fragmentation of the stone, the balloon catheter can be advanced proximal to the stone fragments, and the balloon can be inflated and withdrawn into the duodenum, carrying the stone fragments with it. There have been no serious complications in this small series (Table 11.5).

One patient in our series of 25 patients, a failure, was treated with the probe placed into the gallbladder through a cholecystostomy. A large gallbladder stone was obstructing the neck of the gallbladder, and percutaneous access through the cholecystostomy stoma allowed placement of the probe. However, because a

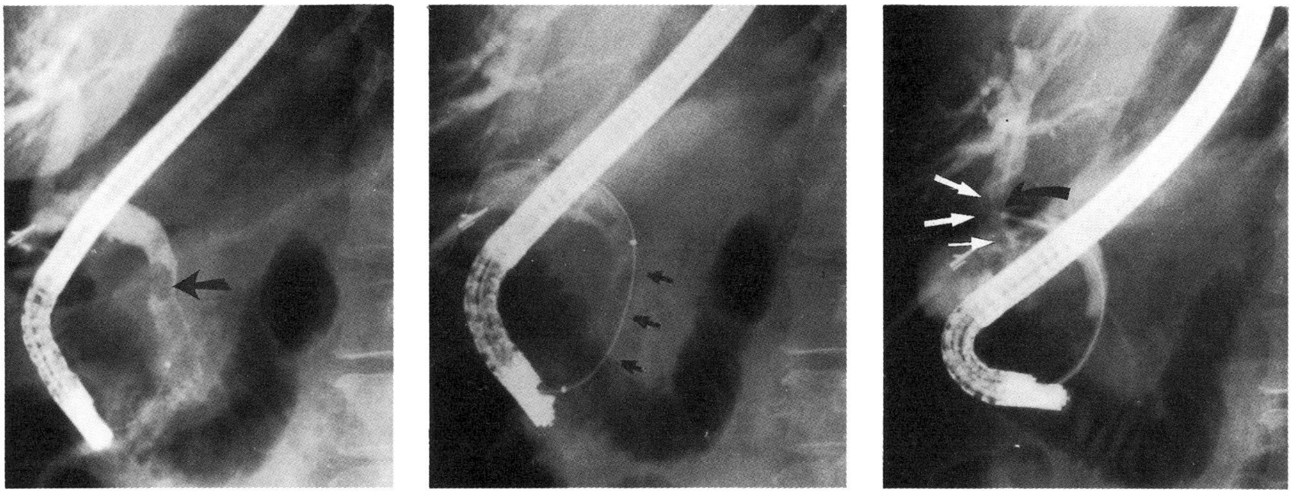

FIG. 11.62. **Left:** A medium-sized stone (*arrow*), which was retained after cholecystectomy and common bile duct exploration, was found on an ERCP performed in a practicing Jehovah's Witness patient. The T-tube is present, and the bile duct is not dilated. **Middle:** To avoid possible bleeding, a sphincterotomy was not performed, but balloon dilatation of the sphincter was performed (*arrows*). **Right:** Dilatation allowed for the introduction of the electrohydraulic probe (*arrow*). The stone migrated to the acutely angulated portion of the bile duct, which is a commonly found deformity created by a T-tube. Despite this angulation, the probe was discharged, fragmenting the stone into smaller pieces (*small arrows*). All fragments were removed.

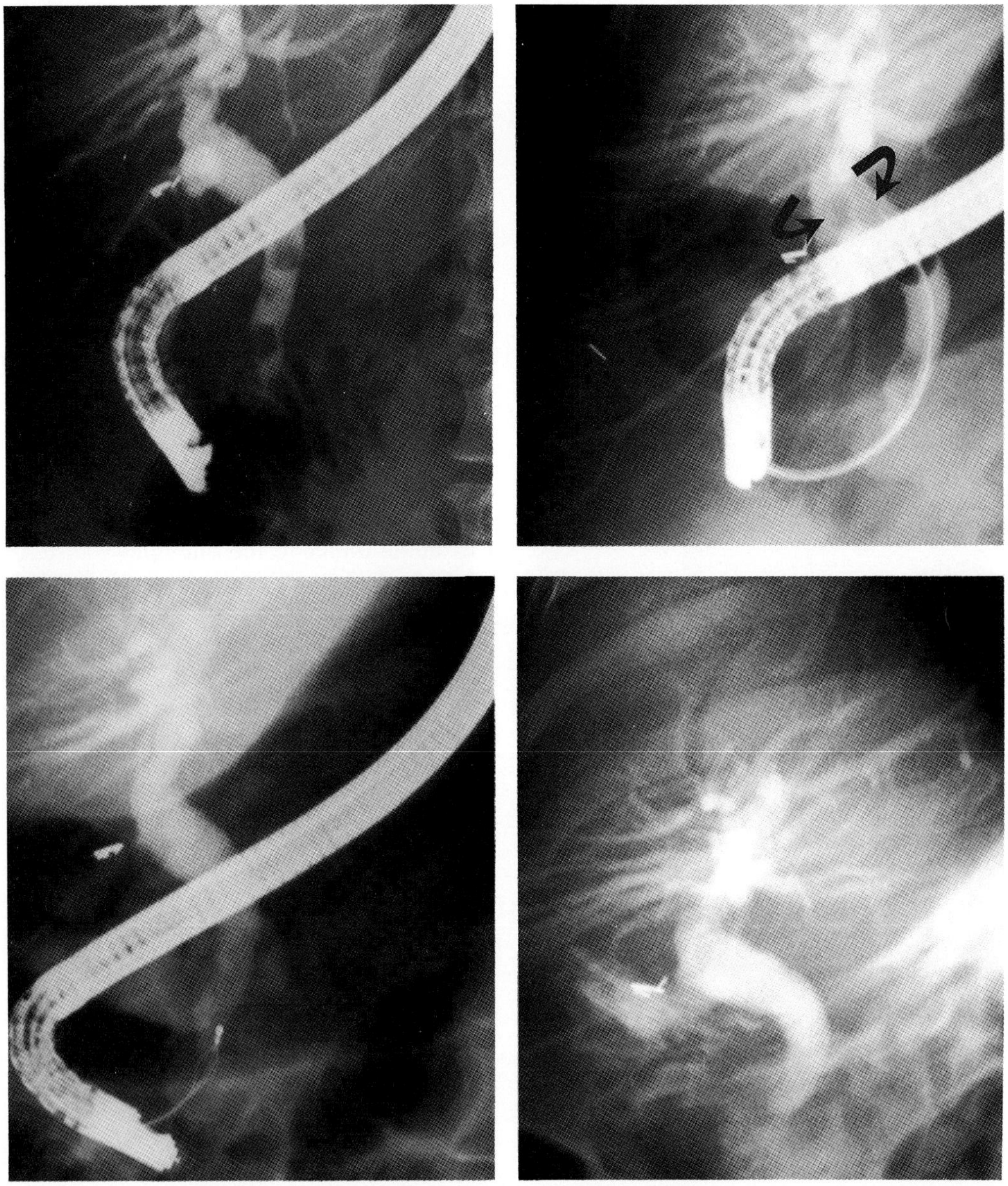

FIG. 11.63. Top left: Medium-sized stones are visible in a nondilated bile duct, and a small drainage tube is entering the bile duct near the metal clips. **Top right:** After dilating the sphincter, the electrohydraulic probe is advanced into the bile duct, and discharged, fragmenting the stones (*arrows*). The balloon of the probe is seen as a lucency just inferior to the endoscope. **Bottom left:** Extraction of a stone fragment with a small stone retrieval basket. **Bottom right:** The cholangiogram confirms that all stone fragments were removed.

liquid interface was not maintained in the gallbladder, the stone was not fragmented. Another patient was treated per orally using an endoscope that was advanced through a choledochoduodenostomy, and the probe was passed directly into the bile duct toward the stone in the left hepatic duct. Again, a liquid interface was not maintained, and fragmentation was unsuccessful. Failure may result when attempts are made to fragment calcified stones or stones composed of calcium bilirubinate because these mixed-composition stones will usually not fragment. A stone composed predominantly of cholesterol may fragment more quickly than one of mixed composition. Unfortunately, we usually do not know the composition of bile duct stones unless they are directly visible on endoscopy or an accompanying stone is removed. Most primary bile duct stones are composed of cholesterol and should fragment with EHL; we usually find out by trial and error. No serious complications have occurred with this technique (one patient had mild pancreatitis) so treating as many patients as possible to determine the success of this technique is justifiable.

Other Uses of Electrohydraulic Lithotripsy

The placement of the electrohydraulic probe through a T-tube tract accessing the bile duct has been previously described (48), and percutaneous advancement of the probe through a percutaneous fistulous tract that is enlarged using dilating catheters has also been described (49), again with success. Using the mother-daughter endoscope system to deliver electrohydraulic charges is another option currently being utilized (50).

These procedures therefore offer options to the endoscopist for the successful management of retained common bile duct stones.

Laser Lithotripsy, Electrohydraulic Techniques, Ultrasonic Lithotripsy, and Extracorporeal Shockwave Lithotripsy (ESWL)

I have not participated in the fragmentation of retained stones using pulsed dye or Q-switch lasers or ultrasonic generators. Early results indicate that these systems are effective and have been universally adapted by other endoscopists (52–56). The major single drawback of the laser procedure is the start-up cost for the purchase of the laser generator. The principle of laser lithotripsy is similar to that of the electrohydraulic lithotripsy, of vaporization of the liquid interface between the probe and the stone producing a forceful shock wave. Currently both EHL and laser lithotripsy are being utilized by a small number of investigators. Adjustments and alterations of the protocols will be necessary before sufficient data are available to compare efficacies. At this time it appears that the results of EHL lithotripsy are comparable to those of the laser techniques. The electrohydraulic technique is more readily available (many hospitals already have the generator available for urologists treating bladder stones), is adaptable,and is considerably cheaper than the laser techniques. This availability obviates an additional purchase deficit. As investigations continue and the results of EHL and laser lithotripsy are analyzed, electrohydraulic lithotripsy will probably be more universally accepted because of its portability and its reduced cost. The use of ultrasound lithotripsy has been limited but deserves mention in the approach to the retained stone (57–59).

In truth, the approach to the retained common bile duct stone is multidisciplinary (60). All physicians approaching this problem are working in concert in an effort to pulverize (61), remove (62–72), dissolve (73–86), or crush the stones with extracorporeal systems (87–93). This cooperative effort has enabled us to manage this problem efficiently and effectively. The least expensive method that requires minimal manipulation, pain, and complications and reduces hospital stays is of course desirable.

TABLE 11.6. *Stents and stones*

No. patients	189
Women	113
Men	76
Age range	62–101 yrs
Mean age	79 yrs
Duration—range	3–87 mos
Mean	47 mos

STENTS AND STONES

My colleague and I originally described the technique of placing biliary prostheses into the bile duct of patients with retained stones that could not be extracted as an option for the management of large or multiple common duct stones and unretrievable intrahepatic stones (94). A time interval preceded subsequent reports of the technique, which corroborated our earlier results (95–99). Over the past eight years, I have placed more than 180 prostheses in patients with retained stones (Table 11.6). Most of these patients were followed for complications during the interval after stent placement, and complications were infrequent (Table 11.7). As part of the follow-up, several patients with stents and stones were recalled for lithotripsy if they were available and agreed to further manipulation. Many patients were elderly and frail and preferred not to undergo further therapeutic manuevers; by serendipity, this led to the establishment of our large series of patients.

The placement of a prosthesis in the bile duct of a patient with retained stones has proved to ameliorate an acute situation and to prevent recurrences of cholangitis and cholestasis. In more than 180 stent placements, only five patients developed recurrent cholangitis with the stent in place, and in only three other patients did the prosthesis actually fracture and result in recurrent cholangitis (Table 11.7). One of these patients underwent surgery elsewhere for removal of the fragments and the formation of a choledochoduodenostomy, one underwent endoscopic removal of the fragments and stone removal, and the other opted to have an additional stent placed. Three other patients underwent stent replacement. Overall, the results are

TABLE 11.7. *Complications with stents and stones*

Fever	5
Fractured or dislodged stent[a]	3
Replacement	4
Surgery	1
Follow-up	
range	9–37 mos
Mean	26 mos

[a] 2 7Fr, 1 10Fr, all straight

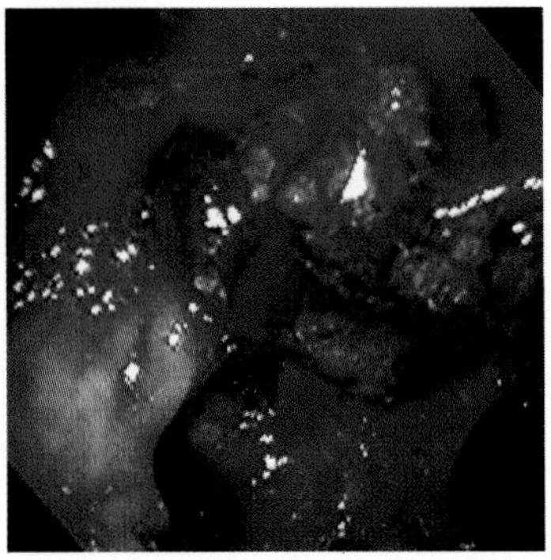

FIG. 11.64. A videoendoscopic image demonstrating the presence of stone material in the duodenum found on repeat endoscopy, which was being performed for removal of a prosthesis. The prosthesis may have contributed to the spontaneous passage of the stones.

somewhat remarkable when one considers the natural history of stone disease, the placement of a foreign object into the bile duct, and the potential complications associated with retained bile duct stones.

It is thought in the case of stents and stones that the prosthesis functions as a "wick," permitting bile to flow through it as well as around it. It is obvious that after a short period of time, the prosthesis will occlude; however, bile continues to flow around the prosthesis without resultant obstruction. The lack of complications is attributed to the fact that in most cases, a wide-open sphincterotomy has been formed, permitting the free flow of bile. The prosthesis also maintains the integrity of the sphincterotomy while it holds the stones in place, thus preventing migration of the stone and recurrent obstruction. Occasionally, because of the presence of the prosthesis and/or reflux of gastrointestinal contents, stones may fragment and pass spontaneously or may pass intact if the sphincterotomy is large enough to accommodate them (Figs. 11.64, 11.65). *Caution*: If a patient is considering surgery for removal of the retained stone after stent placement, I advise obtaining a preoperative cholangiogram. The stone may actually have passed, and surgery will be redundant and embarrassing (this has happened more than once in my experience). The thought of using oral dissolution agents to enhance fragmentation of the stone has been entertained, and several patients have been placed on chenodeoxycholic acid, urosodeoxycholic acid, or a combination of both. Some reports have indicated that after a treatment period with oral dissolution agents, retained stones disappeared from the bile duct; presumably they either dissolved or became smaller, permitting migration out of the bile duct. On follow-up examination, if no stone is found, or if it is smaller and can be retrieved or fragmented by lithotripsy, the prosthesis can be removed. To date,

Text continues on page 265.

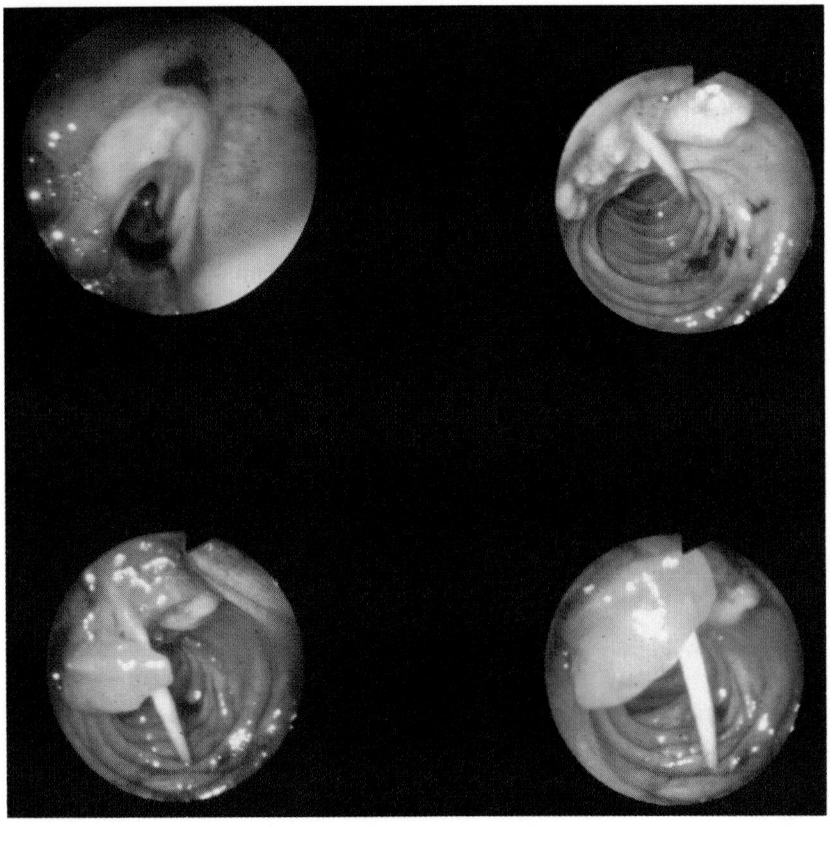

FIG. 11.65. Top left: A healing sphincterotomy. **Top right:** The presence of a stent in the bile duct. **Bottom left, bottom right:** During observation of the sphincterotomy site, several stones passed spontaneously alongside the stent into the duodenum.

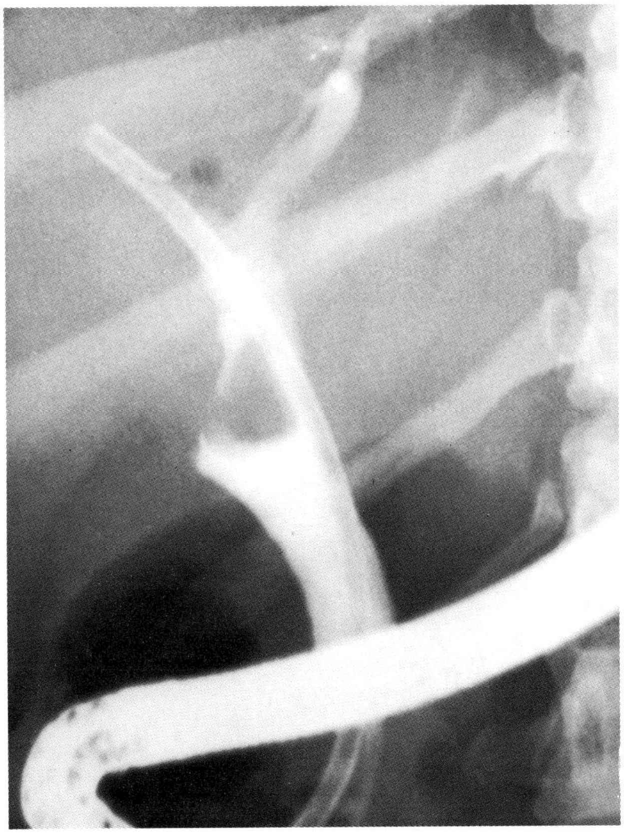

FIG. 11.66. This cholangiogram shows a solitary, triangular stone that could not be entrapped for removal. A large-caliber prosthesis was placed temporarily before the patient underwent electrohydraulic lithotripsy.

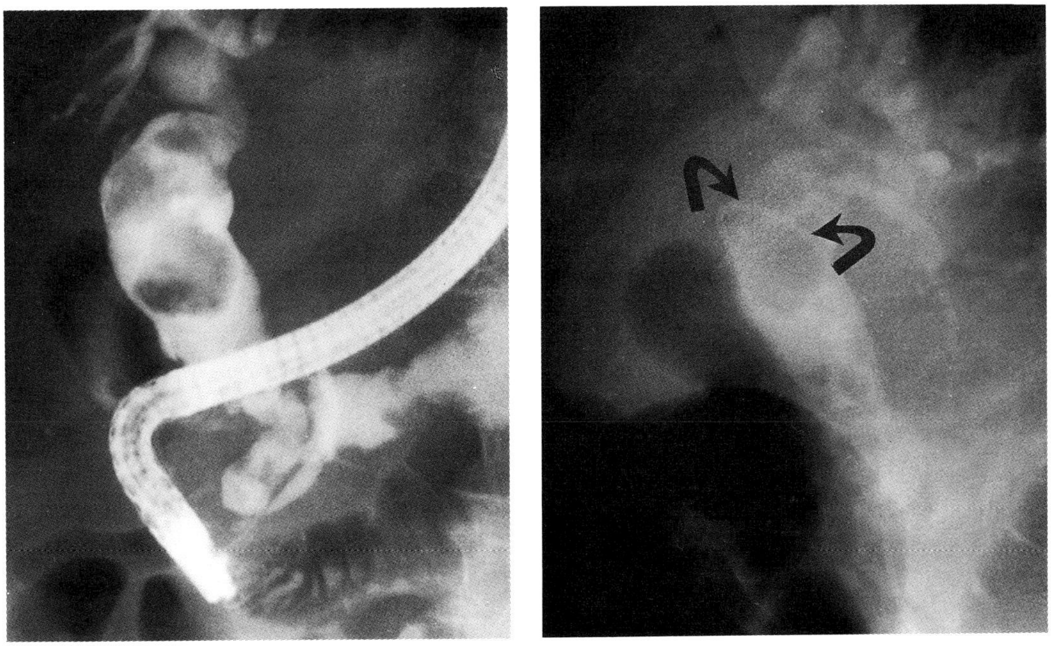

FIG. 11.67. Left: Multiple large stones are seen in this cholangiogram. Because of the narrowed intrapancreatic segment of the bile duct, extraction was not possible. **Right:** A small-caliber prosthesis was placed (*arrows at pigtail*) to avoid cholangitis.

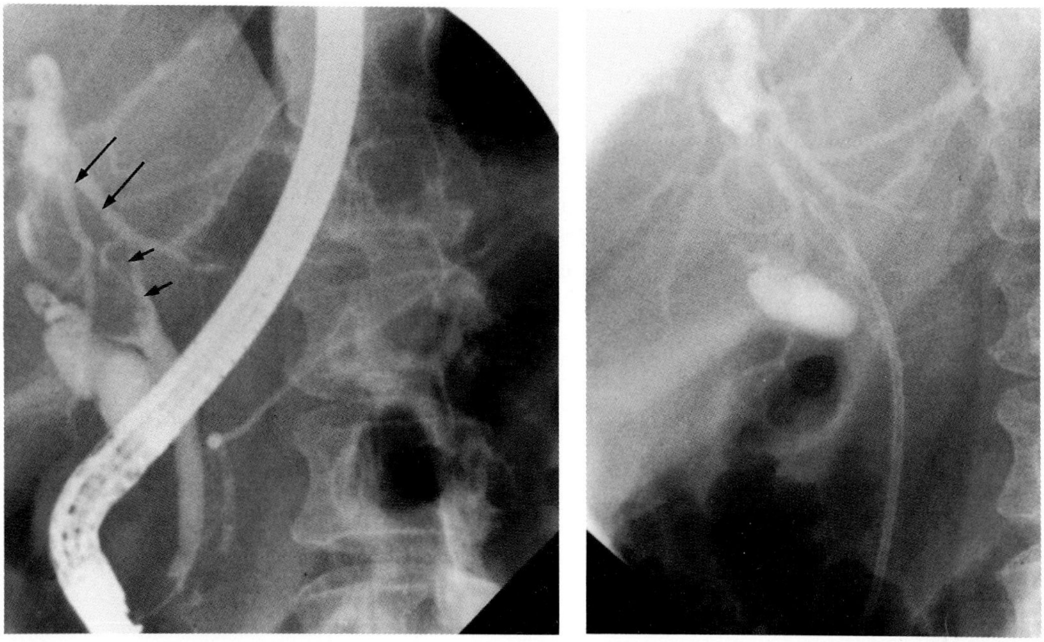

FIG. 11.68. Left: A large common hepatic duct stone (*arrows*), which obviously could not be extracted through the narrowed common bile duct. Note the prominent cystic duct remnant. **Right:** A pigtail stent was placed.

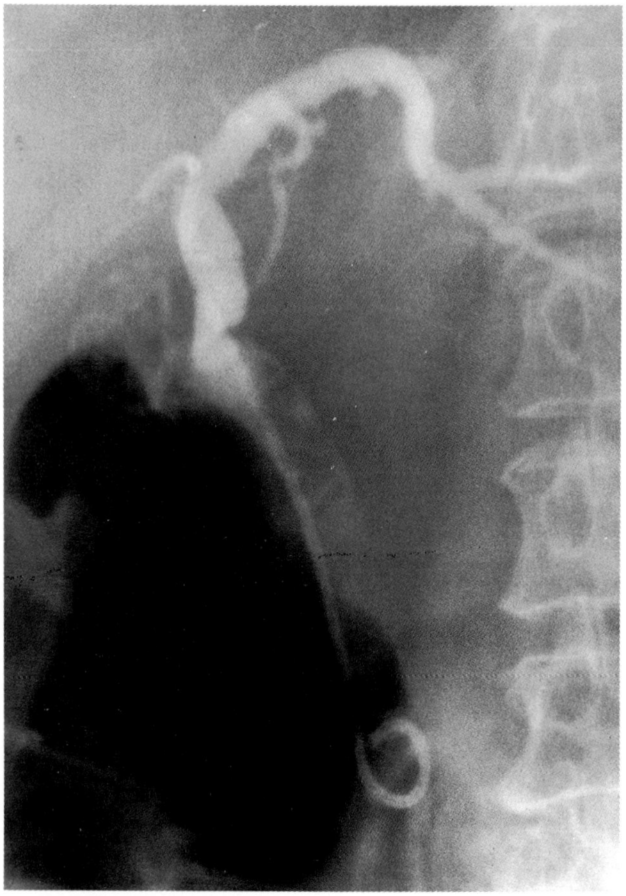

FIG. 11.69. Multiple small stones are evident in this cholangiogram, and a double pigtail catheter was placed before the patient underwent further intervention.

Text continued from page 262.
the follow-up of patients with stents and stones in my series ranges from 3 months to 7 ½ years, with a mean of nearly 4 years (47 months). Figures 11.66 through 11.74 are radiographs of specific situations in which stents were placed for retained stones.

The option of placing prostheses for either temporary or permanent management of retained stones, especially in patients at risk, is viable and has become an acceptable entity utilized by many endoscopists today (94–99).

TABLE 11.8. *Stent size*

No. patients	Stent size	Configuration
119	7FR	91 pigtail, 28 straight
43	10Fr	5 pigtail, 38 straight
27	5Fr	27 pigtail, 0 straight

Table 11.8 identifies the sizes and configurations of the stents I have used for stone disease. There is a preponderance of 7Fr single- and double-pigtail stents.
Text continues on page 268.

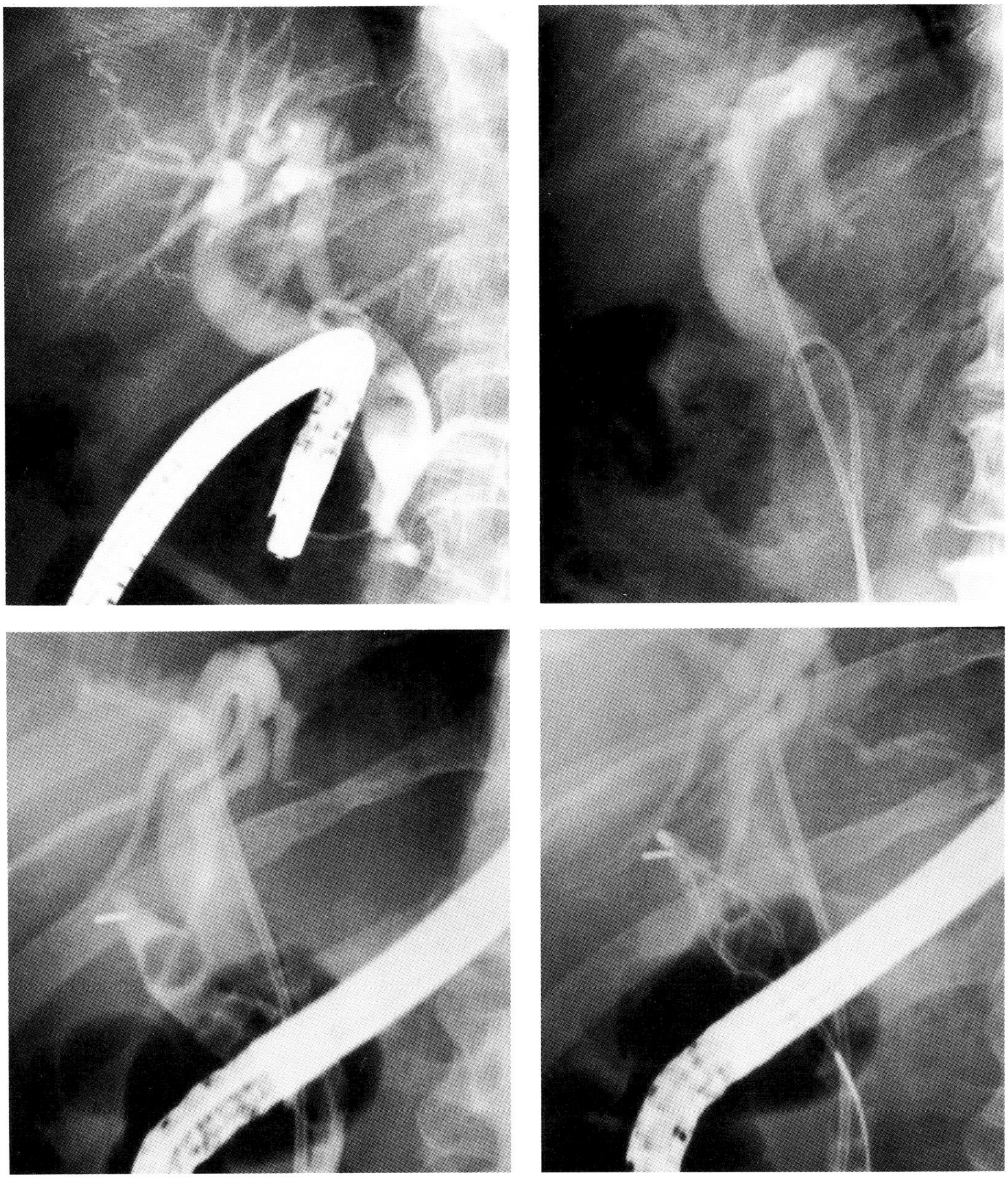

FIG. 11.70. A: A common duct stone migrated into the cystic duct remnant in this patient, producing recurrent cholangitis as the stone moved intermittently into the bile duct. **Left:** The stone is visible (*arrows*) but could not be retrieved. **Right:** Stents were placed into both the bile duct and the cystic duct to prevent further episodes of recurrent infection. **B: Left:** A stone is evident in the cystic duct remnant, and a stent is in the bile duct. **Right:** A basket has captured the stone for removal.

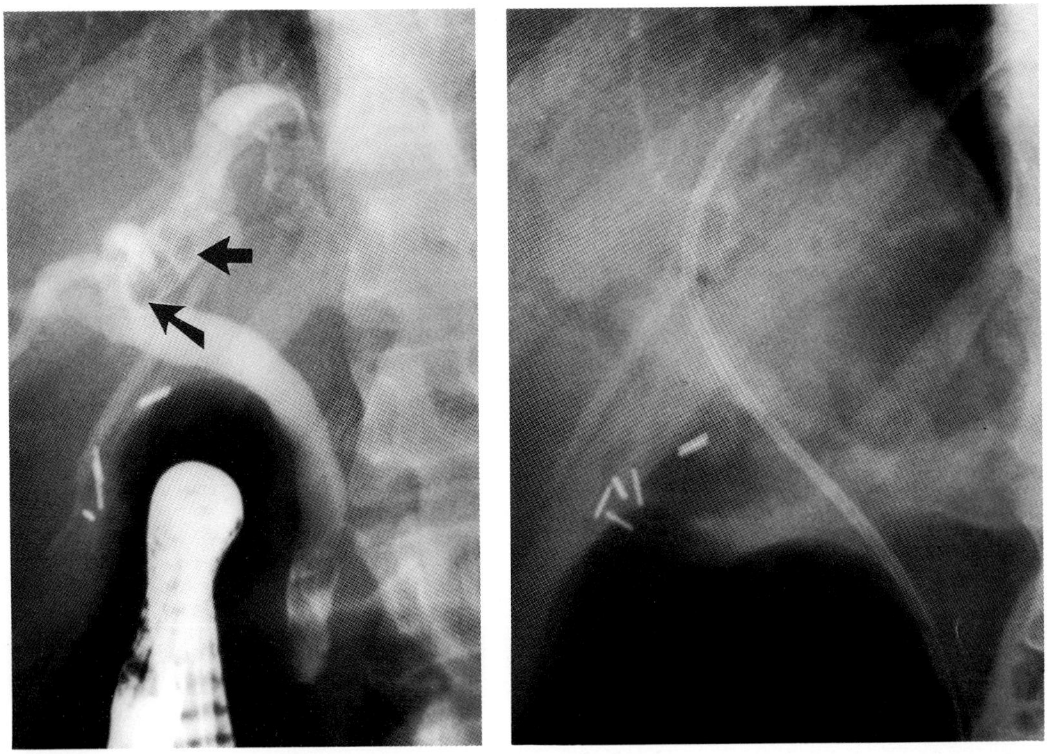

FIG. 11.71. Left: Retained stones are noted in the left hepatic duct (*arrows*) in this patient, who experienced recurrent pain, fever, and chills. **Right:** A prosthesis was selectively placed into the left hepatic duct for drainage. The patient was started on ursodeoxycholic acid, and a balloon catheter was subsequently advanced into the affected duct over a guidewire. The stones, which were smaller, were retrieved.

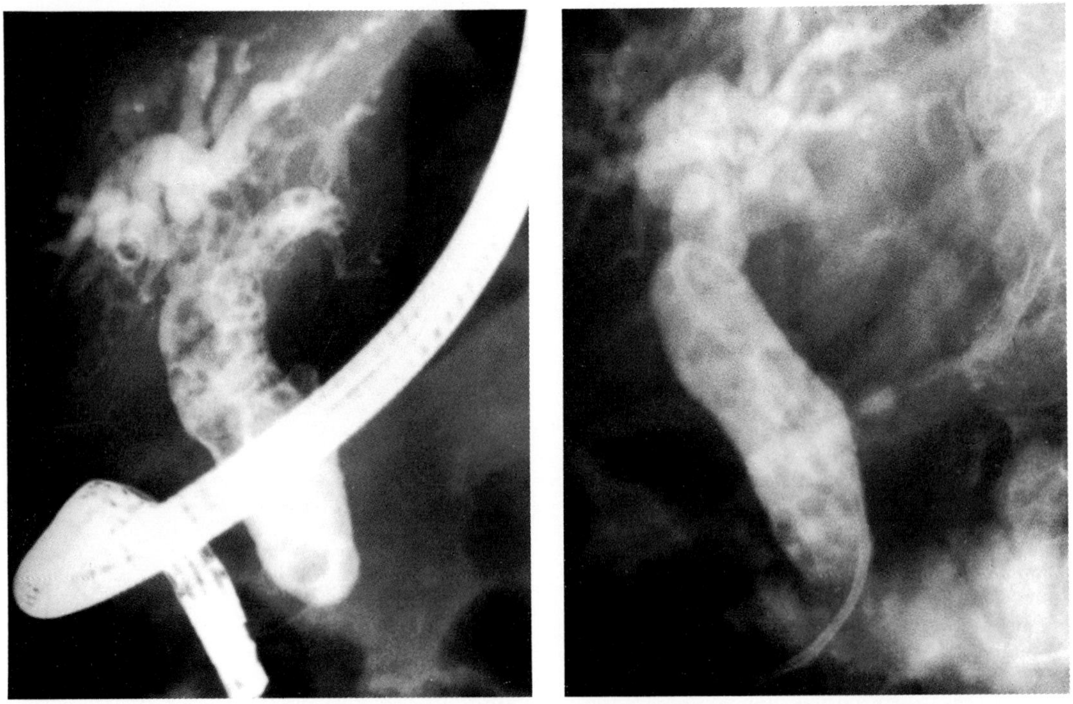

FIG. 11.72. A classical example for which "stents and stones" is indicated. **Left:** This patient had too many stones for mechanical extraction and was too feeble for surgery. **Right:** The decision was made to place a prosthesis for immediate and, possibly, long-term decompression.

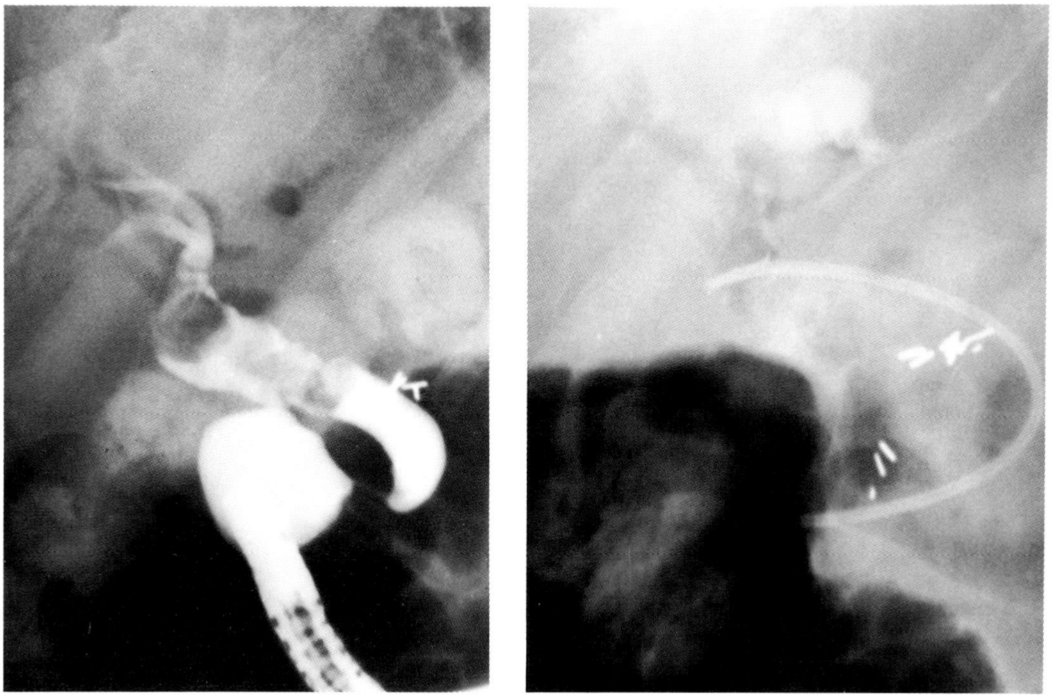

FIG. 11.73. If possible, stents can also be placed for treatment of retained stones in patients who have undergone a Bilroth II gastric resection. **Left:** A large stone and several smaller ones are evident in the common hepatic duct and common bile duct in a patient who had previously undergone a gastric resection, Bilroth II. **Right:** A long stent was placed for decompression. The patient will be recalled for an attempt with mechanical therapy, either extraction or lithotripsy.

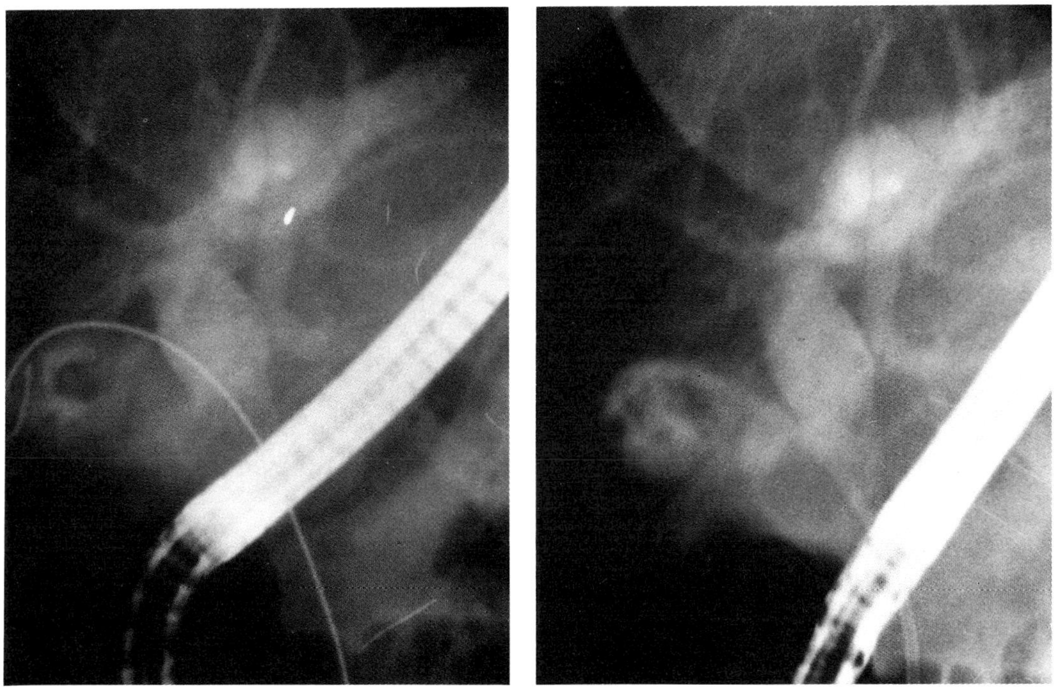

FIG. 11.74. Stents have even been placed into the gallbladders of some patients to provide drainage and prevent cholecystitis after manipulation of the bile duct and gallbladder. **Left:** A guidewire is visible in the gallbladder, looping a stone. **Right:** A pigtail stent may be seen in position in the gallbladder. I have performed this technique only twice without untoward effects.

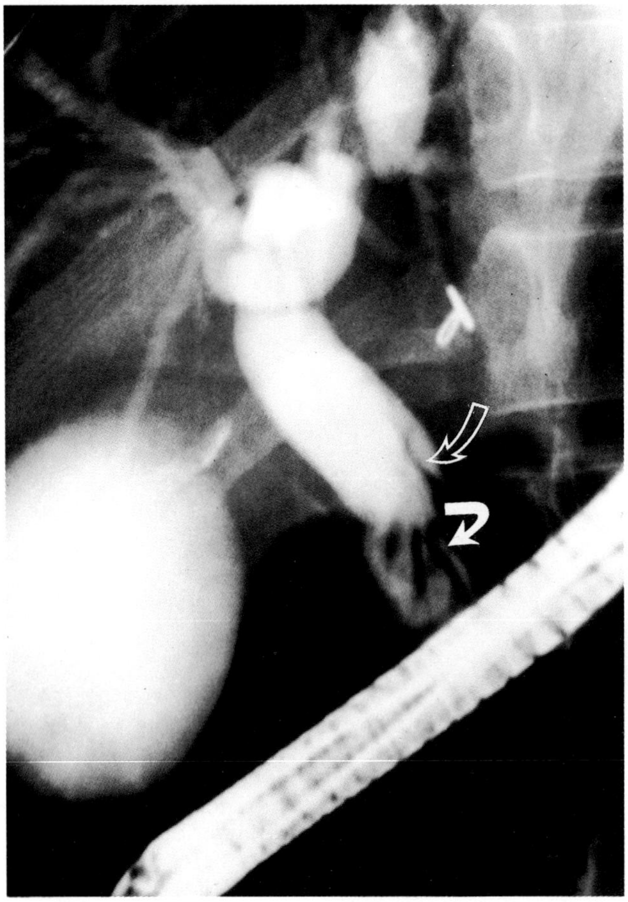

FIG. 11.75. This cholangiogram was obtained in patient who had experienced a 10-year history of right upper quadrant and epigastric pain, which was preceded by an acute episode of abdominal pain, fever, and joint aches. Note the curvilinear lucencies in the distal common bile duct (*arrows*). (From ref. 100, with permission.)

Text continued from page 265.

I do not believe that a straight 10Fr stent offers any advantage over the 7Fr pigtail in the management of stone disease. In fact, a straight stent may migrate out of the bile duct and impact or become imbedded in the bowel wall where a generous sphincterotomy has been formed because no stricture is present to hold the "flap." A pigtail stent, on the other hand, is less likely to migrate because the pigtail occupies more space in the bile duct. Again, the wick effect in the presence of stones and the absence of malignant obstruction prolongs the effectiveness of the stents.

CONCLUSION

This chapter has described the different techniques for extracting stones, fragmenting stones, or leaving them in place while treating them either temporarily or permanently with the placement of prostheses. These extraction techniques have also been employed in the management of foreign bodies and parasites (Figs. 11.75–11.77) (100–106).

An ERCP may occasionally reveal unusual findings, including linear filling defects located within the biliary tree or pancreas. Figures 11.75 through 11.77 illustrate the presence of *Fasciola hepatica* liver flukes, which were extracted live from the bile duct of a 43-year-old Haitian man who had complained of chronic abdominal pain for 10 years following an acute abdominal event. He had even undergone surgery for a suspected perforated ulcer. The classical curvilinear lucent defects in the distal bile duct were diagnostic, and, after a sphincterotomy was performed, the flukes were extracted. Ascariasis, clonorchiasis, and hydatid disease have been recognized and confirmed by ERCP performed in affected persons usually residing in endemic areas (99–107). Our case of *Fasciola* is the first report

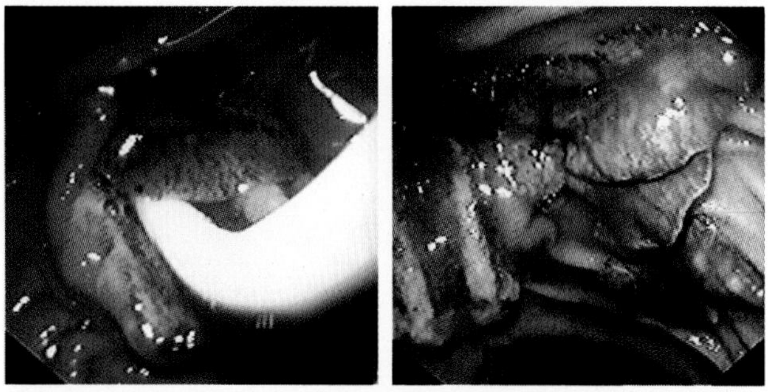

FIG. 11.76. Left: A live *Fasciola hepatica* fluke being extracted with a balloon catheter after performance of a sphincterotomy. **Right:** Other live flukes are being extracted from the bile duct. (From ref. 100, with permission.)

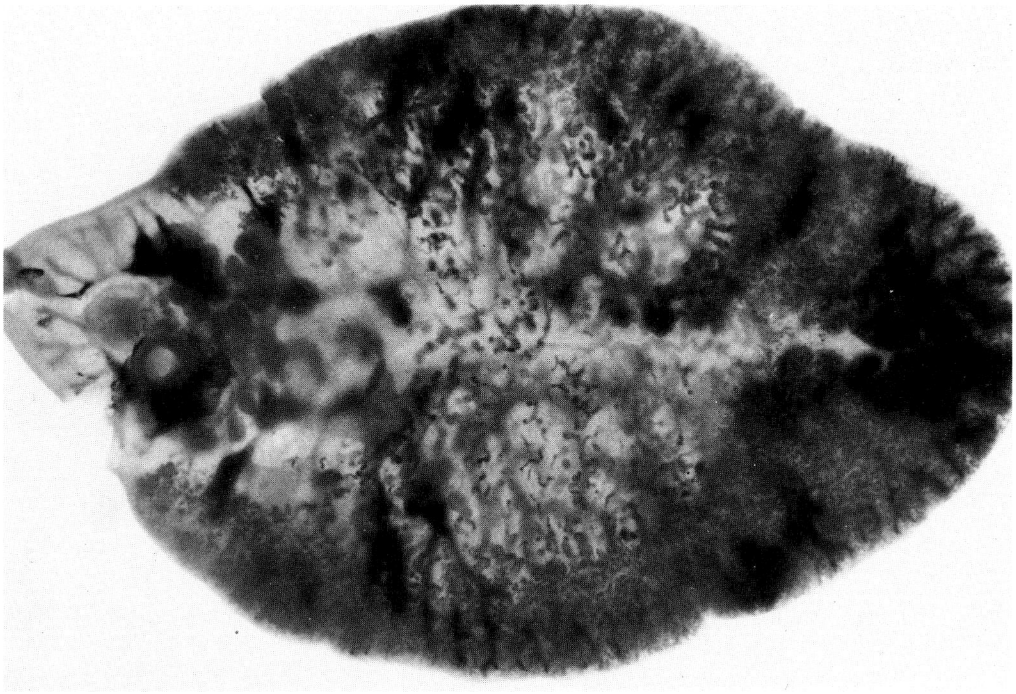

FIG. 11.77. One of the *Fasciola hepatica* flukes retrieved and sent for fixation and identification. (From ref. 100, with permission.)

of the endoscopic extraction of live liver flukes from the biliary tree. The fact that this parasite was detected live after 10 years in a foreign national residing in a nonendemic environment is unique.

I favor a more aggressive approach for the management of retained bile duct stones, but the experience of the endoscopist and the availability of specific devices predicates the ultimate results. The less experienced endoscopist should attend postgraduate courses and/or visit centers where these procedures are being performed. I do not recommend a "do nothing; let the stone pass" approach because the patient may present with acute, life-threatening cholangitis. For the elderly, compromised patient, the latter approach could be fatal. If lithotripsy is not available or the endoscopist is inexperienced, I advise placing a stent.

REFERENCES

1. Way LW. Retained common duct stones. *Clin North Am* 1973;53:1139.
2. Walker JW. The removal of gallstones. *Lancet* 1981;1:874.
3. Broughan TA, Sivak MV, Hermann RE. The management of retained and recurrent bile duct stones. *Surgery* 1985;98:746–51.
4. Way LW, Pellegrini C. *Surgery of the gallbladder and bile duct.* Philadelphia: WB Saunders, 1987.
5. Kawai K, Akasaka Y, Murakami K, et al. Endoscopic sphincterotomy of the ampulla of Vater. *Gastrointest Endosc* 1974;20:148–151.
6. Classen M, Safrany L. Endoscopic papillotomy and removal of gallstones. *Br Med J* 1975;4:371–4.
7. Koch H. Endoscopic papillotomy. *Endoscopy* 1975;7:89.
8. Zimmon DS, Falkenstein DB, Kessler RE. Endoscopic papillotomy for choledocholithiasis. *N Engl J Med* 1975;293:1181.
9. Cotton PB. ERCP. *Gut* 1977;18:316.
10. Cremer M, et al. La sphincterotomie endoscopique: experience europeene actuelle. Proceedings, La Brussels 3rd International Symposium of Digestive Endoscopy. Brussels, Brussels Hilton, 1977.
11. Safrany L. Duodenoscopic sphincterotomy and gallstone removal. *Gastroenterology* 1977;72:338–43.
12. Geenen JE, Hogan J, Shaffer RD, et al. Endoscopic electrosurgical papillotomy and manometry in biliary tract disease. *JAMA* 1977;237:2075–8.
13. Siegel JH. ERCP update: diagnostic and therapeutic applications. *Gastrointest Radiol* 1978;3:311–8.
14. Siegel JH. Endoscopic management of choledocholithiasis and papillary stenosis. *Surg Gynecol Obstet* 1979;148:747–52.
15. Stewart ET, Vennes JA, Geenen JE. *Atlas of endoscopic retrograde cholangiopancreatography.* St. Louis: CV Mosby, 1977.
16. Siegel JH. Endoscopic retrograde cholangiopancreatography (ERCP): present position, and papillotomy. *NY State J Med* 1978;78:583–91.
17. Weizel A, Stiehl A, Raedsch R. Passage of a large bilirubin stone through a narrow papillotomy. *Endoscopy* 1980;12:191–3.
18. Staritz M, Ewe K, Meyer zum Buschenfeld KH. Endoscopic papillotomy dilation (EPD) for the treatment of common bile duct stones and papillary stenosis. *Endoscopy* 1983;15:197–8.
19. Cotton PB. Endoscopic management of bile duct stones (apples and oranges). *Gut* 1984;25:587–97.
20. Staritz J, Poralla T, Dormeyer HH, Meyer zum Buschenfelde KH. Endoscopic removal of common bile duct stones through the intact papilla after medical sphincter dilation. *Gastroenterology* 1985;88:1807–11.
21. Siegel JH, Ben-Zvi JS, Pullano WE. Mechanical lithotripsy of common duct stones. *Gastrointest Endosc* 1990;36:351–6.

22. Irvin TT, Arnstein PM. Management of symptomatic gallstones in the elderly. *Br J Surg* 1988;75:1163–5.
23. Dowsett JF, Vaira D, Polydorou A, Russell RO, Salmon PR. Interventional endoscopy in the pancreatobiliary tree. *Am J Gastroenterol* 1988;83:1328–36.
24. Ikeda S, Tanaka M, Matsumoto S, Yoshimoto H, Itoh H. Endoscopic sphincterotomy: long-term results in 408 patients with complete follow up. *Endoscopy* 1988;20:13–7.
25. Simon DM, Brooks WS Jr, Hersh T. Endoscopic sphincterotomy: a reappraisal. *Am J Gastroenterol* 1989;84:213–9.
26. Matsumoto S, Ikeda S, Tanaka M, Yoshimoto H, Nakayama F. Nonoperative removal of giant common duct calculi. *Am J Surg* 1988;155:780–2.
27. Riemann JF, Seuberth K, Demling L. Clinical application of a new mechanical lithotripter for smashing common bile duct stones. *Endoscopy* 1982;14:226–30.
28. Frimberger E, Weingart J, Kuhner W, et al. Eingeklemmter Papillenstein: mechanische Lithotripsie moglichkeit (letter). *Dtsch Med Wochenschr* 1983;108:38.
29. Riemann JF, Seuberth K, Demling L. Clinical application of a new mechanical lithotripor for common bile duct stones. *Scand J Gastroenterol* 1982;17(suppl)78:378.
30. Riemann JF, Seuberth K, Demling L. Mechanical lithotripsy of common bile duct stones. *Gastrointest Endosc* 1985;31:207–10.
31. Staritz M, Ewe K, Meyer zum Buschenfelde KH. Mechanical gallstone lithotripsy in the common bile duct—in-vitro and in-vivo experience. *Endoscopy* 1983;15:316–8.
32. Halver B. Endoscopic mechanical crushing of calculi in the common bile duct. *Ugeskr Laeger* 1986;148:3306–8.
33. Ho CS, Yee AC, McLoughlin MJ. Biliary lithotripsy with a mechanical lithotriptor. *Radiology* 1987;165:791–3.
34. Yoshida S, Nakajima M, Fujimoto S, Yoshinaka M, Kimoto K. New therapeutic methods—technique, application, efficiency and problems—endoscopic lithotripsy. a) Mechanical lithotripsy. *Nippon Rinsho* 1987;45:1494–500.
35. Liguory C, Lefe, Beaugeri L, Canard JM, Etienne JP. Mechanical lithotripsy of calculi of the common bile duct. *Chirurgie* 1987;113:556–61.
36. Higuchi T, Kon Y. Endoscopic mechanical lithotripsy for the treatment of common bile duct stones. Experience with the improved double sheath basket. *Endoscopy* 1987;19:216–7.
37. Schneider MU, Matek W, Bauer R, Domschke W. Mechanical lithotripsy of bile duct stones in 209 patients: effect of technical advances. *Endoscopy* 1988;20:248–53.
38. Koch H, Stolte M, Walz V. Endoscopic lithotripsy in the common bile duct. *Endoscopy* 1977;9:95–8.
39. Siegel JH, Pullano W, Ramsey WH. Lithotripsy—to crush or explode? State of the art. *Gastrointest Endosc* 1986;15:191.
40. Burhenne HJ. Electrohydraulic fragmentation of retained common duct stones. *Radiology* 1975;117:721–2.
41. Lear JL, Ring EA, Macoviak JA, Baum S. Percutaneous transhepatic electrohydraulic lithotripsy. *Radiology* 1984;150:589–90.
42. Martin EC, Wolff M, Neff RA, et al. Use of the electrohydraulic lithotriptor in the biliary tree in dogs. *Radiology* 1981;139:215–7.
43. Frimberger E, Kuhner W, Weingart J, et al. Eine neue Methode der elektrohydraulischen Cholelithotripse (Lithoklasie). *Dtsch Med Wochenschr* 1982;107:213–5.
44. Tanaka M, Yoshimoto H, Ikeda S, et al. Two approaches for electrohydraulic lithotripsy in the common bile duct. *Surgery* 1985;98:318–9.
45. Manegold BC, Memicken G, Jung M. *Endoscopic electrohydraulic disintegration of common bile duct concrements*. World Congress of Gastroenterology. Abstract 573, Stockholm, 1982.
46. Silvis SE, Siegel JH, Hughes R Jr, Katon RH, Sievert CE, Sivak M. Use of electrohydraulic lithotripsy to fracture common bile duct stones. *Gastrointest Endosc* 1986;32:155–6.
47. Sievert CE Jr, Silvis SE. Evaluation of electrohydraulic lithotripsy as a means of gallstone fragmentation in a canine model. *Gastrointest Endosc* 1987;33:233–5.
48. Picus D, Weyman PJ, Marx MV. Role of percutaneous intracorporeal electrohydraulic lithotripsy in the treatment of biliary tract calculi. Work in progress. *Radiology* 1989;170:989–93.
49. Ponchon T, Valette PJ, Chavallon A. Percutaneous transhepatic electrohydraulic lithotripsy under endoscopic control. *Gastrointest Endosc* 1987;33:307–9.
50. Ponchon T, Chavaillon A, Ayela P, Lambert R. Retrograde biliary ultra thin endoscopy enhances biopsy of stenoses and lithotripsy. *Gastrointest Endosc* 1989;35:292–7.
51. Siegel JH, Ben-Zvi JS, Pullano WE. Endoscopic electrohydraulic lithotripsy. *Gastrointest Endosc* 1990;30:134–6.
52. Ell CH, Hochberger J, Muller D, et al. Laser lithotripsy of gallstones by means of a pulsed neodymium YAG laser in vitro and in animal experiences. *Endoscopy* 1986;18:92.
53. Lux G, Ell CH, Hochberger J, Muller D, Demling L. The first successful endoscopic retrograde laser lithotripsy of CBD stones in man using the pulsed neodymium YAG laser. *Endoscopy* 1986;18:144–5.
54. Ell CH, Lux G, Hochberger J, Muller D, Demling L. Laser lithotripsy of common bile duct stone. *Gut* 1988;29:746–51.
55. Kozarek RA, Low DE, Ball TT. Tunable dye laser lithotripsy: in vitro studies and in-vivo treatment of choledocholithiasis. *Gastrointest Endosc* 1988;34:418–21.
56. Cotton PB, Kozarek RA, Schapiro RH, et al. Endoscopic laser lithotripsy of large bile duct stones. *Gastroenterology* 1990;1128–33.
57. Hwang MH, Yang JC, Lin J. The treatment of retained intrahepatic stones with electrohydraulic and ultrasonic shock waves. *Dig Dis Sci* 1986;31(Suppl):10.
58. Nichioka NS, Levins PC, Murray SC, Parrish JA, Anderson RR. Fragmentation of biliary calculi with tunable dye lasers. *Gastroenterology* 1987;93:250–5.
59. Bean WJ, Daughtry JD, Rodan BA, Mullin D. Ultrasonic lithotripsy of retained common bile duct stone. *AJR* 1985;144:1275–6.
60. Chespak LW, Ring EJ, Shapiro HA, Gordon RL, Ostroff JW. Multidisciplinary approach to complex endoscopic biliary intervention. *Radiology* 1989;170:995–7.
61. Wholey MH, Smoot S. Choledocholithiasis: percutaneous pulverization with a high-speed rotational catheter. *AJR* 1988;150:129–30.
62. Mazzariello RM. Removal of residual biliary tract calculi without reoperation. *Surgery* 1979;67:566–73.
63. Bean WJ, Smith SL, Mahorner HR. Equipment for nonoperative removal of biliary tract stones. *Radiology* 1973;107:452–3.
64. Burhenne HJ. Nonoperative retained biliary tract stone extraction, a new roentgenologic technique. *AJR* 1973;117:388–99.
65. Clouse ME, Stokes KR, Lee RGL, Falchuck KR. Bile duct stones: percutaneous transhepatic removal. *Radiology* 1986;169:525–9.
66. Stokes KR, Falchuck KR, Clouse ME. Biliary duct stones: update on 54 cases after percutaneous transhepatic removal. *Radiology* 1989;170:999–1001.
67. Burhenne HJ. Complications of nonoperative extraction of retained common duct stones. *Am J Surg* 1976;131:260–2.
68. Latshaw RF, Kadir S, Witt WS, Kaufmann SL, White RI Jr. Glucagon-induced choledochal sphincter relaxation: aid for expulsion of impacted calculi into the duodenum. *AJR* 1981;137:614–6.
69. Meranze SG, Stein EJ, Burke DR, Hartz WH, McLean GK. Removal of retained common bile duct stones with angiographic occlusion balloons. *AJR* 1986;146:383–5.
70. Perez MR, Oleaga JA, Freiman DB, McLean GL, Ring EJ. Removal of a distal common bile duct stone through percutaneous transhepatic catheterization. *Arch Surg* 1979;114:107–9.
71. Fernstrom I, Delin NA, Sundblad R. Percutaneous transhepatic extraction of common bile duct stones. *Surg Gynecol Obstet* 1981;153:405–7.
72. Ellman BA, Berman HL. Treatment of a common duct stone via transhepatic approach. *Gastrointest Radiol* 1981;6:357–9.
73. Haskin PH, Teplick SK, Sammon JK, Gambescia RA, Zitomer N, Pavlides CA. Monooctanoin infusion and stone removal

through the transparenchymal tract: use in 17 patients. *AJR* 1987;148:185–8.
74. Brandon JC, Teplick SK, Haskin PH, et al. Common duct calculi: updated experience with dissolution with methyl tertiary butyl ether. *Radiology* 1988;166:665–7.
75. Van Sonnenberg E, Casola G, Zakko SF, et al. Gallbladder and bile duct stones: percutaneous therapy with primary MTBE dissolution and mechanical methods. *Radiology* 1988;169:505–9.
76. Sadek S, Cuschieri A. Efficacy of ceruletide controlled saline infusion for retained ductal stones after cholecystectomy and exploration of the common bile duct. *J Hepatol* 1987;5:288–91.
77. Tritapepe R, diPadova C, diPadova F. Non-invasive treatment for retained common bile duct stones in patients with T-tubes in situ: saline washout after intravenous ceruletide. *Br J Surg* 1988;75:144–6.
78. Gardner B, Ostrowitz A, Masur R. Reappraisal of the possible role of heparin solution of gallstones: a clinical extension of laboratory studies in removal of retained common duct stones. *Surgery* 1971;69:854–7.
79. Teplick SK, Pavlides CA, Goodman LR, Babayan VK. In vitro dissolution of gallstones: comparison of monooctanoin, sodium dehydrocholate, heparin, and saline. *AJR* 1982;138:271–3.
80. Velasco N, Brashetto I, Osendes A. Treatment of retained common bile duct stones: a prospective controlled study comparing monooctanoin and heparin. *World J Surg* 1983;7:266–70.
81. Wurbs D, Phillip J, Classen M. Experiences with the longstanding nasobiliary tube in biliary diseases. *Endoscopy* 1980;12:219–23.
82. Thistle JL, Carlson GL, LaRusso NF, Hofmann AF. Effective dissolutions of biliary duct stones by intraductual infusion of monooctanoin. *Gastroenterology* 1978;74:1103.
83. Hofmann AF. Medical treatment of cholesterol gallstones by bile desaturation agents. *Hepatology* 1984;4:1995–2085.
84. Mack E, Crummy AB, Babayan VK. Percutaneous transhepatic dissolution of common bile duct stones. *Surgery* 1981;90:584–7.
85. Brandon JC, Teplick SK, Haskin PH, et al. Common bile duct calculi: updated experience with dissolution with methyl tertiary butyl ether. *Radiology* 1988;166:665–7.
86. Murray WR, LaFerla G, Fullarton GM. Choledocholithiasis: in vivo stone dissolution using methyl tertiary butyl ether (MTBE). *Gut* 1988;29:143–5.
87. Sauerbruch T, Stern M. Study group for shock-wave lithotripsy of bile duct stones. Fragmentation of bile duct stones by extracorporeal shock waves. *Gastroenterology* 1989;961:146–52.
88. Bland KI, Jones RS, Maher JW, et al. Extracorporeal shockwave lithotripsy (ESWL) of bile duct calculi: an interim report of the Dornier U.S. bile duct lithotripsy prospective study. *Ann Surg* 1989;209:743–55.
89. Drach GW, Drother S, Fair W, et al. Report of the United States cooperative study of extracorporeal shock wave lithotripsy. *J Urol* 1986;135:1127–33.
90. Delius M, Mueller A, Vogel A, Brendel W. Extracorporeal shock waves: properties and principles of generation. In: Ferrucci JT, Delius M, Burhenne JH, eds. *Biliary lithotripsy*. Chicago: Year Book Medical Publishers, 1989:9–21.
91. Sauerbruch T, Holl J, Sackmann M, et al. Treatment of bile duct stone by extracorporeal shock waves. *Semin Ultrasound CT MR* 1987;8:155.
92. Johlin FC, Loening SA, Maher JW, Summers RW. Electrohydraulic shock wave lithotripsy (ESWL) fragmentation of retained common duct stones. *Surgery* 1988;104:592–8.
93. Taylor MC, Marshall JC, Laszlo AF, et al. Extracorporeal shock wave lithotripsy (ESWL) in the management of complex biliary tract stone disease. *Ann Surg* 1988;208:586–92.
94. Siegel JH, Yatto RP. Biliary endoprostheses for the management of retained common bile duct stones. *Am J Gastroenterol* 1984;79:50–4.
95. van den Brandt Gradel V, Scheurer U, Halter F. Endoscopic insertion of endoprostheses in benign bile duct calculi. Description of 4 cases. *Schweiz Rundsch Med Prax* 1986;75:260–2.
96. Cotton PB, Forbes A, Leung JWC, Dineen L. Endoscopic stenting for longterm treatment of large bile duct stones: 2 to 5 year followup. *Gastroint Endosc* 1987;33:411–3.
97. Kiil J, Kruse A, Rokkjaer M. Large bile duct stones treated by endoscopic biliary drainage. *Surgery* 1989;105:51–6.
98. Foutch PG, Harlan J, Sanowski RA. Endoscopic placement of biliary stents for treatment of high risk geriatric patients with common duct stones. *Am J Gastroenterol* 1989;84:527–9.
99. Soomers AJ, Nagengast FM, Yap SH. Endoscopic placement of biliary endoprostheses in patients with endoscopically unextractable common bile duct stones. A long term followup study of 26 patients. *Endoscopy* 1990;22:24–6.
100. Veerappan A, Siegel JH, Podany J, Prudente R, Gelb A. *Fasciola hepatica* pancreatitis: endoscopic extraction of live parasites. *Gastrointest Endosc* (In press).
101. Jassen K, Al Mofleh I, Al-Mofarreh M. Endoscopic treatment of ascariasis causing acute obstructive cholangitis. *Hepatogastroenterology* 1986;33:275–7.
102. Sahel J, Bastid C, Choux R. Biliary ascariasis combined with a villous tumor of the papilla. Diagnostic and therapeutic value of endoscopy. *Endoscopy* 1987;19:243–5.
103. van-Severen M, Lengele B, Dureuil J, Shapira M, Dive C. Hepatic ascaridiasis. *Endoscopy* 1987;19:140–2.
104. Leung JW, Sung JY, Chung SC, Metreweli C. Hepatic clonorchiasis—a study by endoscopic retrograde cholangiopancreatography. *Gastrointest Endosc* 1989;35:226–31.
105. Al-Karawi MA, Mohamed AR, Yasawy I, Haleem A. Nonsurgical endoscopic transpapillary treatment of ruptured echinococcus liver cyst obstructing the biliary tree. *Endoscopy* 1987;19:81–3.
106. Van-Steenbergen W, Fevery J, Broeckaert L, et al. Hepatic echinococcosis ruptured into the biliary tract. Clinical, radiological and therapeutic features during five episodes of spontaneous biliary rupture in three patients with hepatic hydatidosis. *J Hepatol* 1987;4:133–9.
107. Lee SH, Scudamore CH. Combined radiologic and endoscopic management of biliary obstruction from ruptured hydatid disease. *Gastrointest Endosc* 1991;37:73–4.

CHAPTER 12

Decompression Techniques: Nasobiliary Catheters and Endoprostheses

The capability of providing drainage and decompressing an obstructed biliary tree with endoscopic techniques has provided the endoscopist with an efficacious, therapeutic resource. With the introduction of nasobiliary drainage catheters, the endoscopist entered a new area of therapy, decompression, providing effective treatment of obstructive jaundice, cholangitis, and pancreatic disorders (1–13). Access to the biliary tree provided by a nasobiliary catheter enables the endoscopist to perform serial cholangiograms without having to reintubate with an endoscope, and, with the catheter in place, therapeutic options such as perfusion of dissolution agents, antibiotics, and steroids can be utilized (14–21). Endoprostheses, on the other hand, provide a relatively permanent treatment modality that is more convenient than the nasobiliary catheter and is safer and more comfortable than percutaneous drains, which are encumbered by their external hardware (22–32).

The morbidity associated with insertion of nasobiliary catheters and endoprostheses is much lower than that of percutaneous interventional techniques and is significantly below the rates of surgical decompression. The lower morbidity rate for the endoscopic techniques is even more significant when either percutaneous decompression or surgery are performed in patients at risk or when either is performed in an emergency (33–39). Incidently, the morbidity associated with endoscopic stents is more commonly related to the performance of sphincterotomy.

Placement of a nasobiliary catheter is easier than placement of an endoprosthesis. The nasobiliary catheter is a continuous tube, which allows it to be both advanced and withdrawn, a factor that facilitates its placement. This fact becomes clearer to the less experienced endoscopist when the technique of insertion of an endoprosthesis is described. The insertion of an endoprosthesis is more difficult because, by virtue of its design (separate components and discontinuous catheter), the prosthesis can only be pushed, not withdrawn. Therefore, the length of a prosthesis is critical, and because it cannot be withdrawn, proper placement is important to its function. These points will be clarified in later discussions regarding the techniques.

TECHNIQUE—NASOBILIARY CATHETERS

An ERCP is performed in order to demonstrate the cause of obstruction to the bile duct (i.e., stricture or stone), which is identified on the radiographs obtained during the procedure. If retained stones are responsible for the obstruction, and, for some reason, the stones are not removed, insertion of a nasobiliary tube can be considered a therapeutic option providing decompression and access to the biliary tree (39). As an alternative, insertion of a prosthesis can be considered a viable option (40). After performing the diagnostic cholangiogram, I usually perform a sphincterotomy to facilitate access of the nasobiliary catheter or endoprosthesis. A sphincterotomy is carried out in the usual manner, but the incision does not have to be as long as the one required for the removal of a stone. *However, I prefer a maximum sphincterotomy in most situations because it facilitates manipulation of the bile duct.* The sphincterotomy should permit easier insertion of a large catheter, nasobiliary catheter, or endoprosthesis and separate the bile duct orifice from the pancreas, thus preventing occlusion of the pancreatic duct and avoiding manipulation of the pancreatic duct on subsequent examinations. For the latter reason, I routinely perform a standard or long sphincterotomy, not a papillotomy as others have suggested. In placing more than 1,000 prostheses, I have not encountered severe bleeding from the performance of a long sphincterotomy. Only 11 patients were noted to have experienced bleeding significant enough to delay discharge from the hospital for monitoring, and only five required transfusions.

There are cannulas available that will accept a 0.035″ guidewire made by Microvasive (Bilitrac 35), Olympus Corporation, and Wilson-Cook. Advancing a guidewire through an existing catheter is advantageous because the cannula can be placed, the cholangiogram can be obtained, and if the cannula has already traversed the area of stricture, the guidewire can be advanced through the cannula without having to remove or exchange the catheter and risk the possibility of failing to traverse the stricture on a repeat attempt. A standard nipple-tip cannula will not accept a guidewire unless the tip has been dilated using either an 18 g or a 19 g needle (4). If the endoscopist anticipates placing a guidewire, he or she should check the cannula before inserting it to determine if the wire can be passed through the tip. Another option I often use to access the bile duct and traverse a stricture is to insert a 7 French Van Andel dilating catheter, into which the guidewire has already been placed, to facilitate access across the sphincter into the bile duct. Once it is in position, the guidewire can be advanced into the proximal biliary tree to be anchored before removal of the catheter (41). This dilating catheter, Van Andel or Sohendra by Wilson-Cook, permits an easier exchange or removal of the guidewire because it is shorter (180 cm) than the cannula (220 cm). It is also larger in diameter than the cannula (5Fr versus 7Fr), and, being larger, the dilating catheter eliminates friction and drag.

Once the catheter-guidewire assembly is positioned in any duct, the endoscopist has control of that duct and the stricture, and the wire provides access for any accessory. With the technique described by Seldinger (42), a radiologist, for exchanging catheters using a wire-guided system, the guidewire is left in place while the cannula or dilating catheter is removed. This is accomplished by having an assistant feed the guidewire into the catheter as the endoscopist slowly withdraws it while continuously observing the guidewire's position both endoscopically and fluoroscopically and preventing dislodgment. After the catheter is removed and the guidewire is in place, the appropriate accessory can be advanced over the guidewire. These accessories include occlusion balloons, the newer wire-guided baskets, dilating balloons, wire-guided sphincterotomes, nasobiliary catheters, and endoprostheses.

With the guidewire in place, the nasobiliary catheter may be advanced over the guidewire while its position is observed through the endoscope. Fluoroscopic control ensures its proper location. I prefer the pigtail type of nasobiliary catheter (Fig. 12.1) to the type that maintains a loop configuration in the duodenum. Either type is effective, but in most situations, my preference is the pigtail type (Fig. 12.2) unless a large-caliber 10Fr nasobiliary tube is used for insertion of radioactive materials. In this case I use a straight tube with side flaps only (Chapter 14). Advancing a 5Fr pigtail nasobiliary catheter is easier than placing a 7Fr pigtail because the stiffness of the pigtail, which must be straightened in order to be placed onto the guidewire, may produce crimping of the catheter, resulting in increased friction and difficulty in pushing the catheter.

The wire is maintained in a straight position by the assistant while light pull tension is placed on the wire

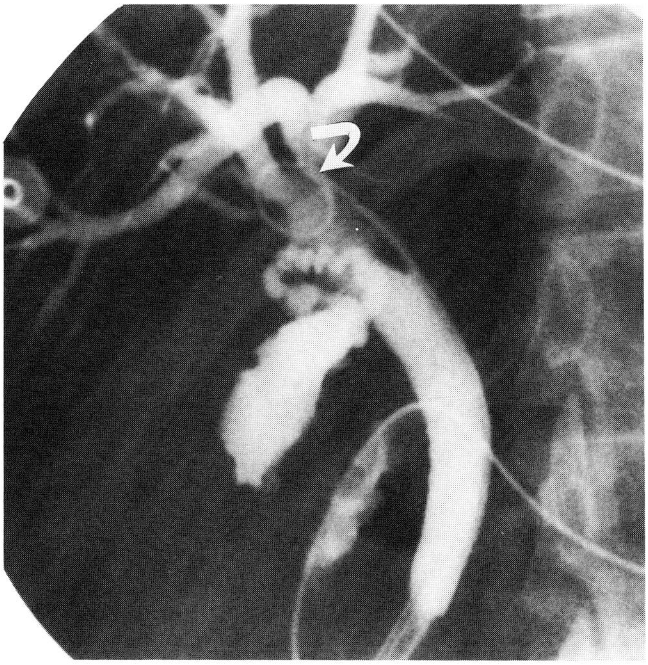

FIG. 12.1. A radiograph showing the pigtail (*arrow*) of a nasobiliary tube in position in the common hepatic duct near the bifurcation of the right and left hepatic ducts.

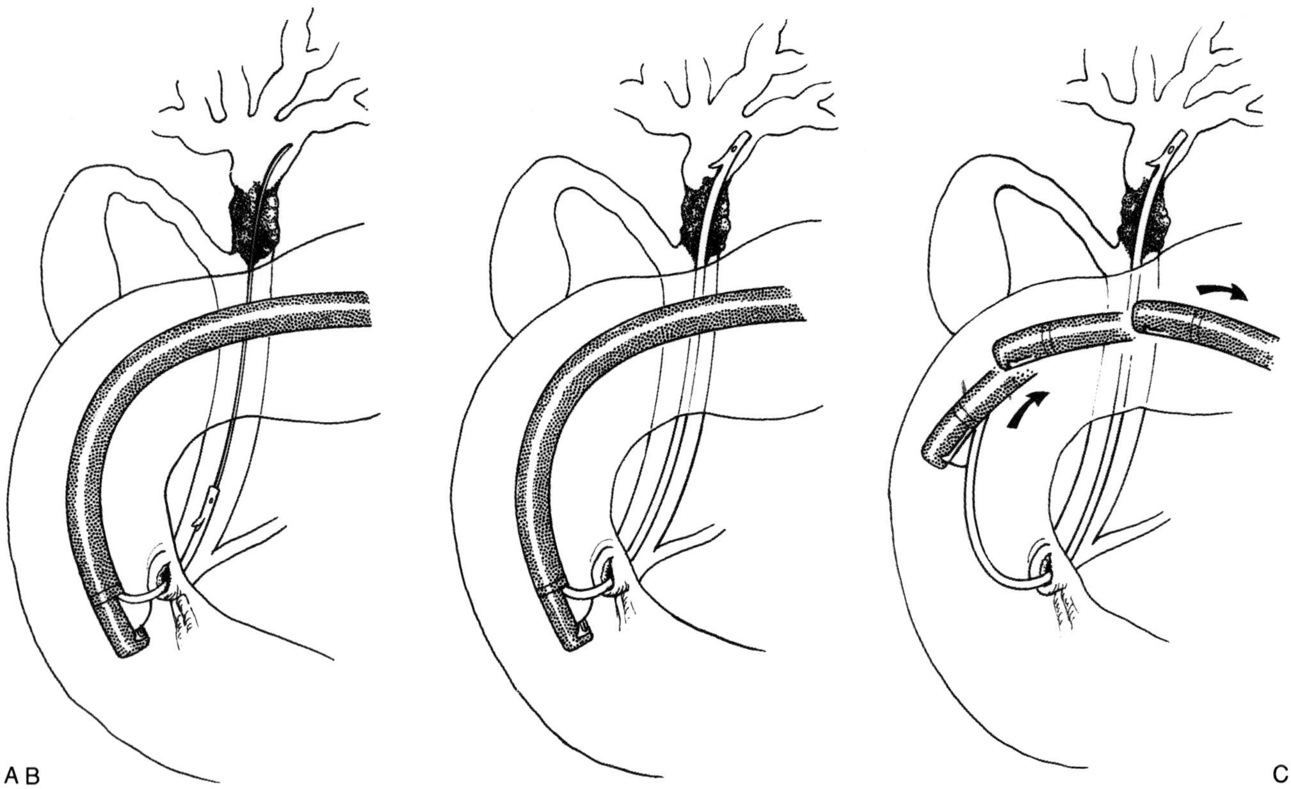

A B C

FIG. 12.2. A: A lesion in the common hepatic duct near the bifurcation (Klatskin type I). A guide catheter and guidewire have been advanced through the obstructing lesion. A sphincterotomy is evident, and a large caliber (10Fr) nasobiliary catheter is being pushed into the common bile duct through the sphincterotomy. **B:** The nasobiliary catheter being advanced through the stricture while the guidewire and guide catheter have been pulled back more proximally. **C:** The withdrawal of the endoscope.

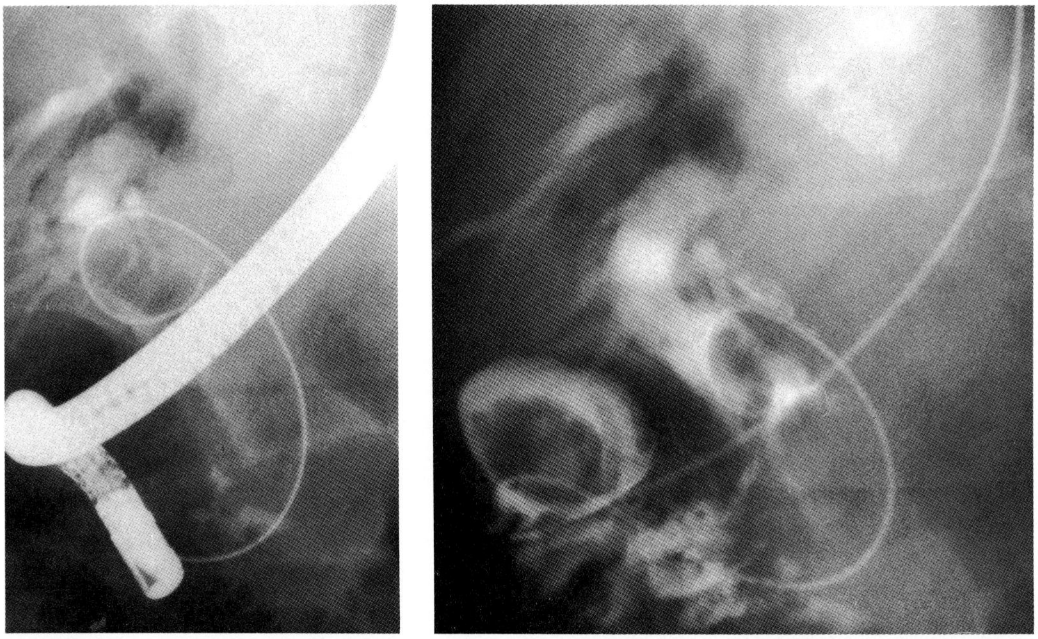

FIG. 12.3. Left: The endoscope in position, and a nasobiliary catheter and guidewire in place in the common hepatic bile duct. **Right:** The endoscope has been removed off the nasobiliary catheter, and the guidewire has been removed as well. Contrast material is being injected through the nasobiliary catheter to determine its position while providing a cholangiogram.

to reduce the slack in the wire. This maneuver minimizes friction and permits an easier advance or glide of the catheter over the wire and into position. While advancing the nasobiliary catheter, the endoscopist should keep the guidewire, which is visible in the duodenum through the endoscope, under continuous observation to prevent looping and dislodgment. Once the nasobiliary tube is in position in the proximal biliary tree above the stricture or stone, the guidewire may be withdrawn so that the pigtail is formed. This procedure may be visualized on the fluoroscope screen. As an alternative technique, which some endoscopists prefer, the nasobiliary tube can be preloaded onto the guidewire before inserting it into the endoscope. It may then be advanced as a single unit through the sphincterotomy, bile duct, and stricture (Figs. 12.3, 12.4). This method avoids the multiple steps of prior placement of the guidewire, subsequent removal of the cannula or dilating catheter, and advancement of the nasobiliary catheter.

The technique for maintaining the position of the nasobiliary catheter while removing the endoscope again requires cooperation between the endoscopist and the assistant. Experience in performing these procedures is necessary to avoid dislodging the wire or the nasobiliary catheter. Once the nasobiliary catheter and wire are in position, the endoscope may be removed over the assembly, leaving it in place (Fig. 12.5A). While the endoscopist advances the guidewire and nasobiliary catheter into the biopsy port of the endoscope, the assistant carefully and slowly withdraws the endoscope from the patient. Intermittent fluoroscopic monitoring ensures the position of the catheter. Once the endoscope has exited from the mouth, the assistant firmly grasps the nasobiliary catheter and wire and completely removes the endoscope from the catheter-guidewire, leaving the catheter exiting from the mouth. The guidewire is then removed completely from the nasobiliary catheter, reducing its stiffness. The nasobiliary catheter must then be exchanged from the mouth to the nose to complete the nasobiliary portion of the procedure. The softer catheter, without the wire, is easier to manipulate and much safer to use. A shortened nasogastric catheter or nasopharyngeal tube (a short, 16Fr, clear polyethylene tube) is then advanced into the patient's nose;

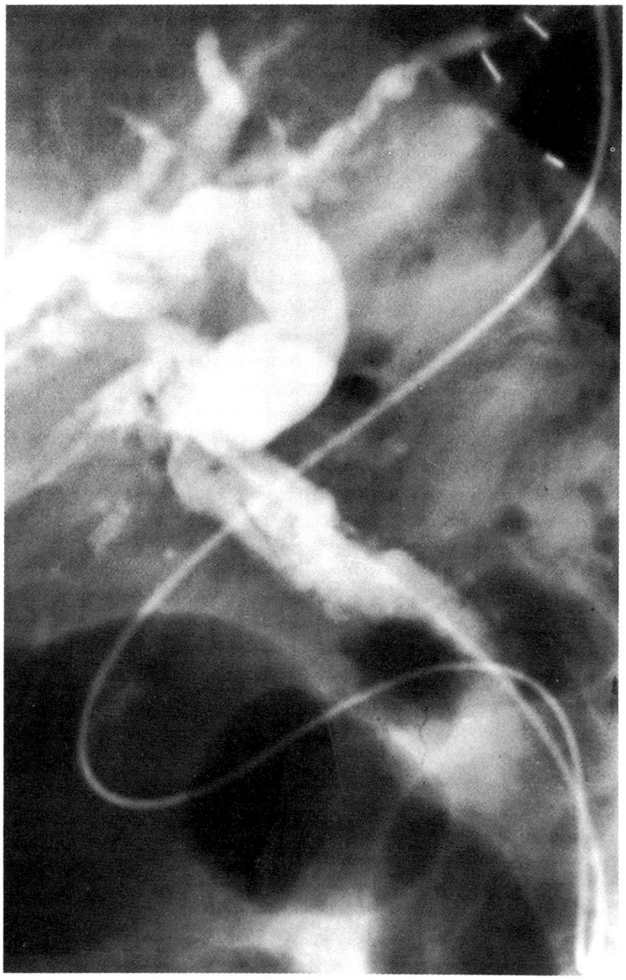

FIG. 12.4. A cholangiogram provided by injection of contrast material through a nasobiliary tube.

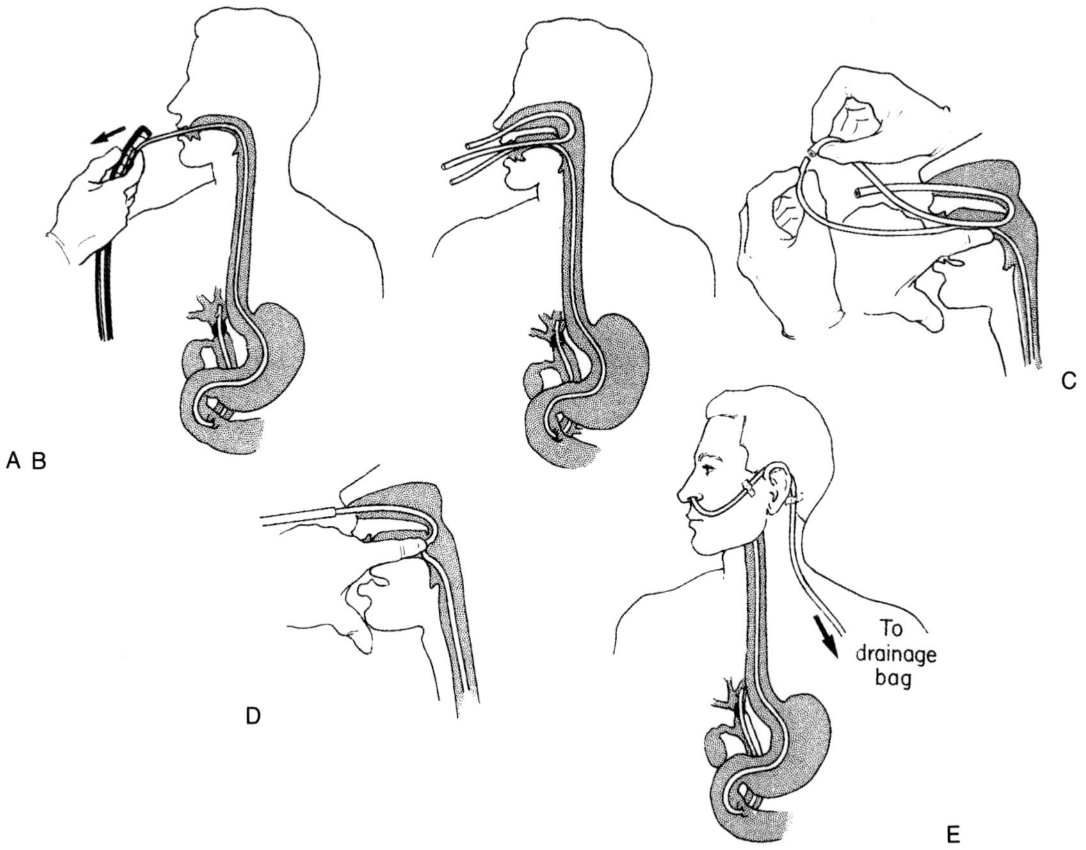

FIG. 12.5. A: The endoscope has been removed from the patient leaving the nasobiliary tube extending from the mouth. The tube is continuously advanced into the biopsy channel while the endoscope is removed. This maneuver is necessary to maintain the position of the tube. **B:** A short nasopharyngeal tube has been advanced through the patient's nose, grasped in the posterior pharynx by the endoscopist or the assistant, and the distal end has been pulled out of the patient's mouth. Now the nasopharyngeal tube enters the patient's nose and exits the mouth. **C:** The proximal portion of the tube is now fed into that portion of the nasopharyngeal tube which exits the mouth. The nasobiliary tube is compressed against the patient's lower jaw to fix its position and prevent movement or dislodgment. **D:** The nasopharyngeal tube is being pulled out the patient's nose while the endoscopist or assistant maintains the position of the nasobiliary tube by compressing the tube against the lower jaw. Following this maneuver, the tube becomes a nasobiliary tube. **E:** The nasobiliary tube is shown in its most distal position in the bile duct, traversing the upper gastrointestinal tract and exiting the nose. The proximal portion of the nasobiliary tube is connected to a gravity-type drainage bag.

when the distal end reaches the posterior pharynx, it is grasped by the endoscopist and pulled out of the patient's mouth (Fig. 12–5B). The patient is left with the nasopharyngeal catheter entering the nose and exiting from the mouth. The nasobiliary catheter is then fed through the distal portion of the nasopharyngeal catheter and is advanced through this nasopharyngeal catheter until it is seen exiting from the nasal portion of this catheter (Fig. 12–5C). The exchange of position from the mouth to the nose is carried out in the following manner: The endoscopist places his or her finger onto the nasobiliary catheter, which is present in the pharynx, and presses the catheter against the lower dental molars or lower jaw to affix its position as the catheter is pulled through the nose (Fig. 12–5D). With the nasobiliary catheter fixed in position by the endoscopist's finger, the proximal portion of the nasobiliary catheter, which is contained in the nasopharyngeal tube, is pulled through the nose. The excess catheter exiting from the mouth is pulled up into the posterior pharynx and out the nose. Once the catheter is straight (that is, from the pharynx to the nose), the endoscopist can release the hold against the molars or jaw and permit the catheter to stabilize in the posterior pharynx. The nasobiliary catheter is then in place, exiting from the nose (Fig. 12–5E). The catheter can be shortened, taped to the patient's cheek, and placed behind his or her ear. The catheter is then connected to a Tuohy-Borst adapter, which accepts a syringe. It can also be connected to a gravity-type bile drainage bag for collection of bile (Fig. 12–5E), which ultimately decompresses the biliary tree. The tube's position and function can then be assessed by injecting contrast through the nasobiliary catheter opacifying the biliary tree. This latter procedure is monitored on the fluoroscope (Fig. 12.5).

The patient is then returned to his or her hospital room, and appropriate orders are given to the staff nurses to ensure that the nasobiliary catheter remains taped to the patient's face and does not become dislodged. The appropriate type of gravity drainage bag can be attached and decompression accomplished.

Periodically, during the course of follow-up, the patient can be brought to a fluoroscopic unit to have contrast injected and serial cholangiograms obtained to document decompression. The versatility of the nasobiliary catheter allows the physician to attach this catheter to an infusion pump for perfusion of monooctonoin or other therapeutic agents or to use it primarily as a drainge system.

Another distinct advantage of a nasobiliary catheter is the fact that it provides noninvasive cholangiography (intubation with an endoscopy is not necessary). This fact should be considered in the follow-up of patients with obstructive jaundice (43).

Sclerosing Cholangitis

Nasobiliary catheters have been used effectively in the treatment of diseases or conditions that produce biochemical cholestasis and jaundice. An example of such a disease is sclerosing cholangitis (20–22). I have placed 5Fr pigtail nasobiliary catheters into the bile ducts of patients with sclerosing cholangitis, positioning the catheter above the dominant stricture (Fig. 12.6) and leaving it in place for up to 4 months. Leaving this catheter in place was intended to provide access for perfusing saline and medicaments to offer more definitive treatment for this ubiquitous but progressive disease. The patients were given instructions for the manual perfusion of saline using a 30 cc syringe filled with saline, steroids, or antibiotics to be implemented after discharge from hospital. While they were still hospitalized, however, the nasobiliary tube was used to perfuse steroids and antibiotics, the latter specifically selected after cultures of the bile were obtained from the nasobiliary catheter drainage. Subsequent to discharge, the patients continued instilling an appropriate antibiotic for 1 to 2 weeks and then perfused saline 4 times a day for up to 4 months (Fig. 12.7). The nasobiliary catheter was removed in 4 months and was replaced with an endoprosthesis. Obviously, in order to continue this method of treatment for the allotted duration, the patients had to be cooperative. These patients were compliant and, despite the presence of the nasal catheter, carried on their usual activities, including work.

Some data suggest that perfusion of the biliary tree of patients with sclerosing cholangitis has positively affected its prognosis, but because of the natural history of the disease (exacerbations and remissions), non-

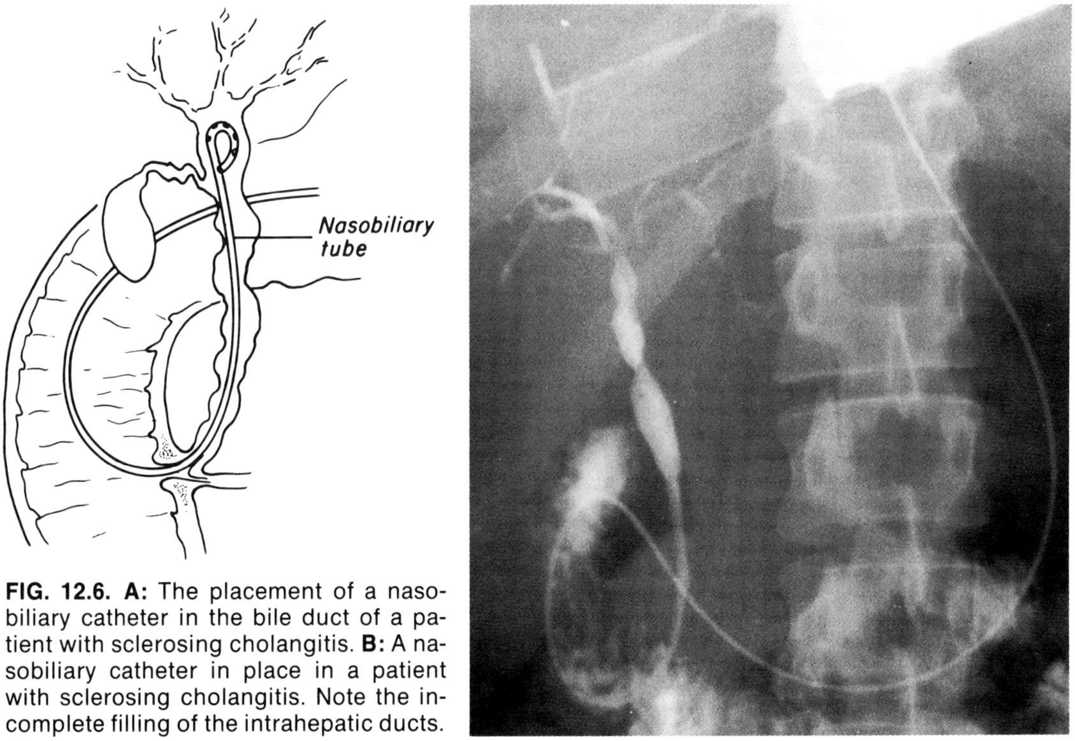

A

B

FIG. 12.6. A: The placement of a nasobiliary catheter in the bile duct of a patient with sclerosing cholangitis. **B:** A nasobiliary catheter in place in a patient with sclerosing cholangitis. Note the incomplete filling of the intrahepatic ducts.

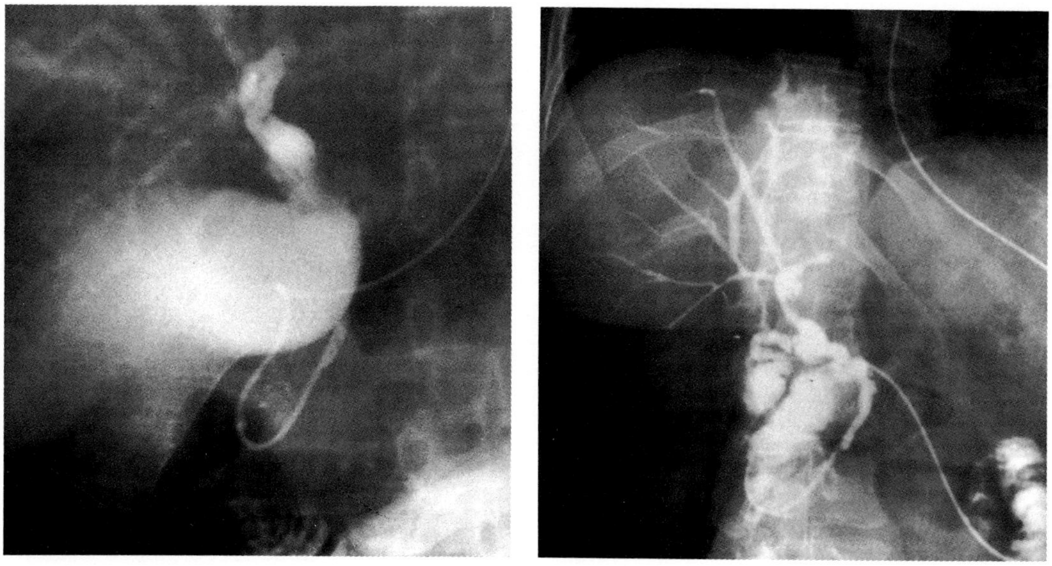

FIG. 12.7. Left: The presence of a nasobiliary tube placed into the bile duct of a patient with sclerosing cholangitis. **Right:** The same patient 4 months later, after the biliary tree is perfused with antibiotics and saline. Note the better definition of the duct morphology on the right after therapy.

randomized results lack credibility. Long-term randomized trials comparing treatment modalities are needed. Endoscopists should be familiar with the multiple uses for the nasobiliary catheters, and this essential technique should be a component of the endoscopists' armamentaria. Endoscopists who wish to become involved in interventional procedures should have a complete understanding of the risk and benefits of these important decompression techniques because they are cost effective as well as beneficial to the patient.

ENDOPROSTHESES

Small and Medium-Sized Endoprosthes

The most outstanding achievement endoscopists have made for patients presenting with obstructive jaundice is the capability of placing endoprostheses. These prostheses remain functional for long periods of time, depending on the type of obstruction treated and the size and numbers of prostheses placed (44–46). Small and medium-sized endoprostheses range in diameter from 5Fr to 8Fr, which may be inserted through endoscopes with a channel size of 2.8 mm to 3.2 mm. A 9Fr can be inserted through the 3.2 mm channel instrument with some difficulty. These endoprostheses are available in variable lengths and configurations conforming to specific strictures in the biliary tree (Figs. 12.8 and 12.9). The technique for inserting endoprostheses is similar to that of the nasobiliary catheter, but there are significant differences.

After completing an ERCP and identifying the stricture or obstruction responsible for cholestasis and/or jaundice, the endoscopist should attempt to decompress the biliary tree. A sphincterotomy should then be performed for the reasons previously specified. Whereas a nasobiliary catheter can be preloaded onto a guidewire and inserted directly into the bile duct and stricture, for insertion of endoprostheses, the guidewire must be in place before the prosthesis is advanced. If a small- to medium-caliber prosthesis is being used, 5Fr to 9Fr, the prosthesis can be advanced

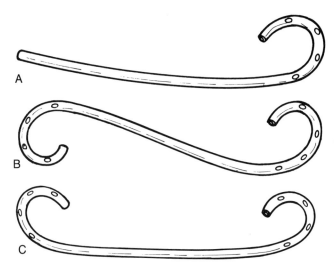

FIG. 12.8. A: A single-pigtail catheter. **B:** A double pigtail with the pigtails located at opposing angles on the catheter. **C:** A double-pigtail catheter with both loops in the same axis of the catheter.

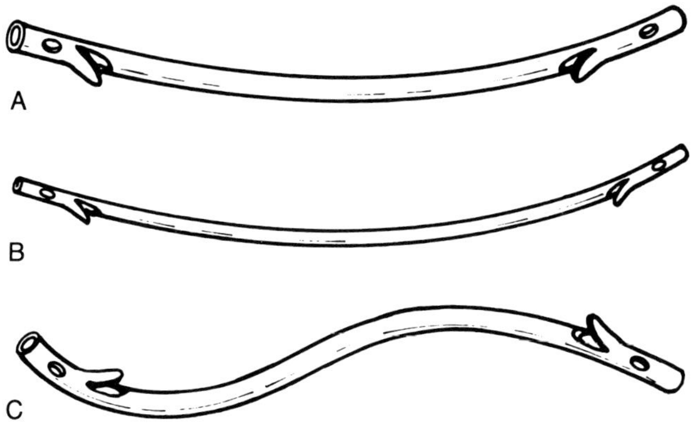

FIG. 12.9. The straight, Amsterdam-type prosthesis. **A:** A large straight prosthesis. **B:** A smaller diameter catheter. **C:** A curved, large-caliber prosthesis. The latter configuration is designed to conform to the tortuous shape of a dilated bile duct, which often occurs in patients with distal bile duct obstruction such as carcinoma of the pancreas.

directly over the guidewire using the pusher catheter. Placement of a 10Fr or 12Fr prosthesis is facilitated by using both a guidewire and a guiding catheter. The guiding catheter fills the void within the large-caliber prosthesis, reducing unnecessary friction or drag while facilitating advancement of the prosthesis over this Teflon or polyethylene tubing (Fig. 12.10). As previously described, the stricture is traversed using either a cannula, which accepts a 0.035″ wire, or a 7Fr dilating catheter, which I frequently use. For smaller diameter prostheses, the dilating catheter or cannula is removed from the guidewire prior to insertion of the prosthesis in the same manner as described; the assistant advances the wire as the endoscopist withdraws the catheter, leaving the guidewire in place while maintaining a visual fix on the wire through the endoscope and the fluoroscope. When the guidewire is in position proximal to the stricture, the prosthesis is placed over the guidewire, advanced to the biopsy port, and fed into the endoscope. The proximal flap of the straight stent is compressed flat against the stent by using the thumb of either hand and then pushing the stent into the port. One can also use an introducer tube, which is initially placed into the port to facilitate the passage of the stent. The pusher catheter is then placed over the guidewire and is advanced up to the biopsy port. Once the pusher catheter is at the biopsy port, the endoscopist advances the pusher catheter, which, obviously, pushes the prosthesis down the biopsy channel. In order to avoid unnecessary friction produced by slack on the guidewire, which results in looping of the guidewire in the duodenum and may lead to dislodgment of the wire, the assistant must apply gentle traction or pull on the guidewire. This action allows the pushing catheter and prosthesis to glide more easily through the endoscope toward the duodenum. The preferred position of the endoscope should be one that has close proximity to the sphincterotomy to avoid looping of the wire and prosthesis in the duodenum, which may lead to dislodgment. While the assistant applies traction to the guidewire, the endoscopist gently pushes the pusher catheter and stent down the channel of the endoscope. The elevator is held in an upward position so the wire does not slip. When the stent strikes the elevator, the endoscopist intermittently releases the elevator. This should permit easier passage of the prosthesis while maintaining pressure or friction on the stent and wire to prevent the wire from slipping and the stent and wire from dislodging. This up-then-down action helps to push and advance the stent while maintaining the wire's position. Care should be taken to observe the position of the prosthesis in the duodenum through the endoscope while simultaneously observing the fluoroscope to maintain the position of the guidewire. The prosthesis should be advanced into position. To avoid advancing the prosthesis too deeply into the duct, the prosthesis and pusher catheter should have contrasting colors, which will allow the endoscopist to appreciate the proximal end of the prosthesis and its position in the sphincter. When the prosthesis is in the correct position both fluoroscopically and endoscopically, the assistant can withdraw the guidewire as the endoscopist maintains the position of the pusher onto the prosthesis to prevent dislodgment of the prosthesis. Minor adjustments of the prosthesis can be

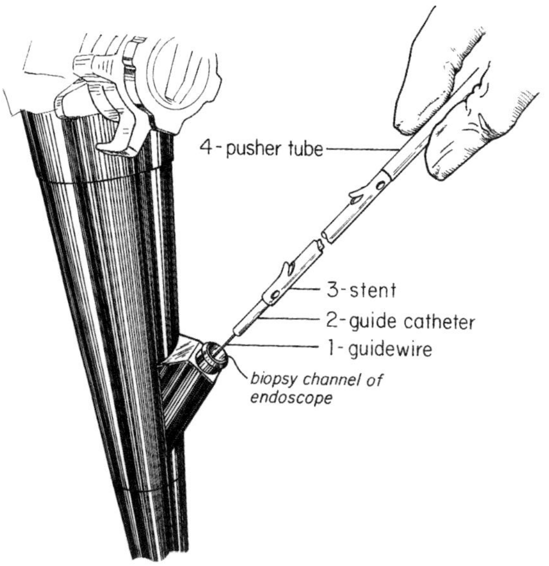

FIG. 12.10. The technique for placing a large-caliber prosthesis. **1:** The guidewire, which was placed into the bile duct, is seen extending from the endoscope biopsy channel port. **2:** The guide catheter is advanced over the guidewire into the bile duct. **3, 4:** Tension is maintained on both so that the stent can be advanced over the assembly using the pusher catheter to push the stent into place.

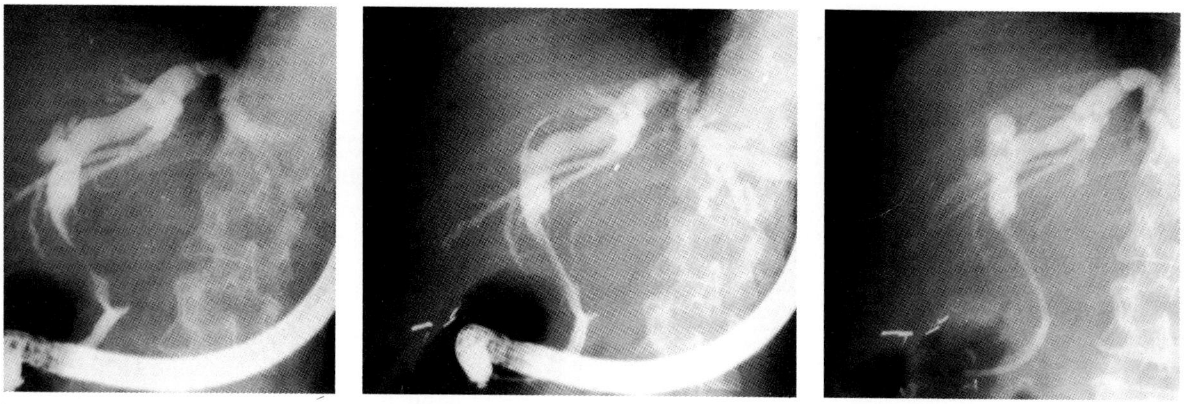

FIG. 12.11. The technique of advancing a medium-size prosthesis, in this case a 7Fr stent, through a stricture produced by cancer of the pancreas. **Left:** A stricture extending from the distal common bile duct to the mid-common hepatic duct. **Middle:** The guidewire and dilating catheter have been advanced into the proximal biliary tree. **Right:** After removal of the dilating catheter, the prosthesis is positioned. Once the prosthesis is positioned correctly for maximum function, the guidewire is removed while holding the pusher catheter in position to prevent movement of the stent.

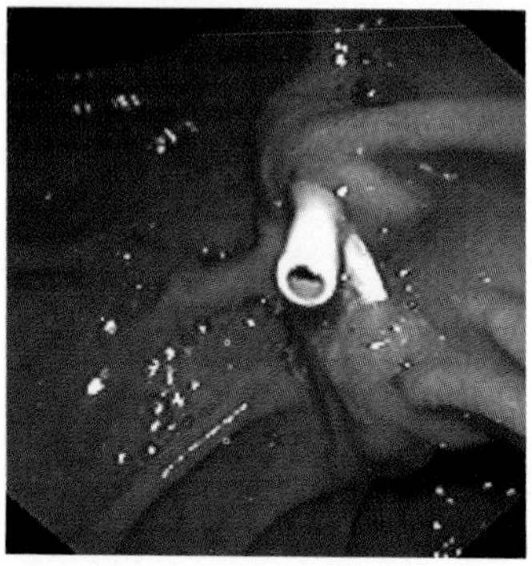

FIG. 12.12. This videoimage shows a 7Fr stent in a papilla that has not been sphincterotomized. It is not difficult to place medium-sized prostheses through an intact papilla. In fact, at times, because of restrictions (e.g., abnormal coagulation profile or patient's refusal to accept transfusions) a 10Fr prosthesis can be placed through an intact papilla. However, performing a sphincterotomy facilitates the placement of any size prosthesis, especially a large-caliber one.

made using the pushing catheter, and if the prosthesis is inserted too deeply, a biopsy forcep or snare can be used to capture the proximal end of the prosthesis and gently withdraw it into proper position. A series of videoendoscopic pictures of medium-sized prostheses is presented in Figs. 12.11 through 12.24. These images illustrate the many situations in which stents are used. Figures 12.25 through 12.33 are radiographs of ERCPs that illustrate obstruction of the biliary tree treated with medium-sized stents.

Large-Caliber Endoprostheses

Insertion of a large-caliber prosthesis, 10Fr and 12Fr, is performed in a similar manner except that the guidewire is contained within a 6Fr guiding catheter. This guiding catheter reduces the friction of the large-cali-
Text continues on page 287.

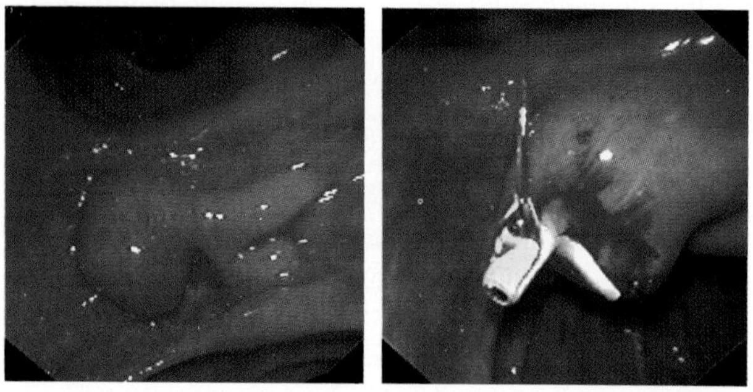

FIG. 12.13. Left: A bulging papilla with the opening dislocated inferiorly. **Right:** A small sphincterotomy is performed, a medium-sized prosthesis is placed into the bile duct. Note the presence of bile flowing from the distal opening.

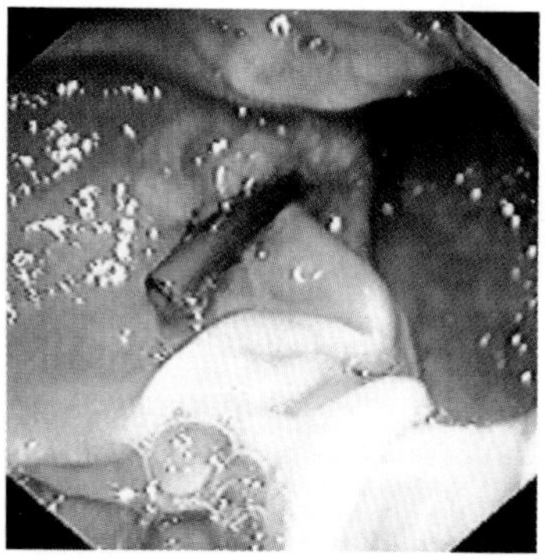

FIG. 12.14. A medium-sized prosthesis exiting from the papilla, which is located on the medial wall of a periampullary diverticulum.

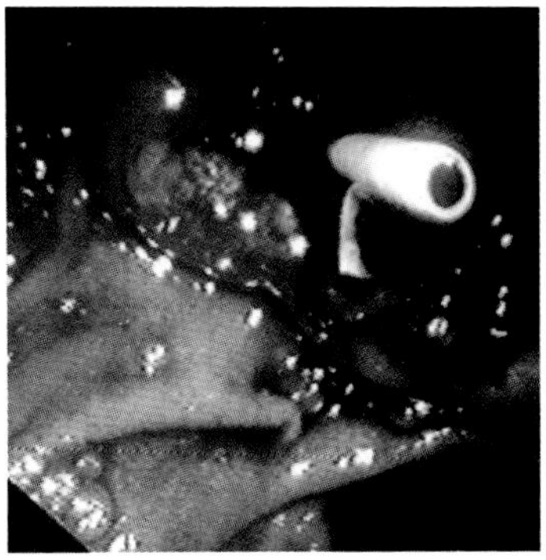

FIG. 12.15. This medium-sized prosthesis was placed into a bile duct obstructed by an ampullary carcinoma. Note the edges of the sphincterotomy and the copius amounts of dark bile flowing through the side opening created by the retaining flap.

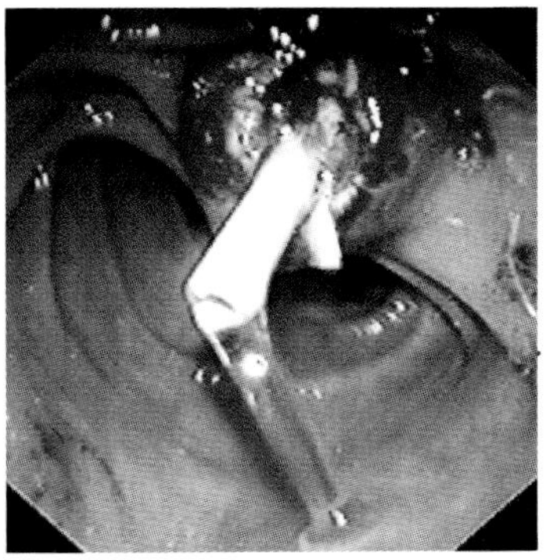

FIG. 12.16. A sphincterotomy has been performed in the papilla, and a medium-sized stent has been placed. A stream of clear fluid is pouring through the distal stent opening.

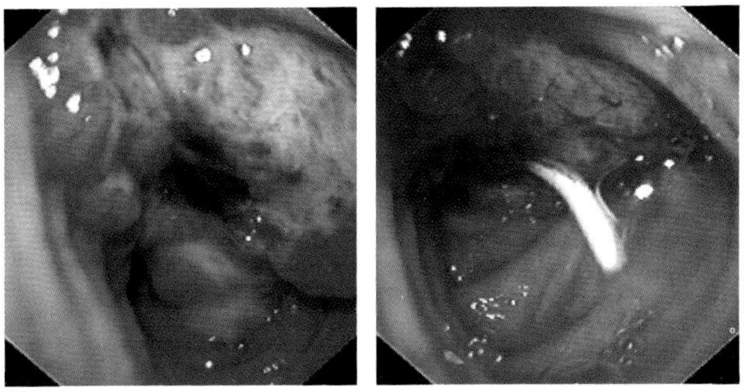

FIG. 12.17. **Left:** An invasive carcinoma of the pancreas partially obstructing the duodenal lumen. **Right:** A small sphincterotomy was created and a medium-sized stent was placed through the obstruction into the bile duct. A large-caliber prosthesis could not be placed because the large-channel endoscope could not be advanced into the duodenum.

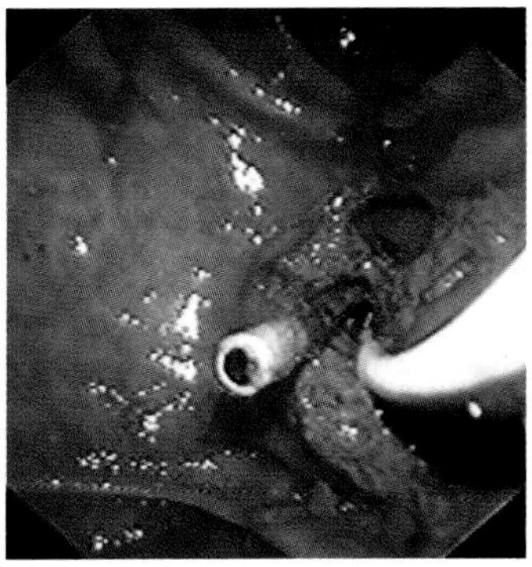

FIG. 12.18. A stent in place with stone sludge being extracted by a balloon and the white catheter to the right of the stent.

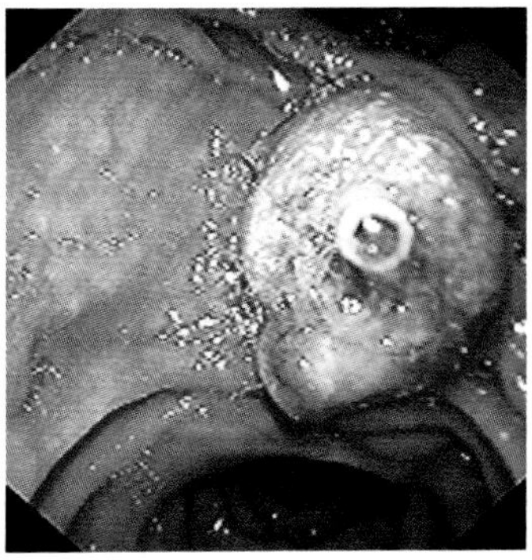

FIG. 12.19. A functioning prosthesis that is in place through an ampullary carcinoma.

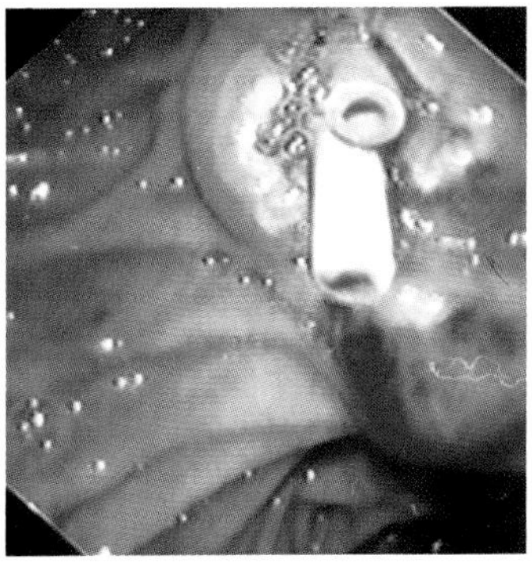

FIG. 12.20. Two prostheses are in place in a papilla after the performance of a sphincterotomy. In general, I use two prostheses when the common hepatic duct is affected and requires selective drainage of both major hepatic ducts.

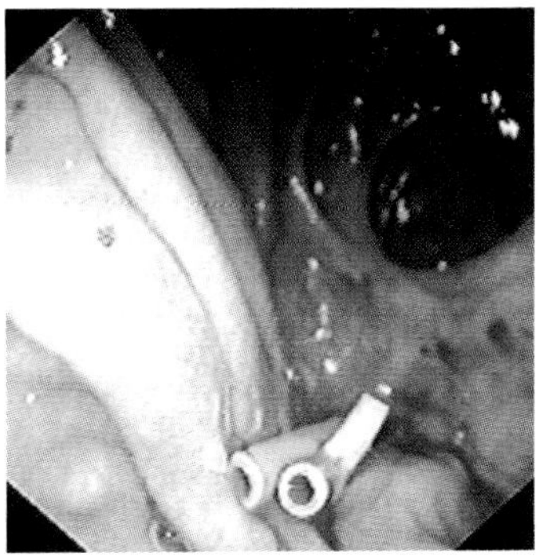

FIG. 12.21. Two prostheses. The papilla is located proximally in the duodenum, and this image shows the retroflexed endoscope in the distance.

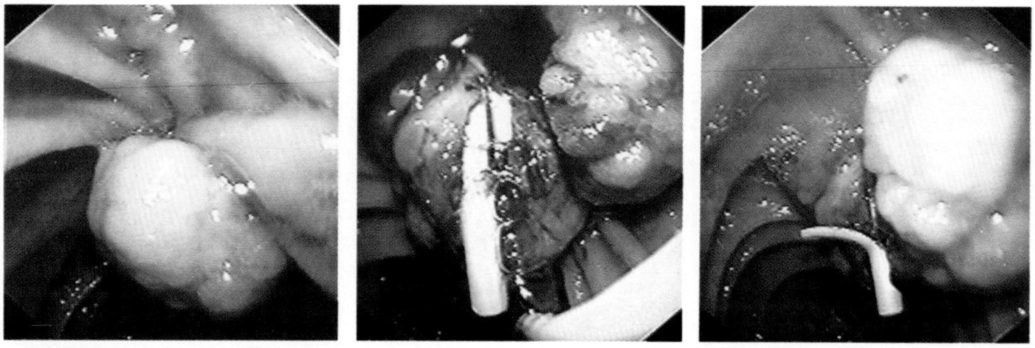

FIG. 12.22. Left: An obstructing ampullary carcinoma. **Center:** Two prostheses have been placed through a sphincterotomy that has been made in the lesion. **Right:** Only a single prosthesis is visible because the shorter prosthesis of the two is hidden by the mass.

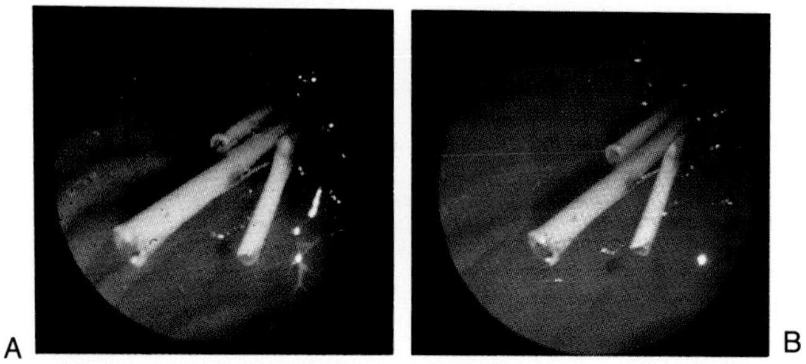

FIG. 12.23. A & B: These endoscopic photographs demonstrate the capability of placing three prostheses into the biliary tree for selective drainage and decompression.

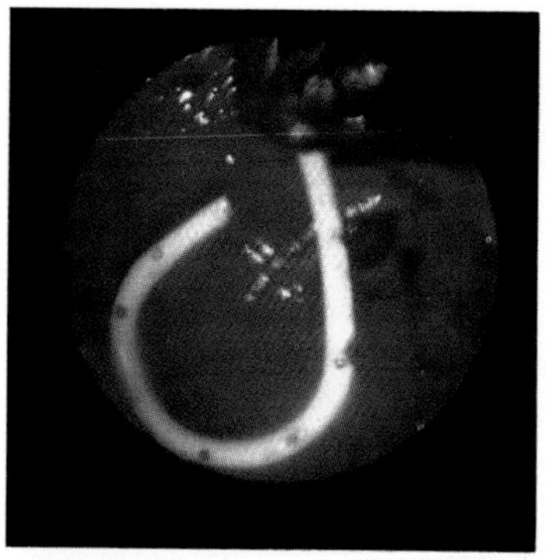

FIG. 12.24. An endoscopic photograph of a pigtail prosthesis. Note the correct placement of the pigtail in the duodenum.

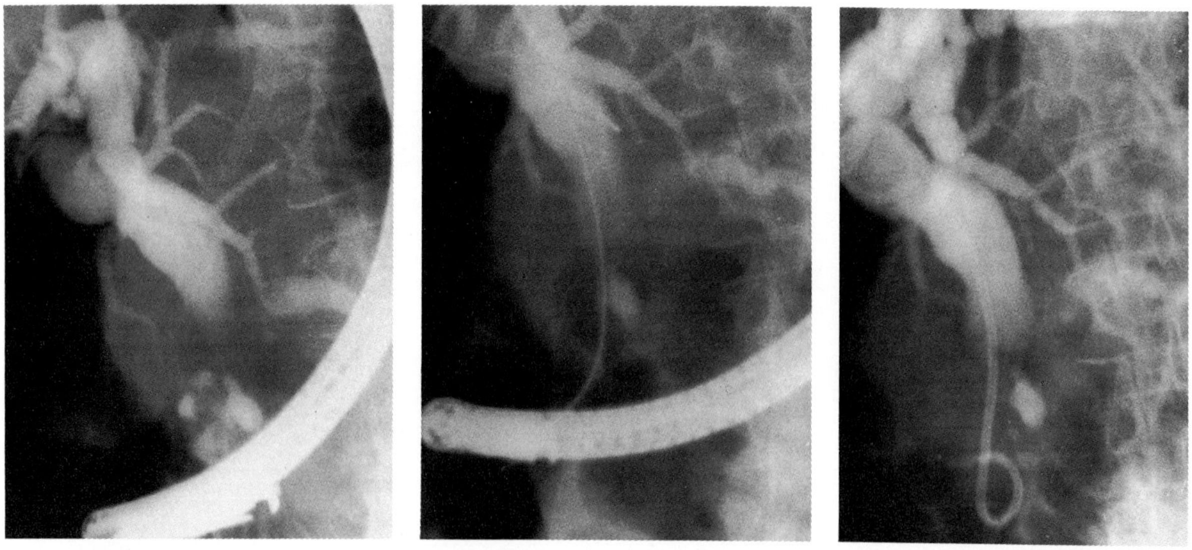

FIG. 12.25. Left: A stricture of the distal common bile duct and incomplete filling of the pancreatic duct, but with dilatation of that duct confirmed. These findings are consistent with carcinoma of the pancreas. **Middle:** A catheter-guidewire assembly has been advanced through the sphincter and distal stricture into the proximal biliary tree. **Right:** A double pigtail catheter is seen in position providing drainage to the obstructed system.

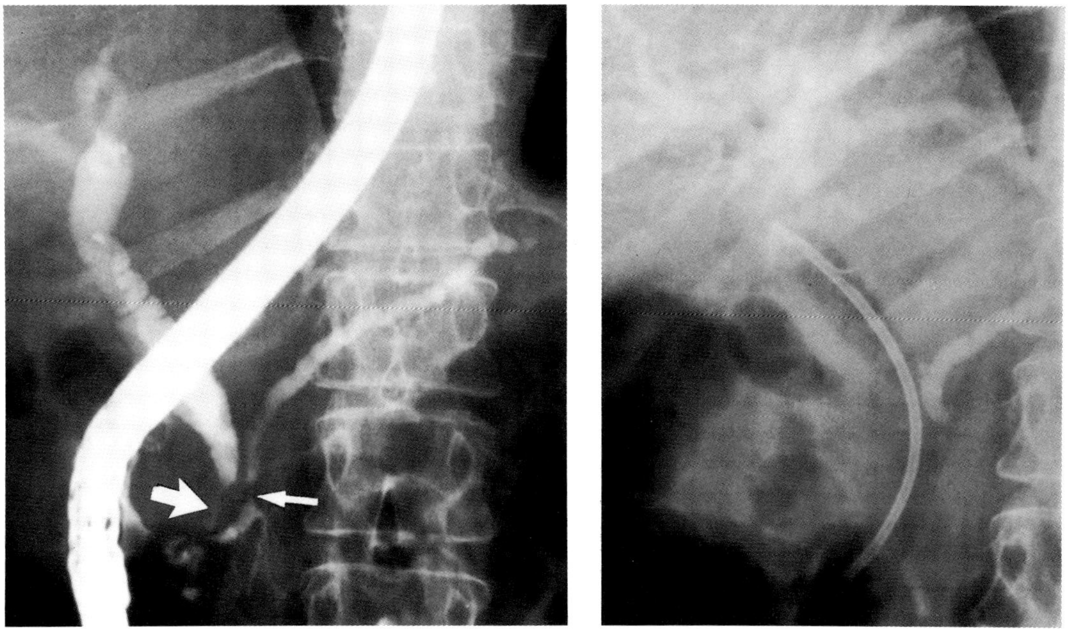

FIG. 12.26. **Left:** A small lesion in the head of the pancreas involving both the pancreatic (*small arrow*) and bile duct (*large arrow*). **Right:** A 7Fr stent is shown in position in the bile duct. Air in the biliary tree indicates that a sphincterotomy has been performed.

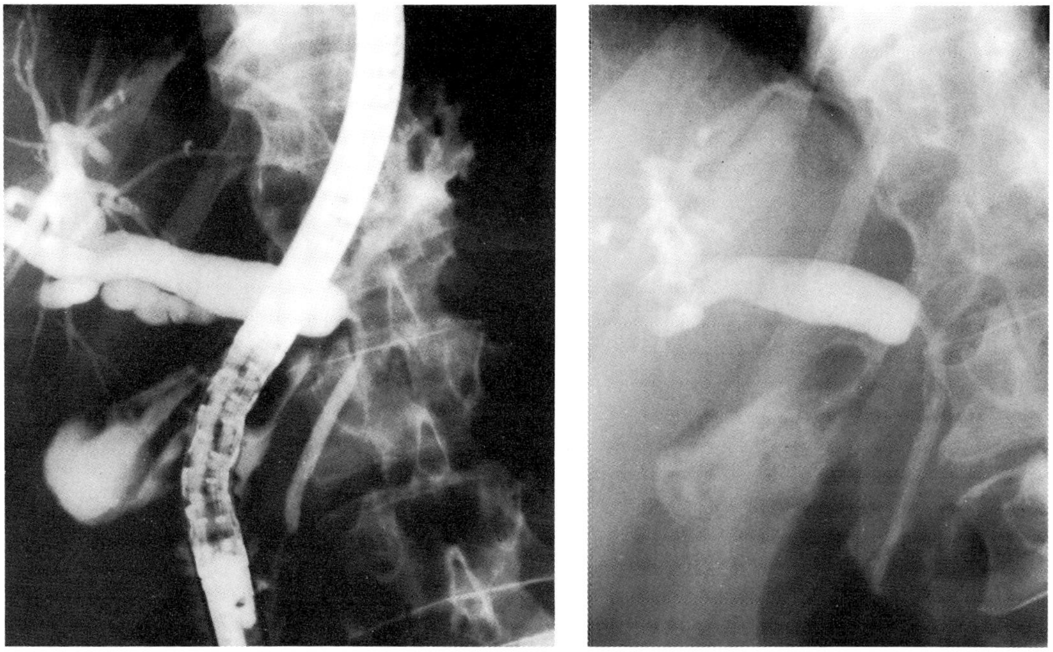

FIG. 12.27. **Left:** A long stricture of the distal common bile duct. **Right:** A 7Fr stent was placed through the stricture.

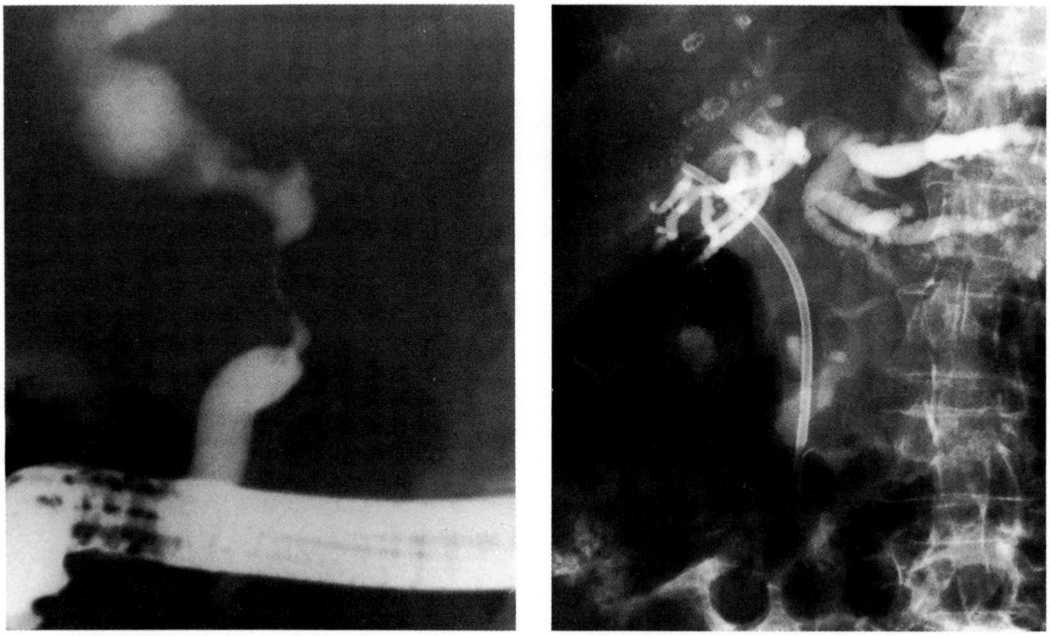

FIG. 12.28. Left: A long, irregular stricture, probably from either a pancreatic lesion with local extension or a cholangiocarcinoma. **Right:** A long 7Fr stent has been placed for decompression. Note the dilated intrahepatic ducts not seen on the close-up on the left.

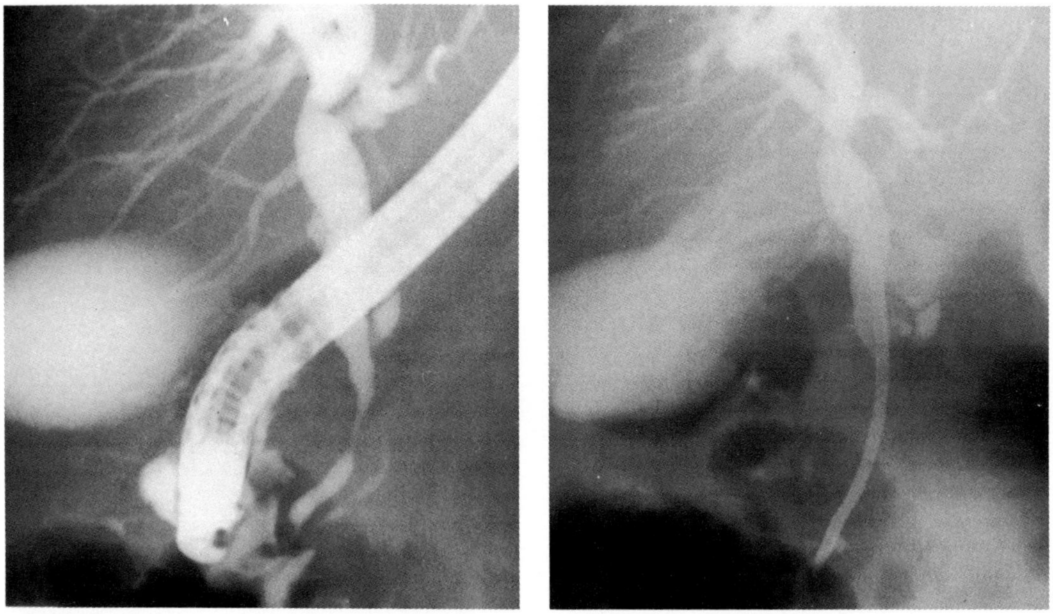

FIG. 12.29. Left: Another example of a pancreatic carcinoma extending into the distal bile duct. **Right:** A medium size stent.

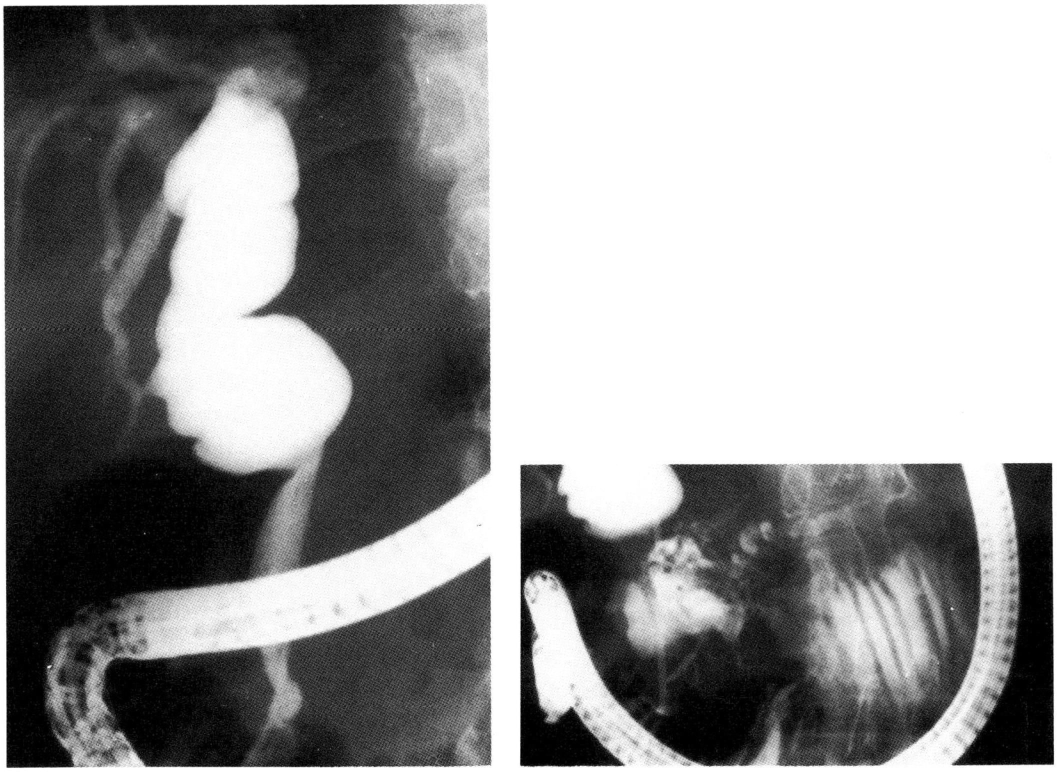

FIG. 12.30. Left: A markedly dilated proximal biliary tree and a long, narrow segment of the distal common duct. **Right:** A cystic lesion of the pancreas proved to be cystadenocarcinoma. The bile duct was temporarily drained before surgery with an 8Fr stent, shown extending from the dilated bile duct through the cystic mass.

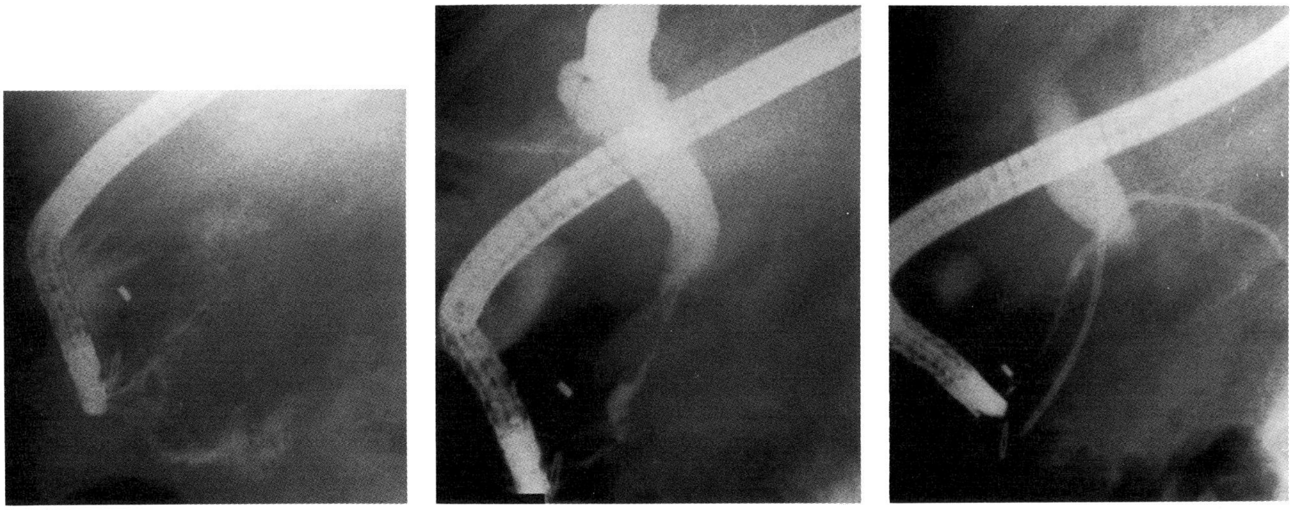

FIG. 12.31. Left: The ventral duct of a pancreas divisum. Note the branching, which is a classical finding for pancreas divisum. **Middle:** A stricture of the distal common bile duct is compatible with carcinoma. **Right:** A 7Fr stent extends from the bile duct; contrast has already drained from the biliary tree. Opacification of the dorsal pancreatic duct shows a stricture of the duct in the head of the gland and represents the primary lesion.

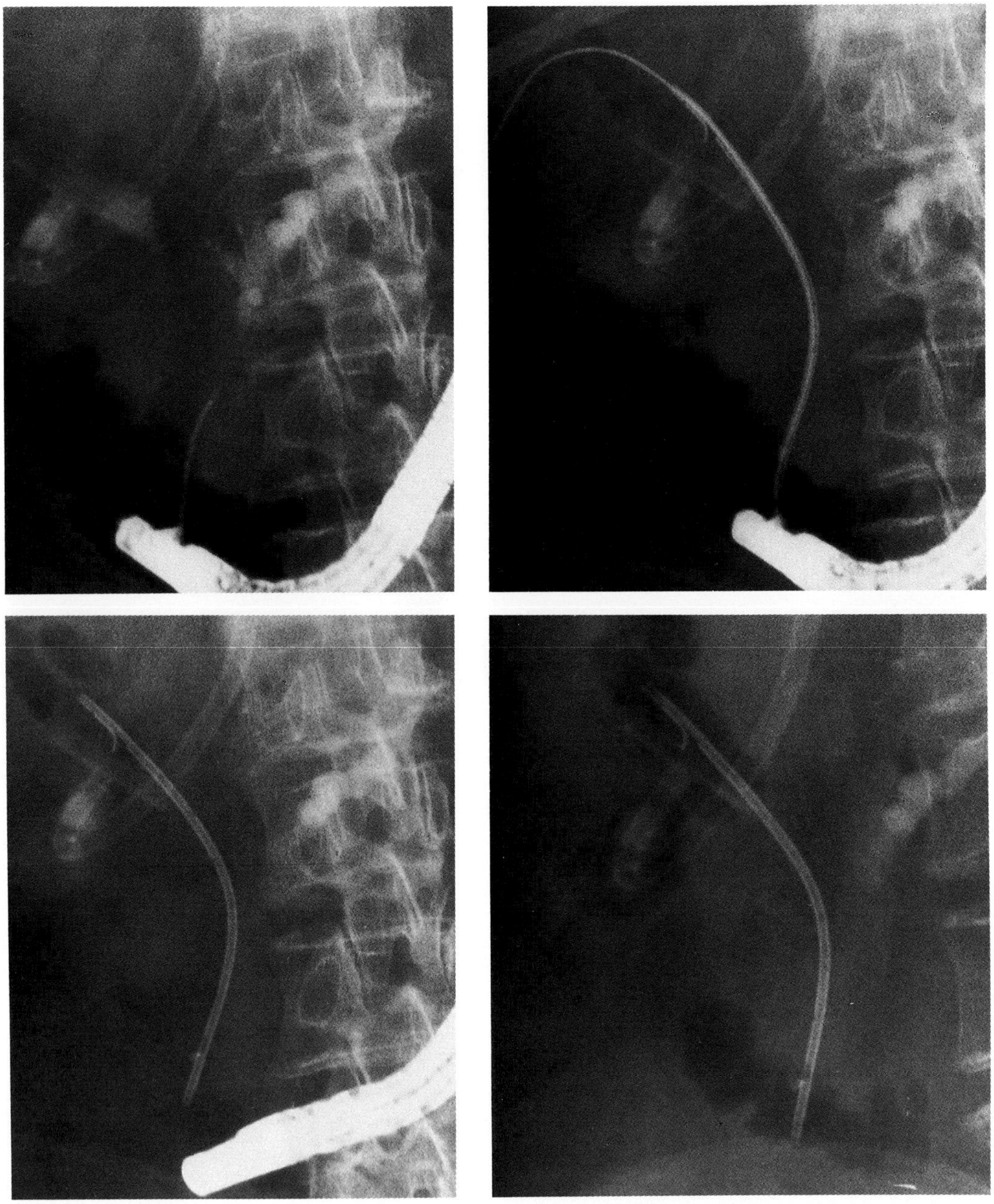

FIG. 12.32. This four-picture series describes the placement of a prosthesis into the bile duct of a patient, who had previously undergone a Bilroth II gastric resection, for decompression of an obstructed system secondary to carcinoma of the pancreas. **Top left:** A T-tube is visible at the top and the endoscope at the bottom in the reversed position because of the gastrectomy. A catheter extending from the endoscope facilitated cannulation of the pancreatic duct. The pancreatic duct is tortuous and dilated and a stricture is noted near the catheter tip. **Top right:** A guidewire in the right hepatic duct system and a 7Fr prosthesis being placed into the bile duct. **Bottom left:** The guidewire has been removed. **Bottom right:** The stent is correctly positioned, and the endoscope has been removed. Note the presence of contrast in the pancreatic duct throughout the procedure.

FIG. 12.34. The method employed for placing a large caliber stent, 10Fr or 12Fr. **A:** A distal lesion of the pancreas encroaching upon the bile duct, producing obstruction to the biliary tree. After dilating the stricture with a catheter or balloon, a guide catheter and guidewire are advanced through the sphincterotomy and stricture into the proximal bile duct. **B:** With the guide catheter and guidewire in place, the large-caliber prosthesis is pushed through the stricture into position. The pusher catheter is seen exiting the endoscope abutting the stent. **C:** The guide catheter, wire, and endoscope are removed, leaving the stent in position.

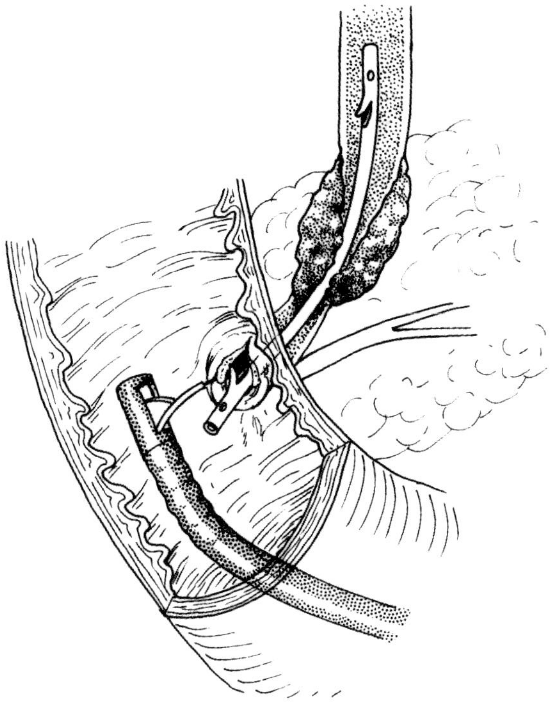

FIG. 12.33. The technique for performing a sphincterotomy in a patient who has previously undergone a Billroth II gastric resection. This technique was employed in Fig. 12.32. After a prosthesis is placed, especially if a Billroth II sphincterotome could not be placed, a needle-knife sphincterotome is used to cut down onto the prosthesis, creating a substantial sphincterotomy and avoiding potential complications such as perforation and pancreatitis.

Text continued from page 280.
ber prosthesis and facilitates advancement of the prosthesis with minimal resistance (Fig. 12.34) (47–49). A similar system is used when inserting 14Fr and 15Fr prostheses, but these stents, which are used infrequently, require a 5.5 mm channel instrument. The more commonly used endoscope for inserting 10Fr and 12Fr prostheses is the 4.2 mm channel endoscope, the TJF-1T20, and V-10, or V-100 (video). The catheter-guidewire assembly can be placed directly into the sphincterotomy and through the stricture into the proximal biliary tree, where it should be anchored (Fig. 12.34A). If the guidewire has been previously placed through a cannula or dilating catheter, the guiding catheter can be advanced over the guidewire similar to placement of a nasobiliary catheter. Once the guidewire and guiding catheter are in position, the appropriate large-caliber prosthesis is advanced over this assembly using a 10Fr pusher catheter (Fig. 12.34B). Gentle traction on the guidewire, and in this instance, the guiding catheter, permits easier advancement of the prosthesis and avoids looping in the duodenum as well as dislodgment of the assembly from the bile duct. When the prosthesis is in view in the duodenum, the endoscope should be placed as close to the sphincterotomy as possible to avoid looping of the guidewire-catheter assembly and prosthesis. Traction exerted by the assistant and intermittent pushing of the prosthesis by the endoscopist with alternate lifting of the elevator to anchor the prosthesis will permit insertion of the

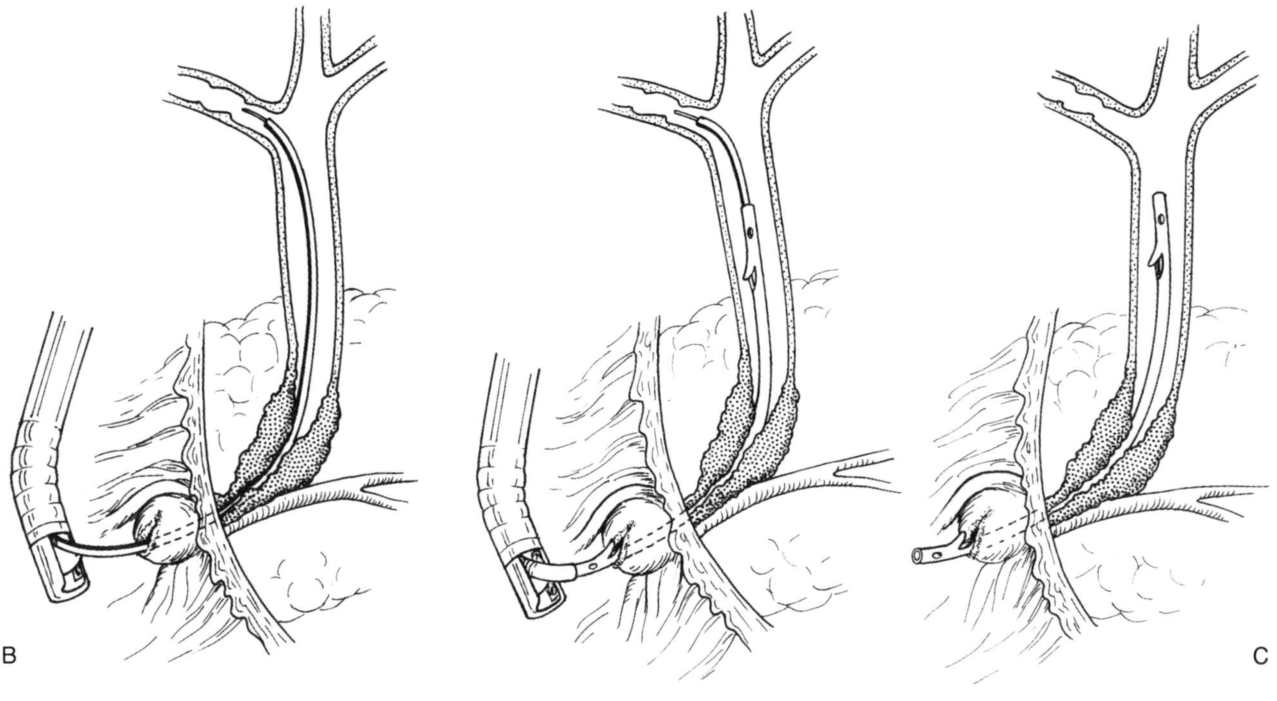

A,B

C

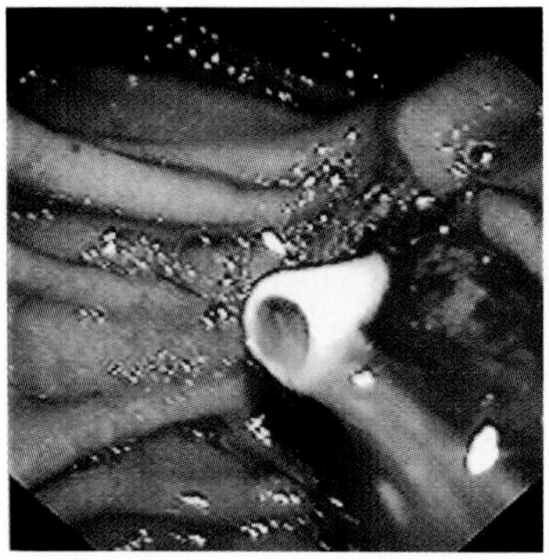

FIG. 12.35. A large-caliber prosthesis shortly after placement, illustrating the free flow of bile into the duodenum.

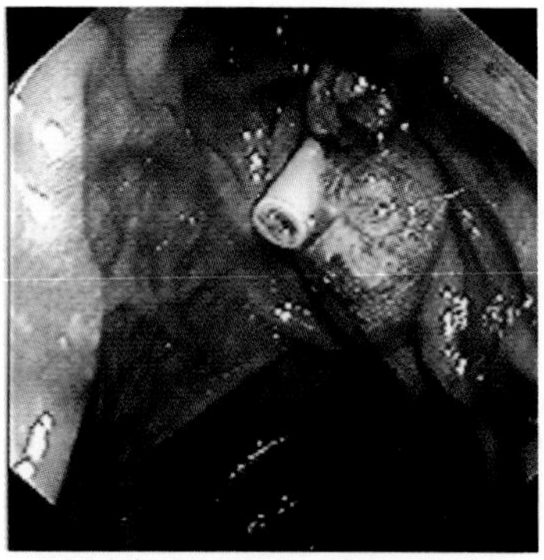

FIG. 12.36. A large-caliber prosthesis that has been in place for at least 4 weeks. This patient has sclerosing cholangitis and has been treated intermittently with stents. The hyperplastic area adjacent to the stent has recently developed. Biopsies were negative for tumor.

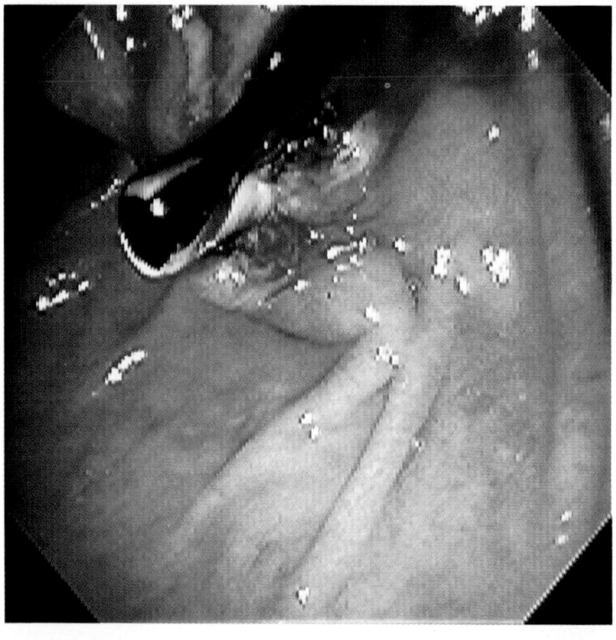

FIG. 12.37. The flow of dark bile from a large-caliber prosthesis into the duodenum shortly after separation of the guide catheter, guidewire, and pusher catheter.

prosthesis through the stricture and into the appropriate position. Again, the pushing catheter and prosthesis should have constrasting colors so that when the proximal end of the prosthesis is visualized, its color prevents the endoscopist from advancing the prosthesis too deeply into the bile duct (Fig. 12.34C). Once the guidewire and guiding catheter are removed and the pushing catheter is separated, a free flow of bile should be observed, especially if the prosthesis is placed into a dilated biliary tree that is filled with both

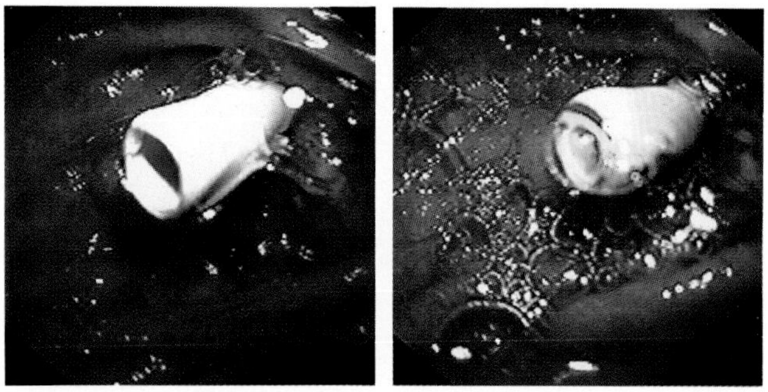

FIG. 12.38. **Left:** The large-caliber prosthesis immediately after separation from the pusher. **Right:** The flow of bile.

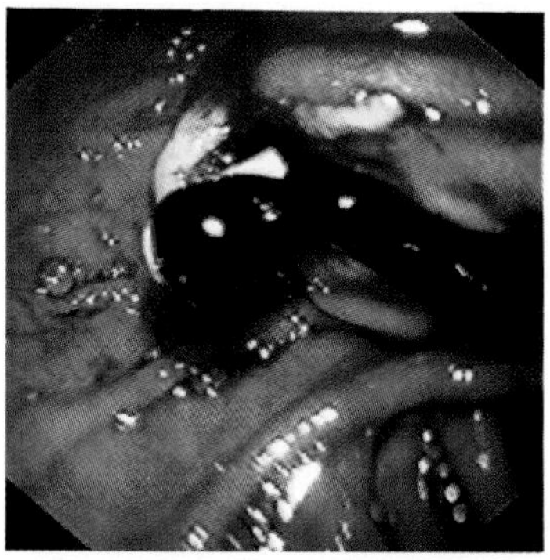

FIG. 12.39. The heavy flow of dark bile, which has been held under pressure, secondary to obstruction.

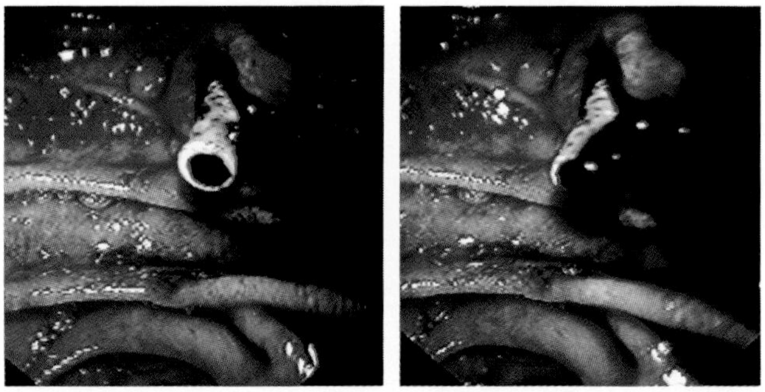

FIG. 12.40. The high rate of flow of bile seen immediately after placement of a large caliber prosthesis. **Left:** Bile begins to flow into the duodenum. **Right:** During observation, the visual field is almost obliterated by the large volume of bile entering the duodenum.

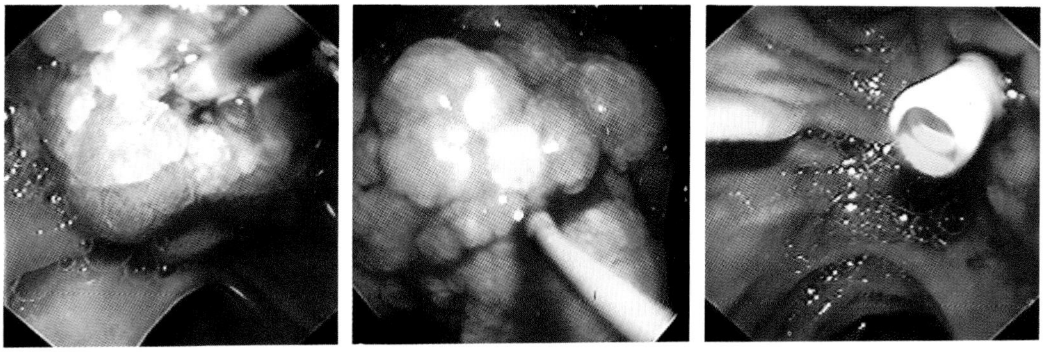

FIG. 12.41. Placement of a prosthesis when the bile duct orifice is nearly totally obliterated by an ampullary tumor. **Left:** The cannula is placed into the bile duct orifice. **Center:** Following the performance of a sphincterotomy, the guidewire is placed. **Right:** The stent is inserted. The stent is visualized beneath the mass.

bile and contrast (Figs. 12.35–12.45). Figures 12.46 through 12.56 are radiographs obtained at ERCP that demonstrate insertion of large-caliber prostheses in patients with distal obstruction of the bile duct. Figure 12.47 is presented for historical purposes. I initially used pigtails that were available in the angiography special procedures room in the radiology department. Endoprostheses were not commercially available when endoscopists began inserting stents, and we utilized materials that were available. The FDA had not approved some endoscopic devices, and, because stents were considered devices, special approval was necessary before manufacturers could produce stents for general use. This prohibition was ultimately circumvented because these devices were not considered

Text continues on page 293.

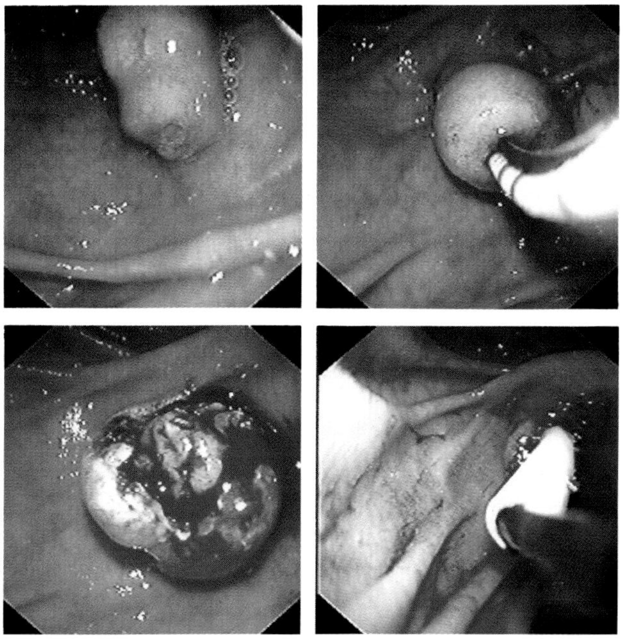

FIG. 12.42. This series of videoimages is important because it demonstrates the full range of therapeutic maneuvers that may be necessary to reveal an obstructing lesion of the bile duct that was not identified or confirmed until a sphincterotomy was performed. **Top left:** A bulging papilla. **Top right:** The sphincterotome is placed. **Bottom left:** The sphincterotomy is completed. Note the mass filling the ampulla which was adenocarcinoma on biopsy. **Bottom right:** A large-caliber stent was placed, and a steady stream of bile and contrast flow into the duodenum.

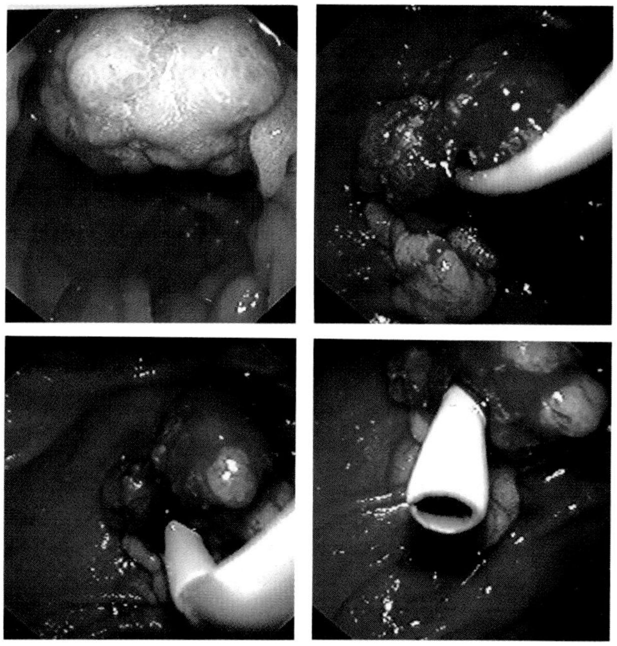

FIG. 12.43. Often the papilla is obscured by an ampullary mass and is difficult to localize. **Top left:** A large, nodular mass. **Top right:** The papillary orifice was identified and cannulated using a guidewire-catheter system. **Bottom left:** A wire-guided sphincterotome was used to open the papilla, and a large-caliber prosthesis is being pushed into place. The stent and pusher are different colors which helps to avoid pushing the stent in too deeply. **Bottom right:** The large-caliber prosthesis is in place.

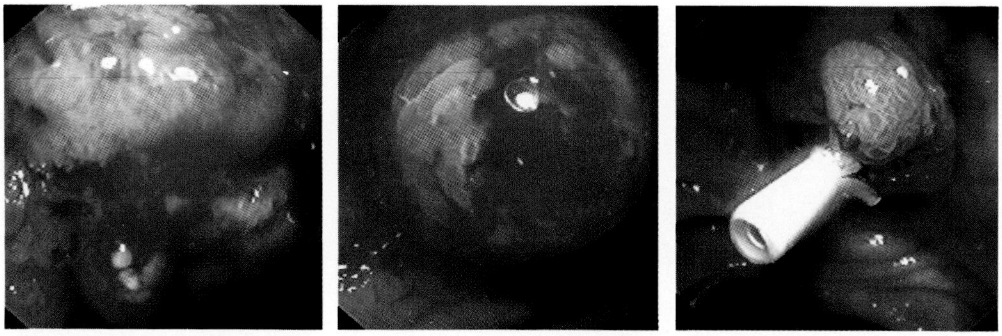

FIG. 12.44. An obscure papillary opening was localized after closely inspecting the papilla and the ampullary mass. **Left:** A friable nodular mass is partially occluding the lumen of the duodenum. **Middle:** Beneath the mass, the edematous, infiltrated papilla is visible. **Right:** A large-caliber stent has been placed after a sphincterotomy was performed.

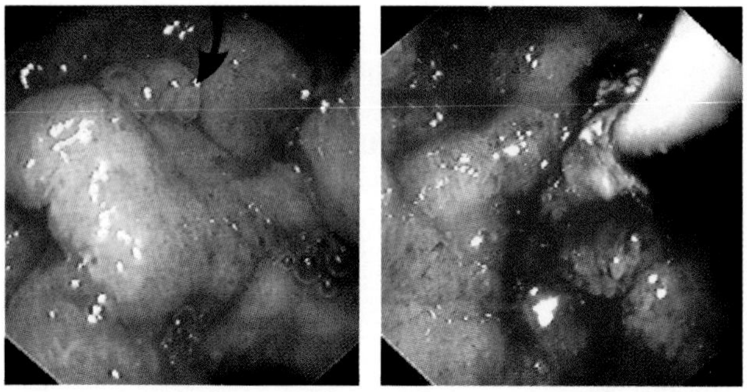

FIG. 12.45. Left: Again an obscured papilla is identified within a malignant mass (*arrow*). **Right:** A sphincterotomy was performed and a large-caliber prosthesis is being placed.

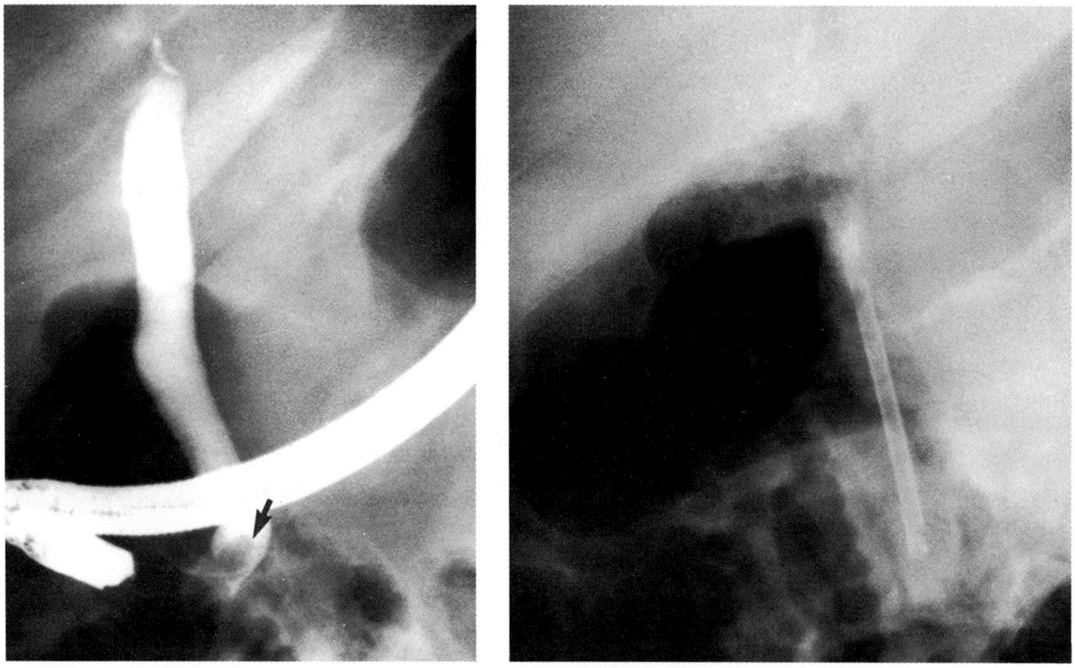

FIG. 12.46. Left: Distal obstruction of the bile duct. A filling defect seen (*arrow*) proved on biopsy to be an adenocarcinoma, either a periampullary or an ampullary carcinoma. **Right:** A 12Fr stent has been placed for drainage. Note that all contrast has drained from the bile duct.

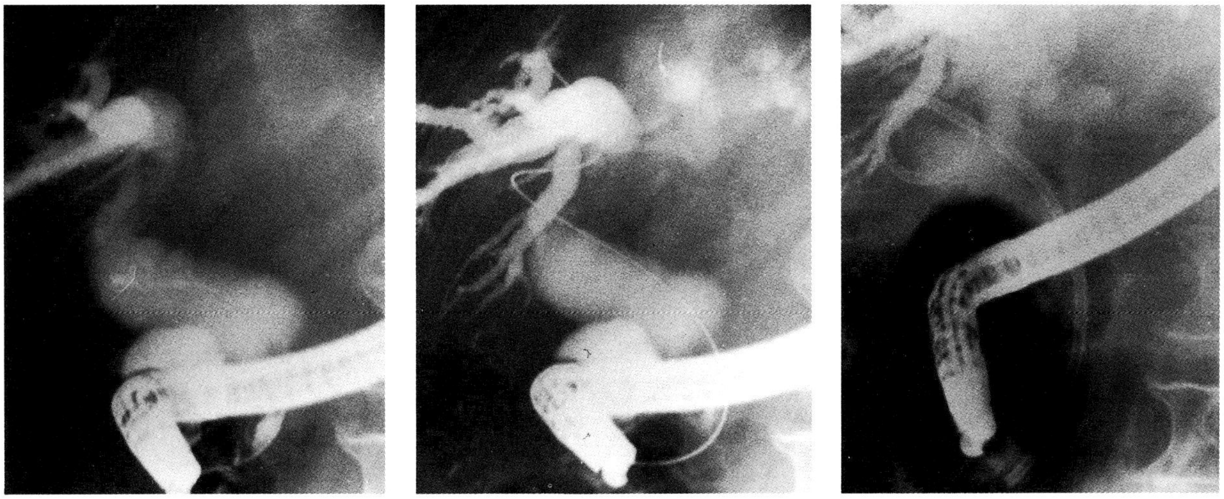

FIG. 12.47. Left: A high-grade stricture of the distal common bile duct (behind endoscope). **Middle:** A catheter-guidewire assembly is advanced through the stricture into the proximal biliary tree. **Right:** A large-caliber single-pigtail stent is visible in the bile duct.

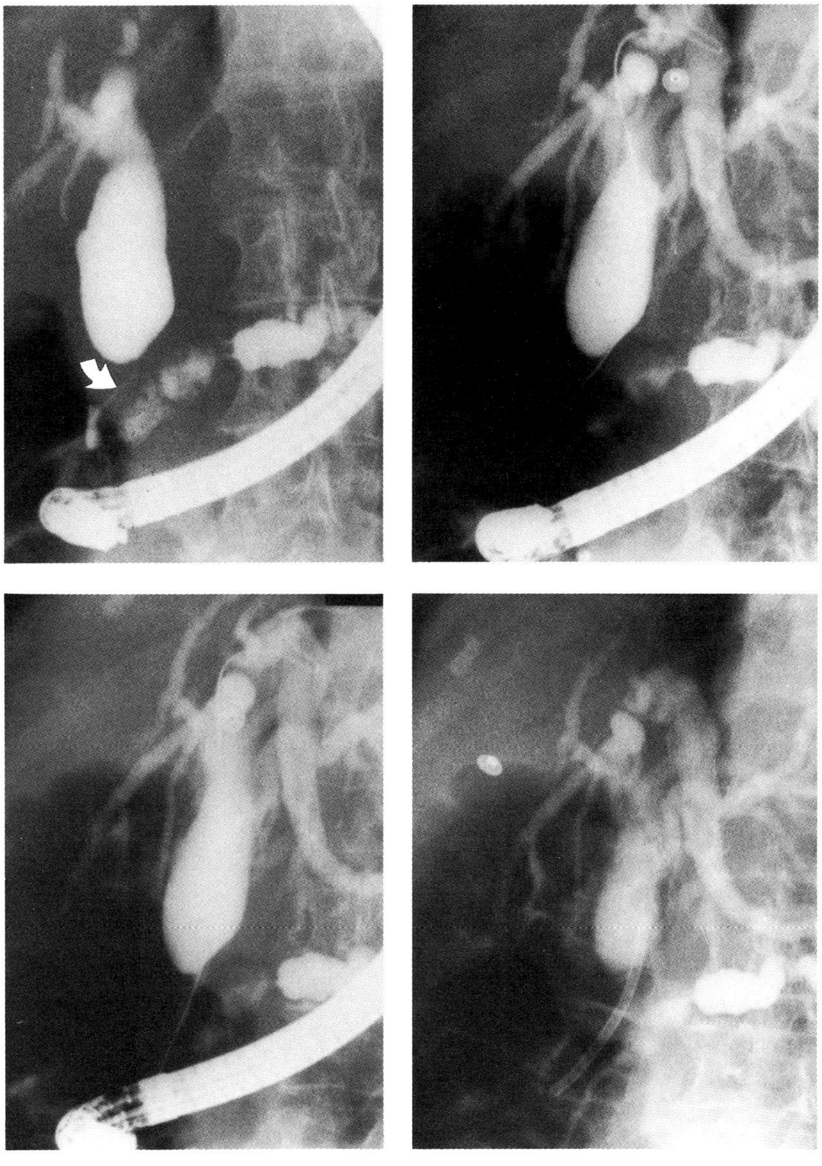

FIG. 12.48. Top left: Placement of a large-caliber prosthesis is accomplished despite the high-grade distal common bile duct stricture (*arrow*) secondary to carcinoma of the pancreas. Note the dilated pancreatic duct. **Top right:** A guidewire has passed through the stricture. **Bottom left:** A dilating catheter has advanced through the stricture. **Bottom right:** A large-caliber prosthesis is in place.

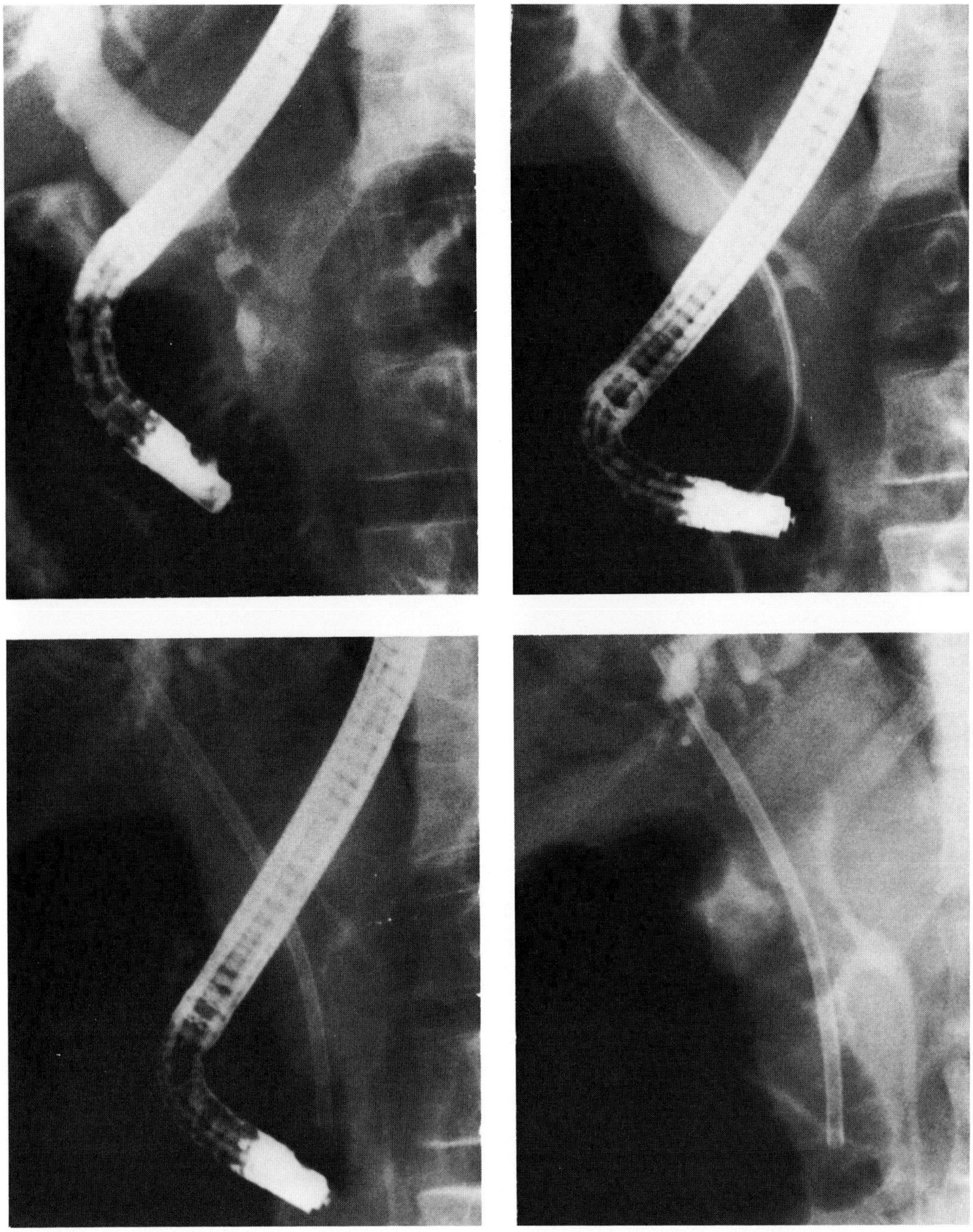

FIG. 12.49. Another example of the technique of placing a large-caliber prosthesis. **Top left:** A high-grade stricture secondary to carcinoma of the pancreas. **Top right:** A dilating catheter and guidewire are seen in the bile duct traversing the stricture. **Bottom left:** A large-caliber prosthesis is seen being placed within the bile duct. **Bottom right:** After removal of the endoscope, the prosthesis is visible in its proper position. Note that a pyelogram resulted from absorption of the contrast medium. This phenomenon was commented on in Chapter 2 and most likely results from absorption of contrast through the pancreatic parenchymal venous system. In this case, contrast was probably absorbed because of extravasation of the material through a neoplastic ductal rupture.

Text continued from page 289.
permanent and could be removed. The accessory manufacturers soon gained FDA approval, and stents were manufactured in all sizes and shapes. (Prior to the commercial availability of stents, we either "borrowed" pigtails from the special procedures room or made our own. I ordered polyethylene tubing in rolls of 7Fr, 8Fr, and 10Fr diameters, purchased pigtail formers and hole punchers, and made my own.) Subsequently, the Amsterdam group designed the straight configuration stent that I use exclusively for obstructive biliary disease, except stone disease. I then place pigtails as discussed in Chapter 10.

Expandable Mesh Stents

In our quest to place large prostheses that remain patent for longer periods or never occlude, the search for different materials continues. One of these prostheses, the expandable mesh stent, has recently been introduced. I have no personal experience using the wire mesh expandable stents. A special mechanism that contains the stent on a catheter is inserted through a standard duodenoscope. This mechanism is manipulated to release the stent when it has been placed into position in the bile duct and stricture. The stent then

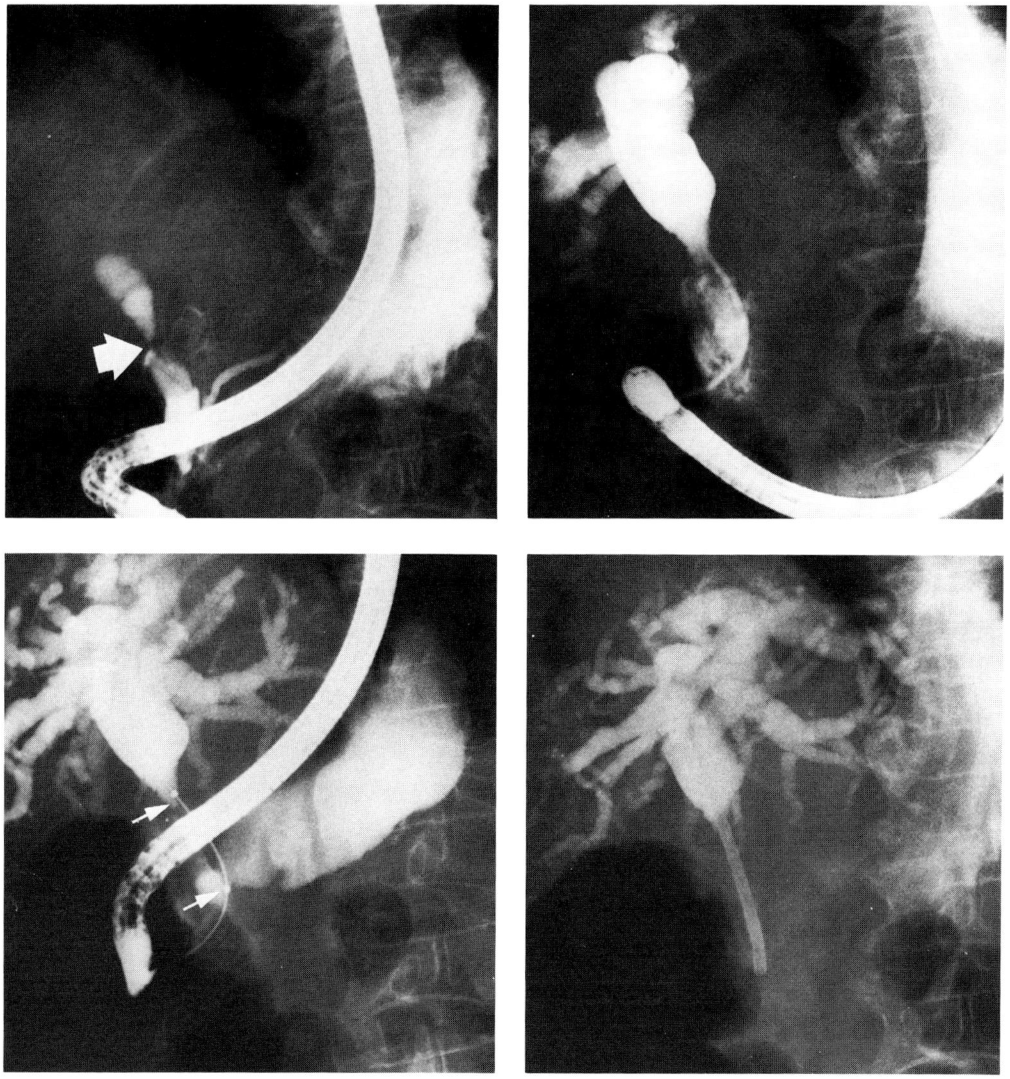

FIG. 12.50. In the next two series, prior to insertion of a large-caliber prosthesis, the technique of balloon dilatation of malignant strictures is illustrated. **Top left:** A high-grade malignant stricture (*arrow*). **Top right:** The stricture was traversed with a catheter-guidewire system, and the proximal biliary tree was entered and opacified, demonstrating a markedly dilated system. **Bottom left:** A balloon catheter has been placed, and its length and position are outlined by the arrows. **Bottom right:** The large-caliber prosthesis is in place through the strictures.

slowly expands to 1 cm over the course of 1 or 2 days, dilating the stricture. Most experience with this stent has been accumulated in Europe, and data are being collected to determine the stent's long-term effectiveness (50, 51).

In treating tumors the stent slowly occludes with tumor ingrowth of the neoplasm through the wire mesh. Because of the large diameter of the stent, a daughter endoscope can be inserted, and a laser can be used to recanalize the lumen. Alternatively, balloons can be inserted to dilate the occluded lumen.

In benign disease, if the stent occludes, is misplaced, or dislodges, it cannot be removed endoscopically; its removal requires surgery. Therefore, the indications are currently strict. The stent is mostly being used for malignant disease in patients not expected to survive long. The concept of this stent is exciting, however, and we hope to have the opportunity to use it soon.

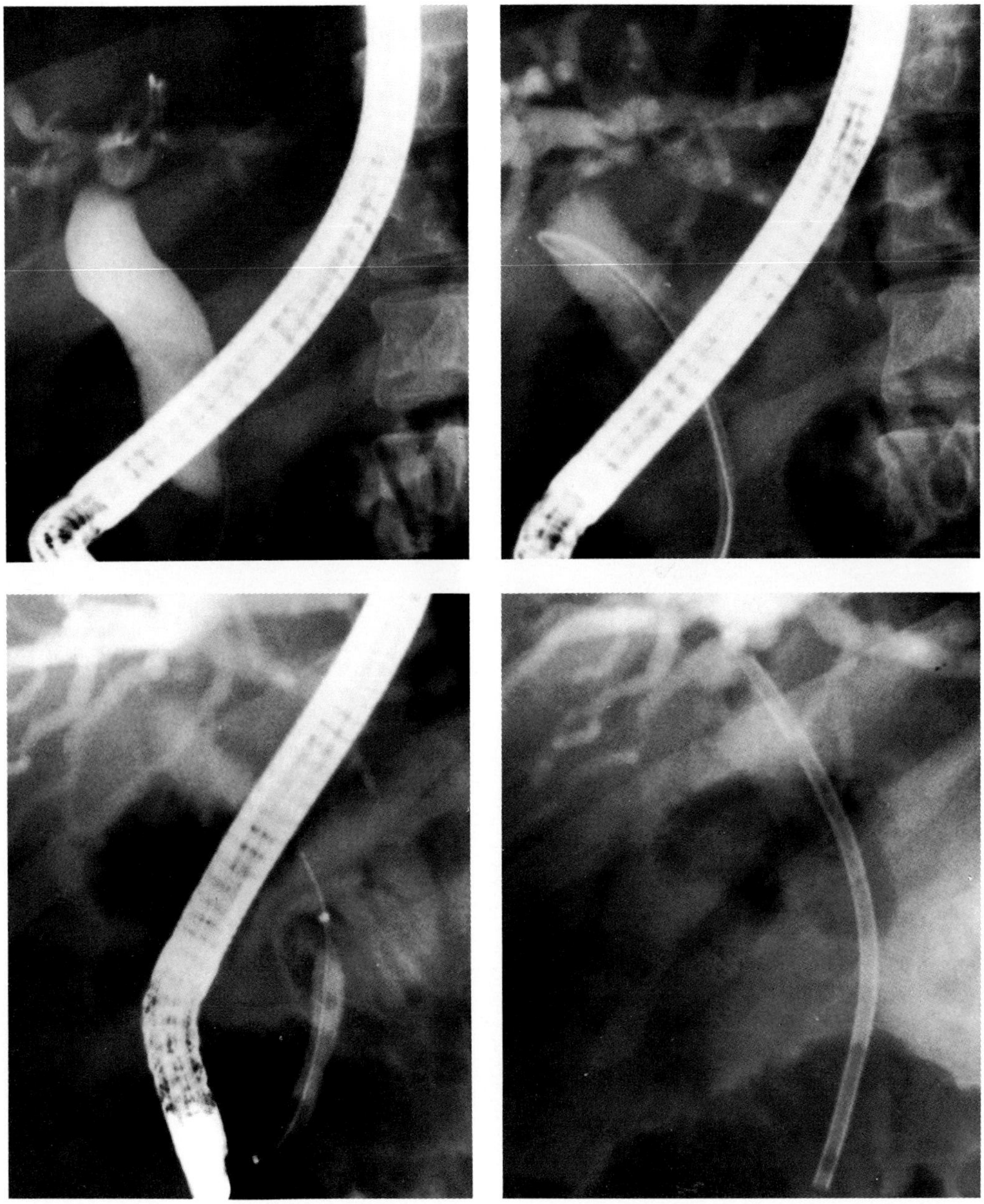

FIG. 12.51. Top left: A dilated biliary tree with a high-grade stricture seen affecting the distal common bile duct. **Top right:** A dilating catheter and guidewire. **Bottom left:** A balloon dilator is seen opacified with contrast material, dilating the stricture produced by carcinoma of the pancreas. **Bottom right:** The prosthesis in place. Most of the contrast has drained, and one can appreciate air in the bile duct secondary to a biliary enteric shunt created by the large-caliber prosthesis.

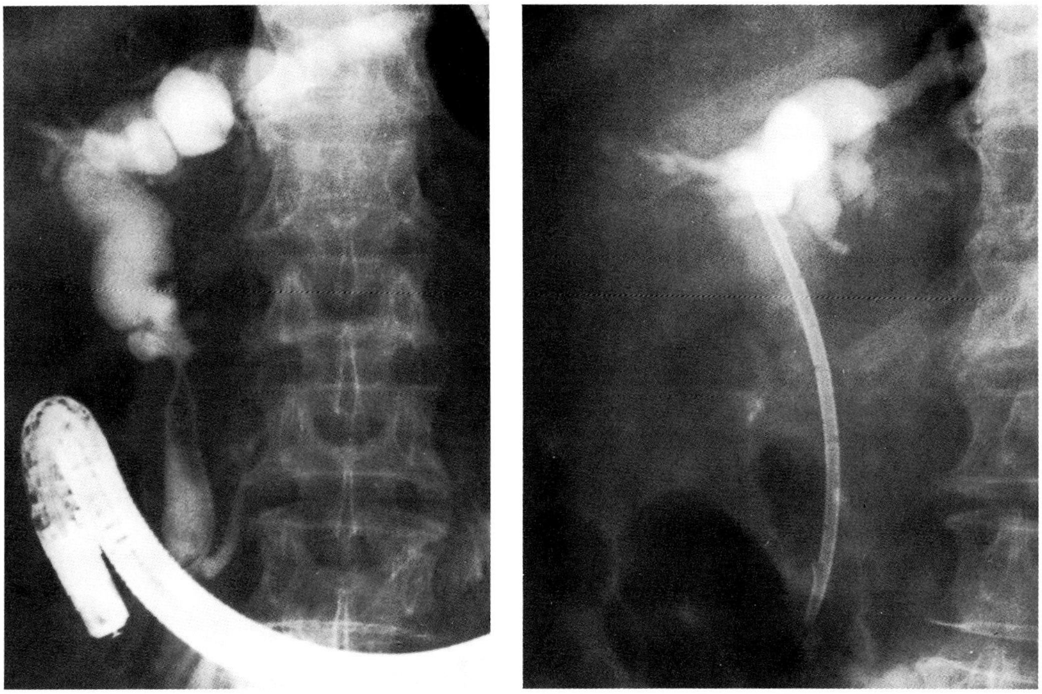

FIG. 12.52. Left: An obstructed pancreatic duct and a high-grade obstruction of the bile duct at the junction of the mid and lower bile duct. These findings are consistent with carcinoma of the pancreas. **Right:** A 10Fr prosthesis, which has a tapered tip and too many side holes. This configuration leads to earlier obstruction of the stent because of the diffusion or dissipation of flow through too many holes. Fewer holes permit a steadier flow of bile under greater pressure through the prosthesis, retarding a biofilm formation and prolonging patency.

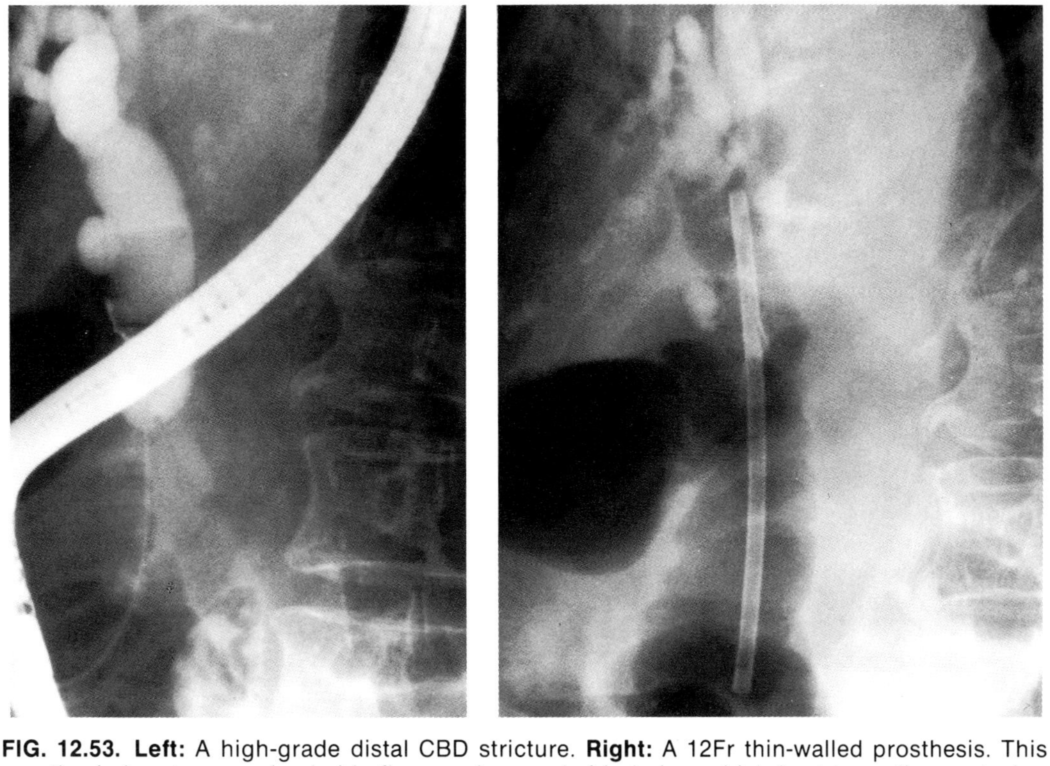

FIG. 12.53. Left: A high-grade distal CBD stricture. **Right:** A 12Fr thin-walled prosthesis. This prosthesis has two proximal side flaps and several side holes, which lead to earlier occlusion despite its large size. Again, fewer side holes permit flow of bile through the prosthesis under greater pressure, whereas too many holes dissipate the pressure, leading to earlier occlusion.

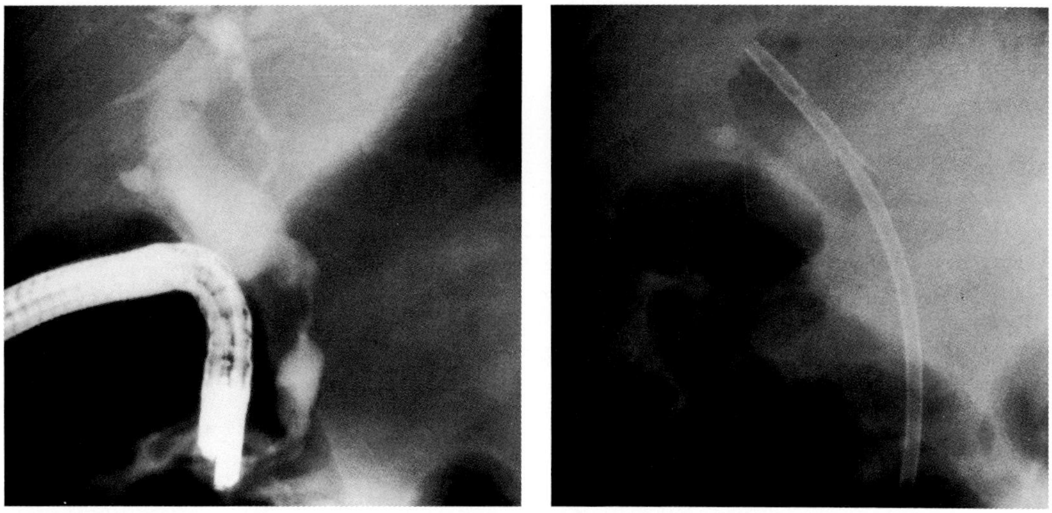

FIG. 12.54. Another example of the double-flap, double–side hole stent. **Left:** High-grade distal obstruction. **Right:** The stent. Despite the large diameter of the stent, it is soft enough to conform to the bile duct wall, which curves laterally.

Large-Caliber Prosthesis Insertion—Alternate Techniques

A procedure that is gaining popularity, the "rendezvous" procedure (52–55), is being performed more frequently because of the numbers of experienced interventional radiologists and less experienced endoscopists. The so-called rendezvous procedure is instituted by the radiologist, who performs a percutaneous cholangiogram and advances a guidewire into the duodenum. The endoscopist then passes an endoscope into the duodenum, captures the wire with a snare or basket, and pulls the wire out either through the mouth or through the endoscope. The patient is ostensibly impaled on the wire; in other words, the wire enters the patient's body through the right flank, is passed through the liver into the bile duct, and is passed out into the duodenum, where it is captured by

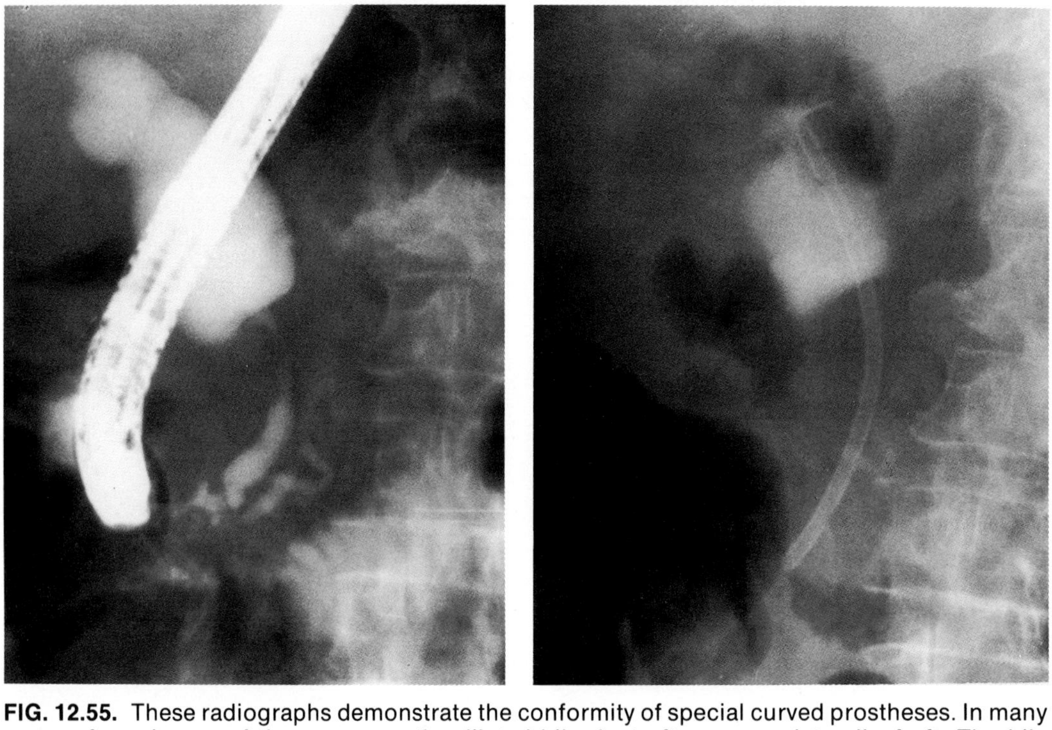

FIG. 12.55. These radiographs demonstrate the conformity of special curved prostheses. In many cases of carcinoma of the pancreas, the dilated bile duct often curves laterally. **Left:** The bile duct curves laterally as it becomes more dilated, and the large-caliber prosthesis conforms to this deviation. **Right:** Precurved stents can be procured from the manufacturer.

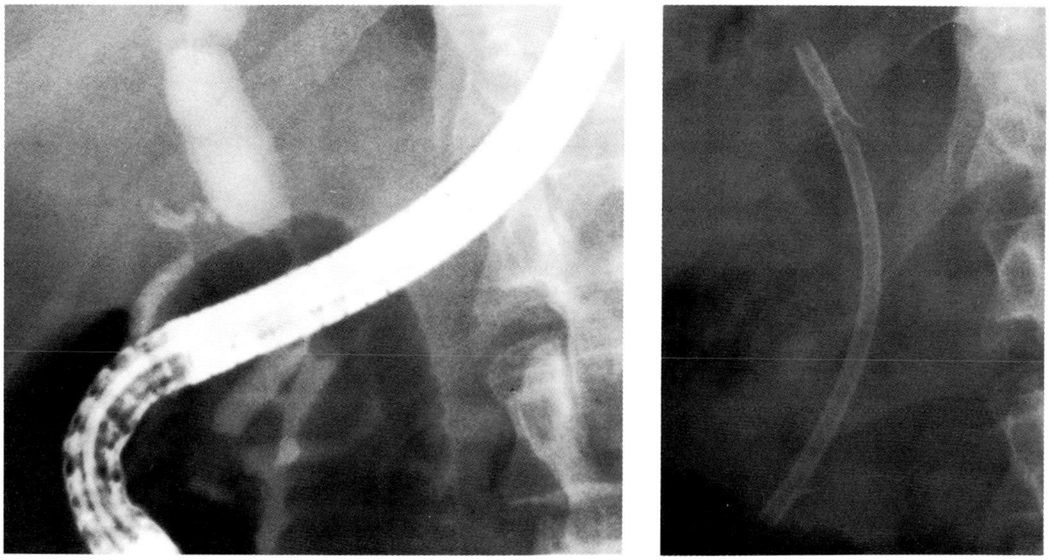

FIG. 12.56. Left: A stricture of the distal common bile duct. The proximal duct curves laterally. **Right:** A large-caliber prosthesis conforms to the curves of the bile duct.

the endoscopist. After retrieval the wire is pulled out the stomach and esophagus and exits through the mouth. Once the wire is in position, a large-caliber prosthesis can be advanced over this wire into the bile duct. Placement of the stent using this technique is inaccurate. Because the procedure is usually monitored fluoroscopically and not endoscopically, one may need to reinsert the endoscope to confirm its position. The patient is most uncomfortable while impaled, especially while tension is placed on the wire to facilitate passage of the stent.

The advantages of this procedure are indirectly economic for the endoscopist or the hospital because the purchase of a large-channel endoscope is obviated. Because the stent can be advanced over the guidewire (onto which the patient is impaled), a larger channel endoscope is not required. This approach is limiting. The endoscopist must always work in tandem with a radiologist in order to place a large-caliber stent, so the endoscopist loses his or her independence and does not gain valuable experience with the larger endoscope.

The disadvantages include greater patient discomfort; increased complications—those associated with percutaneous transhepatic procedures (28); and the lack of experience in developing ERCP and stent insertion skills.

I have found that the need for percutaneous cholangiography has decreased with time and that a combined approach may be necessary for about 7% of patients. In fact, I have replaced percutaneous stents endoscopically without performing a rendezvous because of recurrent infection and pain and the inability of the patient or attendant to manage the hardware. Figures 12.57 through 12.61 illustrate the endoscopic conversion of percutaneous stents to large-caliber endoprostheses accomplished in a standard fashion without performing the rendezvous procedure.

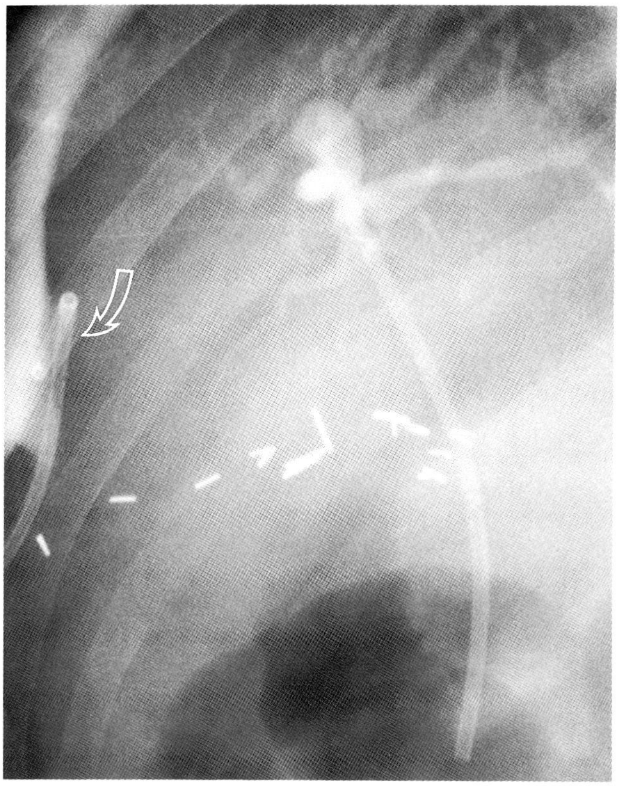

FIG. 12.57. A large-caliber endoprosthesis in position in the bile duct. A percutaneous catheter (*arrow*) had been inserted for decompression but became dislodged, migrating to the right upper quadrant outside the liver capsule. Contrast material can be seen outlining the liver. Internal drainage was reestablished with the endoprosthesis.

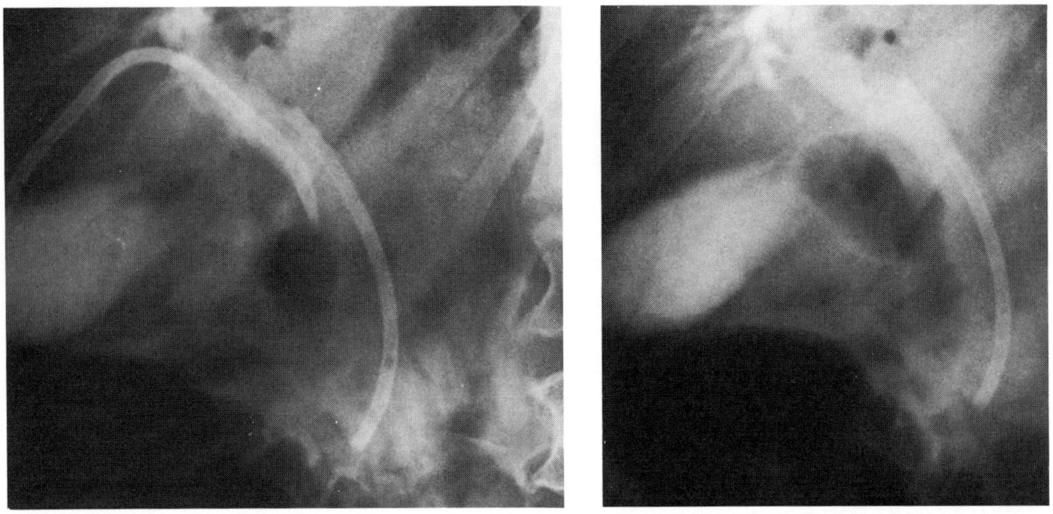

FIG. 12.58. Left: This percutaneous stent was being replaced because the patient experienced recurrent fever, continuous pain, and pain on respiration. A comparable-sized endoprosthesis was advanced into the bile duct after the endoscopist performed a sphincterotomy and placed a guide catheter and guidewire into the biliary tree. This radiograph shows the percutaneous stent being withdrawn after the endoprosthesis was placed. **Right:** The percutaneous stent has been removed, and the internal stent remains.

Other Large-Caliber Prostheses and Use of a Special Guidewire

A system for placing larger caliber prostheses, 15Fr and 24Fr, was introduced in Germany several years ago by Kautz (56). A colleague and I subsequently reported the first use of the system in the United States (57), but since the introduction of the large-channel (4.2 mm) endoscope, we have abandoned this system in favor of using large-caliber 12Fr stents when possible, which are introduced in the more standard fashion.

The German system requires the use of a special guidewire that is introduced through either a 2.8 mm or a 3.2 mm channel endoscope. Once this guidewire enters the liver (biliary radicals), the handle is removed (the handle is used to flex the guidewire in the liver to anchor it), and the endoscope is removed from the pa-

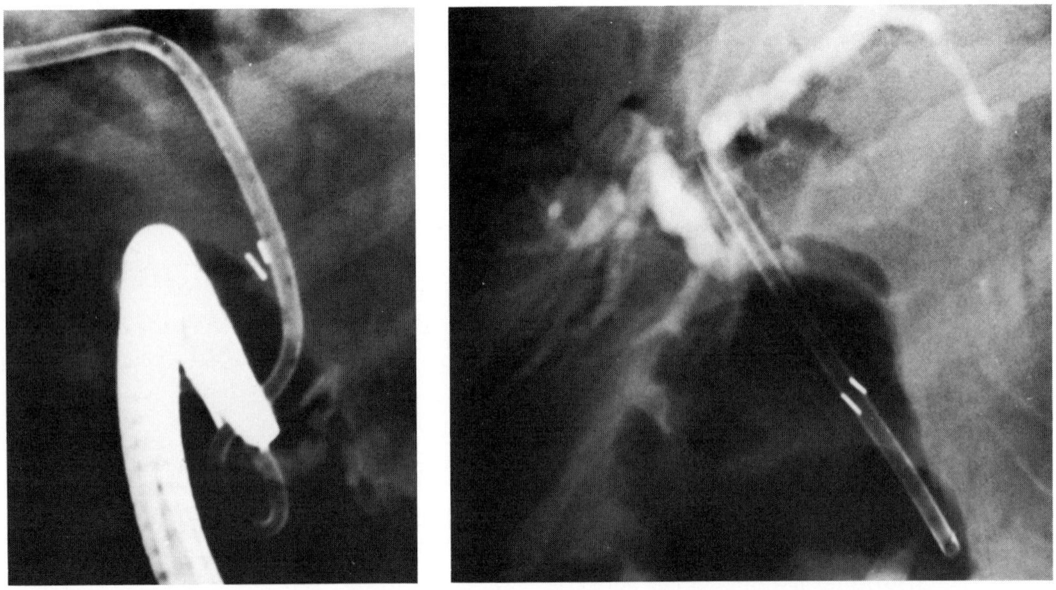

FIG. 12.59. Left: An internal-external prosthesis extending into the duodenum. **Right:** After a needle-knife sphincterotomy, a guide catheter and guidewire were placed. The large-caliber endoprosthesis is in place.

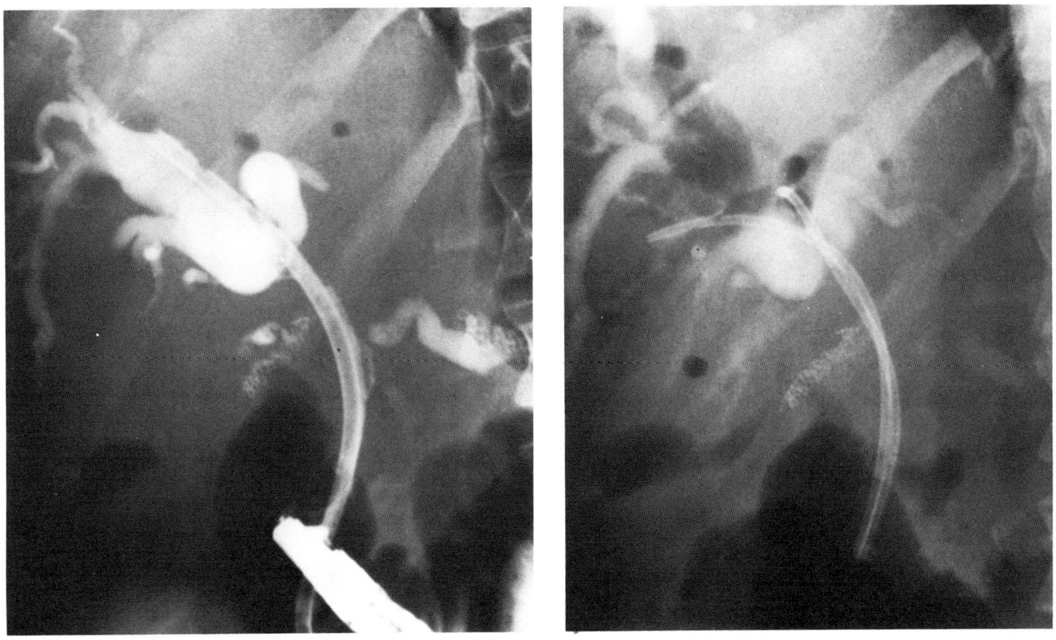

FIG. 12.60. Left: In this series, a long, large-caliber prosthesis, which was placed at surgery, is seen extending into the duodenum in a patient with a Bilroth II gastrectomy. The cholangiogram reveals evidence of a dilated intrahepatic biliary tree, which is secondary to metastatic carcinoma of the stomach (the reason for the gastrectomy). **Right:** Since the obstruction was at the portahepatis, medium-sized stents were placed into each main bile duct branch.

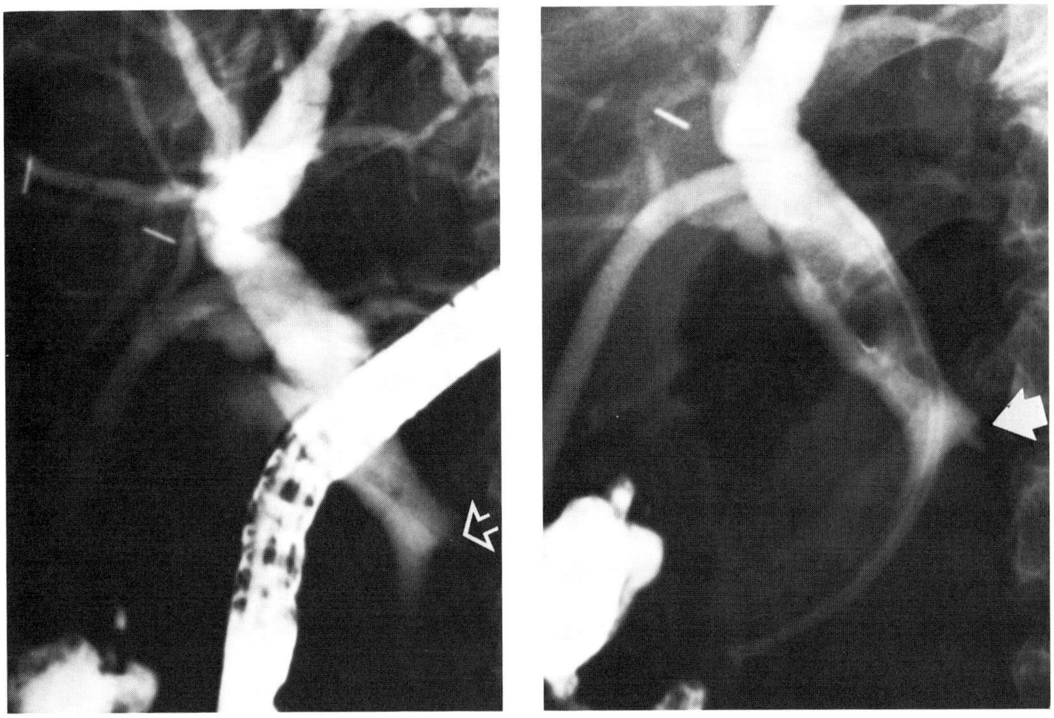

FIG. 12.61. This patient had experienced recurrent pancreatitis following the placement of a T-tube. **Left:** At ERCP, the distal limb of the T-tube had penetrated the bile duct wall into the parenchyma of the pancreas. (*arrow*). **Right:** An endoscopic prosthesis has been placed into the bile duct, and the T-tube is seen penetrating the pancreas (*arrow*). The patient improved, and the T-tube was removed.

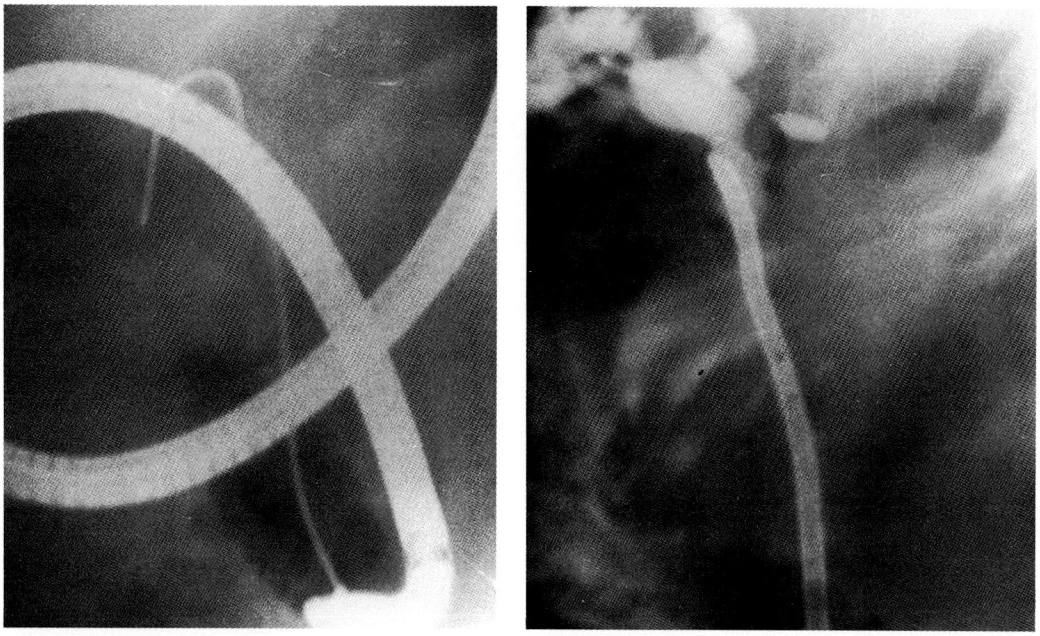

FIG. 12.62. Left: In a patient with a Klatskin tumor, cholangiocarcinoma of the bifurcation, and a Bilroth II gastric resection, a special guidewire is seen extending from the endoscope and anchored in the liver. **Right:** With this special system, the endoscope is removed and a straight 15Fr stent can be pushed into the right hepatic duct system.

tient over this wire. The large-caliber stent is placed onto this guidewire system, the pusher catheter is placed, and the stent is passed down the wire. The guidewire handle is reattached, the wire is flexed to anchor it, and the stent is pushed into place under fluoroscopic control (without an endoscope). Figures 12.62 and 12.63 illustrate the system and the stent configurations. The system can also be used to place a 12Fr stent, which may be more readily available, without the need for a large-caliber endoscope or a ra-

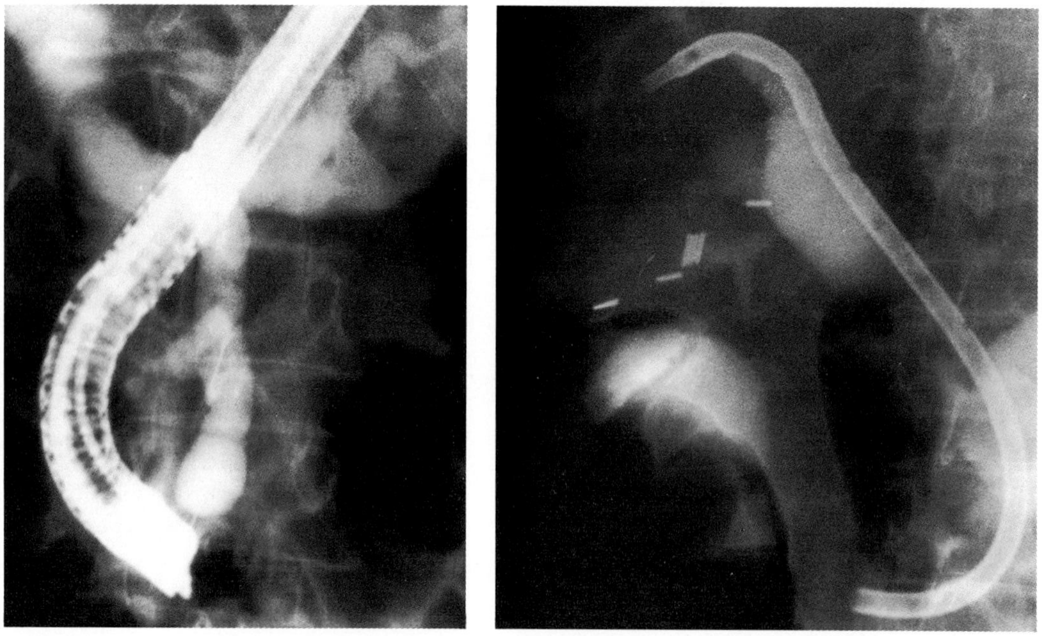

FIG. 12.63. Left: This high-grade distal bile duct obstruction was traversed with the special guidewire. **Right:** The endoscope was removed, and a 15Fr curved stent was placed into the proximal biliary tree.

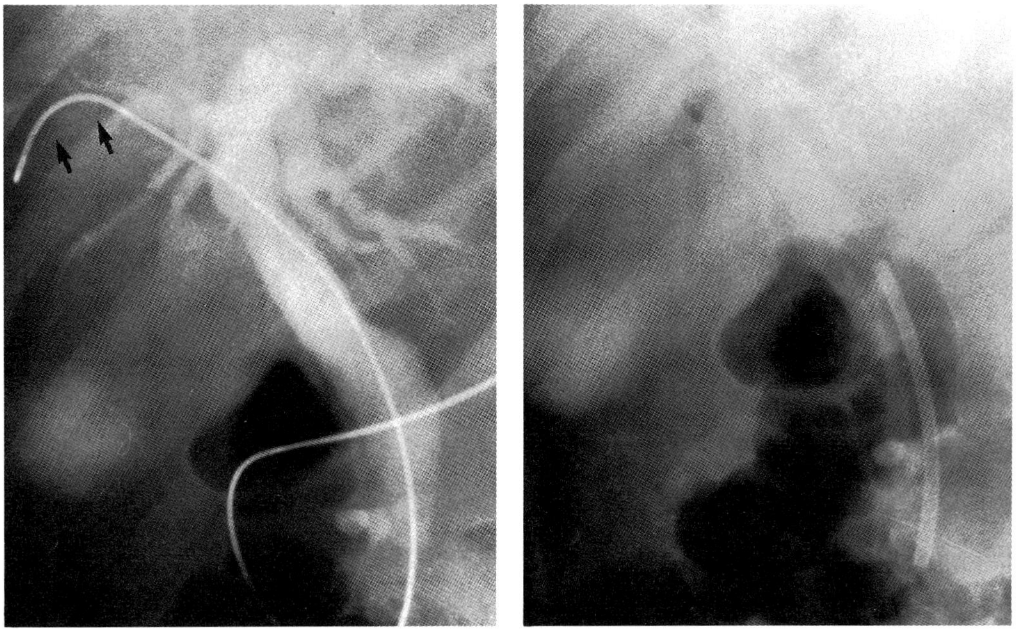

FIG. 12.64. **Left:** In this distally obstructed bile duct, the special guidewire is visible in the right hepatic duct in a flexed configuration. The position is held by pulling tension on the proximal wire, which flexes a distal cable tip (*arrows*). **Right:** A large-caliber 12Fr stent is in position, having already decompressed the biliary tree.

diologist to assist in a rendezvous (Fig. 12.64). The single disadvantage of the system is dislodgment of the guidewire, which occurred about 40% of the time in our experience, requiring repeat intubation. The morbidity associated with this system was reported to be slightly higher than that associated with routine placement of large-caliber prostheses. Hemobilia was the most frequent complication and was attributed to liver laceration, which is another reason this system is used less frequently than the standard techniques for placing large-caliber prostheses. Obviously, the financial advantage of not having to purchase a large-channel endoscope was cancelled out because of the higher morbidity rates associated with this system.

PERIAMPULLARY TUMORS—SYMPTOMATIC OBSTRUCTION TO BOTH THE BILIARY TREE AND PANCREAS

A patient with cholestasis and jaundice caused by bile duct obstruction from a periampullary mass, polyp, or ampullary carcinoma (58–64) may occasionally present with obstruction of the pancreatic duct and clinical pancreatitis, which might necessitate decompression of both duct systems. I have placed stents into both duct systems to relieve symptoms of obstruction (Figs. 12.65–12.72), with relief of pancreatitis as well as obstructive jaundice. In my experience, obstructive symptoms of pancreatitis were dramatically relieved after stent placement. One patient who presented with jaundice and pancreatitis owing to an ampullary carcinoma stent and was treated with decompression of both ducts has been free of obstructive symptoms for more than 3 years and has not required stent exchange. Some patients in my series who had resectable ampullary lesions did not undergo surgery because of intercurrent medical problems such as cardiac disease (i.e., low ejection fraction), myasthenia gravis, and severe chronic obstructive pulmonary disease (COPD). Fortunately, in patients at greater risk, frequent manipulation and stent exchange has not been necessary, which has had a positive effect on reduction of procedure-related morbidity.

Decompression of pancreatic duct obstruction

Text continues on page 304.

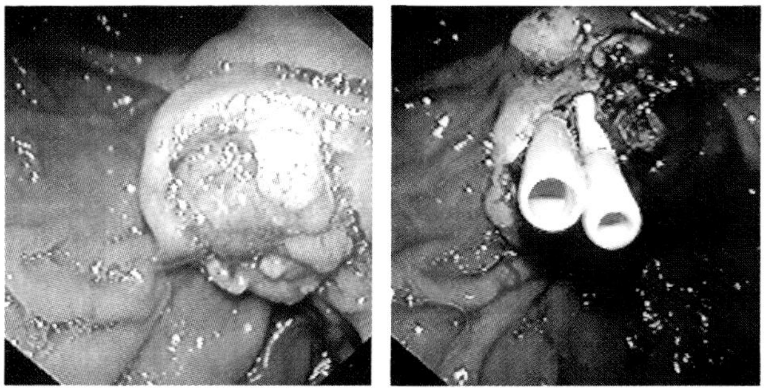

FIG 12.65. **Left:** An ampullary lesion. **Right:** Its appearance after sphincterotomy and placement of a large-caliber prosthesis into the bile duct, the stent may be seen on the left. A 7Fr catheter was placed into the pancreatic duct, the stent on the right.

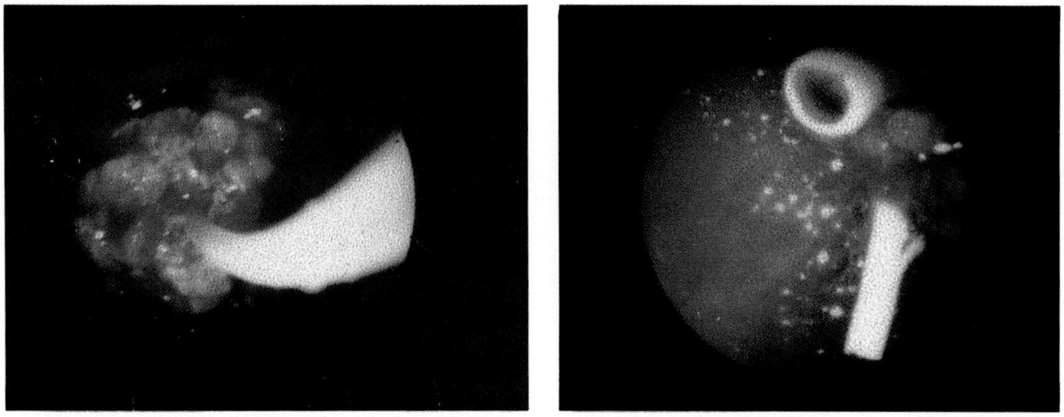

FIG. 12.66. This endoscopic picture illustrates an ampullary mass with two stents in place. **Left:** The larger stent is in the biliary tree. **Right:** The smaller 7Fr stent is in the pancreatic duct.

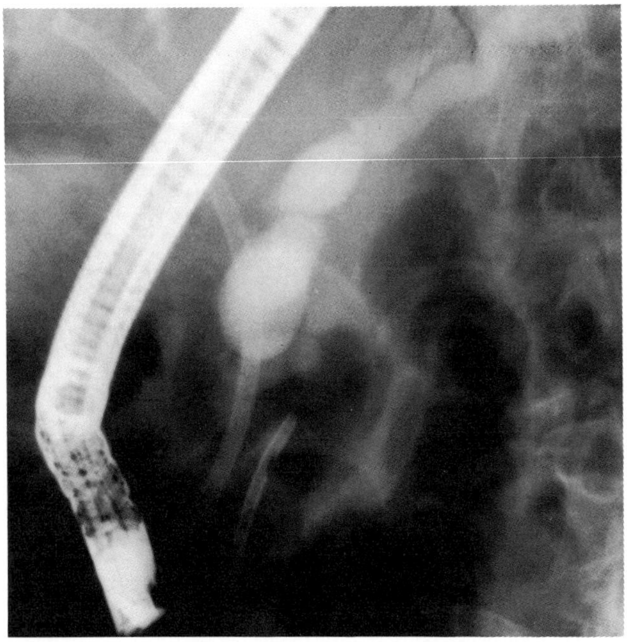

FIG. 12.67. This radiograph shows a large-caliber prosthesis in the bile duct and a medium-sized prosthesis in the pancreatic duct.

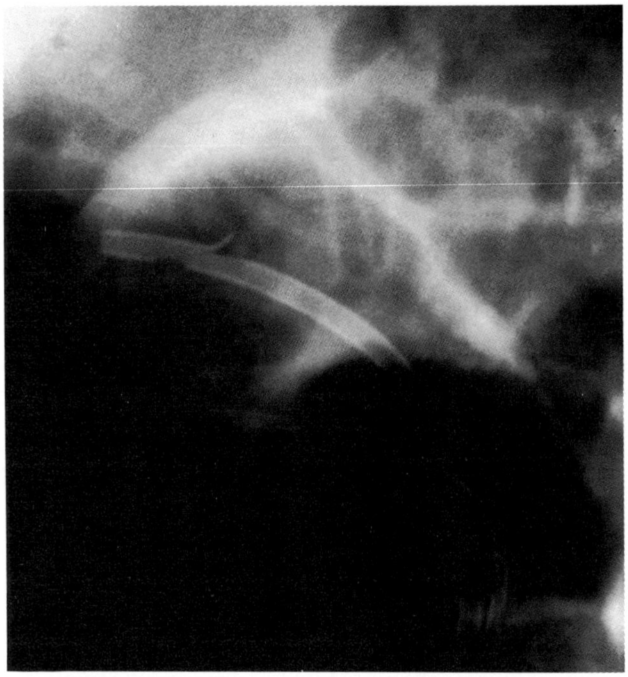

FIG. 12.68. Two stents are shown on this radiograph. The larger one is in the bile duct, and the smaller one is in the pancreatic duct. Both stents were placed because of obstruction to both the biliary and the pancreatic ductular systems produced by an ampullary tumor.

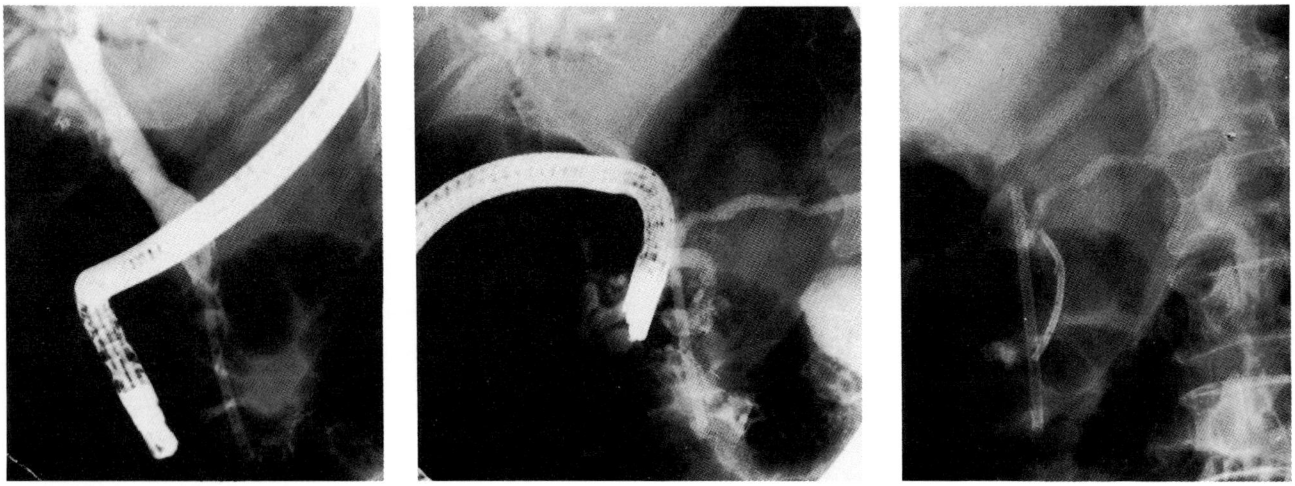

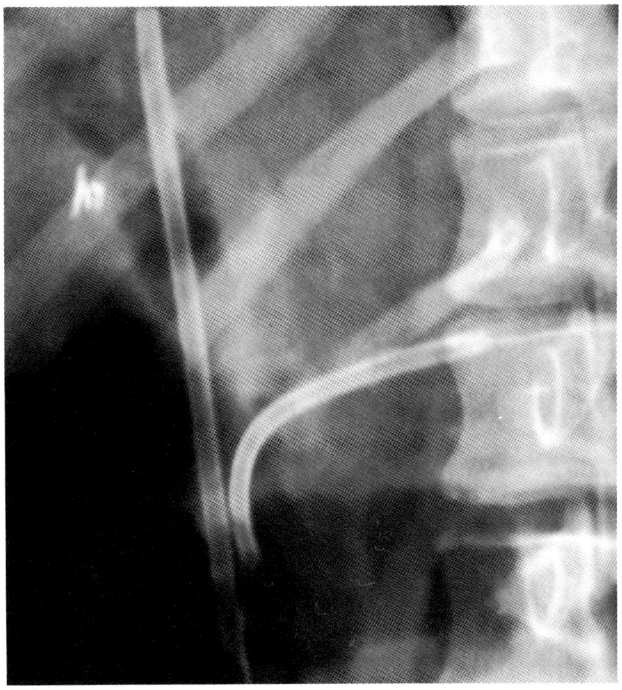

FIG. 12.70. Two stents in position in the bile duct and pancreatic duct. These positions are the usual configuration, but when the tumor creates distortion and displacement of the ducts, the stent positions may vary, as seen in the preceding figures.

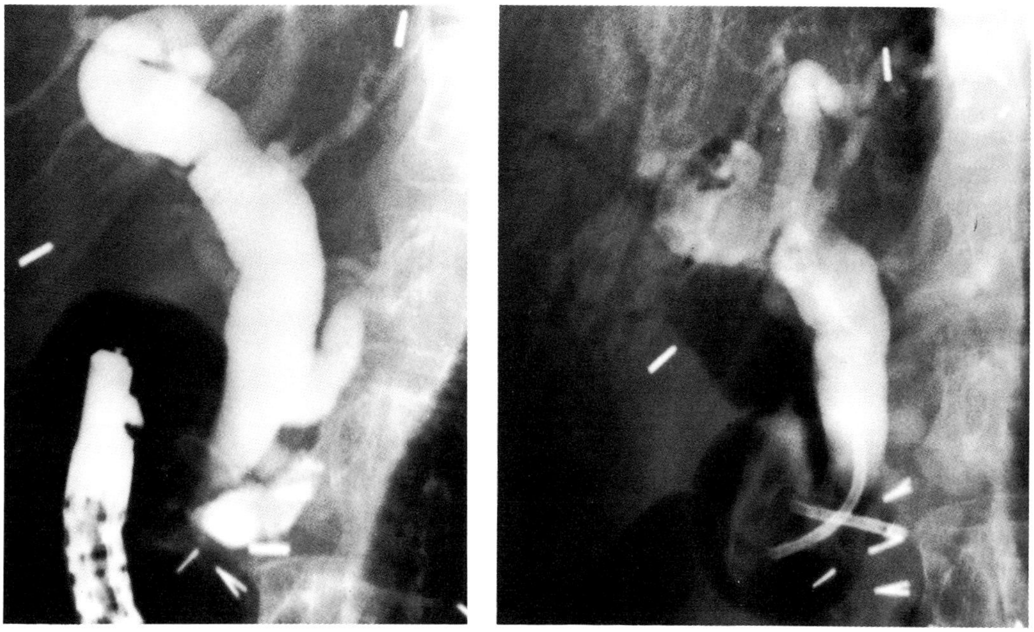

FIG. 12.71. Occasionally the author has treated ampullary tumors in patients who have undergone Bilroth II gastric resections. **Left:** Dilatation of both duct systems is confirmed. **Right:** A stent has been placed into each duct.

FIG. 12.69. Left: A large-caliber prosthesis that has been placed into the bile duct. **Middle:** Parenchymal filling of the pancreas, and a stricture at the ampulla, which was produced by an ampullary tumor. **Right:** Two prostheses, the larger one in the bile duct, the smaller one in the pancreas. The patient did well following stent placement, which has not required replacement for a follow-up period of 3.5 years.

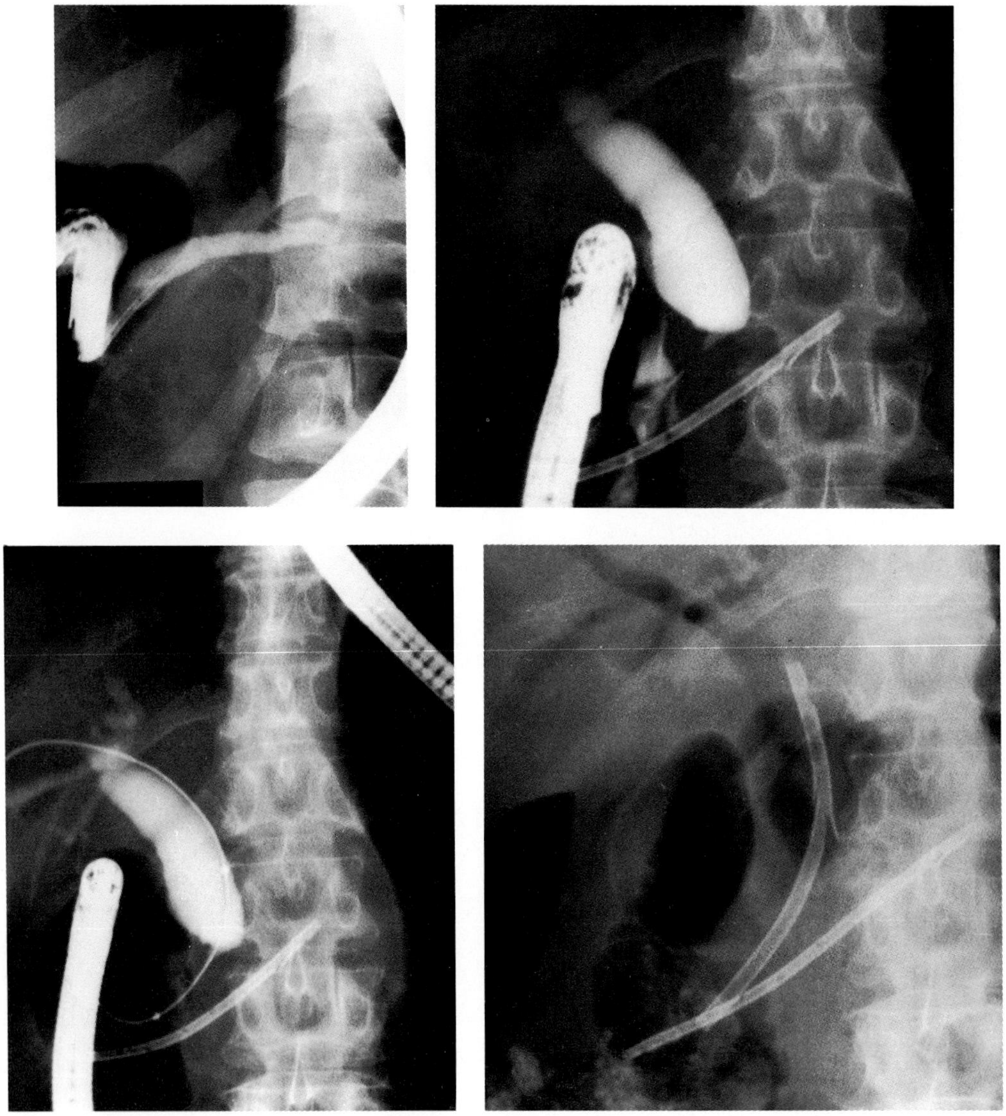

FIG. 12.72. Occasionally prostheses are placed into the pancreatic duct for decompression of the obstructed duct caused by carcinoma. **Top left:** A dilated pancreatic duct. However, this is the dorsal duct of pancreas divisum and was thought to be a benign structure. **Top right:** A large-caliber prosthesis was placed. This second radiograph was taken 3 months after the first. At the initial examination, the bile duct appeared normal. On this study, a high-grade stricture of the bile duct is demonstrated and consistent with carcinoma of the pancreas arising in the dorsal duct of a pancreas divisum. **Bottom left:** A guidewire and balloon catheter in the bile duct and stricture, respectively. **Bottom right:** A 12Fr stent is seen after placement into the bile duct. A 9-10Fr prosthesis is in the dorsal pancreatic duct.

Text continued from page 301.
owing to exocrine carcinoma of the pancreas, in my experience, has not been essential to survival or quality of life, and I routinely attempt to place a prosthesis only into the bile duct under these circumstances, not into the pancreatic duct. Pancreatic enzyme replacement is usually effective in managing steatorrhea caused by pancreatic duct obstruction. Decompression of the biliary tree, however, is more essential for surviving and maintaining fluid and nutritional balance. In addition, internal drainage of the biliary tree, surgical or nonsurgical, is reportedly essential not only to maintaining fluid and electrolyte equilibrium but also to keeping hematopoietic and immunologic balance (65). Therefore, if possible, *external stents should be converted to internal drains because longer survival and improved quality of life are experienced by patients with carcinoma of the pancreas when the enterohepatic circulation is restored and equilibrium is reestablished.*

Assessing Stent Patency and Function

An option for confirming the patency of a prosthesis and its position is to insert a cannula deeply into the prosthesis, beyond the side drainage holes, and to inject contrast material. If the prosthesis is patent and remains in position, contrast should flow through its proximal end (that portion within the bile duct) into the biliary tree, opacifying the ductular system and confirming the position and patency of the prosthesis. This technique may be necessary when it is suspected that a prosthesis has occluded or when the patient's cholestatic picture has not improved several days after insertion of the prosthesis. This early "second look" helps to confirm the position and function of a prosthesis, especially when the patient's obstructive picture remains the same despite the placement of a large-caliber prostheses.

Assessment of the function of an endoprosthesis can be made without further endoscopic manipulation, although the endoscopic techniques are more definitive and accurate. If a patient develops cholestasis subsequent to the insertion of a prosthesis or if the cholestatic picture has not improved sufficiently after several days of observation, scintigraphy procedures (HIDA or Dissida) can be performed if the bilirubin level is not elevated above that acceptable for radionuclide studies. If the radionuclide study demonstrates patency or flow of the medium through the prosthesis into the duodenum, the cholestatic presentation may be attributed to metastatic disease or to deteriorating liver function, which is associated with the malignancy or declining nutritional status and is not a direct result of an occluded prosthesis (Fig. 12.73). If the radionuclide studies cannot be performed because of the elevated bilirubin, a second-look endoscopy should be performed by placing the cannula either into or alongside the prosthesis and injecting contrast material. If it is injected directly into the prosthesis, the contrast will be seen entering the proximal biliary tree if the prosthesis is patent; if injected alongside the stent, contrast will be seen entering the proximal biliary tree and flowing back through the prosthesis into the duodenum. Another alternative method for assessing patency of a large-caliber prosthesis is having the patient swallow either barium or a water-soluble contrast agent (Gastrographin) and observing for reflux of the contrast into the prosthesis (Fig. 12.74A).

Another method for assessing stent patency is a careful evaluation and interpretation of the CT scan. With the patient lying supine, air will rise and enter the left hepatic duct via the large-caliber stent (Fig. 12.74B), confirming patency.

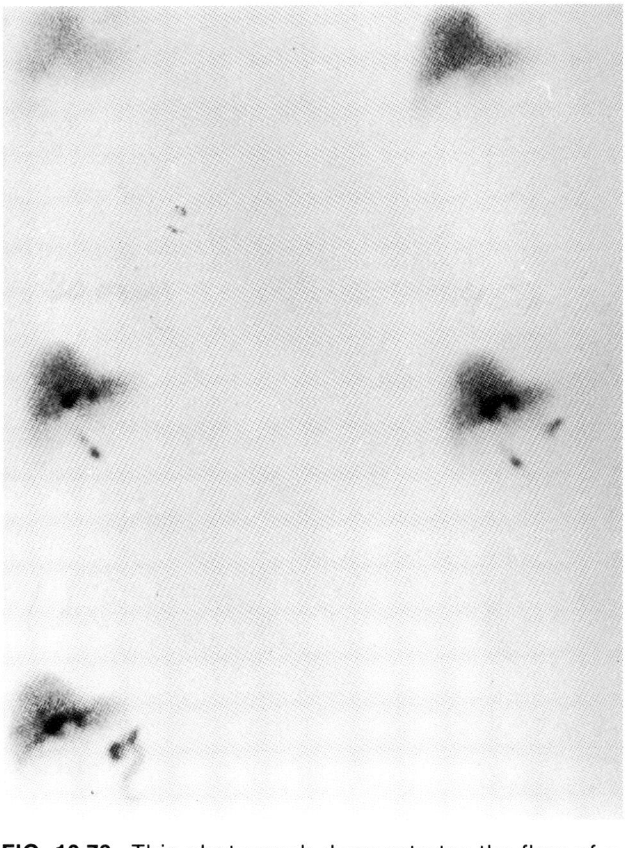

FIG. 12.73. This photograph demonstrates the flow of a radionuclide, HIDA, through a prosthesis into the duodenum. The patient had a stent placed for carcinoma of the pancreas and developed cholestasis and jaundice that were associated with metastatic disease but *not* stent occlusion. It is important to observe such patients expectantly because improvement may occur more slowly in a patient who has impaired liver function owing to high-grade obstruction and/or metastatic disease.

Significance of Prostheses in the Management of Carcinoma of the Pancreas

An interesting study reported by Neff et al. described the prognostic value of bilirubin reduction and patient survival after percutaneous drainage procedures (percutaneous transhepatic drainage—PTHD) that preceded palliative bypass surgery (Table 12.1) (66). The patient population was divided into three groups, each

TABLE 12.1. *Prognostic value of a decrease in bilirubin following percutaneous drainage in patients presenting with obstructive jaundice, carcinoma of the pancreas: results of surgical palliation*

	Decrease in bilirubin	30-day mortality after surgical palliation	Mean survival after palliation (days)
Group 1	Near normal	10%	198
Group 2	50%, not below	33%	72
Group 3	0%	88%	12

From ref. 66.

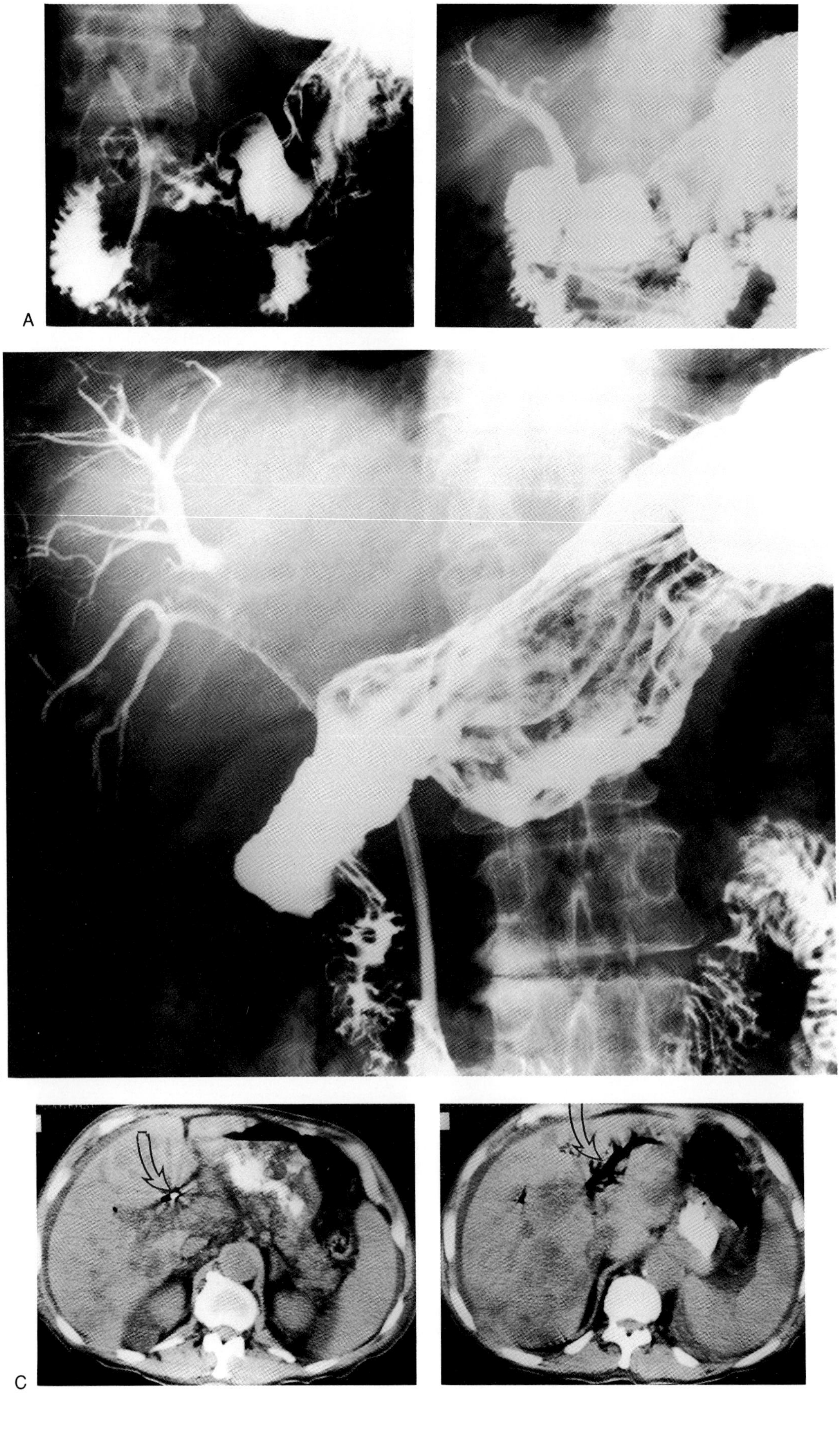
A
B
C

demonstrating different responses to percutaneous drainage. In Group 1, the bilirubin returned to near normal with PTHD, and, after a palliative bypass surgical procedure, the 30-day mortality approached 10%, with a mean survival of 198 days. The second group (Group 2) responded less dramatically to percutaneous drainage. Bilirubin reduction approached 50% but did not fall below the predrainage level. After undergoing biliary bypass surgery, these patients experienced a 30-day mortality of 33% and a mean survival of 72 days. The final group (Group 3) in this series had very little response to the percutaneous drain, with the cholestatic liver function studies and bilirubin remaining approximately the same after placing the drain, even though bile was draining freely into the gravity bag. The 30-day mortality of this last group of patients following biliary bypass surgery was 88%, and the mean survival was only 12 days. This study was extremely important in determining the degree of intervention to which patients should be subjected with unresectable carcinoma of the pancreas. In general, patients in Group 1 were younger, presented with a better nutritional status, and were expected to survive a longer period of time. Such patients may benefit more from a surgical exploration, possible resection or bypass, than from endoscopic or radiologic decompression because the prosthesis inserted by either nonsurgical method would require subsequent changes and several hospitalizations during the patient's remaining lifetime.

I have placed prostheses in more than 1,000 patients with obstructive jaundice (Table 12.2), the majority being patients with carcinoma of the pancreas. Because of this experience and the need to compare endoscopy to other disciplines, radiographic and surgical, H. Snady and I reviewed and compared the results of endoscopic drainage, surgical palliation, and percutaneous techniques. We included more than 200 published articles from the three disciplines in this review (65). The 30-day mortality and survival rates for palliation were essentially the same for all three disciplines: 20 to 21% and 5 to 7 months, respectively. However, procedure-associated morbidity was much lower in the endoscopic series. Comparing different modalities requires a careful evaluation of all parameters. Each discipline offers advantages to the unresectable patient, so each patient should be studied individually.

TABLE 12.2. *Endoscopic prostheses: location of obstructive biliary lesions*

Proximal hepatic duct/bifurcation	294
Malignant	227
Benign	67
Distal CBD	671
Pancreas	577
Periampullary	94
Ampulla of Vater	63
Total	1028

A randomized trial comparing palliative surgery to percutaneous drainage techniques concluded that the nonsurgical, percutaneous method has distinct advantages early in the patient's course. During the immediate perioperative period, hospitalization time was reduced and, to no one's surprise, morbidity and mortality were significantly lower in the percutaneous group (67). The savings in hospitalization times were lost if patients survived 6 months or longer because the nonsurgical group required repeat hospitalizations for exchange of prostheses when they occluded, reducing the earlier cost-conserving advantages.

Other trials have proved the efficacy of endoscopic palliation compared to radiologic techniques, but the efficacy of endoscopic palliation is even more significant when compared to palliative surgery. In a randomized trial, endoscopy proved to be safer and more cost effective than both percutaneous and surgical palliative procedures. It was also shown to be as effective as surgery, especially in patients at greater risk with limited or restrictive survival (68–70). Certainly, the quality of life of these high-risk patients improved with endoscopic palliation. However, the dilemma we face concerns the younger, healthier, and better nourished patients (Neff's Group 1) who may survive a year or longer. Until endoscopists can prolong the patency rate of stents, long-term survivors still require several stent changes during their lifetime. I recommend surgical exploration and possible resection or bypass decompression for these patients because if they are

FIG. 12.74. A: Left: This radiograph illustrates patency of a large-caliber prosthesis. The patient has ingested barium, which is seen in the stomach and duodenum, and this barium is noted to enter the prosthesis. **Right:** Filling of the biliary tree with barium, which has refluxed through the prosthesis. **B:** This radiograph demonstrates patency of a large-caliber prosthesis. Barium has been ingested by the patient, and it refluxes freely into the biliary tree through a patent, large-caliber prosthesis. Note the nondilated intrahepatic radicals. **C: Left:** A CT scan of the abdomen showing multiple defects in the liver secondary to liver metastases. The white density (*arrow*) is a large-caliber stent. **Right:** The large lucent area in the left lobe of the liver (*arrow*) is a dilated bile duct filled with air that has migrated through the large-caliber stent. The air will localize in the left lobe when the stent is patent and the patient is lying supine.

treated endoscopically, they require subsequent hospitalizations for stent changes, thus offsetting the earlier economic advantages of endoscopy. Patients in the other two groups classified by Neff et al. (Groups 2 and 3) derive greater benefits from nonsurgical decompression techniques, and surgery is not recommended unless nonsurgical techniques fail. This conclusion is based on the fact that these higher risk patients usually do not survive more than 4 to 6 months and would not require subsequent stent changes. Therefore, nonsurgical techniques, specifically endoscopy, have an economic advantage because the morbidity associated with their management is lower than that of other disciplines, and they usually do not require prolonged or recurrent hospitalizations. I offer this recommendation for the management of patients with carcinoma of the pancreas and lesions of the lower bile duct. Management of patients with proximal bile duct obstruction requires further assessment, and palliative treatment of bifurcation tumors is problematic and enigmatic. Most methods of treatment, including surgical methods, are associated with serious, recurrent complications such as cholangitis and cholestasis, and these complications often require a multidisciplinary approach.

Bifurcation Tumors

In Chapter 6, the classification of bifurcation tumors (Klatskin tumors, cholangiocarcinoma, gallbladder carcinoma) was presented and discussed. Illustrations and radiographs of these lesions provided examples of the location, degree of obstruction, and extension of these lesions into the liver parenchyma. Because of the extensive nature of these lesions, one can appreciate how difficult it would be to provide adequate decompression for these lesions using a single modality (71–80). It is often necessary to combine disciplines (81,82)—endoscopic, radiologic, and surgical—to decompress the obstructed biliary tree and to avoid complications such as cholangitis (83, 84). Significant reports comparing endoscopic management techniques are emerging and emphasizing the likelihood that a multidisciplinary approach may be the most efficacious. However, some groups report success with a single prosthesis, though others use more than one (85). I have placed single large prostheses (Figs. 12.75, 12.76) through the dominant stricture, and these endoprostheses may function adequately without requiring a second or third stent. I have often attempted and succeeded in placing more than one prosthesis into an

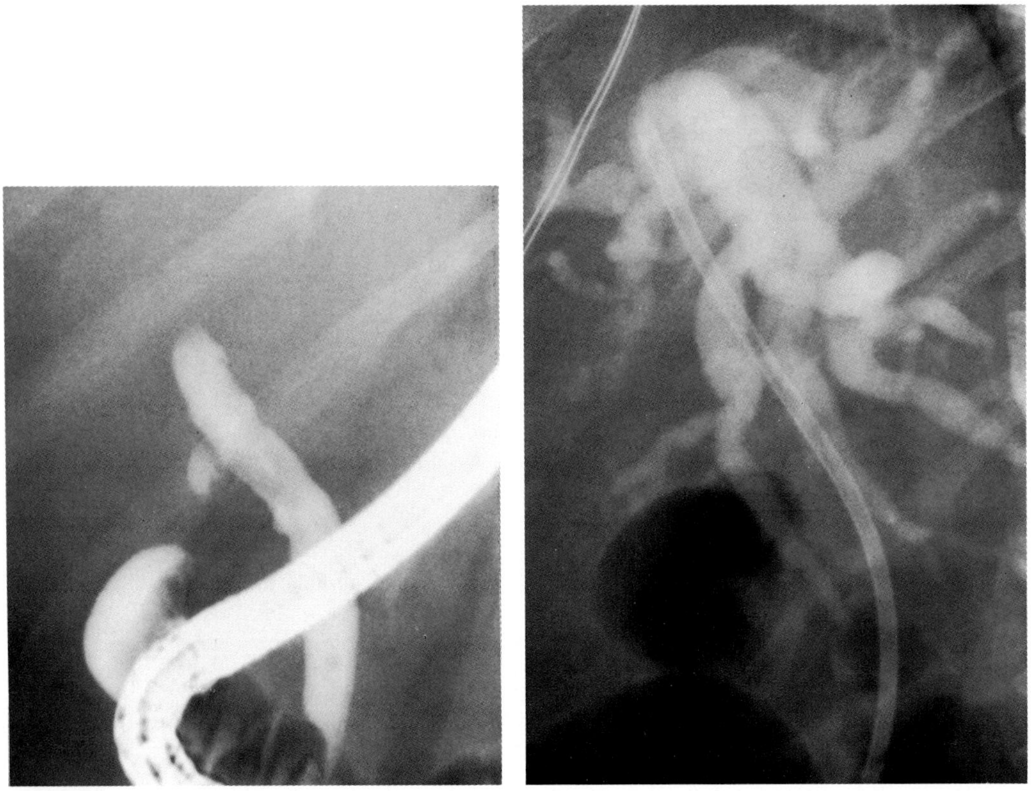

FIG. 12.75. Left: Obstruction of the bile duct is confirmed at the bifurcation. **Right:** A single large prosthesis is placed into the proximal biliary tree.

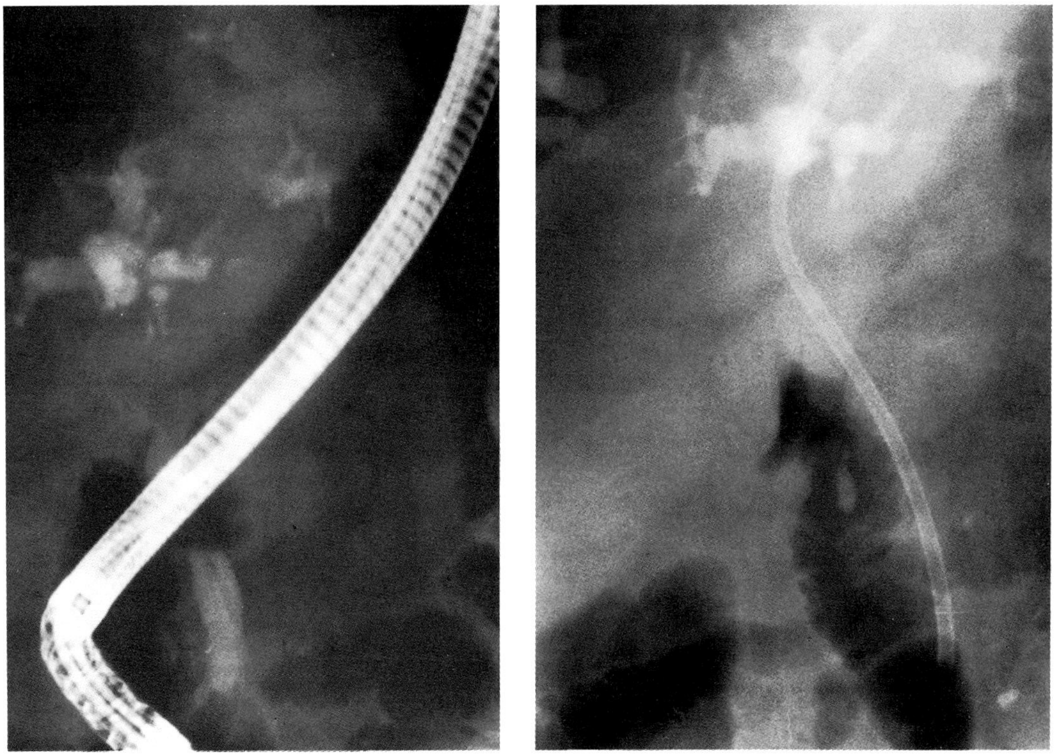

FIG. 12.76. Left: Incomplete opacification of the biliary tree is seen with the common hepatic duct poorly visualized. **Right:** A single large prosthesis is placed through the obstruction into the left hepatic duct system.

obstructed intrahepatic biliary system. In my opinion, if it is possible to place individual large-caliber stents into each major hepatic duct, morbidity associated with endoscopic manipulation will be reduced. Overwhelming life-threatening cholangitis may often occur after stent placement and inadequate drainage simply because many small and large biliary radicals are insufficiently drained. If the patient develops fever shortly after the attempted decompression despite adequate antibiotic coverage, I encourage early consultations with both the interventional radiologist and the surgeon because other prostheses or drainage procedures may be helpful.

Examples of bile duct obstruction located distal to

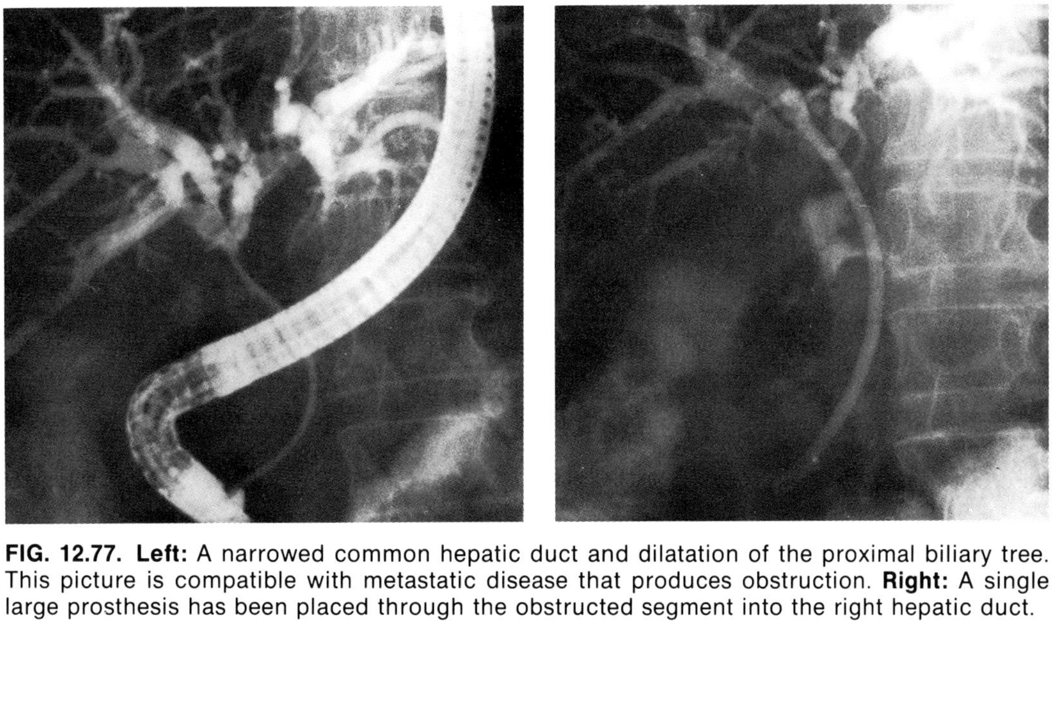

FIG. 12.77. Left: A narrowed common hepatic duct and dilatation of the proximal biliary tree. This picture is compatible with metastatic disease that produces obstruction. **Right:** A single large prosthesis has been placed through the obstructed segment into the right hepatic duct.

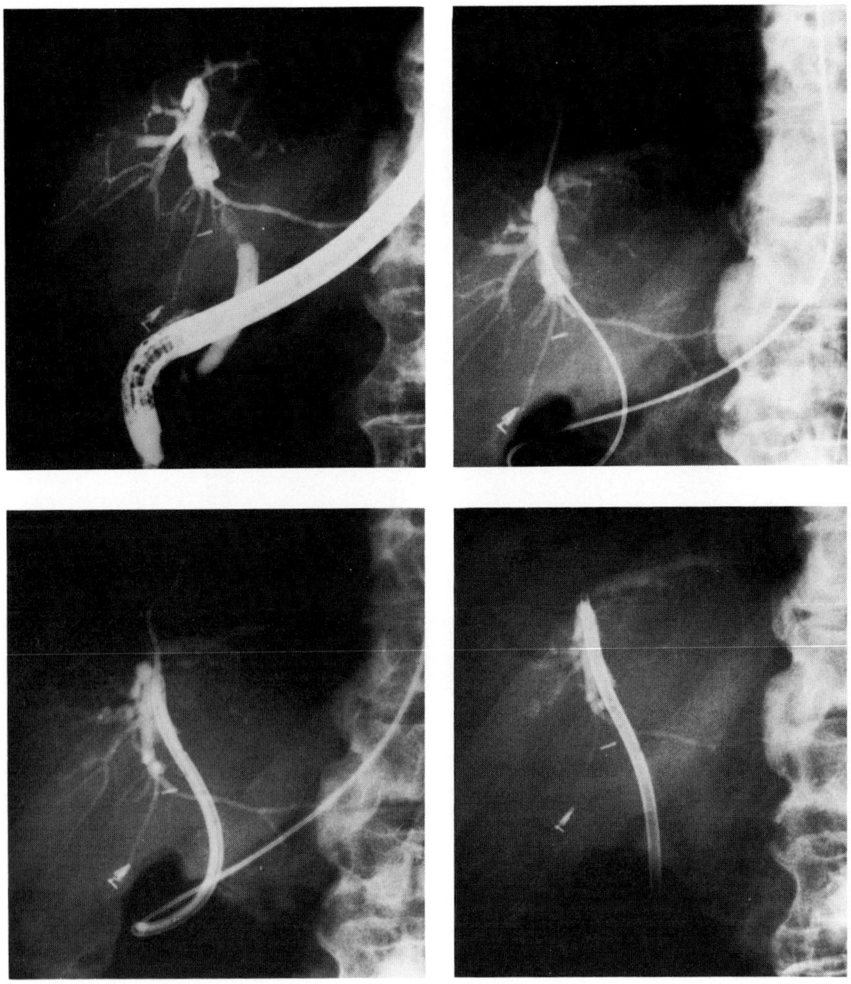

FIG. 12.78. Top left: A cholangiocarcinoma of the common hepatic duct. **Top right:** The special guidewire, which accepts a 15Fr prosthesis, has been introduced through the stricture and into the intrahepatic radicals, and the endoscope has been removed. **Bottom left:** The stent is being inserted into the biliary tree. **Bottom right:** After placement, the guidewire is removed, leaving the stent in place. (From ref. 57, with permission.)

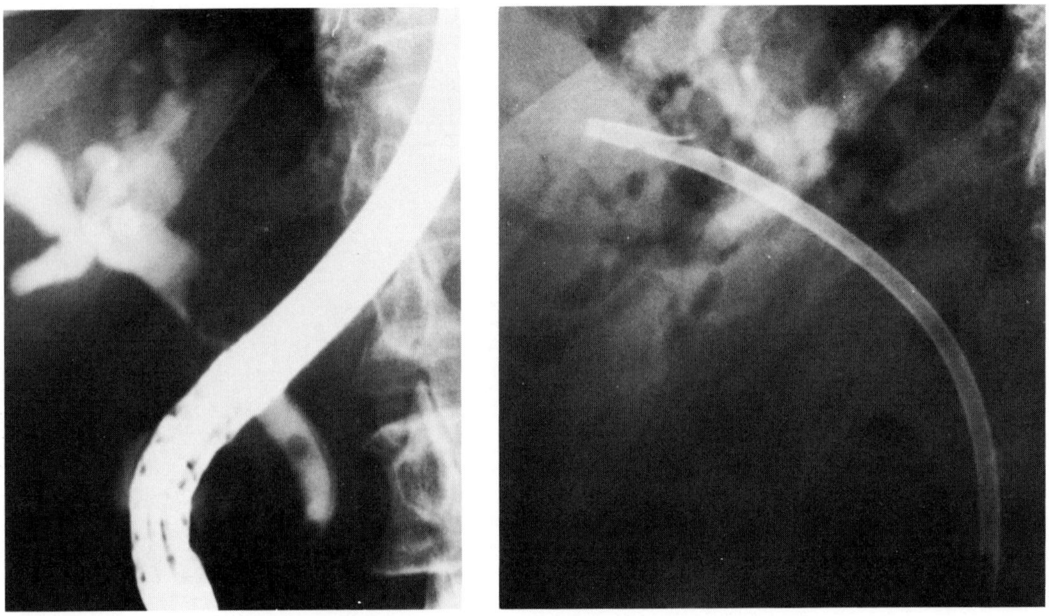

FIG. 12.79. Left: A high-grade stricture with proximal dilatation of the biliary tree. **Right:** A large-caliber prosthesis has been inserted.

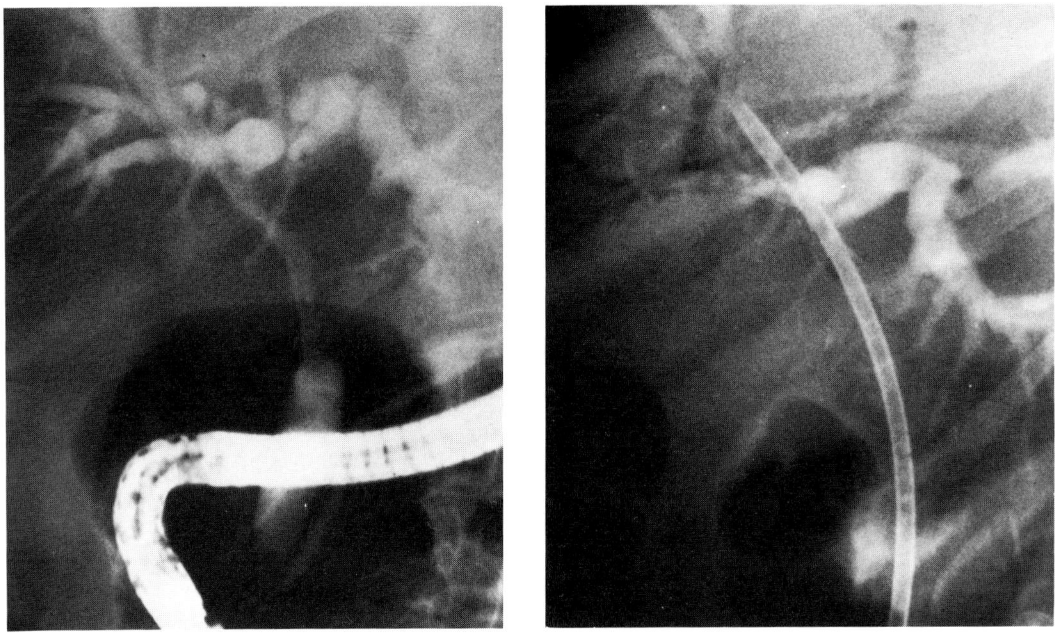

FIG. 12.80. Left: The extrahepatic bile duct is displaced and compressed by infiltrating Hodgkin's disease. **Right:** A large-caliber prosthesis has been placed through the obstruction. The patient can undergo definitive chemotherapy without experiencing increasing clinical jaundice, which may be associated with posttreatment edema.

the bifurcation, which includes primary cholangiocarcinoma, gallbladder carcinoma, and metastatic disease, are shown in Figs. 12.77 through 12.81.

Figures 12.82 through 12.92 illustrate the types of Klatskin tumors I have encountered. An artist's illustration is again used to describe and classify these tumors, and specific radiographs are used to illustrate treatment modalities. As indicated earlier, manipulations of an obstructed biliary tree requires the liberal

Text continues on page 315.

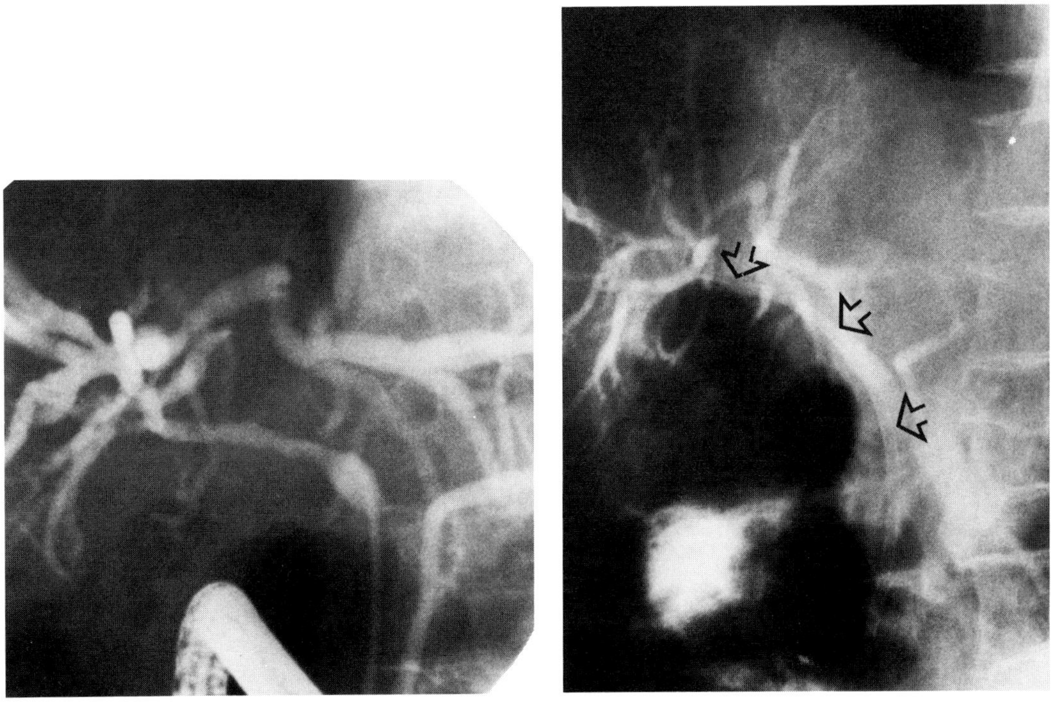

FIG. 12.81. Left: Evidence of diffuse metastatic disease involving the common hepatic duct. **Right:** A large-caliber prosthesis (*arrows*) has been placed through the stricture to provide decompression.

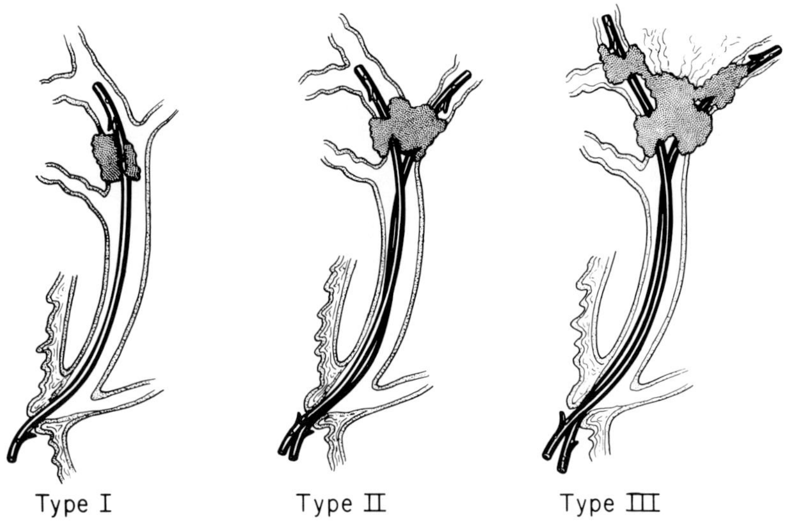

FIG. 12.82. Left: The presence of a tumor near the bifurcation of the bile ducts, Klatskin I, which is treated with placement of a single large-caliber prosthesis to provide decompression. **Middle:** As the tumor encroaches upon both the right and left hepatic ducts, Klatskin II, placement of two prostheses is considered the better way to decompress this lesion. **Right:** More diffuse involvement of the intrahepatic branches by a cholangiocarcinoma (Klatskin III) requires at least one or even two large prostheses. One may have to be satisfied with the largest single prosthesis that can be placed because of the difficulty in inserting more than one prosthesis. Broad-spectrum antibiotics should be started as soon as possible, and, if the patient becomes febrile, the radiologist and/or surgeon should be consulted to provide additional drainage.

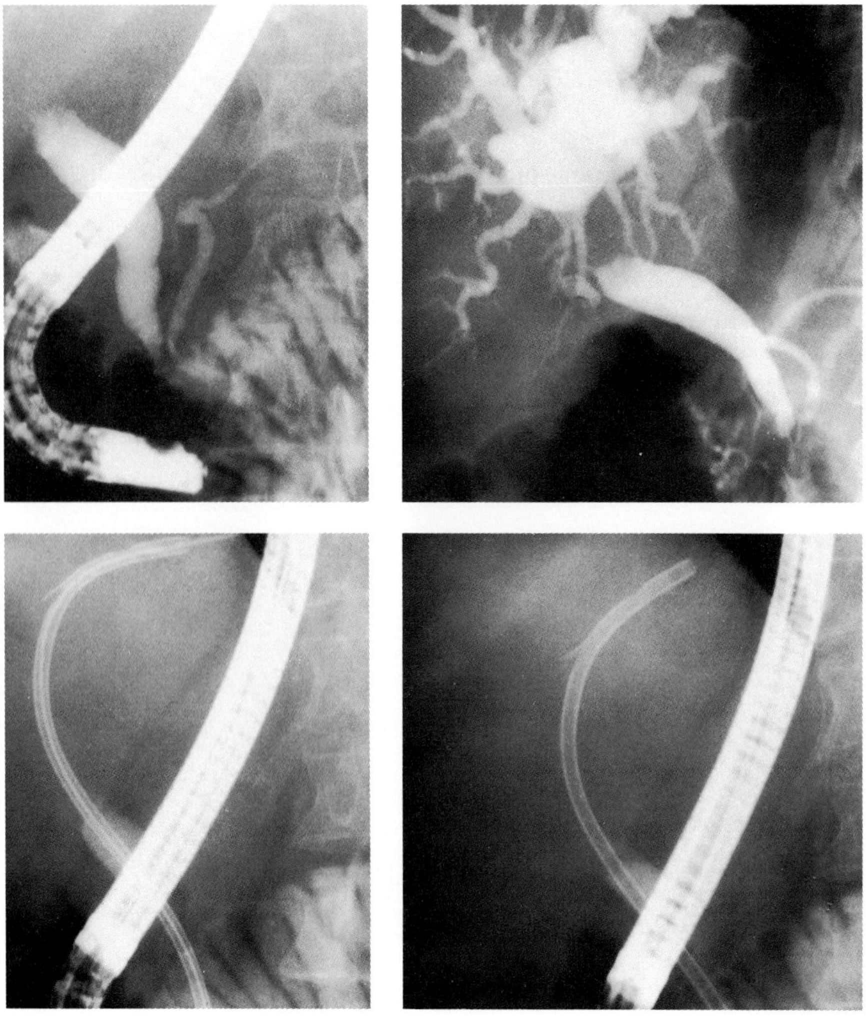

FIG. 12.83. This series of radiographs demonstrates the effectiveness of a single large-caliber prosthesis used in a Klatskin I tumor. **Top left:** No filling of the intrahepatic ducts. **Top right:** Filling of the biliary tree is seen after advancing a catheter-guidewire assembly. Note the high-grade stricture and marked dilatation of the intrahepatic ducts. **Bottom left:** A large-caliber prosthesis is being advanced into the left hepatic system. **Bottom right:** The guidewire has been removed, and the prosthesis is checked for position. Note that all contrast had passed from the intrahepatic ducts during placement of the large-caliber prosthesis.

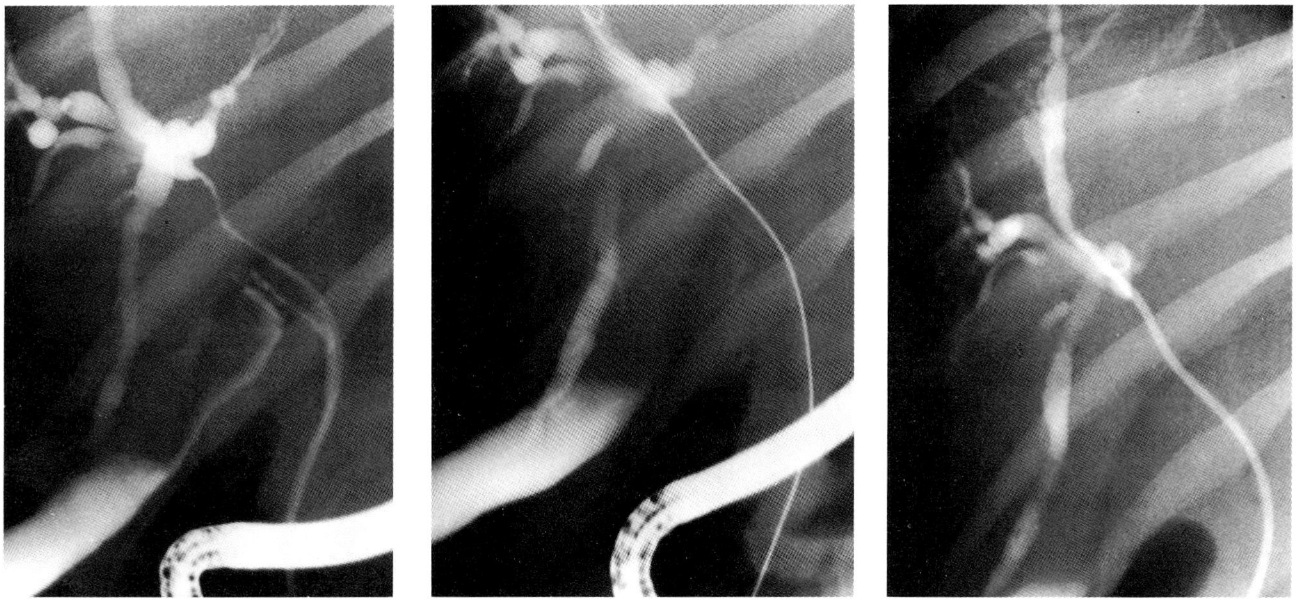

FIG. 12.84. Left: Diffuse involvement of the common hepatic duct, which is seen as a thin, string-like channel. Dilated intrahepatic ducts are noted. **Middle:** A guidewire has been advanced through the stricture. **Right:** A medium-sized prosthesis has been advanced into the biliary tree.

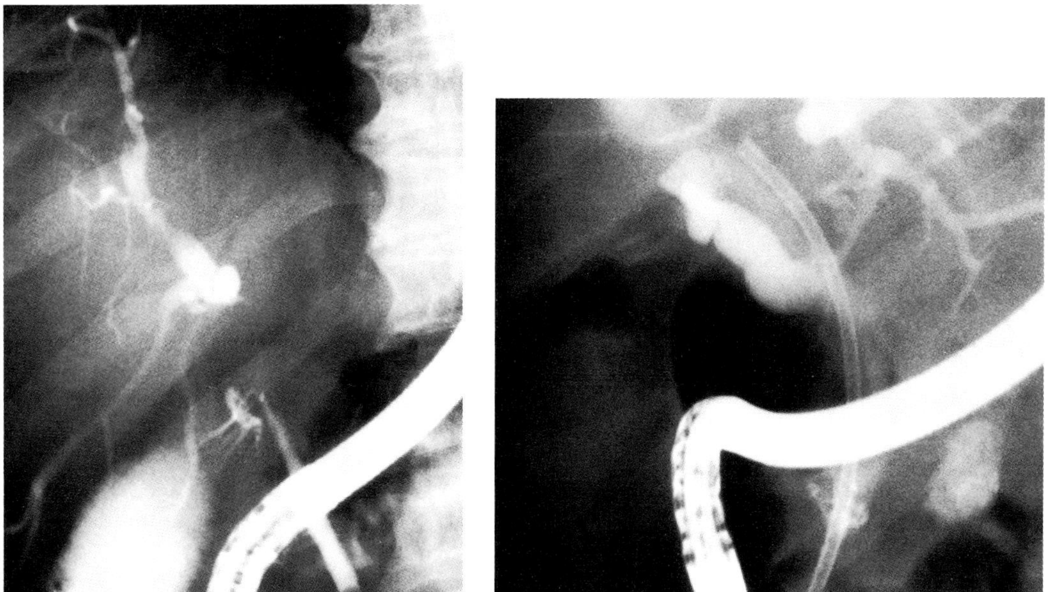

FIG. 12.85. Left: A long high-grade stricture is shown with filling of the right hepatic system as an example of a Klatskin II tumor. **Right:** A single large-caliber prosthesis has been passed into the right system. After the stricture was traversed, filling of the left hepatic duct was accomplished. A single large prosthesis was sufficient for decompression.

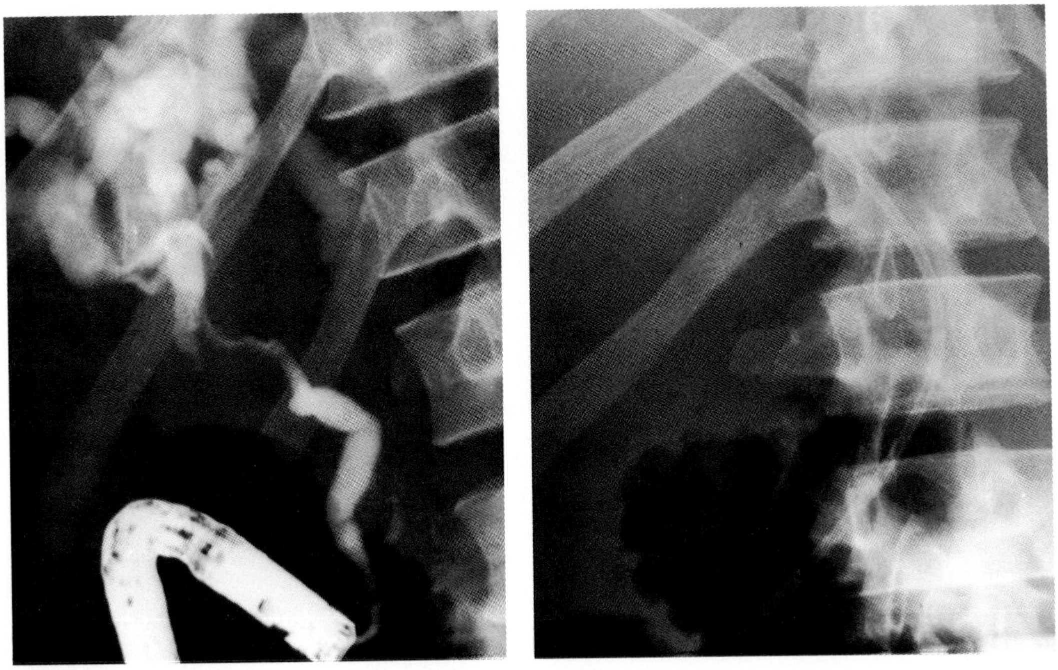

FIG. 12.86. Left: In this example of a Klatskin II lesion, a long stricture is apparent. **Right:** A long, single, medium-sized prosthesis was passed into the biliary tree; no contrast remained after placing the prosthesis.

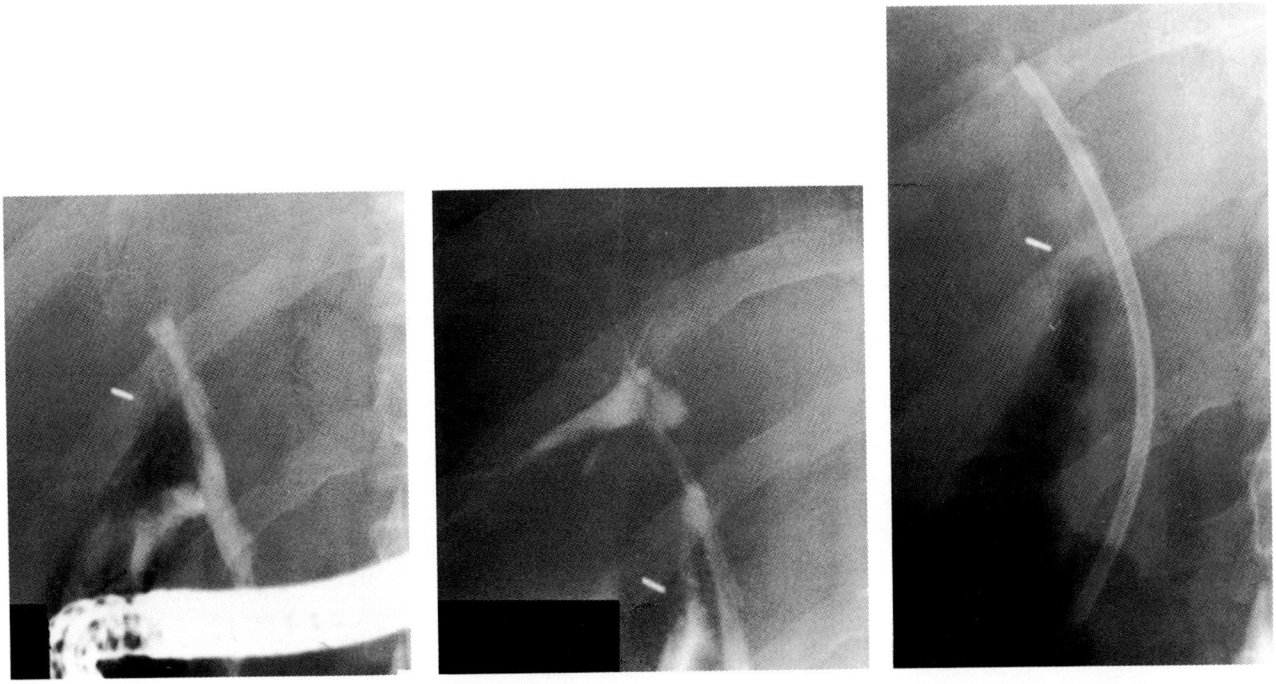

FIG. 12.87. Left: This example of a Klatskin II lesion demonstrates total obstruction of the intrahepatic ducts. **Middle:** Diffuse involvement of the intrahepatic ducts is noted after traversing the lesion and opacifying the ducts. Note that there is poor filling of the intrahepatic ducts. **Right:** A single, large prosthesis was placed.

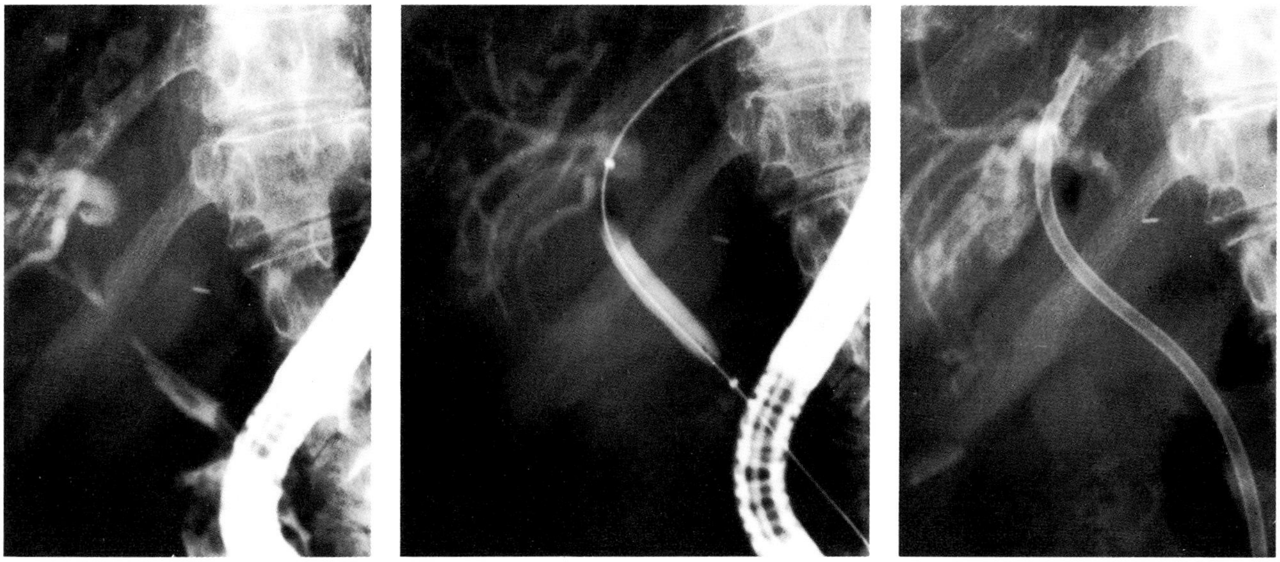

FIG. 12.88. Occasionally, balloon dilatation of a malignant stricture may be necessary to advance a large-caliber prosthesis. **Left:** A long stricture of the common hepatic duct and diffuse intrahepatic disease. **Middle:** A balloon catheter. **Right:** Dilatation of the stricture was accomplished, and a large-caliber prosthesis was inserted.

Text continued from page 311.
but specific administration of broad-spectrum antibiotics, and I often use prophylactic treatment before beginning the procedure. Several antibiotics are recommended to cover the most common opportunistic infections, including, preferably, an antibiotic that is secreted into the bile. My preference for a single agent is a third or fourth generation cephalosporin. If there is evidence of cholangitis that is not controlled with the single antimicrobial agent, I begin triple therapy, incorporating ampicillin, gentamicin, and clindamycin into the treatment regimen. Frequent blood cultures should be obtained to assess treatment results and to determine specific antimicrobial sensitivity in case bacteremia occurs. Appropriate peak and trough blood levels should be collected to determine efficacy of the antibiotic and to avoid toxicity, especially with impending renal failure. If an infection is unremitting, percutaneous drainage of obstructed biliary lobules may be necessary. It may occasionally be necessary to remove or exchange the endoscopic prosthesis to eliminate the source of infection or to improve drainage.

Most experienced endoscopists currently recommend one of two approaches for the palliative management of Klatskin II and III lesions. One group may attempt to place a prosthesis, but, because of the frequency and severity of subsequent infections associ-

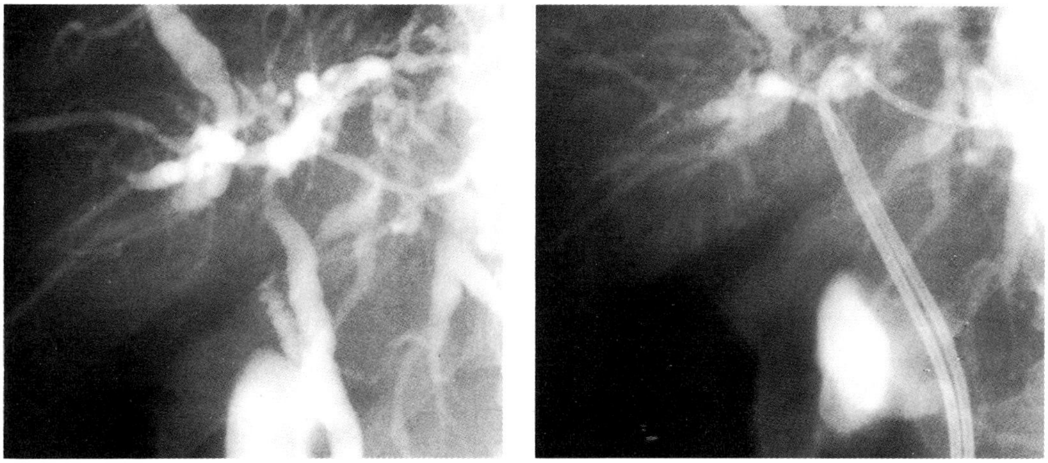

FIG. 12.89. Klatskin II. **Left:** A stricture is appreciated at the bifurcation. **Right:** Two medium-sized prostheses were placed selectively into the right and left hepatic ducts.

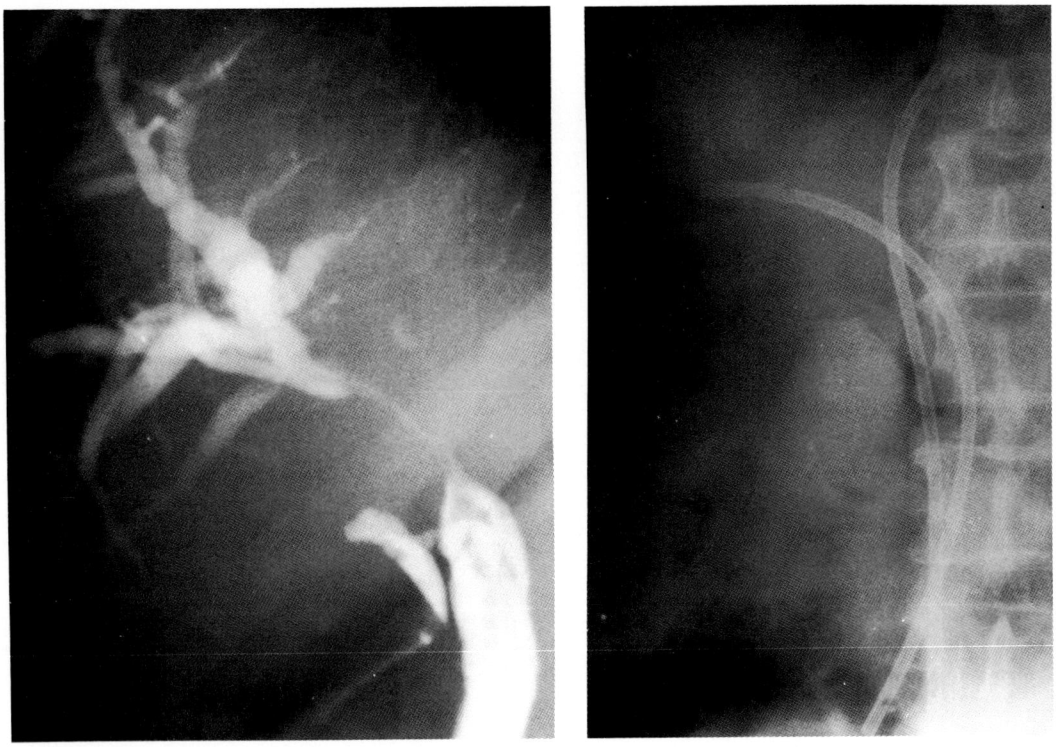

FIG. 12.90. Klatskin III. **Left:** A high-grade obstruction at the bifurcation. No filling of the left hepatic system occurred on the diagnostic ERCP. **Right:** Two prostheses have been selectively placed into each major hepatic duct.

ated with endoscopic stents, it recommends percutaneous or surgical decompression. The other group makes a more aggressive attempt to place as many prostheses as possible and to determine treatment results before making further recommendations. Because of the insidious and progressive nature of bifurcation tumors, and despite the placement of multiple stents, some bile duct radicals and lobules may not drain, and the febrile course may necessitate other types of intervention. The inexperienced endoscopist

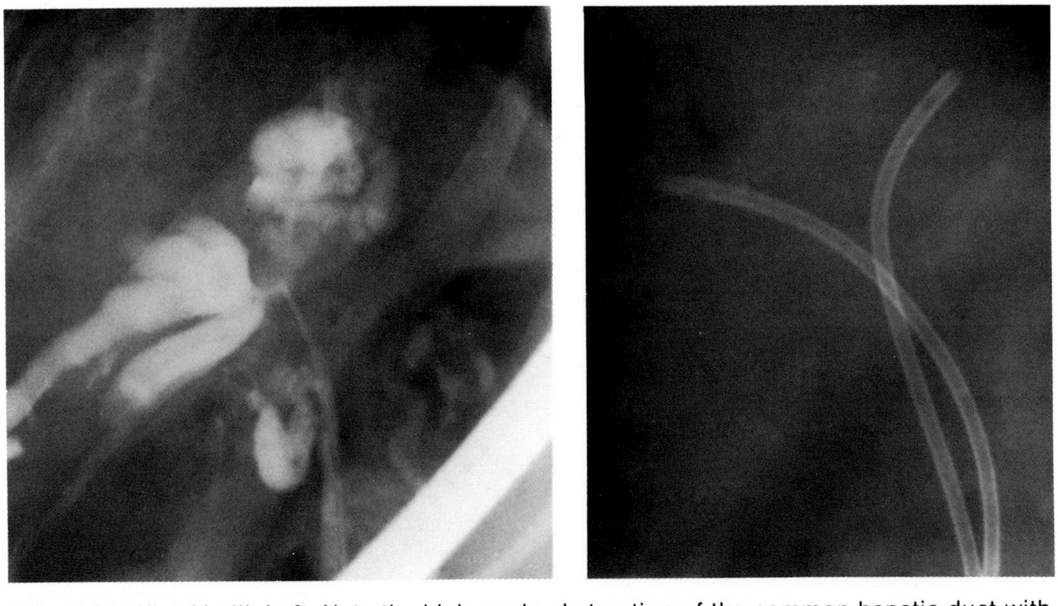

FIG. 12.91. Klatskin III. **Left:** Note the high-grade obstruction of the common hepatic duct with extension of the tumor into both the right and left hepatic duct systems. **Right:** Two large-caliber prostheses have been placed through the strictures to provide decompression.

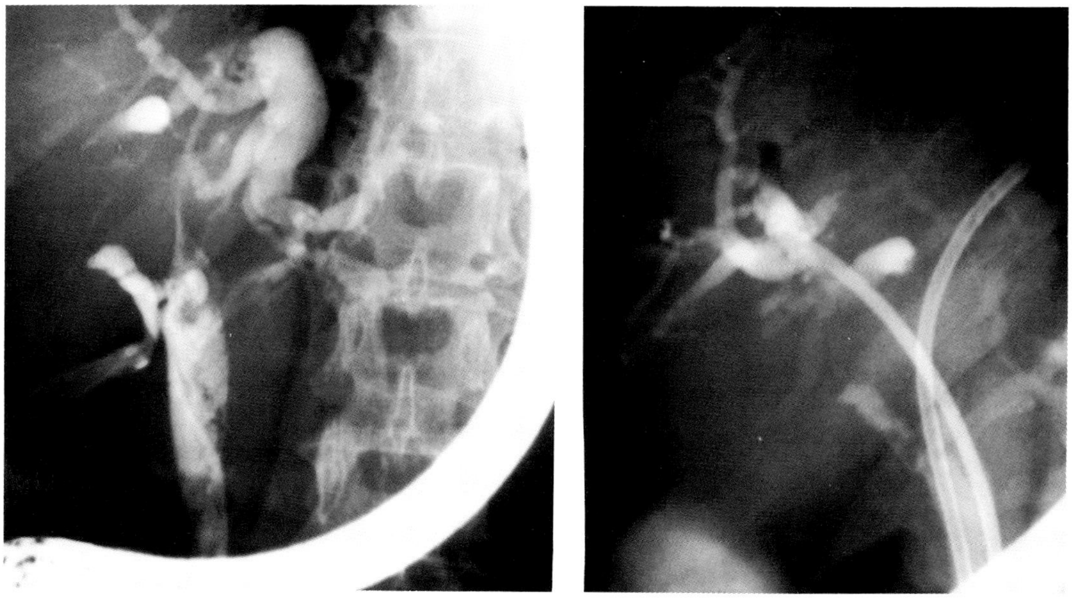

FIG. 12.92. Klatskin III. **Left:** Diffuse involvement of the common hepatic duct and right and left hepatic ducts. **Right:** Two large-caliber prostheses are seen selectively placed into each duct. Note the filling of the right hepatic duct system, which was not seen on the initial injection radiographs.

should refer these difficult management problems to a more experienced endoscopist or an interventional radiologist.

Table 12.3 describes the results of decompression using 363 12Fr stents, and Table 12.4 lists the complications associated with the procedure of inserting 12Fr stents. The results are generally excellent and the complications few, so the rate of success for insertion is high and the patency is longer than for smaller stents. Table 12.5 summarizes the biochemical parameters influenced by biliary stents and the mean survival of patients with malignant diseases. The hospital stay of 3.5 days has greatly influenced our management of patients with unresectable disease.

Cholestasis and/or Jaundice Following Hepatic Resection

I have had the opportunity of evaluating patients who have undergone liver resection, limited or extensive, for either primary biliary malignancies or metastatic disease. Endoscopic evaluation and management of these problems is, to say the least, very challenging. Examples of the endoscopic evaluation are illustrated in Figs. 12.93 through 12.97. Patients presenting with recurrent jaundice were evaluated by either ERCP or percutaneous cholangiography. In some cases, an interventional radiologist placed percutaneous cathe-

Text continues on page 320.

TABLE 12.3. *12 French stent placement (N = 363)*

Results	
Hospital stay	
Mean	3.5 days
Range	1–23 days
Patency	
Mean	210 days
Range	2–477 days
Deaths	1
Surgery	1

TABLE 12.4. *Complications with 12Fr stents (29 of 363, 8%)*

Transient fever	19 (5%)
Bleeding	5 (1.3%)
Pancreatitis	1 (0.3%)
Dislodgment	4 (1%)
Occlusion rate	
Mean	210 days
Range	3–477 days

TABLE 12.5. *Stent placement for malignant obstructive jaundice*

Results	
Laboratory	
Bilirubin (total)	Down 2–3 mg %/day
Alkaline phosphatase	Down 30–70%
Survival	
Mean	210 days
Range	2–540 days
Hospital stay	
Mean	3.5 days
Range	1–23 days

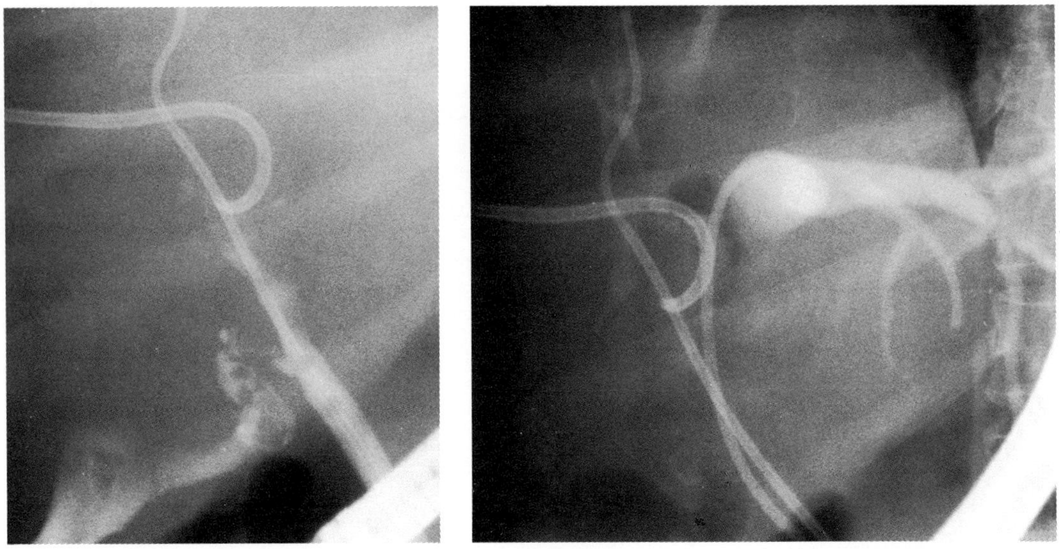

FIG. 12.93. Left: This patient had previously undergone a right lobectomy for treatment of cancer. A percutaneous catheter is visible in this radiograph on the left side of the picture. This catheter was placed at the porta. Also seen in this picture is a single endoscopic prosthesis, which was passed into the posterior lobe. No opacification of the left hepatic system was noted. **Right:** The remaining left hepatic duct system is opacified, and another endoscopic prosthesis was selectively placed into that segment for drainage.

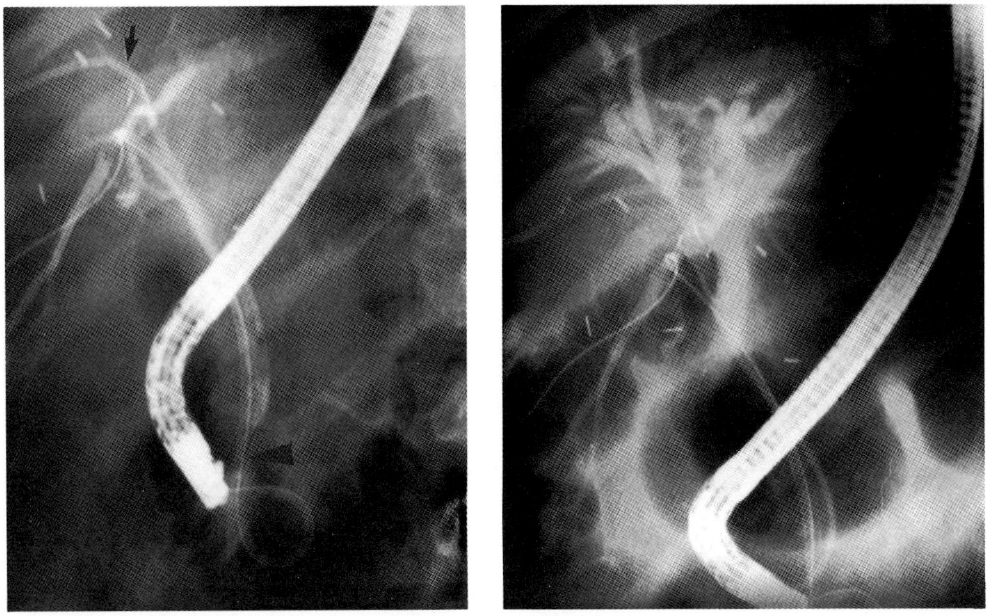

FIG. 12.94. Left: This patient had previously undergone a partial resection of the right hepatic lobe. Because of recurrent jaundice, percutaneous evaluation of the biliary tree was performed first. Two percutaneous prostheses were placed through the upper segments into the duodenum (*arrows*), and another prosthesis, which contained a metal core, was also passed into the duodenum. Opacification of the biliary tree was provided by ERCP. **Right:** Complete opacification of the remaining biliary radicals was accomplished.

FIG. 12.96. Left: Opacification of the right hepatic system following resection of the left lobe. **Middle:** A guidewire being inserted into the right hepatic duct. **Right:** A prosthesis has been placed for decompression.

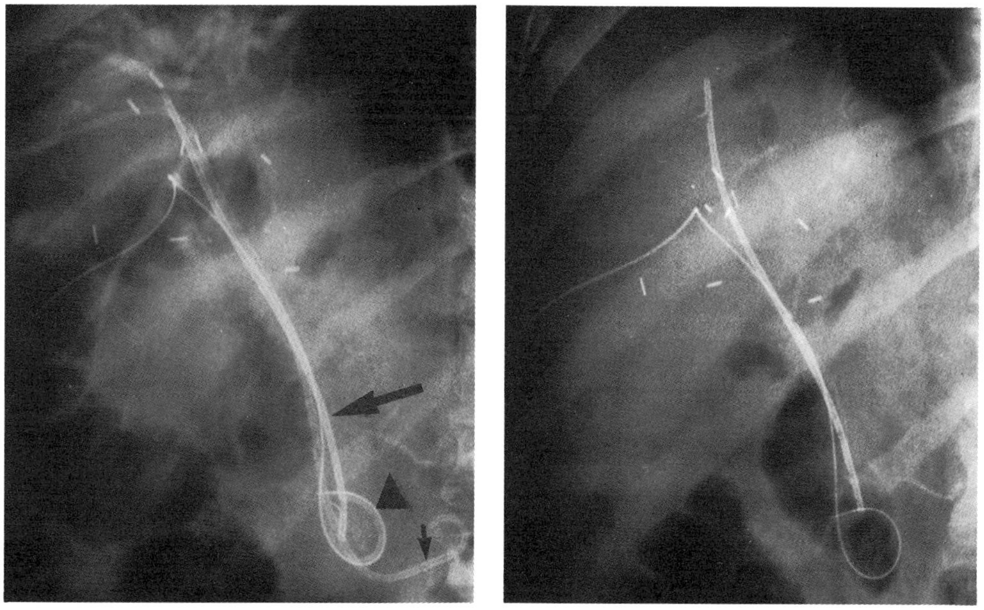

FIG. 12.94. (*Continued*). **Left:** The two percutaneous catheters are visible in the duodenum (*small arrow*) and (*arrow head*). An endoscopic stent is also visible (*large arrow*). **Right:** Only the endoscopic stent and a percutaneous wire remain. The other prostheses were occluded.

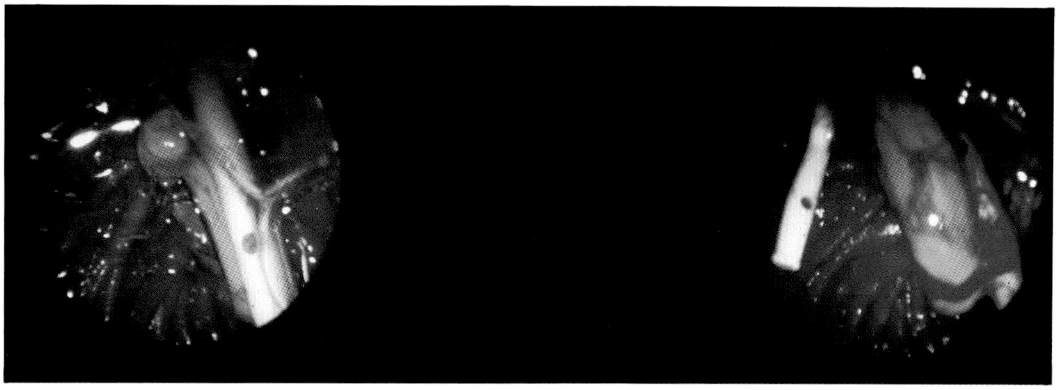

FIG. 12.95. Left: The occluded percutaneous prosthesis in the duodenum. **Right:** The endoscopic stent has been placed before removal of the percutaneous stents.

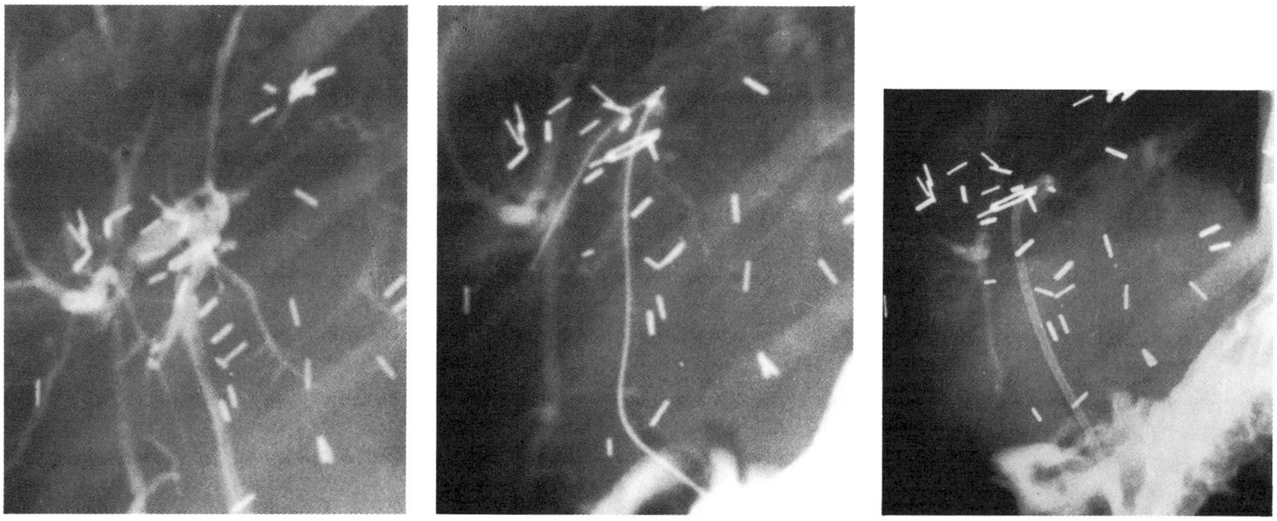

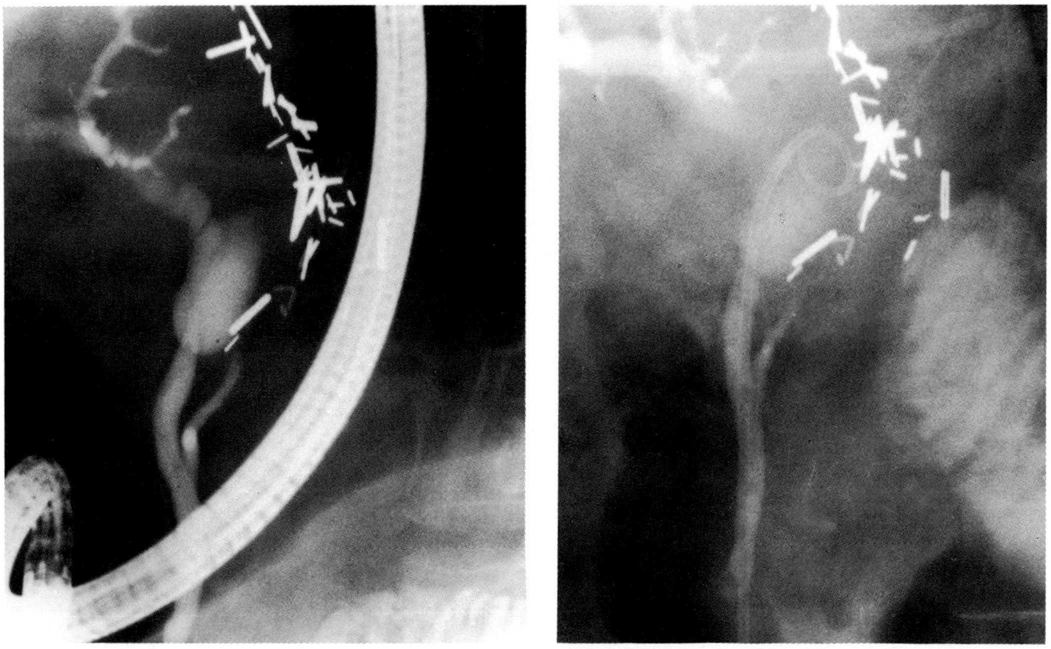

FIG. 12.97. Left: This patient had previously undergone a left hepatic resection. The right hepatic duct system is opacified, and a cystic area at the porta hepatis is noted. The cystic duct remnant is visible. **Right:** A pigtail prosthesis has been placed into the cystic area. This patient did well for nearly 2 years before experiencing recurrent symptoms of cholestasis and jaundice.

Text continued from page 317.
ters. An ERCP was subsequently performed to internalize or exchange the percutaneous catheters or to approach the obstructed area from another axis and insert additional prostheses. Many patients temporarily did well following the insertion of multiple prostheses, but most ultimately succumbed to the malignancy.

STENTS AND BENIGN BILIARY DISEASE

The utility of managing stone disease by placing stents (40) is discussed in Chapter 11. To reiterate, long-term management of patients with retained stones using indwelling prostheses is clearly an efficacious and safe method for the conservative management of stone disease. Other idiopathic benign disease states, including complications of surgical exploration, fistulas, and strictures, have responded to conservative management utilizing sphincterotomy alone; sphincterotomy and balloon dilatation; sphincterotomy and stent placement; or sphincterotomy, balloon dilatation, and stent insertion.

Benign Bile Duct Strictures

Surgical management of bile duct strictures had been the first line of therapy prior to the incorporation of percutaneous and endoscopic therapeutic modalities (86–100). Although surgical techniques for the management of strictures are usually technically successful, recurrent strictures or complications subsequent to surgery may occur in as many as 25% of cases. A primary anastomosis may restenose despite intraductual stenting and may ultimately require elaborate hepaticojejunal anastomoses. If these recurrent strictures are not interrupted or stented, the patient may succumb to severe complications associated with obstruction (e.g., cholangitis) or to those associated with chronic cholestasis and obstruction, leading to biliary cirrhosis and its sequelae.

Early recognition and repair of an injury to the bile duct, especially at the time of surgery, may prevent future consequences. Adequate early stenting of the duct at surgery may avoid recurrent stricture formation. However, if the patient presents with injury after surgery, ERCP and/or PTC are preferred for diagnosis; a therapeutic procedure can be performed at the time of the diagnostic procedure. There are enough data to support the nonsurgical approach to benign biliary strictures. Long-term follow-up of patients treated endoscopically has confirmed the efficacy of the procedure, but the age of the stricture is important (98–100). A younger or more acute stricture is more responsive to dilatation and insertion of prostheses than an old stricture. In other words, from our experience, if stents are left in place for 3 to 6 months, or even longer in a young stricture, reformation of the stricture after removal of the stents is unlikely. Older strictures, however, are more likely to recur when the stents are re-

TABLE 12.6. *Benign strictures—patient demographics*

Women	39
Men	15
Age range	27–77 yrs
Mean age	57 yrs

TABLE 12.7. *Benign biliary strictures*

Distribution of strictures (N = 54)	
Upper third	27
Middle third	17
Lower third	10

TABLE 12.8. *Endoscopic treatment of benign biliary strictures (N = 54)*

Successful dilatation	51 (94%)
Insertion of prostheses	46
Removal of prostheses	36 (78%)
Surgery (failure of endotherapy)	2
Permanent stents	8

TABLE 12.9. *Benign strictures (N = 54)*

Complications of endoscopic treatment	
Fever	9 (17%)
Septicemia	2 (4%)
Surgery (failure of endotherapy)	2 (4%)
Deaths	0

moved. If the old stricture recurs and the patient is a candidate for surgery, I recommend a surgical procedure. However, if surgery is contraindicated, I place one or two large-caliber prostheses and leave them in place for about 1 year (and sometimes longer). Prostheses should be changed on an annual basis in order to avoid recurrent cholangitis. It has been my experience that prostheses remain effective and patent longer in benign disease than in malignant disease, and I have left stents in place up to 1 year in this situation with older strictures. The patient is instructed to recognize symptoms of recurrent cholestasis and to return if pruritis, choluria, or acholic stools occur. The patient must contact me immediately if fever is associated with this symptom complex. Cholangitis has been a rare occurrence with benign disease.

I have treated 54 consecutive patients with benign strictures (Tables 12.6–12.9). The patient demographics, location of strictures, method of treatment, and complications associated with this form of therapy are listed in these tables. The technique for balloon dilatation is discussed in Chapter 13. All strictures were successfully negotiated and dilated. Prophylactic intravenous antibiotics are administered prior to the procedure to reduce morbidity associated with infection. Of the group, 36 have had stents removed with no recurrent stricture formation. One patient with a mid-common bile duct stricture ultimately underwent surgery because of recurrence following stent removal (Fig. 12.98). The remaining 19 patients have been carefully monitored either by the primary care physician or by my group to assess their response to therapy and to determine when or if the stents should be removed or exchanged. Figures 12.99 through 12.102 are illustrative examples of benign, iatrogenic strictures found at ERCP. Placement of prostheses for the endoscopic management of benign strictures appears to be an effective method for the treatment of strictures of the bile duct. Balloon dilatation of these strictures may be temporarily effective, but, because of their fibrous

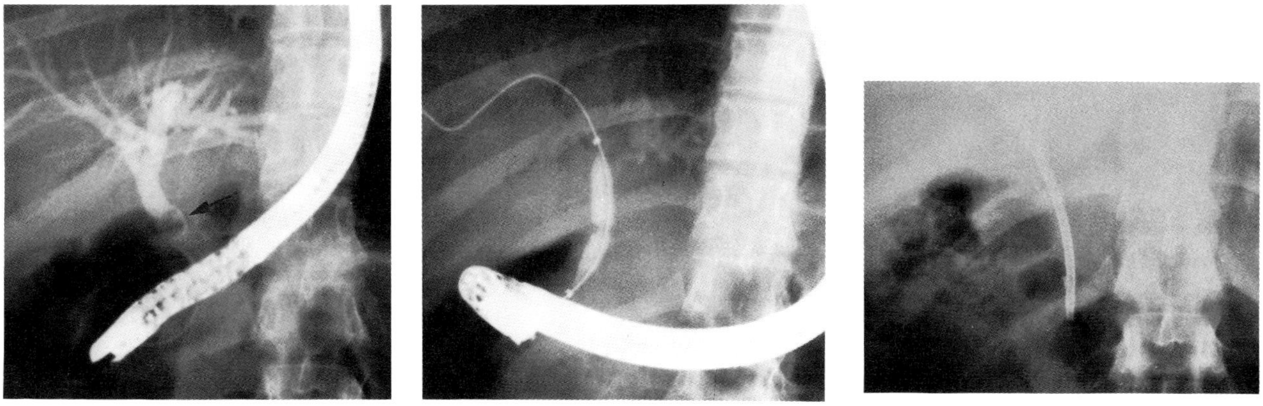

FIG. 12.98. The patient whose ERCP is shown here had a difficult postoperative course following cholecystectomy and was in hospital 3 months. **Left:** A high-grade stricture of the mid common bile duct (*arrow*). **Middle:** An 8 mm balloon dilating the stricture. Note the waist is the middle of the balloon created by the stricture. **Right:** A large-caliber prosthesis is in place.

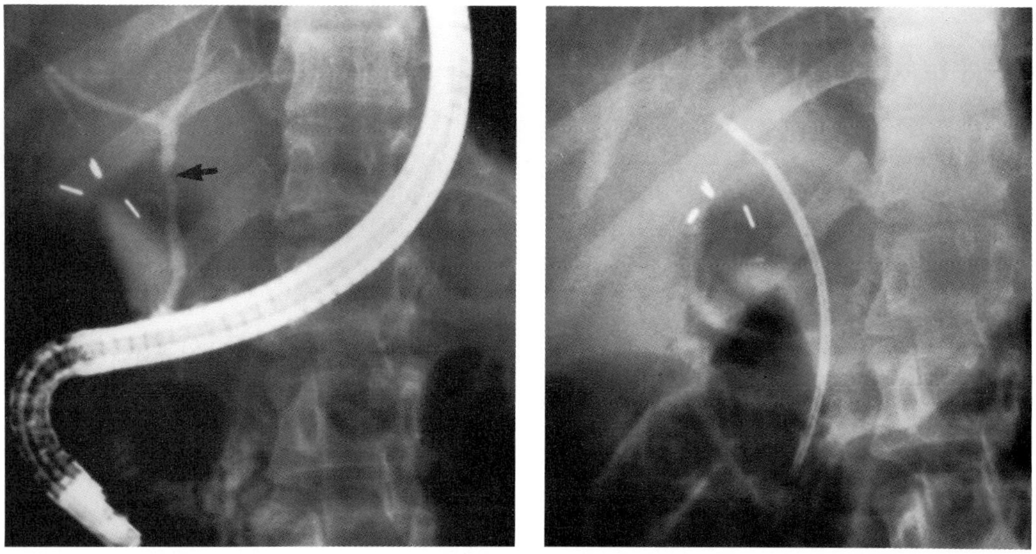

FIG. 12.99. Left: A stricture (*arrow*) in the upper bile duct (common hepatic duct) with no dilatation of the biliary tree proximally, although cholestatic liver tests were obtained. **Right:** A prosthesis traverses the stricture; all contrast has drained from the biliary tree.

composition, the strictures may reform. However, the continuous presence of the prosthesis, preferably a large-caliber one, may exert its effect by maintaining the integrity of the lumen and providing continuous dilatation by its movement (99). Whatever the mechanism, biliary endoprostheses have been effective in this situation, with more than 75% of patients in this series deriving permanent relief and avoiding surgery. The rate of success is as high as 88% in other series (100,101).

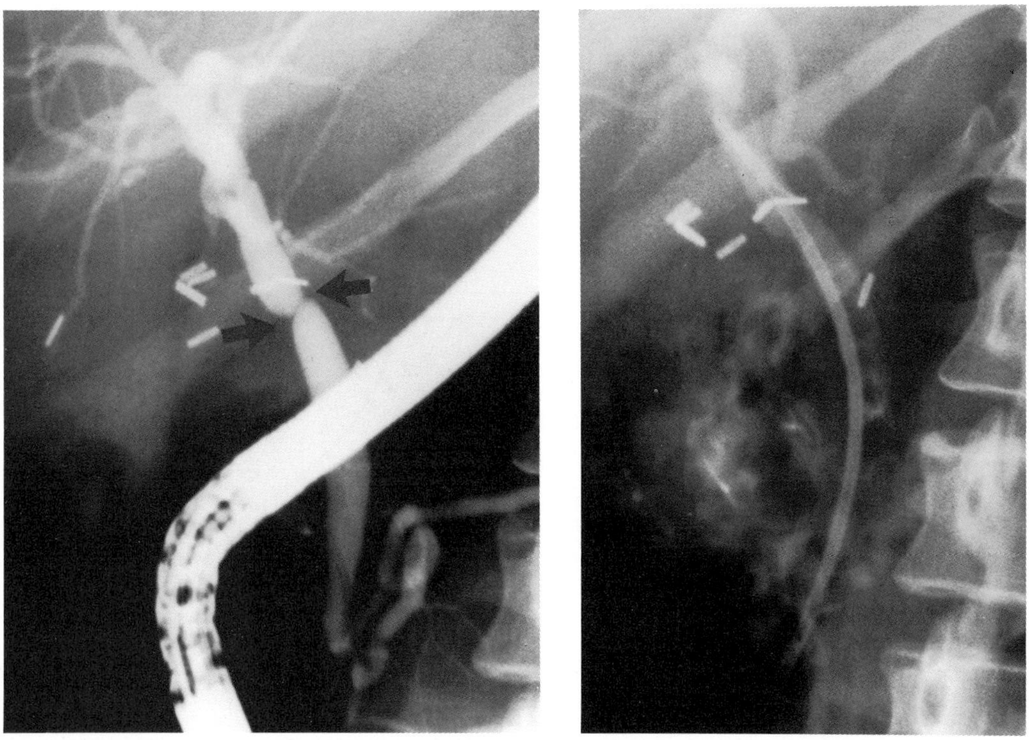

FIG. 12.100. Left: A stricture in the common hepatic duct is visible near the surgical clips (*arrows*) in this patient who has previously undergone a cholecystectomy. Minimal dilatation of the proximal biliary tree is seen. **Right:** A prosthesis has been placed into the proximal duct.

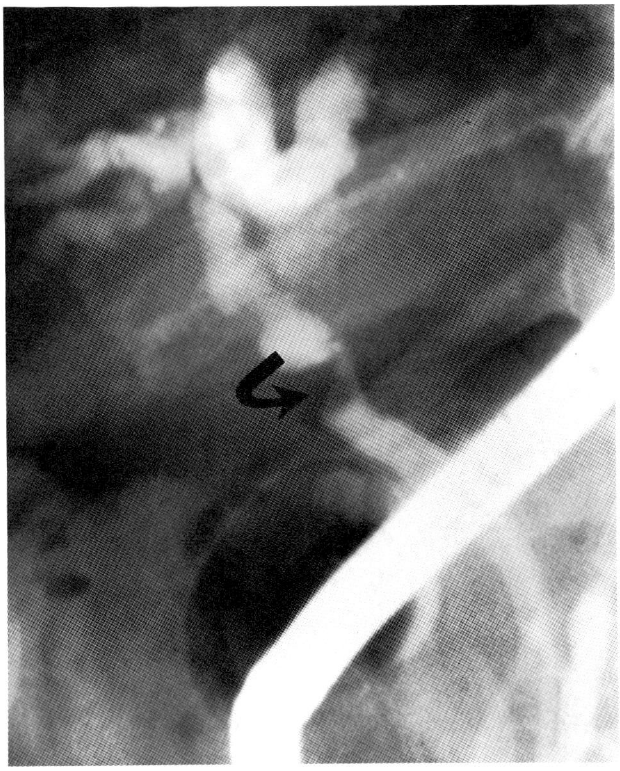

FIG. 12.101. A high-grade stricture of the common hepatic duct (*arrow*) which developed 2 weeks after cholecystectomy and common bile duct exploration.

In my experience, the placement of biliary prostheses for the management of bile duct strictures secondary to chronic pancreatitis are an exception to these results. Figure 12.103 demonstrates the placement of a prostheses in a patient who has experienced recurrent episodes of pancreatitis, the formation of bile duct stricture, cholestasis, and jaundice. The jaundice and cholestasis were relieved, which is often the case, but the patient's pain syndrome remained. Again, others have reported success in this select group (100). Each case of pancreatitis should be individualized, and, if the trial is successful, the stent can remain (otherwise, remove it).

Biliary Fistulas

Prior to nonsurgical manipulation of the biliary tree, iatrogenic fistulae were often difficult to manage and usually required surgery. Fistulae of the common bile duct or hepatic ducts usually result from iatrogenic injury to the duct or ducts, whereas spontaneous rupture of a cystic duct remnant and failure of closure of a T-tube tract usually result from increased pressure within the bile duct produced by a distal obstructing stone, spasm, or stricture. Type 1 fistulae can be adequately managed by performing a sphincterotomy and inserting a prosthesis to divert the flow of bile from the proximal bile duct through the prosthesis and into the duodenum. The diversion of bile flow away from the fistula into the duodenum allows for healing. It has been my experience that most fistulae heal spontaneously, if the stent has occluded or bridged the opening, because the high rate of bile flow through the fistula has been diverted from the hole into the duodenum (20,99,102–105). Type 2 fistulae from distal obstruction, increased pressure, and cystic duct blowout result from distal bile duct obstruction and usually heal after performance of a sphincterotomy and/or removal of the obstructing stone. A stent is usually unnecessary in this latter type of fistula because relieving obstruction promotes the free flow of bile from the bile duct through the sphincterotomy, reducing bile flow through the fistula and allowing spontaneous healing. Figure 12.104 is an artist's drawing of the formation of a biliary fistula and the endoscopic techniques used in managing this complication. These techniques include performing a sphincterotomy and inserting a prosthesis.

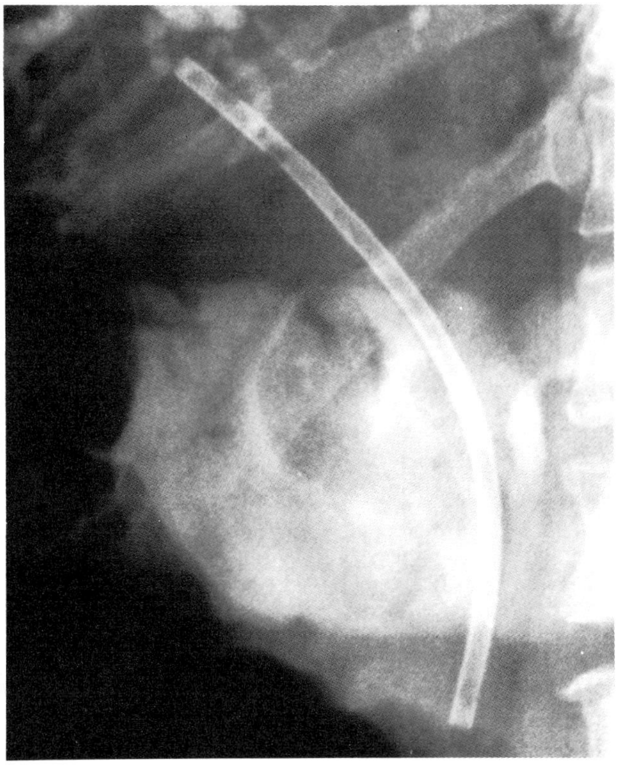

FIG. 12.102. A high-grade benign stricture of the common hepatic duct producing proximal biliary dilatation was traversed with a dilating catheter advanced over a guidewire. A large-caliber prosthesis was then placed through the stricture into the proximal biliary tree.

TABLE 12.10. *Endoscopic management of biliary fistulae (N = 30)*

Type of fistula	
Cutaneous	21
Intraperitoneal	9

TABLE 12.11. *Treatment modalities for biliary cutaneous or peritoneal fistulae (N = 30)*

Sphincterotomy	Spincterotomy—prostheses
13 Cutaneous	11 Cutaneous 6 Peritoneal

I have had the opportunity to manage *30 biliary fistulae: 9 intraperitoneal and 21 cutaneous* (Figs. 12.105–12.110; Tables 12.10, 12.11). All of the fistulae healed spontaneously after sphincterotomy and/or insertion of a prosthesis. Surprisingly, the intraperitoneal fistulae resolved uneventfully. This experience has been shared by other investigators (85,102–104). These fistulae formerly required surgery, but with the therapeutic endoscopic procedures currently available, this potentially dangerous condition can be managed nonsurgically.

I have no personal experience managing fistulae associated with liver transplantation. Reports indicate that endoscopic methods have been effective in the management of many of these fistulae, which arise from breakdown of anastamoses, but some of them may still require surgery. Certainly, endoscopy has begun to make its contributions to this developing field. It is important to remember that intraperitoneal fistulae develop after either resultant injury to the bile duct or leakage from the cystic duct stump because of distal bile duct obstruction. This obstruction is most commonly due to a stone, spasm, or stricture. Sphinc-

Text continues on page 328.

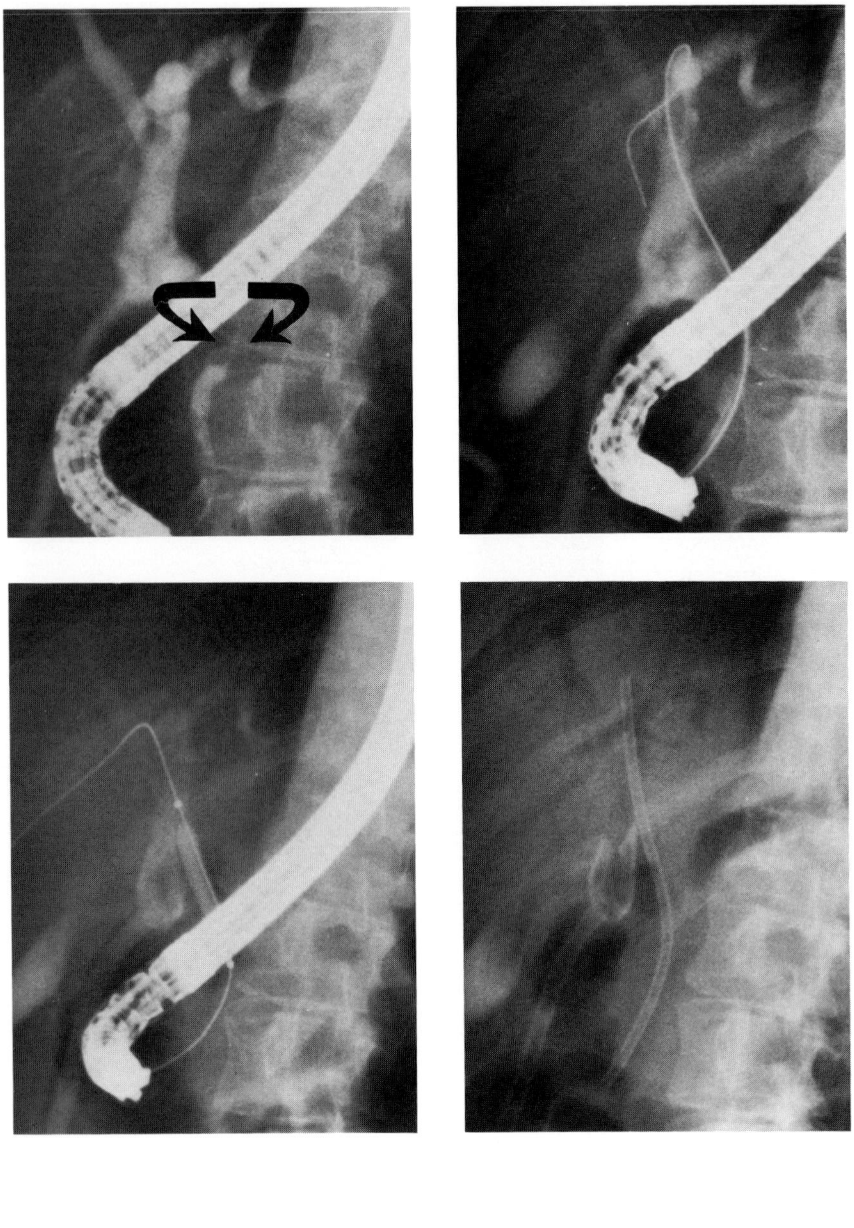

FIG. 12.103. Top left: A cholangiogram obtained at ERCP (a T-tube is also in place) shows a stricture (*arrows*) in the distal bile duct in a patient with recurrent episodes of pancreatitis. **Top right:** A dilating catheter and guidewire have been advanced through the stricture into the proximal bile duct. **Bottom left:** An 8 mm balloon is placed into the stricture, and the stricture is dilated. **Bottom right:** A large-caliber prosthesis has been inserted through the stricture into the bile duct. The T-tube is being removed.

Fistula

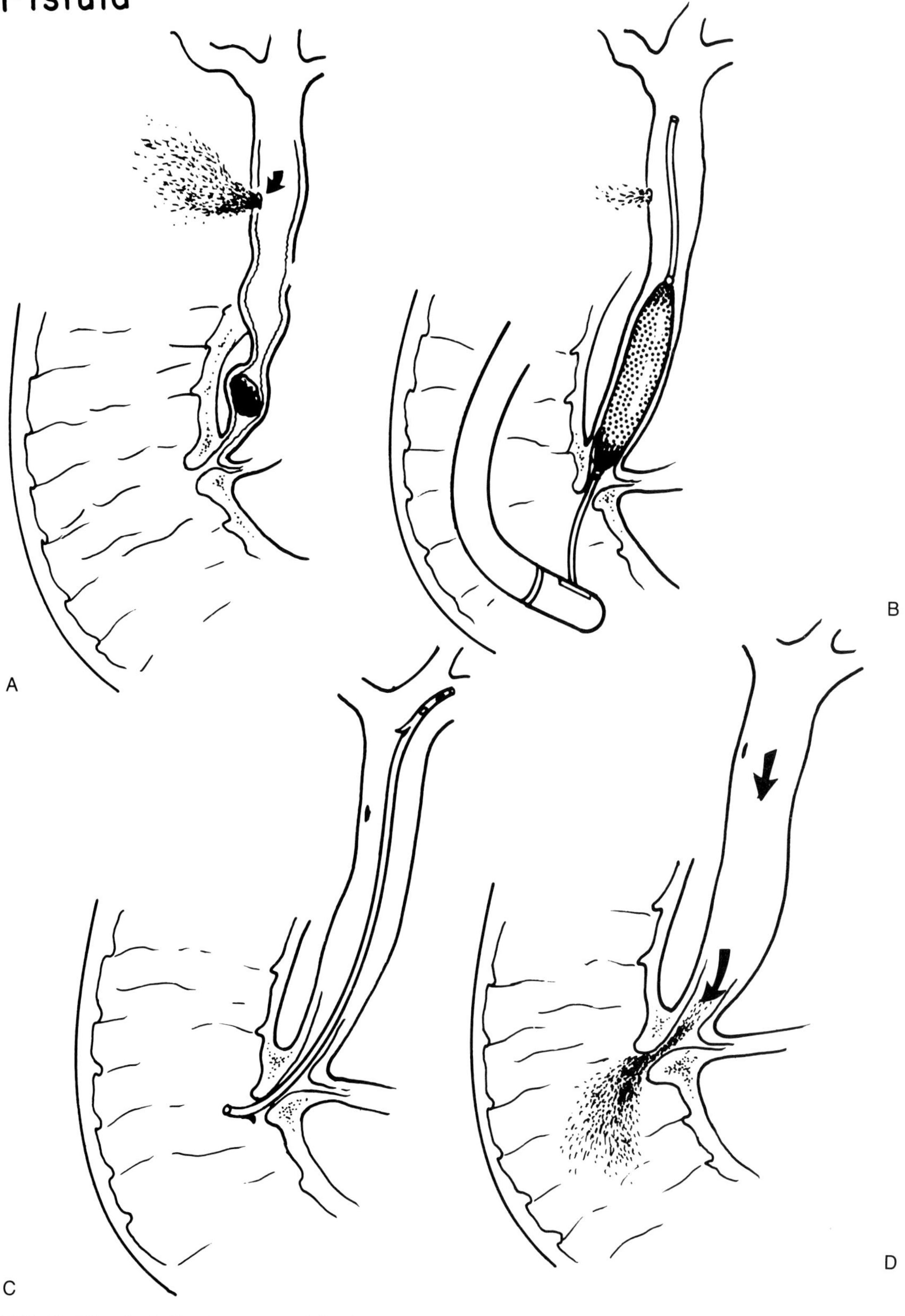

FIG. 12.104. A: A distal common bile duct stone and distal stricture. A fistula has formed at the cystic duct stump (*arrow*). **B:** A balloon catheter is placed into the distal stricture after a sphincterotomy has been performed and the stone has been removed. **C:** Healing of the fistula after a stent has been inserted to permit flow of bile away from the fistula. **D:** After removal of the prosthesis and healing of the fistula, bile flows down the bile duct out into the duodenum (*arrow*).

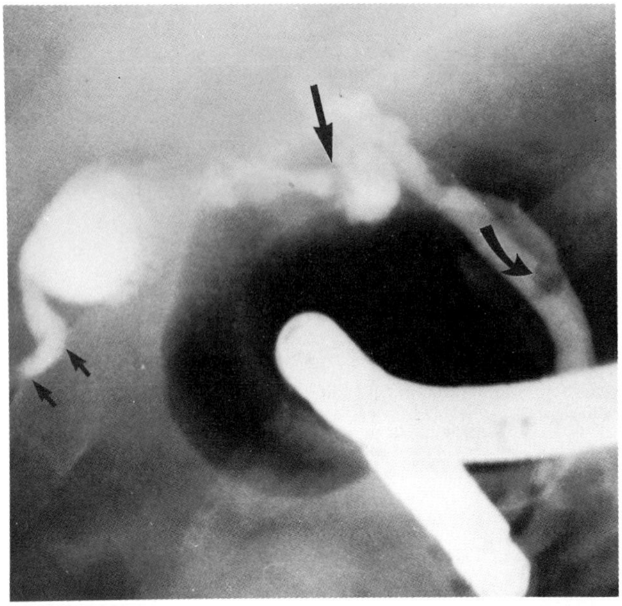

FIG. 12.105. This radiograph demonstrates the presence of a fistula that is shown leaking from the cystic duct stump (*large arrow*). The structure to the far left (patient's right) is a collection in the gallbladder fossa; the continuation of the fistula is shown extending to the far left (*small arrows*). Note the lucency seen in the mid common bile duct (*curved arrow*), a stone, which was displaced from its impaction in the ampulla. A sphincterotomy was performed and the stone removed. The fistula closed spontaneously after removal of the stone.

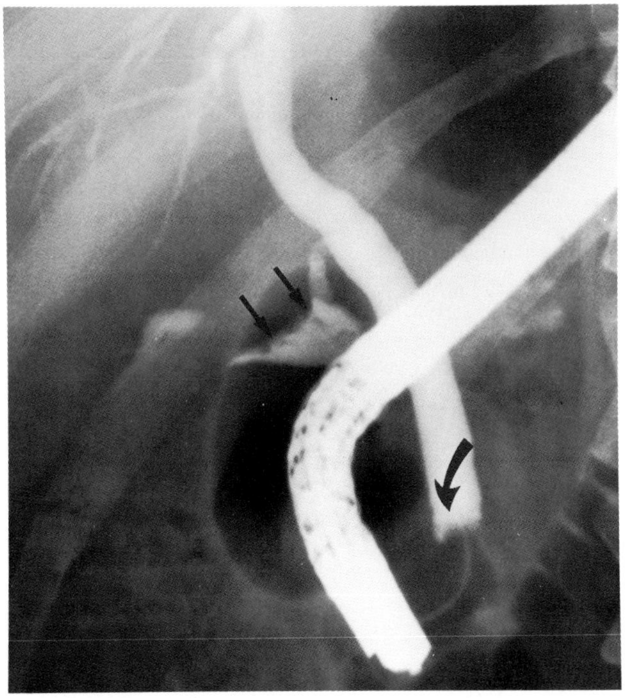

FIG. 12.106. An intraperitoneal fistula (*small arrows*) and a persistent filling defect in the distal common bile duct (*curved arrow*). After performance of a sphincterotomy, a stone was removed, and the fistula closed spontaneously.

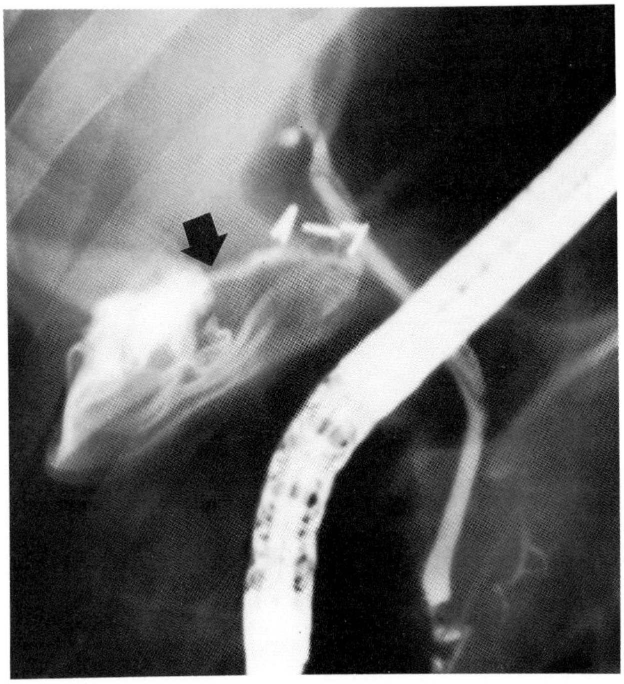

FIG. 12.107. A large collection of contrast material streams into the right upper quadrant (left side of radiograph) arising from the cystic duct stump (*arrow*). Note the persistent spasm or tapering of the distal common bile duct. No stone was found after sphincterotomy, but the fistula slowly resolved when ductal drainage was established.

FIG. 12.110. Left: A fistulous tract arising from the area of the cystic duct. A stone may be seen in the bile duct (*arrow*), and obstruction of the papilla is confirmed. A lucency is visible in the distal bile duct (*curved arrow*). **Middle:** A sphincterotomy was performed, and the stones removed. The bile duct is less dilated, but contrast exits from the fistulous tract (*arrow*). **Right:** A prosthesis was placed into the common hepatic duct (*arrows*) to divert bile flow to the duodenum.

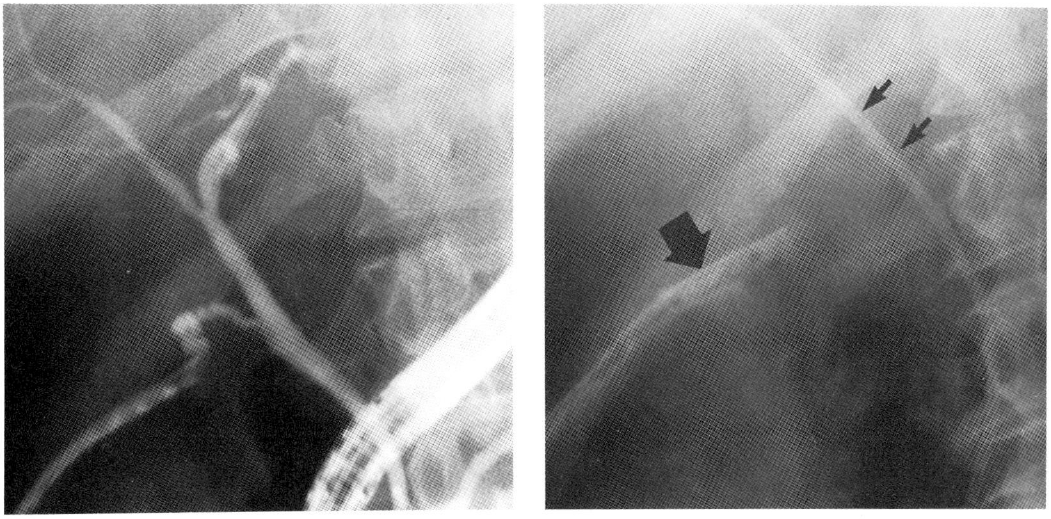

FIG. 12.108. Left: A fistulous tract is shown arising from the cystic duct and flowing toward and through a drain toward the left of the picture. **Right:** A stent is visible in the bile duct (*small arrows*), and the Jackson-Pratt drain appears on the left (*large arrow*). Note that contrast has drained from the biliary tree.

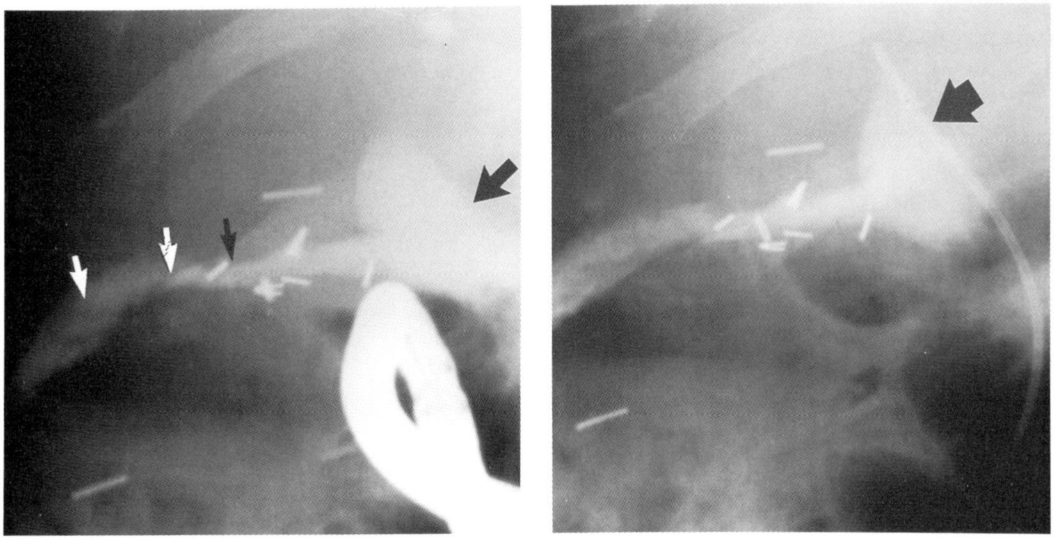

FIG. 12.109. Left: A dilated bile duct (*large arrow*) and a peritoneal-cutaneous fistula (*small arrows*). **Right:** A stent (*large arrow*) after placement above the origin of the fistula.

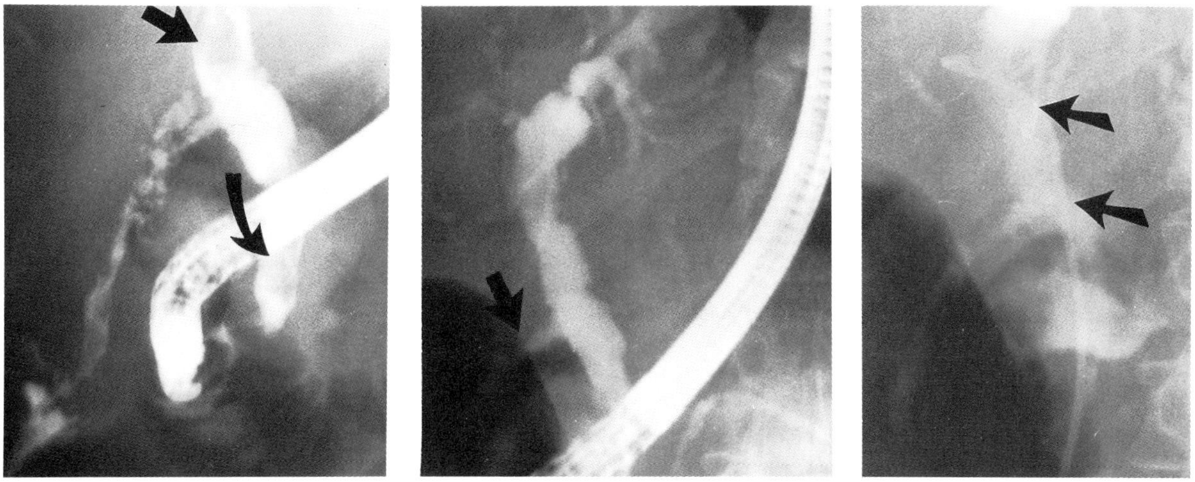

Text continued from page 324.
terotomy often remedies this problem, although earlier reports suggested that sphincterotomy was not necessary if a stent or nasobiliary tube were placed. In our series, like others, sphincterotomy with or without stent placement has been the rule rather than the exception.

A cutaneous fistula commonly develops after removal of a T-tube, especially when a mature tract is present (Type 2 fistula). Suspicion of distal bile duct obstruction is raised when bile is found leaking around a clamped T-tube, soiling the surgical dressing. Before removing a T-tube, one routinely obtains a T-tube cholangiogram to ensure that neither a stone nor another cause of obstruction is found in the distal bile duct. Often an ERCP and sphincterotomy are requested and performed because contrast does not empty into the duodenum on repeat T-tube cholangiography. After demonstrating the cause of obstruction and performing a sphincterotomy, the endoscopist can remove the T-tube because the source of obstruction has been eliminated.

Suspicion of distal obstruction is sustained when persistent flow of bile is appreciated from a T-tube fistula wound after the tube has been removed. If the rate of flow is heavy and the T-tube tract will not heal, a sphincterotomy is indicated to relieve obstruction. After distal drainage is established, the volume of bile flowing from the tract will progressively diminish, and the fistula will close. This is reassuring to the surgeon, and the patient will be grateful to the endoscopist for his or her expertise.

Sclerosing Cholangitis

Over the past 17 years, I have had the opportunity to evaluate patients with radiographic and clinical findings consistent with sclerosing cholangitis and to participate in uncontrolled trials using a variety of medical and endoscopic regimens. My interest in extracolonic manifestations of inflammatory bowel disease, primarily liver disease, was piqued during my special fellowship in liver diseases at The Royal Free Hospital in London, where many patients with this disease were evaluated and treated by Professor Sheila Sherlock. I, like others, have been intrigued with the unusual and varied manifestations of this disease and have observed that it is impossible to correlate the severity of this disease with the cholangiographic, biochemical, or constitutional abnormalities because of the ubiquitous nature of this disease.

Because most treatment regimens, including surgical and pharmacologic, have been universally unsuccessful in inducing morphologic improvement and remissions in this disease (Table 12.12), it seemed appropriate to offer an endoscopic, therapeutic regimen that might prove to be efficacious (99–106). An earlier surgical technique utilizing a drainge-perfusion system suggested that chronic perfusion and irrigation of the affected biliary radicals were directly responsible for improvement in biochemical, constitutional, and morphologic parameters (107). Our initial endoscopic approach to the management of sclerosing cholangitis included the performance of a sphincterotomy followed by balloon dilatation of the dominant strictures affecting the extrahepatic bile duct. We were impressed by the initial encouraging results. We next began to modify and implement the perfusion technique introduced by the Amsterdam group (21) using a different treatment plan. Allison et al. subsequently modified this technique, but their results were less favorable (108). Most investigators have concentrated on dilatation and stenting techniques (109). However, because of the favorable results of endotherapy, we routinely offer these options to patients presenting with symptomatic sclerosing cholangitis.

When beginning our perfusion regimen, we insert a nasobiliary catheter through the dominant stricture in the extrahepatic system. This nasobiliary catheter is perfused automatically using an I-Med controller while the patient is in the hospital. Initially, steroids are perfused alternately with saline and antibiotics, the latter selected after completion of culture and sensitivity tests carried out on aspirates obtained from the nasobiliary catheter. During hospitalization, the steroids are tapered, and the patients are discharged with a supply of syringes, saline, and antibiotics. At home, the nasobiliary catheter is perfused four times per day using a 30 cc bolus of saline each time. After 4 months,

TABLE 12.12. *Therapy employed for sclerosing cholangitis*

Medical	Surgical	Endoscopic
Cholestyramine	Colectomy	Sphincterotomy
Steroids	Cholecystectomy	Cholangioplasty
Azathioprine	Choledochostomy	Endoprosthesis
Penicillamine	T-tube/tube insertion	Nasobiliary tube with irrigation
Colchicine	Sphincteroplasty	
Methotrexate	Biliary-enteric bypass and/or Roux limb placed subcutaneously	
6 Mercaptoprurine		
Ursodeoxycholic acid		

TABLE 12.13. *Patients with sclerosing cholangitis—demographics (N = 42)*

Men	29
Women	15
Age range	17–77 yrs
Mean age	34.5 yrs

TABLE 12.14. *Sclerosing cholangitis: endoscopic treatment results*

Bilirubin	80% decrease
Alkaline phosphatase and gammaglutamyl transpepsidase	60% decrease
Follow-up	
Mean	4.3 yrs
Range	3 mos–7 yrs

TABLE 12.15. *Sclerosing cholangitis patient follow-up (N = 42)*

Patients on medical regimen after endoscopy	31
Interposition bowel loop (surgical)	4
Transplantation	2
Deaths	
Cholangiocarcinoma	2
Sepsis (carcinoma)	1
Lost to follow-up	2

the nasobiliary catheter is removed, and the dominant stricture (if still present) is dilated and an endoprosthesis is inserted at ERCP. As reported previously (101), follow-up of 36 patients (now 42) (Table 12.13) is 7 years, with a mean of 4.3 years. Most patients, 39 of 42, benefitted from this method of treatment (Tables 12.14, 12.15). Two were subsequently found to have cholangiocarcinoma and did not respond favorably to drainage, and one patient ultimately died of sepsis associated with cholangiocarcinoma. Figures 12.111 through 12.118 illustrate the different techniques we have incorporated into our treatment regimen for sclerosing cholangitis.

Because there is no known cure for sclerosing cholangitis and many young patients ultimately become candidates for liver transplantation (two in our series), the least amount of manipulation, especially surgical, should be appreciated by the transplant surgeon. I therefore discourage prior performance of biliary-enteric anastamoses or other complicated surgical procedures, which have been ineffective in this disease, and recommend less invasive procedures to temporize before transplantation. Combined endoscopic, pharmacologic (bile acids), and immunosuppressant therapy may offer the patient a better prognosis, induce remission, and delay transplant surgery. We are cur-

Text continues on page 332.

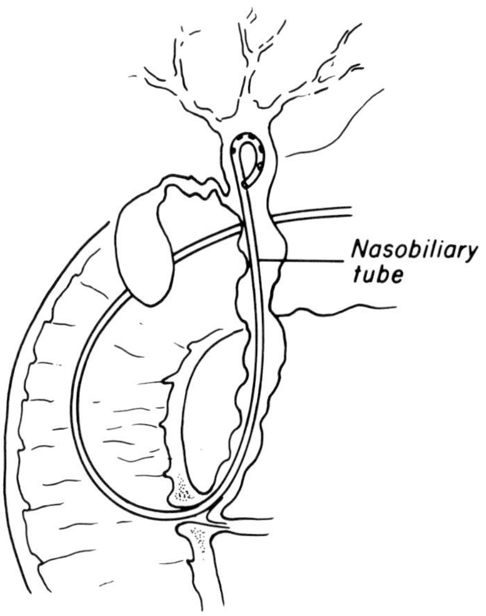

FIG. 12.111. Evidence of diffuse sclerosing cholangitis and the presence of a nasobiliary catheter.

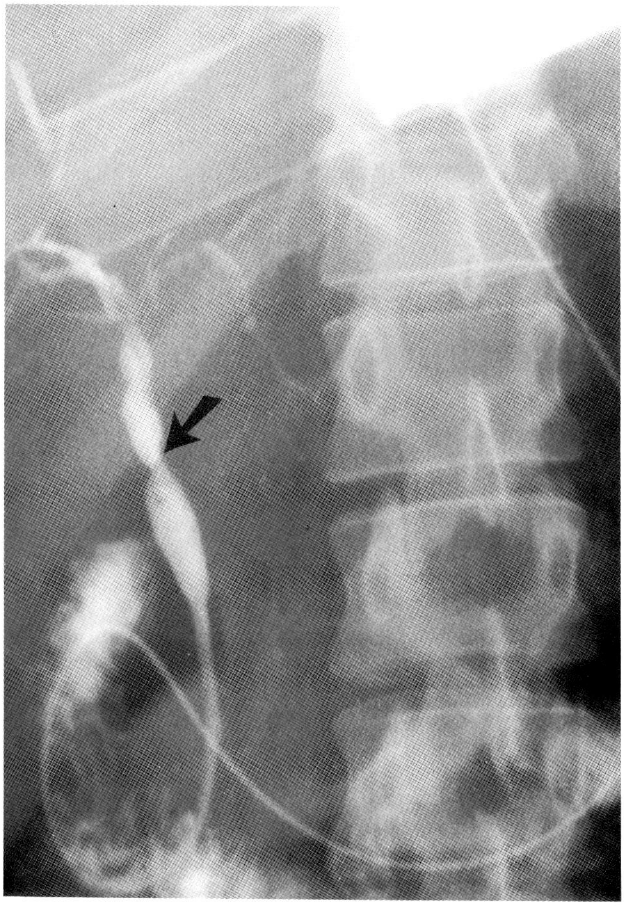

FIG. 12.112. A radiograph illustrating the findings of sclerosing cholangitis affecting both the intra- and extrahepatic ducts. Note the dominant stricture in the mid common bile duct (*arrow*).

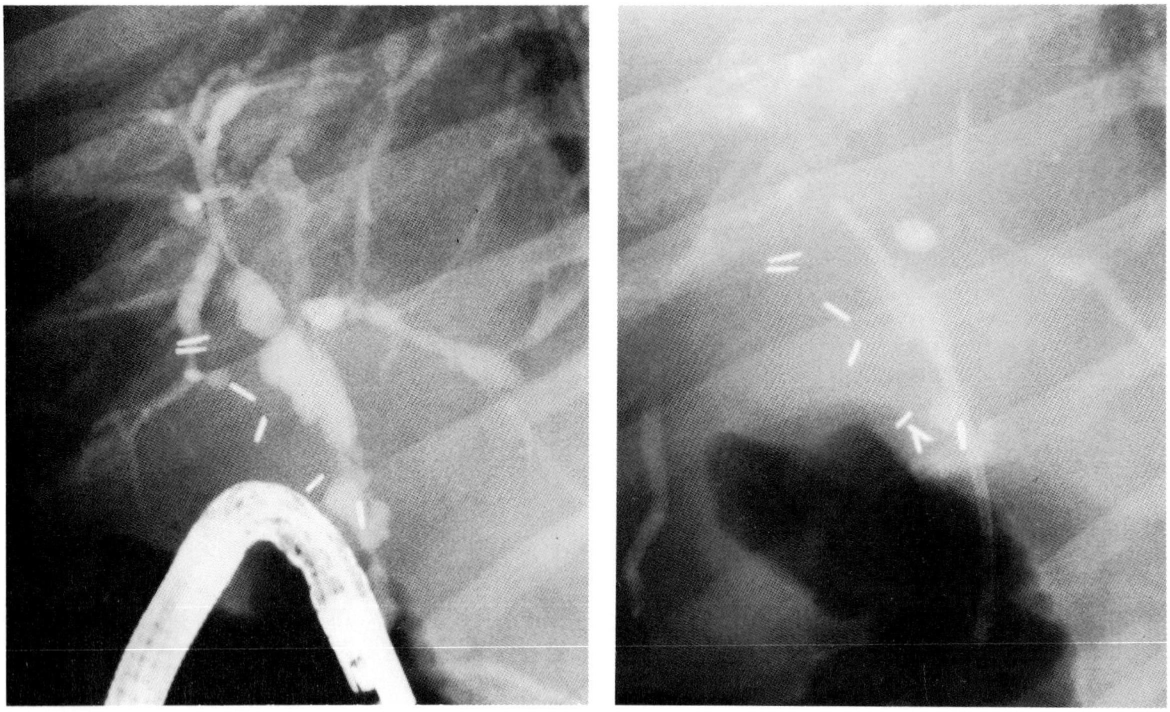

FIG. 12.113. **Left:** Diffuse extra- and intrahepatic disease consistent with sclerosing cholangitis. **Right:** A small-caliber endoprosthesis is shown in the bile duct.

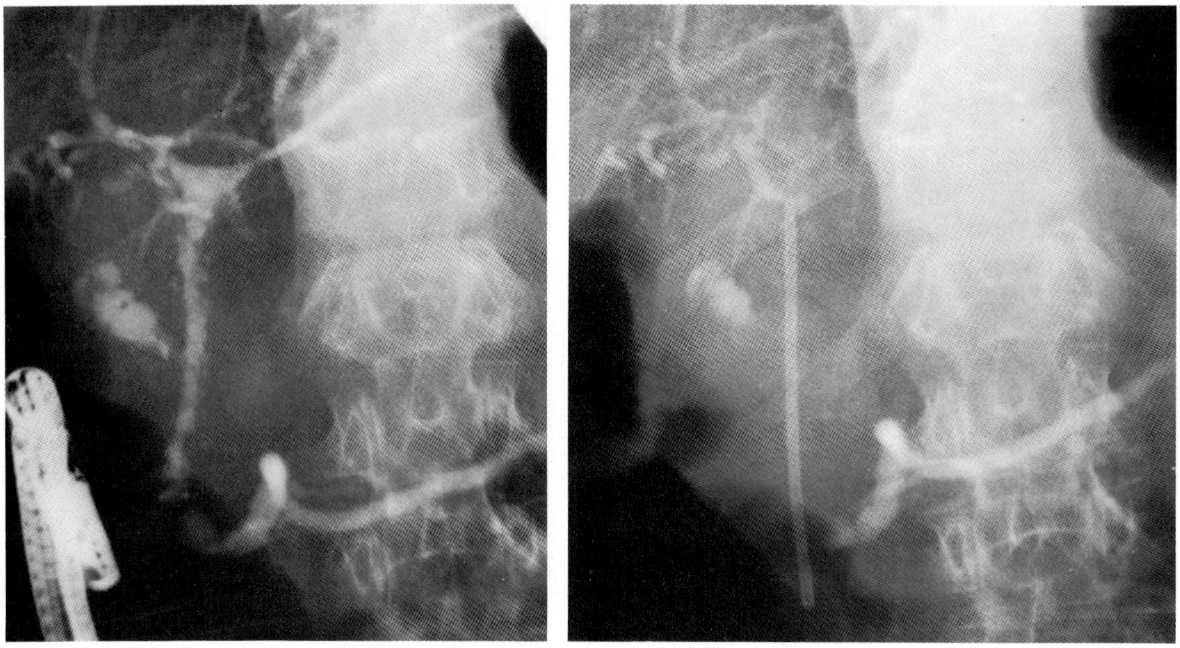

FIG. 12.114. **Left:** Diffuse intrahepatic and extrahepatic disease consistent with sclerosing cholangitis. **Right:** A medium-sized prosthesis was placed in the extrahepatic duct.

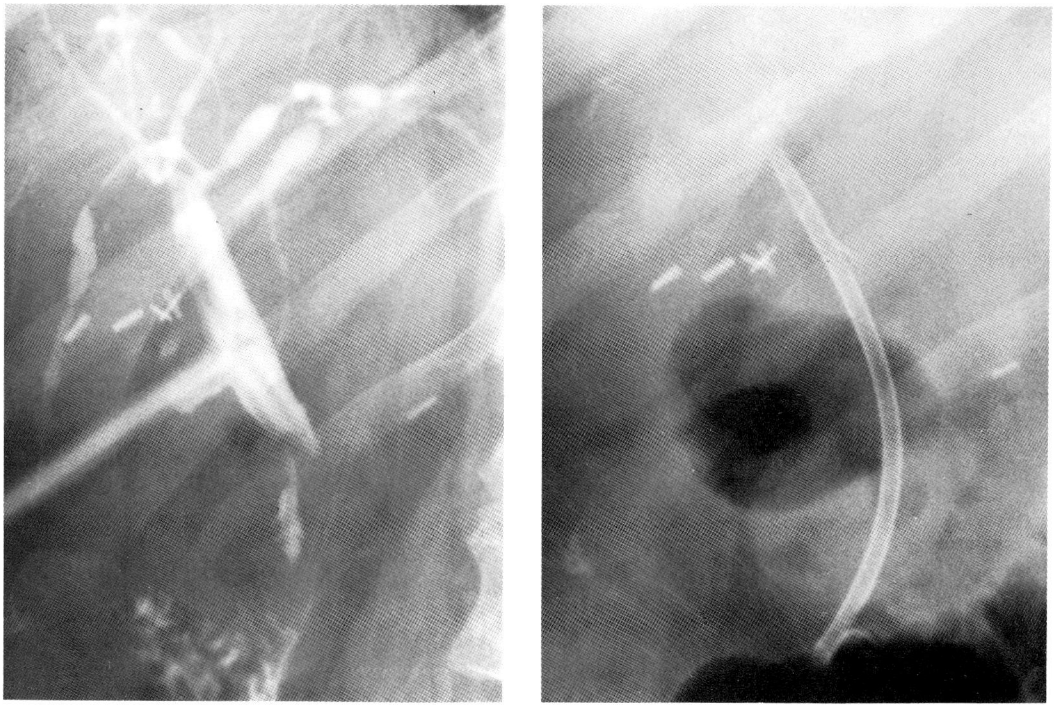

FIG. 12.115. Left: Intrahepatic radicals affected by diffuse sclerosing cholangitis are shown on this T-tube cholangiogram, which was obtained at surgery (cholecystectomy). Note this dominant stricture in the distal bile duct. **Right:** A large-caliber prosthesis was advanced through the dominant stricture after removal of the T-tube 3 months later. This patient did well for 6 months but after repeat stent exchanges was found to have metastatic adenocarcinoma.

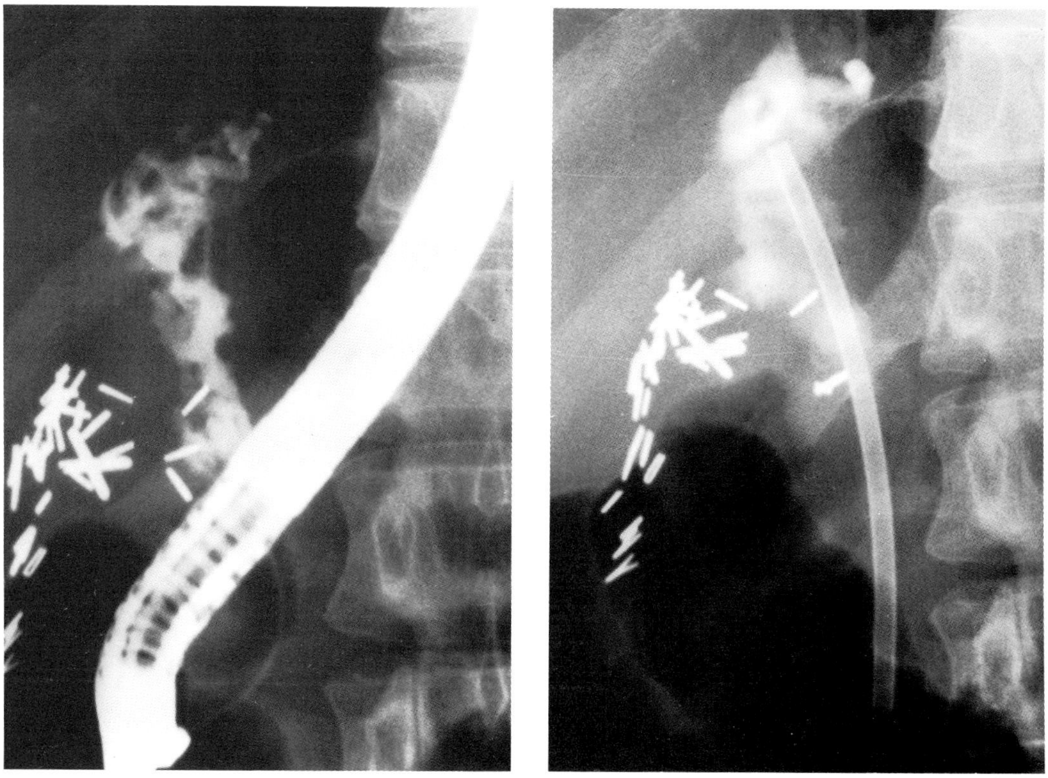

FIG. 12.116. Left: A small amount of contrast fills a few intrahepatic radicals in a patient with sclerosing cholangitis. **Right:** A large-caliber prosthesis was placed into the bifurcation of the main bile ducts.

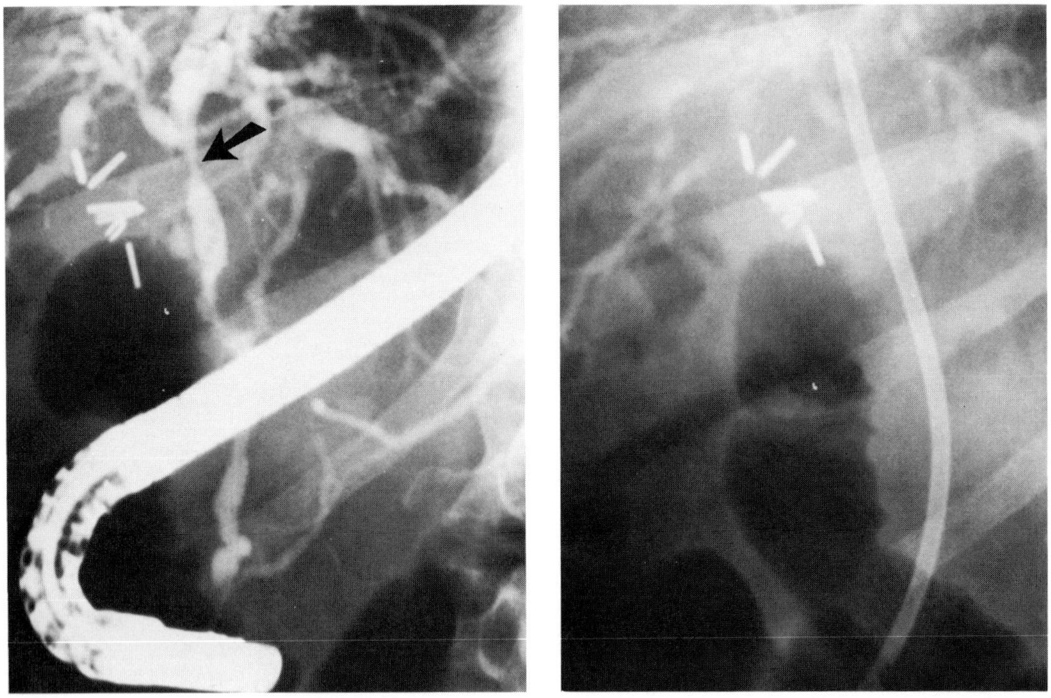

FIG. 12.117. Left: Note the diffuse changes of sclerosing cholangitis (*arrow*). **Right:** A large-caliber prosthesis was advanced through the dominant stricture located at the bifurcation.

Text continued from page 329.

rently engaged in a randomized trial of ursodeoxycholic acid versus placebo. Other trials are also under investigation. Hopefully, one of these drug trials, alone or in combination with endotherapy, will extend the life expectancy of these patients. I support the call for randomized trials comparing endoscopic, percutaneous, surgical, and pharmacologic modalities to determine the effectiveness of these procedures in the management of this debilitating, chronic disease.

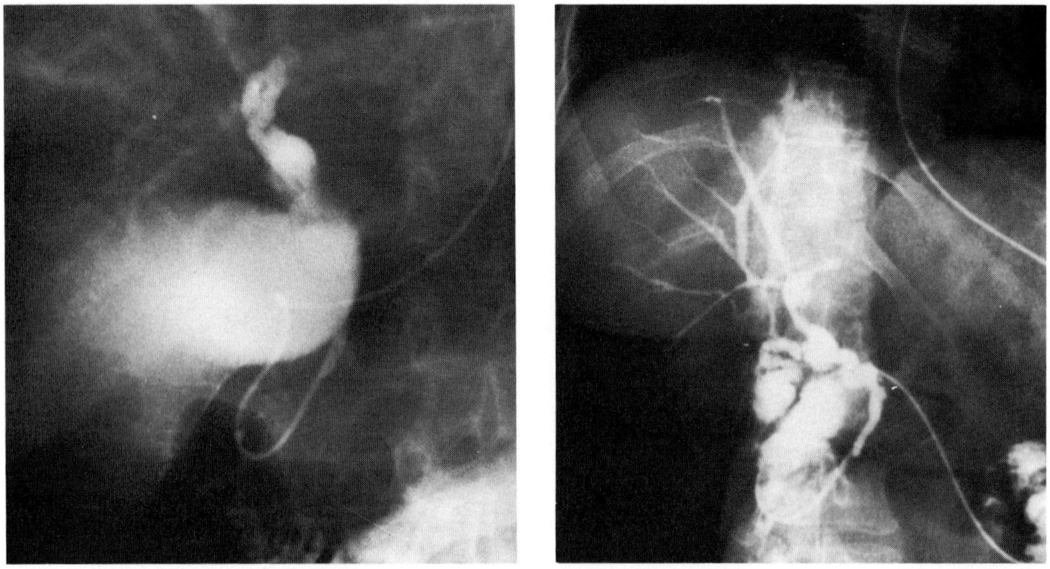

FIG. 12.118. Left: A radiograph obtained through a nasobiliary tube, demonstrating a large gallbladder and diffuse intrahepatic changes consistent with sclerosing cholangitis. This patient was treated with perfusion techniques, which required leaving the tube in place for 4 months. **Right:** A cholangiogram obtained at the end of 4 months after perfusion therapy. Note that the gallbladder is smaller and the intrahepatic ducts appear less affected by the disease process.

ENDOPROSTHESES FOR BENIGN, INFLAMMATORY PANCREATIC DISEASE

The technique for placing endoprostheses into the pancreatic duct is similar to that employed for insertion of biliary prostheses. Sphincterotomy is sometimes obviated in the treatment of pancreatic disorders because its performance may be associated with increased morbidity (when compared to bile duct sphincterotomy), but data are not available to prove or disprove this probability (110–113). However, because bleeding and perforation may occur more frequently during performance of pancreatic sphincterotomy, I have developed a safe technique for the performance of sphincterotomy in patients with pancreatitis, and this technique can be used for both the major and minor papillae (114). This technique requires, first, that a prosthesis, usually 7 French, be inserted into the sphincter of either the

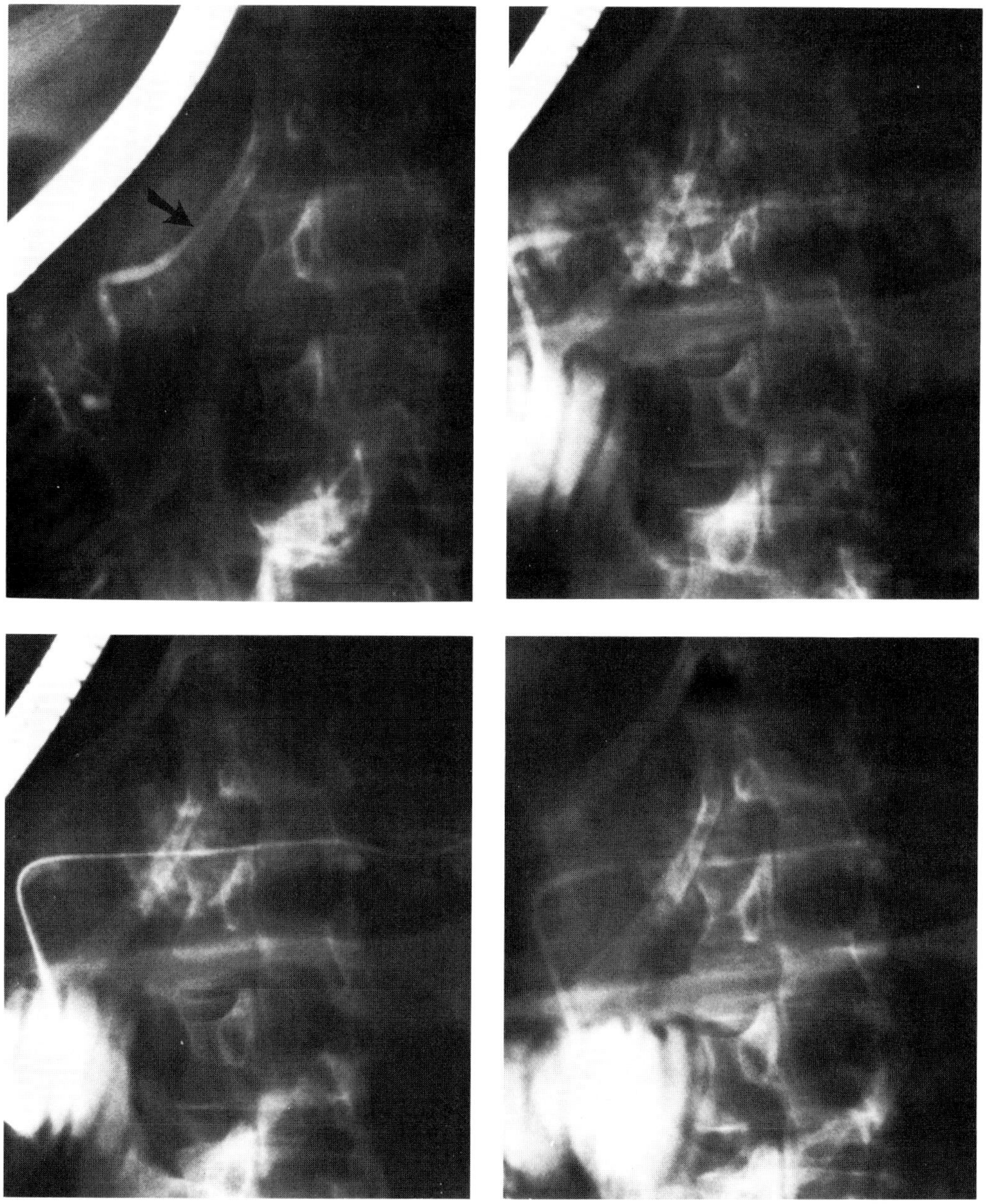

FIG. 12.119. Top left: A pancreatogram showing a stricture of the body of the pancreatic duct (*arrow*). **Top right:** After the stricture is traversed with a catheter-guidewire assembly, a repeat pancreatogram demonstrates diffuse acinar filling resulting from more forceful injection of contrast because of strictures of the main duct. **Bottom left:** A guidewire in place in the pancreatic duct. **Bottom right:** A long 7Fr stent is in place in the pancreatic duct, having traversed the stricture.

TABLE 12.16. *Idiopathic pancreatitis and endoprostheses*[a]

No. patients	40
Women	29
Men	11
Age	
Mean	59 yrs
Range	19–78 yrs

[a] Nonalcoholic pancreatitis

TABLE 12.17. *Idiopathic pancreatitis: results of endotherapy (N = 40)*

No. patients	Duration of relief (mos)
17	<12
6	<24
3	<36
2	<48
2	<60
2	<72
1	>72
Symptoms relieved	33
Duration of relief	11 mos
Range	3–72 mos

duct of Wirsung or the duct of Santorini. After this insertion, a sphincterotomy is performed over the prosthesis using a needle-knife sphincterotome (see Figures 10.37–10.38). The needle knife is either moved downward from the apex of the ampulla to the papillary orifice or moved from the orifice in a cephalad direction. Safety is an advantage of this technique because the overlying mucosa is incised down to the prosthesis, exposing it, while at the same time, a complete sphincterotomy is performed without fear of perforation. Because the pancreatic duct enters the duodenum in a more horizontal attitude than the bile duct does, the intramural segment is shorter than that of the bile duct, and perforation is a more likely complication using a standard sphincterotome. Perforation has not occurred using the needle-knife–prosthesis technique. Bleeding has been minimal, without requiring transfusion, and pancreatitis, if it occurs, is mild and uncomplicated.

A pancreatic prosthesis should decompress the pancreatic duct while dilating the stricture. A larger prosthesis would therefore be optimal. Because a sphincterotomy establishes a larger opening by severing the sphincter fibers, the opening is more likely to remain patent if a large-caliber prosthesis is placed to maintain the luminal integrity. Pancreatic prostheses remain functional for a longer period of time than biliary prostheses but eventually occlude by a process similar to that which occurs in a biliary stent. Concretions enmeshed in a bacterial biofilm begin to accumulate, ultimately occluding the prosthesis. The life expectancy of a 7Fr pancreatic prosthesis approaches 6 months, but I have several patients whose prostheses remained functional for up to 15 months. The reason

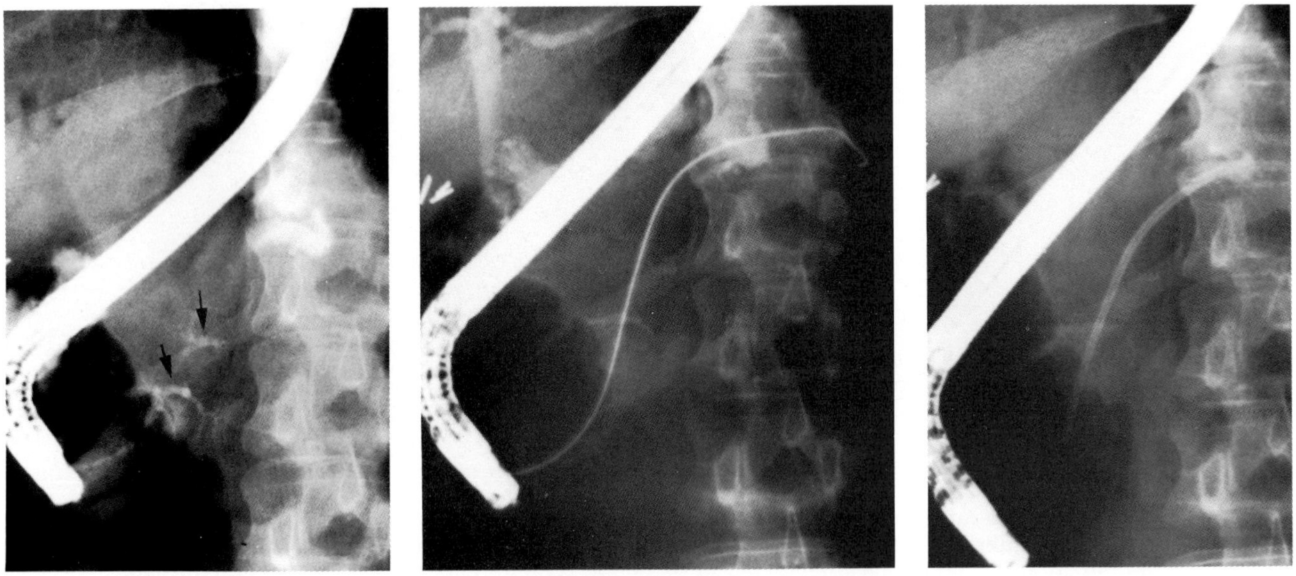

FIG. 12.120. Left: Strictures of the pancreatic duct in the head with no filling of the main duct (*arrows*). **Middle:** A catheter-guidewire assembly has passed through strictures in the duct in the head of the gland and advanced to the tail. **Right:** A 7Fr stent is visible in the duct.

for the increased longevity of pancreatic stents is unclear, but flow through a pancreatic stent, which is under greater pressure than the biliary tree, may retard (but not eliminate) biofilm formation (115).

Figures 12.119 through 12.132 are representative examples of radiographs of pancreatic stenting and demonstrate the types of strictures or disease states involving the pancreas that I treated successfully. Tables 12.16 and 12.17 summarize my experience in placing pancreatic prostheses, and references 116 through 118 detail the favorable results reported by others since my initial description (119). Figures 12.133 through 12.140 are endoscopic videoimages of pancreatic stents placed for treatment of recurrent pancreatitis. Descriptions of these images accompany them.

Text continues on page 343.

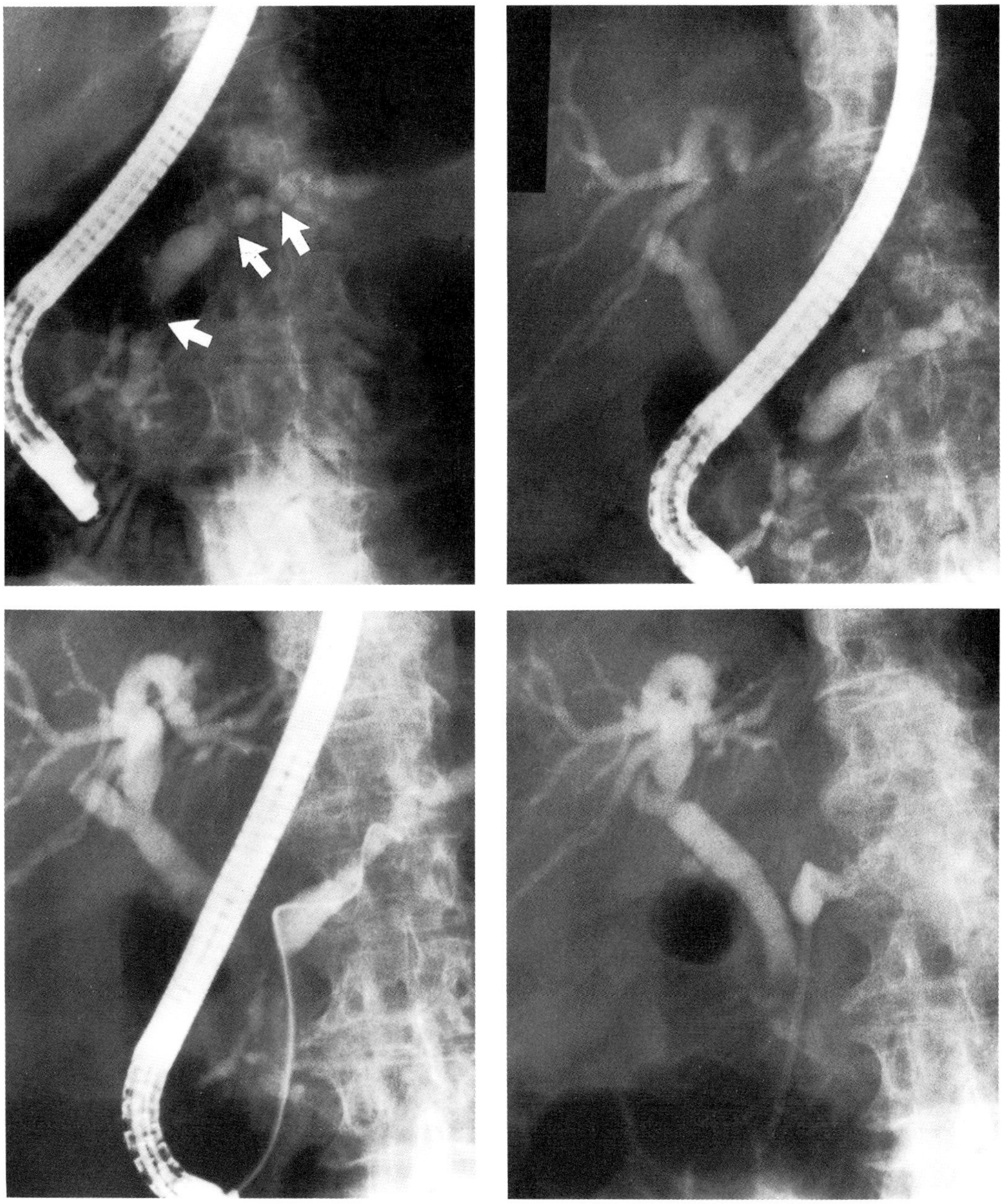

FIG. 12.121. Top left: Evidence of chronic pancreatitis on a pancreatogram obtained in an elderly patient. Note the stricture (*arrows*) and alternating areas of dilatation, the "chain of lakes" or "string of pearls" previously described in senile pancreatitis. **Top right:** The completed ERCP. **Bottom left:** The catheter-guidewire assembly is advanced through the major areas of stricturing in the head of the gland. **Bottom right:** A prosthesis is in place. Note the decreased quantity of contrast remaining in the pancreatic duct.

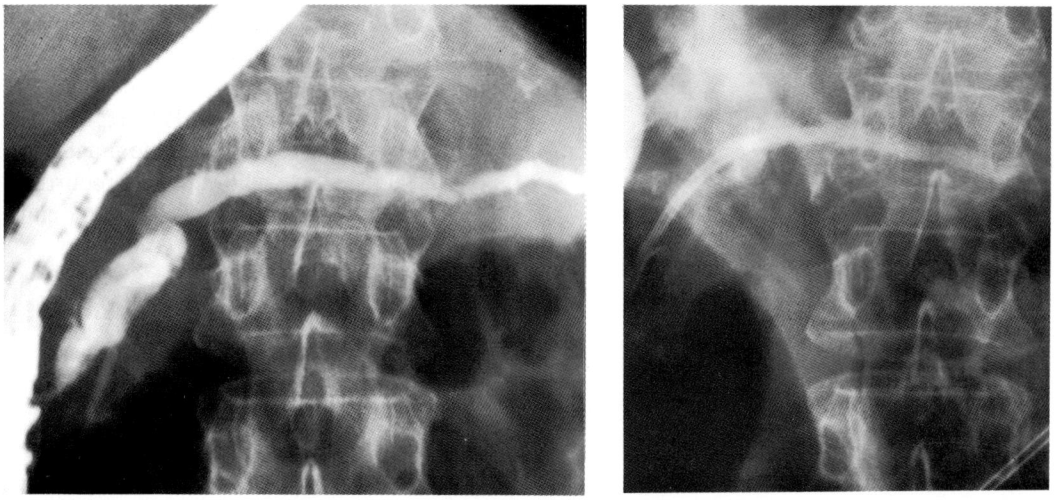

FIG. 12.122. Left: A dilated pancreatic duct. Narrowing of the duct at the sphincter is noted, resulting from papillary stenosis or a hypertensive pancreatic sphincter despite a previously performed bile duct sphincterotomy. **Right:** A 7Fr prosthesis has been placed through the sphincter and the stricture, which was present in the head of the gland.

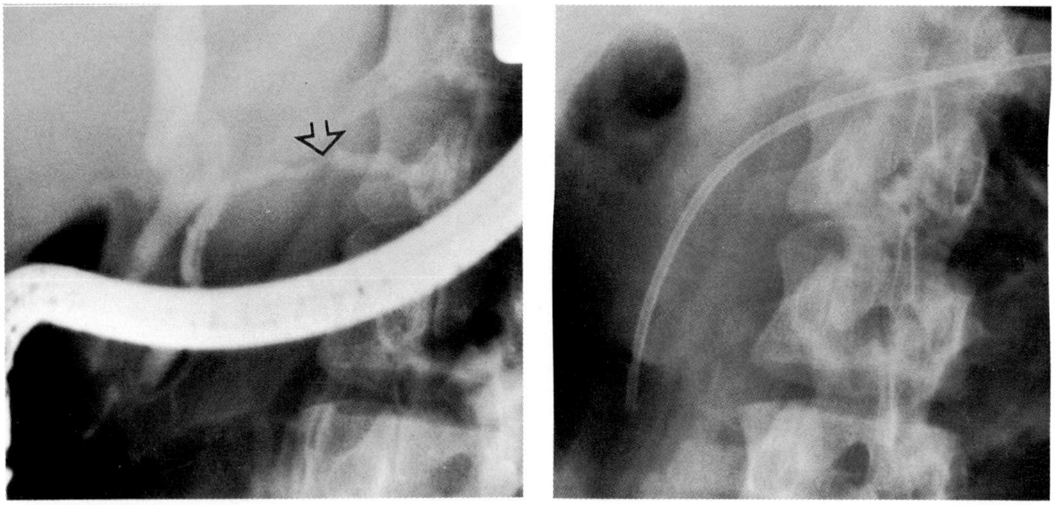

FIG. 12.123. Left: This ERCP demonstrates a stricture in the body of the gland (*arrow*) and proximal dilatation of the duct. **Right:** A long prosthesis has been placed through the stricture into the dilated segment.

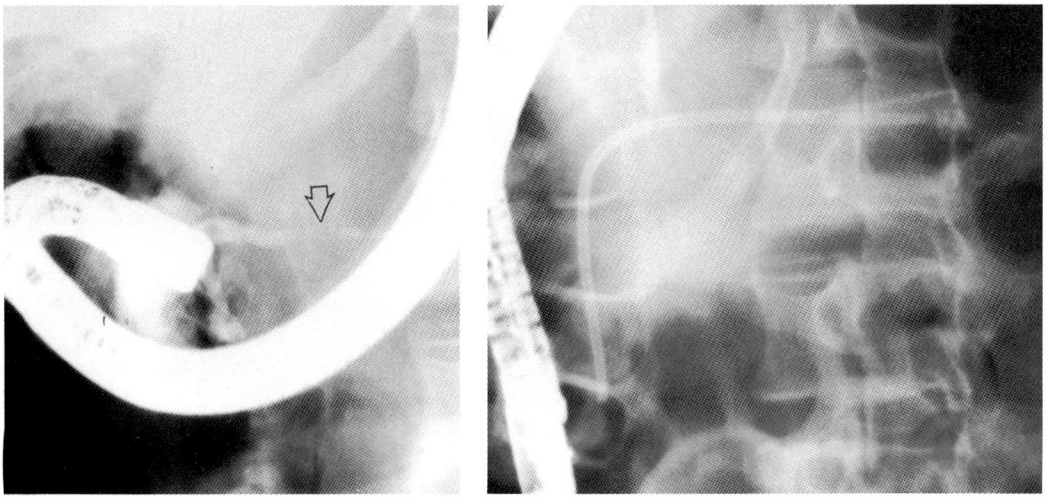

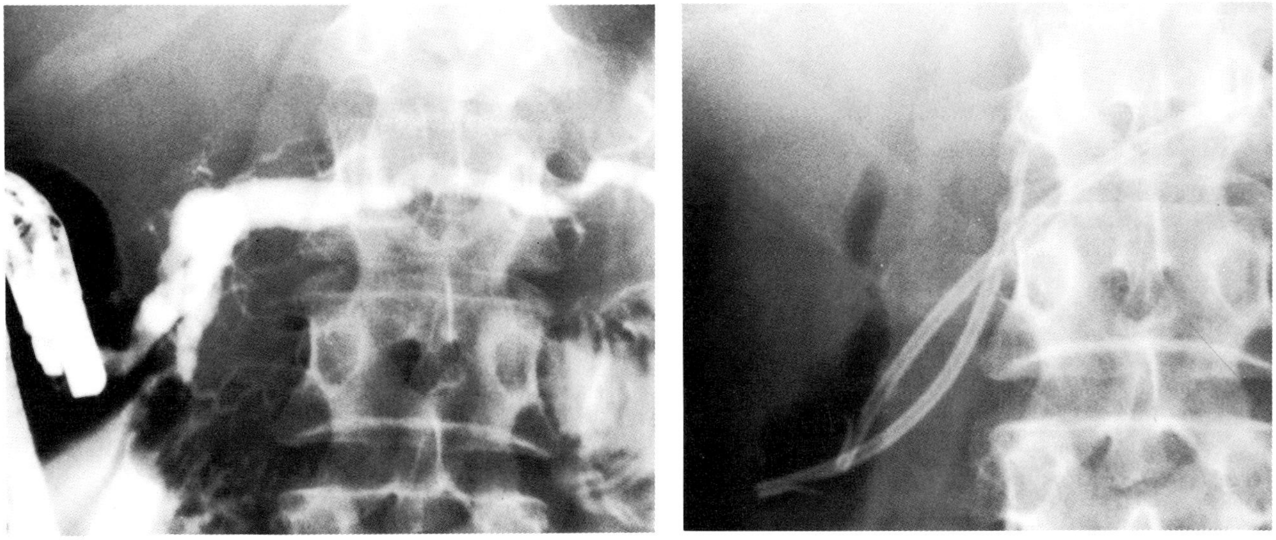

FIG. 12.125. Left: Dilatation of the pancreatic duct secondary to a pancreatic stone (not visible in this picture). The pancreatic duct is opacified from both the major orifice and the minor papilla. **Right:** Pancreatic stents were placed into both the major and minor sphincters to provide adequate decompression.

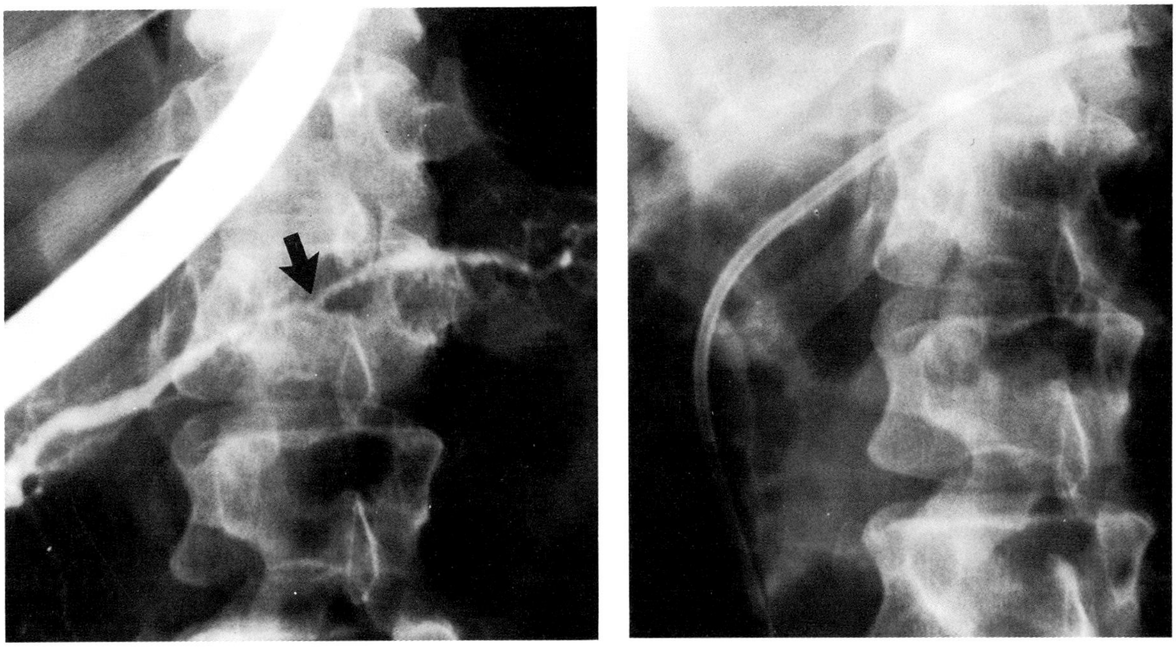

FIG. 12.126. Left: A pancreatogram demonstrating evidence of diffuse pancreatitis with narrowing or stricturing of the duct in the body of the gland (*arrow*). Filling of the side branches is due to increased pressure of injection. **Right:** Because of the proximal stricture, a long stent was necessary in order to traverse the stricture and provide drainage.

FIG. 12.124. Left: A pancreatogram demonstrating a stricture in the body of the pancreas (*arrow*) that resulted from blunt trauma to the abdomen. The patient experienced recurrent episodes of pain consistent with pancreatitis. **Right:** A long prosthesis. The prosthesis should maintain the integrity of the lumen of the duct and can be removed after several months. The pancreatic duct lumen should remain patent after removal of the stent.

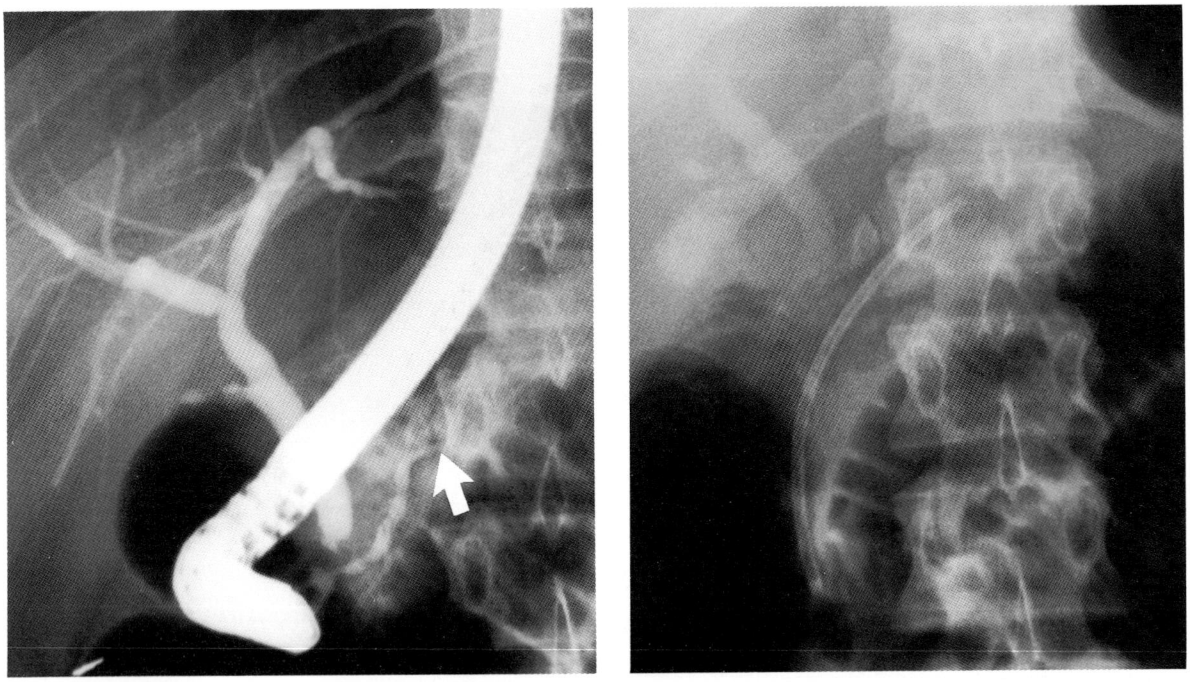

FIG. 12.127. Left: This ERCP demonstrates a tight stricture of the pancreatic duct (*arrow*) and acinar filling resulting from increased injection pressure. No branching of the duct, which is characteristic of divisum, is noted, so this is *not* a divisum. **Right:** A 7Fr stent has been placed for decompression.

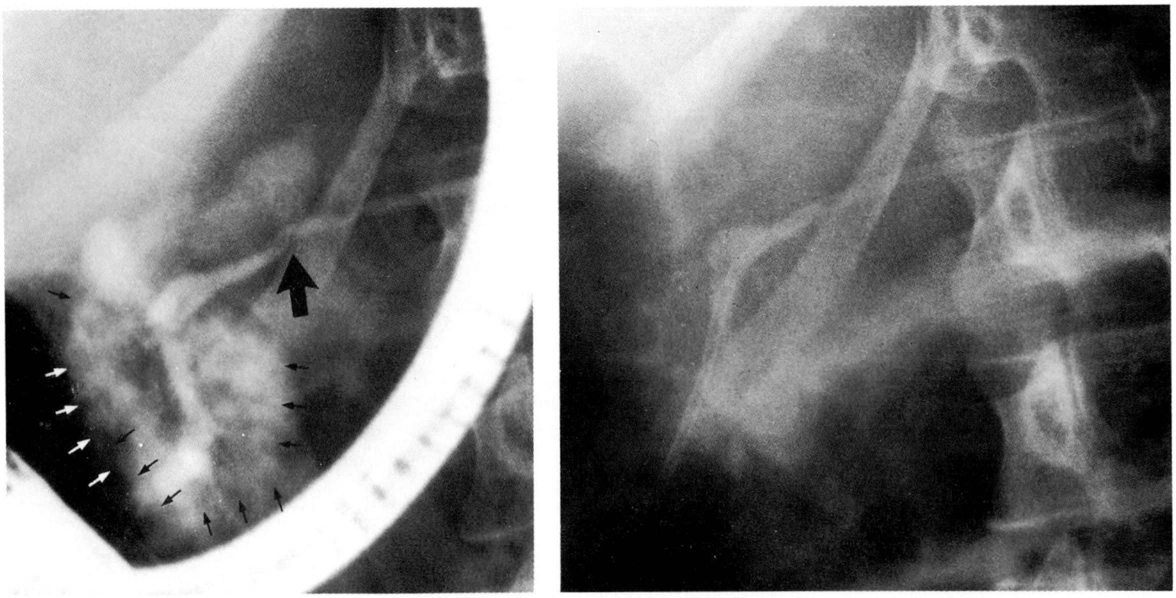

FIG. 12.128. Left: Stricturing of the pancreatic duct proximally (toward tail) (*large arrow*) and acinar filling (*small arrows*) in the head of the gland secondary to increased pressure of injection. **Right:** A long prosthesis has been placed through the stricture into the body of the pancreas.

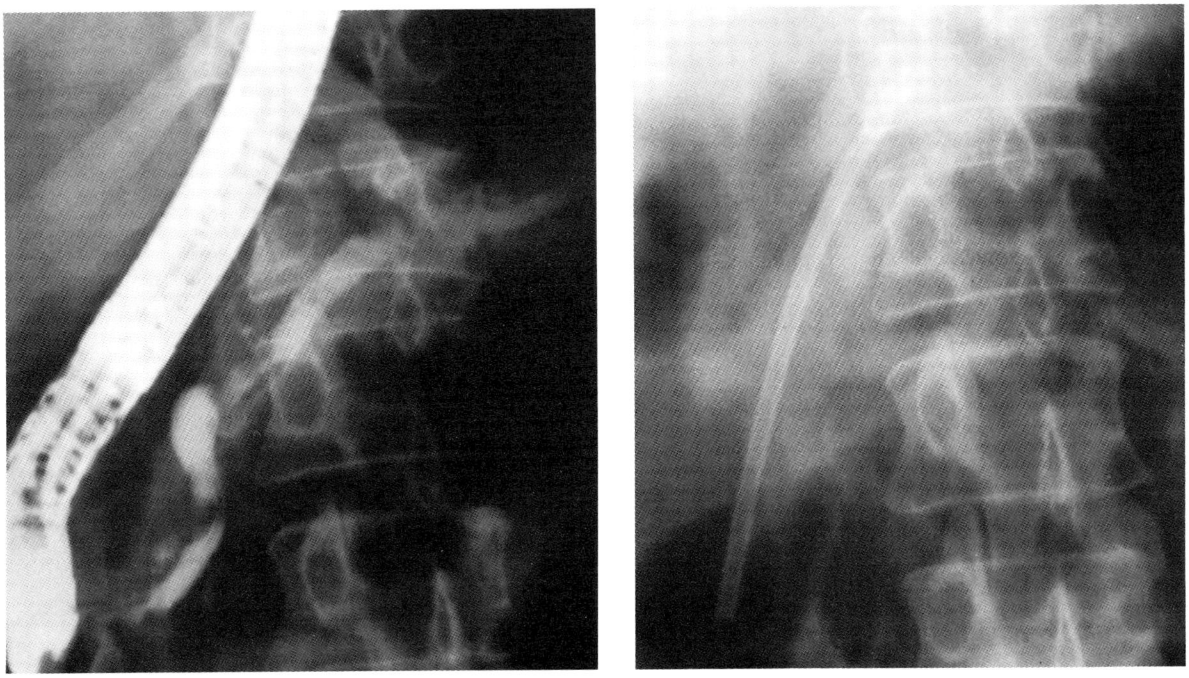

FIG. 12.129. Left: This pancreatogram demonstrates several strictures in the head of the pancreas. **Right:** A 10Fr stent was placed through the head of the gland into the body.

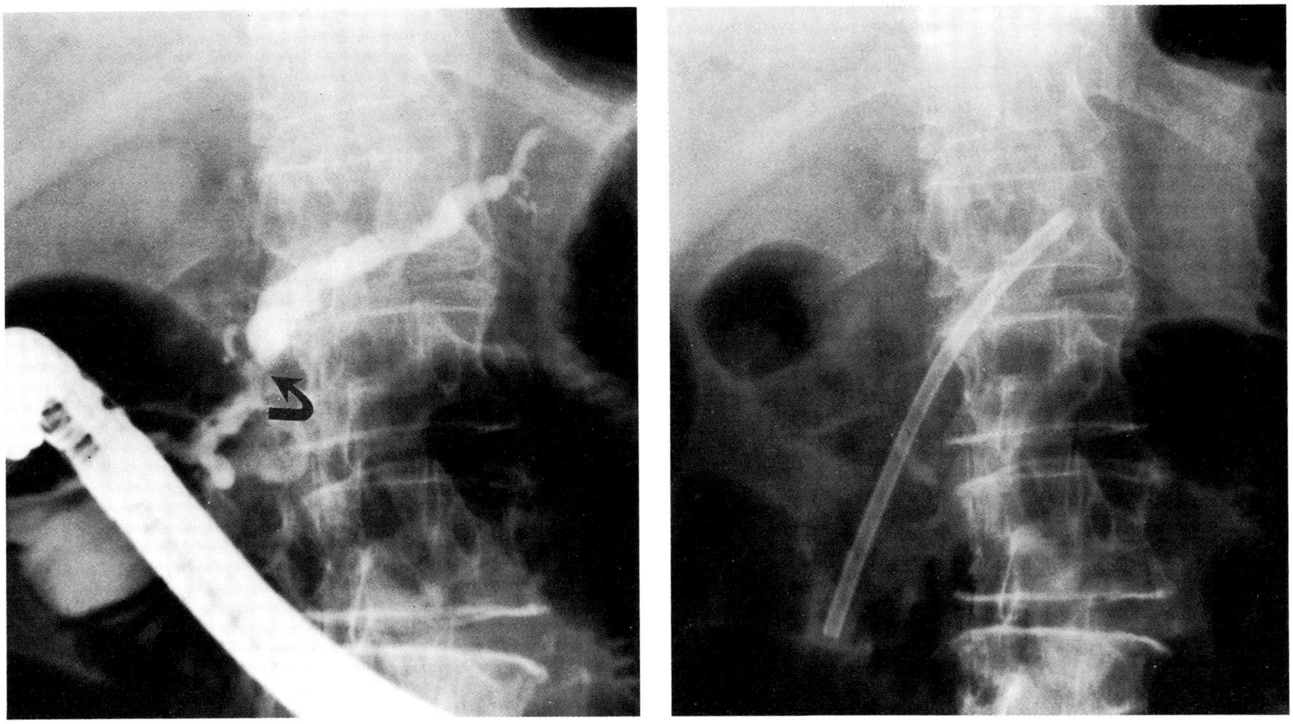

FIG. 12.130. Left: Stricturing of the pancreatic duct in the head of the gland (*arrow*) with dilatation of the duct proximal to the stricture. **Right:** A 10 Fr prosthesis was placed through the strictures into the body of the gland.

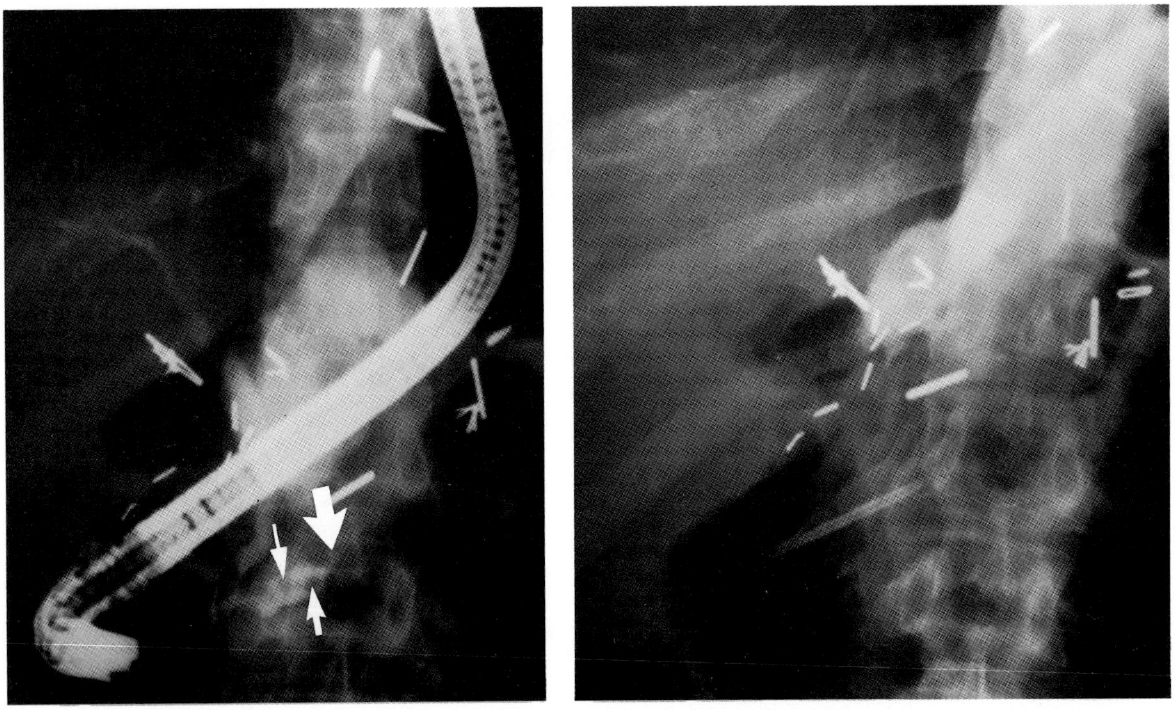

FIG. 12.131. Left: This pancreatogram demonstrates filling of the pancreatic duct in the head of the gland (*large arrow*). The patient underwent a subtotal pancreatectomy previously and experienced recurrent symptoms subsequent to surgery. Stones (*small arrows*) are visible in the residual duct. **Right:** A short prosthesis was placed into the remaining pancreatic duct, traversing the hypertensive sphincter. Subsequently, an endoscopic sphincterotomy was performed over the stent, and the stent and stones were removed. The patient remained asymptomatic.

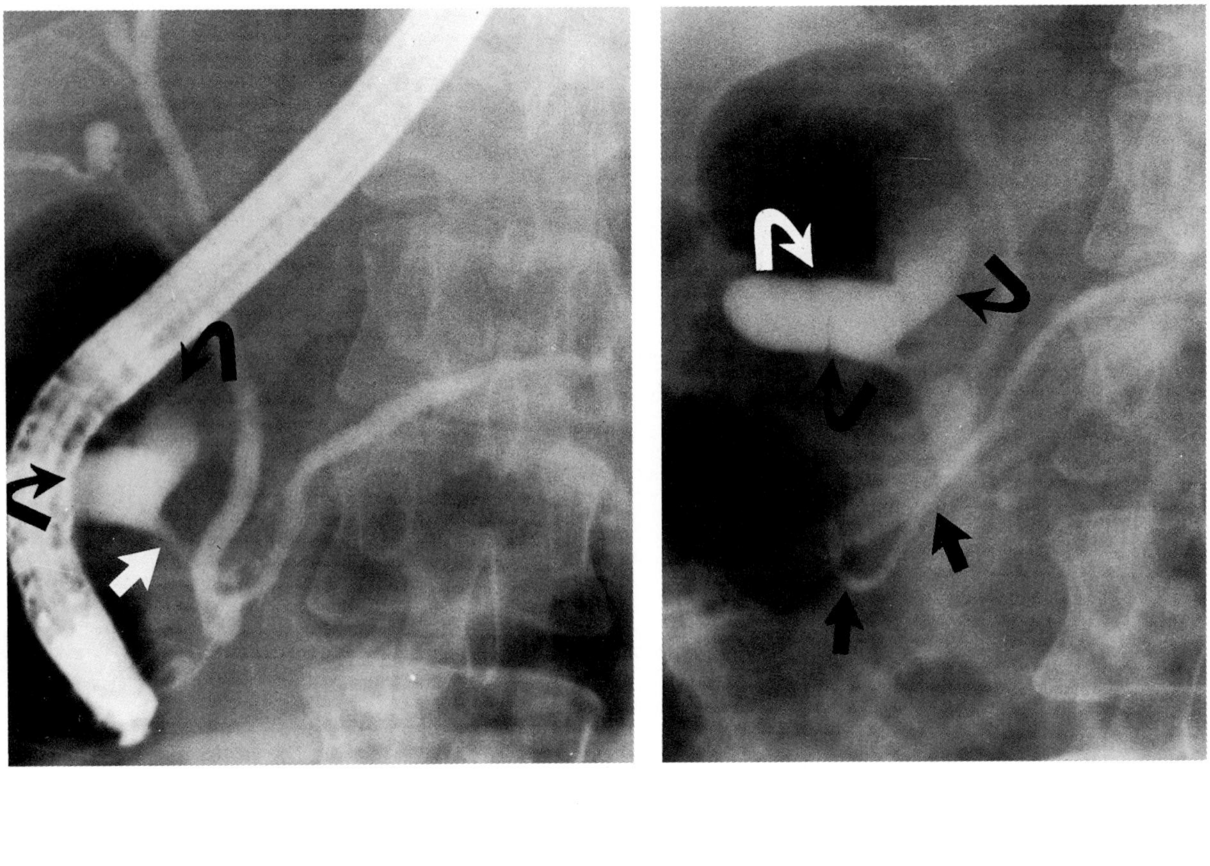

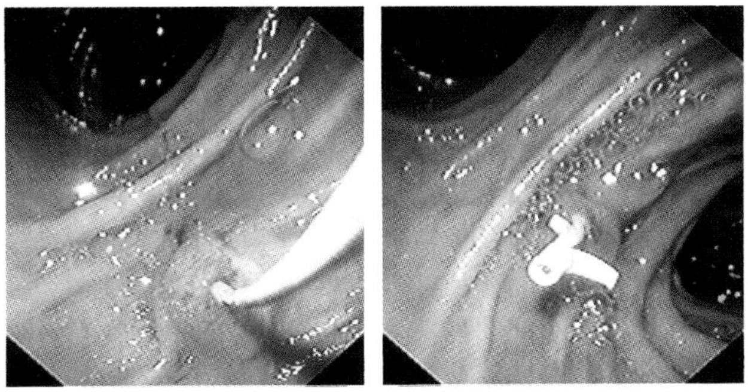

FIG. 12.133. Left: Insertion of a prosthesis into the pancreatic duct. A guidewire is in position in the pancreatic orifice. **Right:** The pancreatic prosthesis has been inserted and is in place.

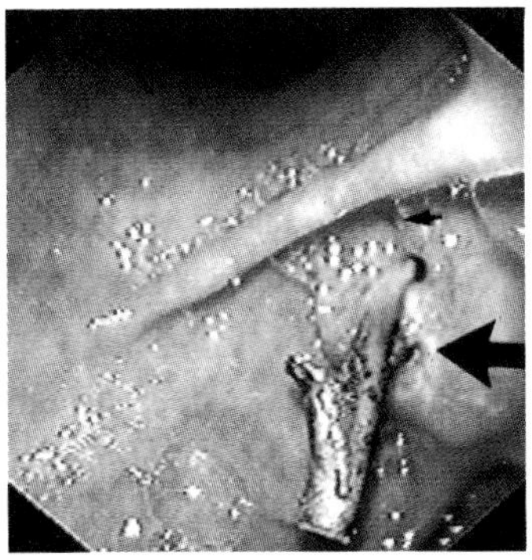

FIG. 12.134. The presence of a pancreatic prosthesis in the pancreatic orifice. This prosthesis has been in place 4 months. Note the color change of the duodenal portion of the stent. This patient has undergone an endoscopic sphincterotomy of the pancreatic duct sphincter, as indicated by the size of the opening. The bile duct sphincter is seen cephalad to the stent (*small arrow*). Also note inflammatory changes of the papilla secondary to abrasions from the extra flap on the stent (*large arrow*).

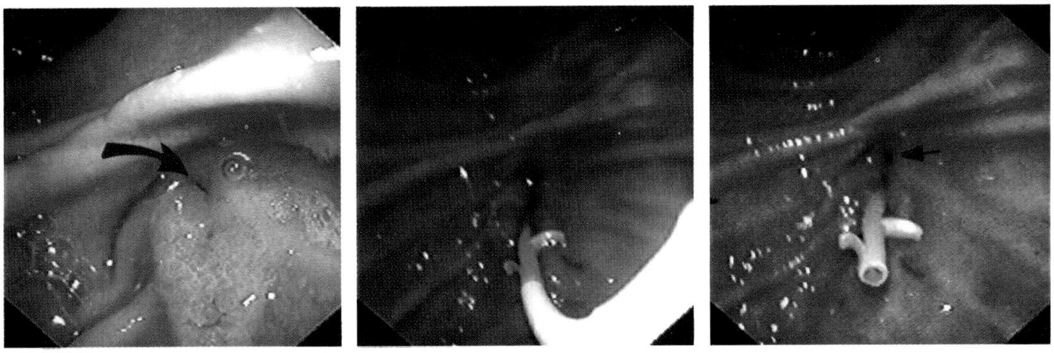

FIG. 12.135. Left: A papilla that shows a small sphincterotomy of the bile duct (*arrow*). **Middle:** A pancreatic prosthesis being pushed into the pancreatic orifice. Note the contrasting colors of the pusher (*white*) and prosthesis (*blue*). **Right:** The pancreatic prosthesis in position. Note the bile duct sphincterotomy cephalad to the stent (*arrow*).

FIG. 12.132. Left: A communicating pseudocyst (*arrows*) of the dorsal aspect of this pancreatic duct. **Right:** A prosthesis (*straight arrows*) has been placed into the pancreatic duct for drainage. Note this better view of the pseudocyst (*curved arrows*).

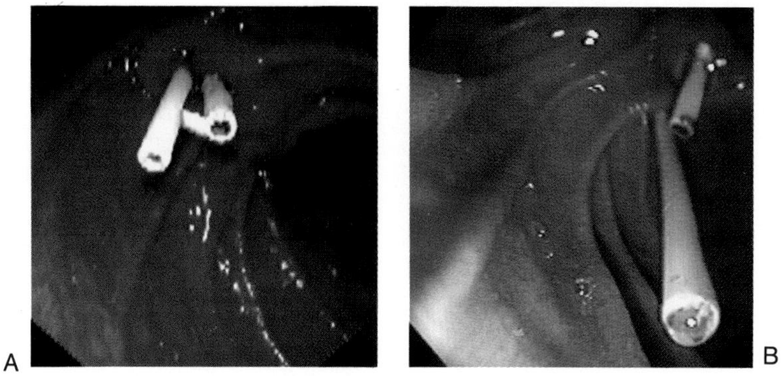

FIG. 12.136. **A:** Two prostheses in position; the upper one is in the bile duct, the lower in the pancreas. Note the septum between the two. **B:** Two endoprostheses seen in videoimage. The upper prosthesis is in the minor papilla, duct of Santorini, the lower in the major papilla, duct of wirsung. These are the same prostheses seen in Fig. 12.125.

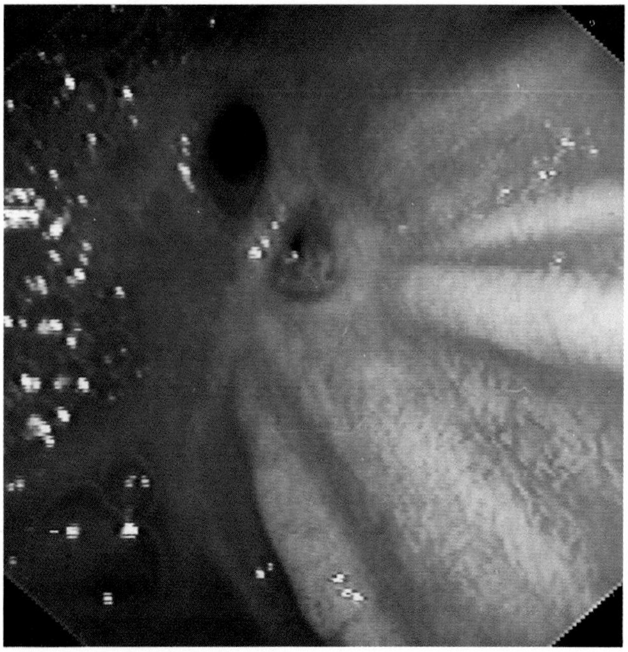

FIG. 12.137. A videoimage showing a surgical sphincteroplasty of the bile duct (upper opening) and pancreatic duct (lower opening).

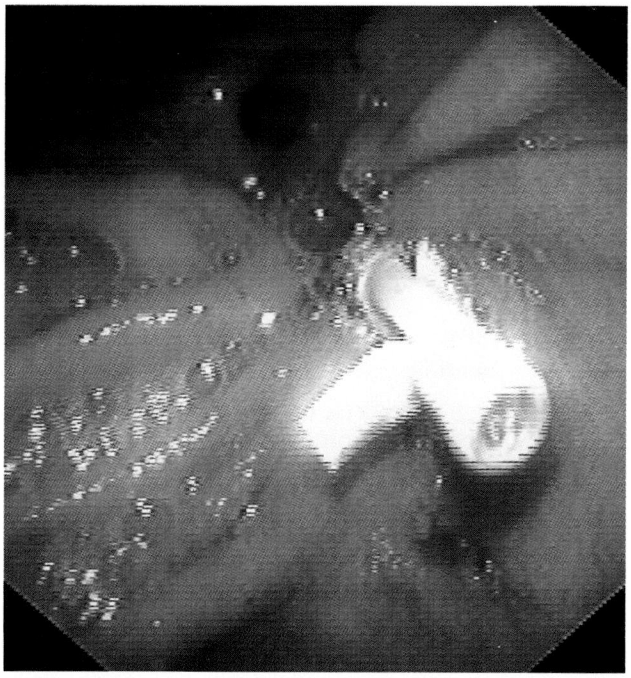

FIG. 12.138. A videoimage of the same patient in Fig. 12.137. A prosthesis has been placed into the pancreatic duct via the sphincterotomy. The bile duct sphincteroplasty is shown cephalad to the stent.

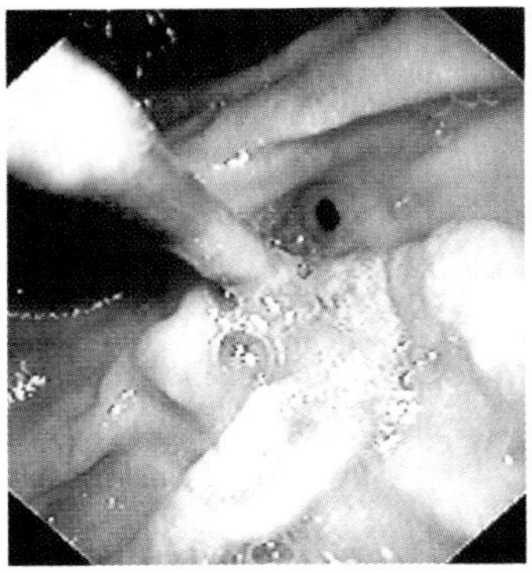

FIG. 12.139. A prosthesis extending from the pancreatic orifice. The bile duct sphincterotomy is cephalad to the stent.

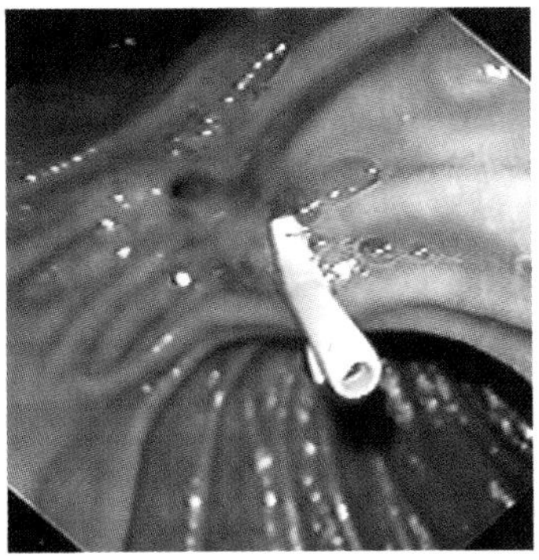

FIG. 12.140. A pancreatic prosthesis extending from the pancreatic duct; the bile duct sphincterotomy is shown cephalad to the stent.

PROSTHESES AND PANCREAS DIVISUM

In pancreas divisum, after cannulating the minor papilla with a needle-tipped catheter and opacifying the dorsal duct (see Chapters 4 and 9), I use a 7Fr Van Andel catheter and a 0.035″ guidewire assembly to

Text continued from page 335.

enter the minor papilla to facilitate insertion of a prosthesis. Once the guidewire is set in place, the guiding catheter or dilating catheter may be removed and either a 5Fr or, preferably, a 7Fr prosthesis may be advanced through the intact papilla into the pancreatic duct beyond the area of stricturing or narrowing (Figs. 12.141–12.153). Balloon dilatation of the stricture or sphincter can be accomplished with the guidewire in place. Sphincteric dysfunction, the cause for symptoms in patients with pancreas divisum, is thought to be responsible for dilatation of the dorsal duct and resultant recurrent pancreatitis (120–123). While the prosthesis is in place, a sphincterotomy of the minor papilla is performed using a needle knife over the prosthesis (114) (see Figs. 10.38, 10.39). Subsequent to the sphincterotomy and replacement of the prosthesis, the prosthesis remains in position for 4 to 6 months, depending on its diameter, and the patient returns for an exchange if and when mild symptoms recur (signs of occlusion). If it is possible to place a larger prosthesis, that will be accomplished during the exchange procedure. Advancement to a larger size is usually carried out when a 5Fr stent has been in place: A 7Fr is inserted on the patient's return. A larger stent, 10Fr, has been placed in only 4 of 35 patients, and in these patients, the dorsal duct was moderately to markedly dilated (124).

Performance of a pancreatic sphincterotomy using the needle knife over a stent technique has been associated with few complications. Rarely does pancreatitis occur, despite manipulation and sphincterotomy, because an indwelling prosthesis provides decompression. Two patients experienced an insignificant bleed, which responded to injections of 1:3,000 epinephrine into the sphincterotomy site using a sclerotherapy needle (see Chapter 10). Figures 12.141 through 12.153 are radiographs taken during the performance of ERCP

Text continues on page 348.

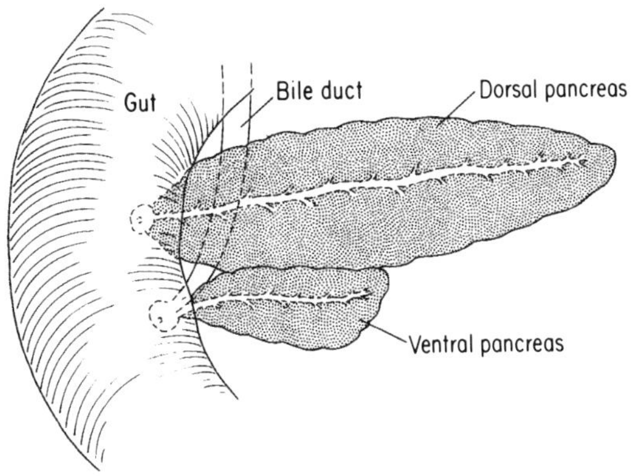

FIG. 12.141. The development of the pancreas at 7 to 8 weeks of gestation. Between 5% and 10% of the population may have pancreas divisum, which is a failure of fusion of the dorsal and ventral pancreatic ducts. Obstruction to flow of pancreatic juice through the small minor papilla is thought to contribute to pain and symptoms of pancreatitis.

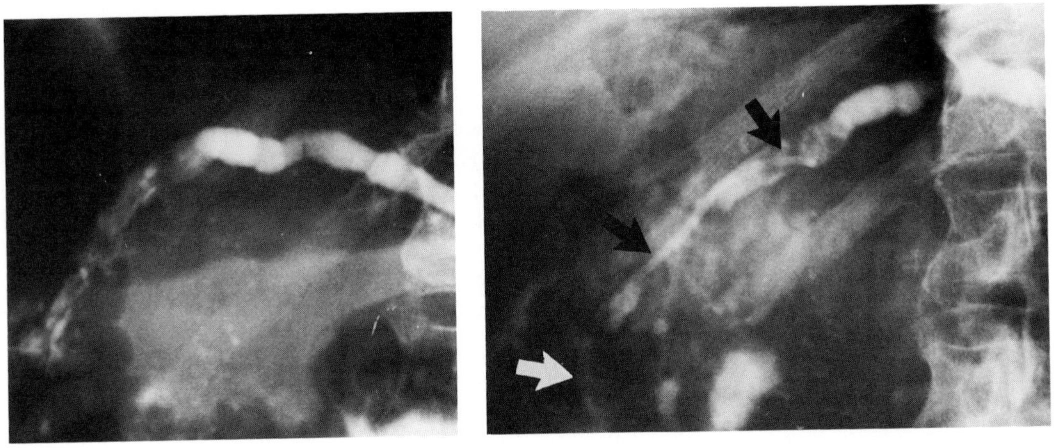

FIG. 12.142. Left: The dorsal duct of the pancreas divisum with evidence of pancreatitis with dilatation and a stricture of the duct in the head of the gland. There are lucencies present in the duct. **Right:** The patient's symptoms were ameliorated after placing a small-caliber prosthesis, which is shown extending from the duodenum to the mid portion of the dilated dorsal duct (*arrows*).

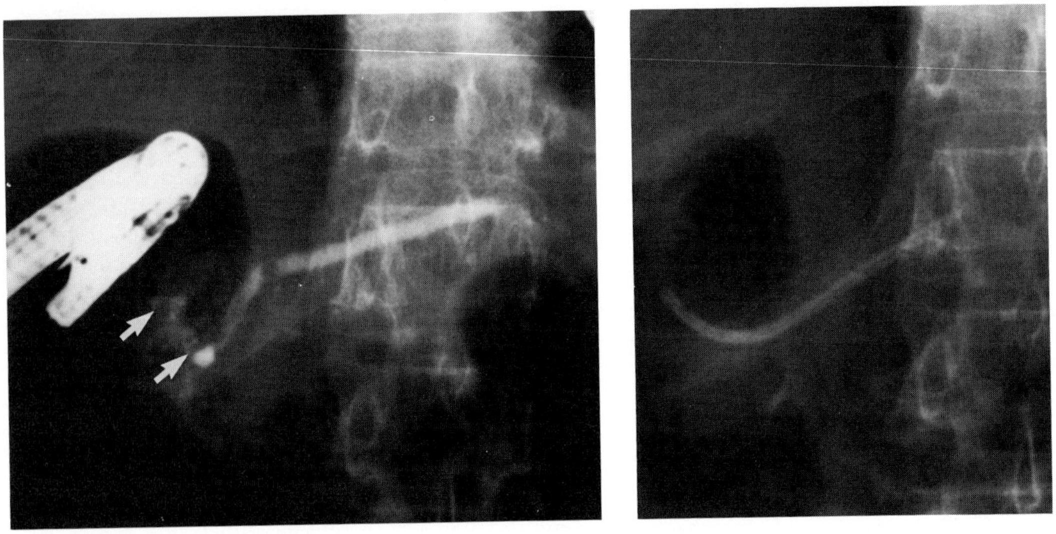

FIG. 12.143. Left: This radiograph shows evidence of pancreatitis of the dorsal pancreatic duct. Note the acutely angulated narrow segment in the head of the gland (*arrows*). **Right:** A prosthesis in the dorsal pancreatic duct. Complete emptying of the duct has occurred after placement of the stent.

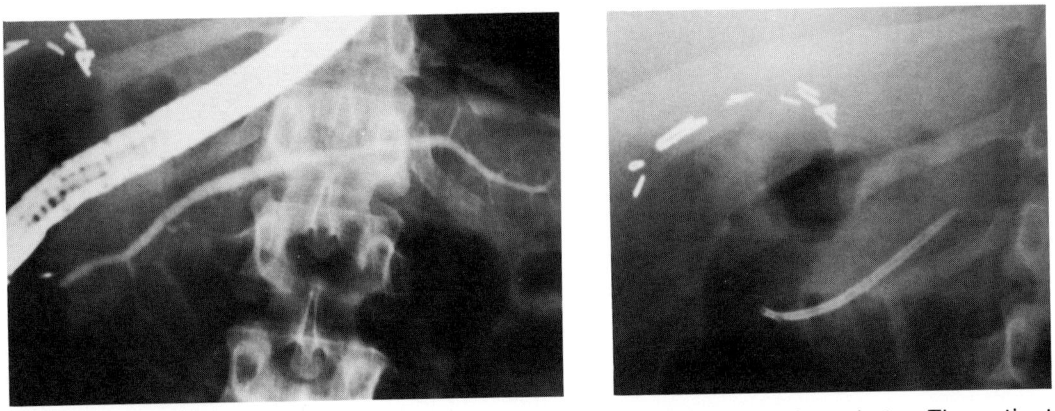

FIG. 12.144. Left: A nondilated dorsal duct is opacified using a needle-tip catheter. The patient presented with recurrent episodes of clinical pancreatitis. **Right:** A prosthesis has been placed for decompression.

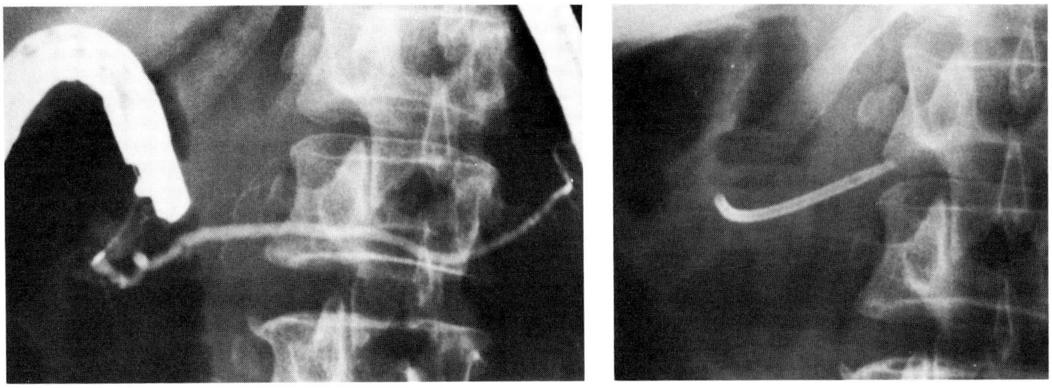

FIG. 12.145. Left: A loop deformity of the dorsal duct in the head of the gland in a patient with pancreas divisum who presented with recurrent pancreatitis. **Right:** A stent has been placed through the area of narrowing to assess the results of decompression.

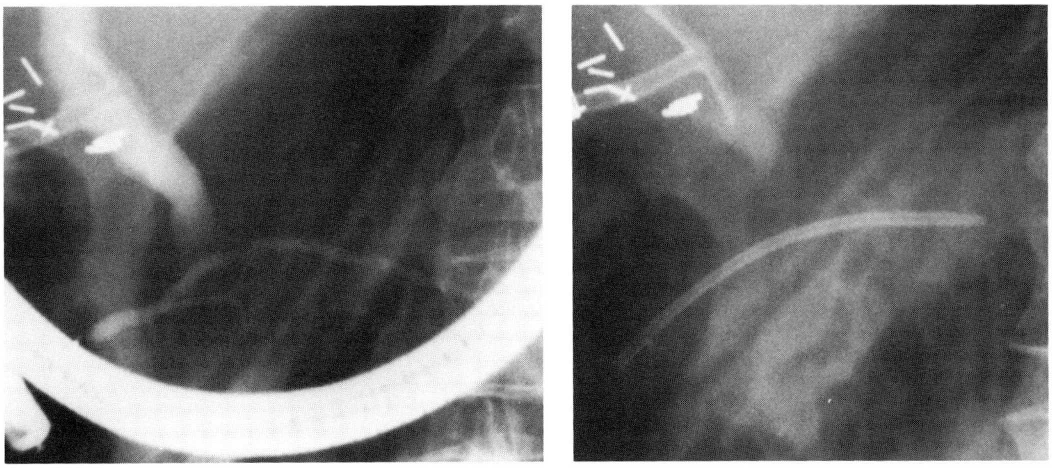

FIG. 12.146. Left: A nondilated dorsal pancreatic duct. Note the dilated ampullary segment, which was corrobrated by a secretin-ultrasound study. **Right:** A prosthesis was placed into the dorsal duct and gave prompt relief of symptoms.

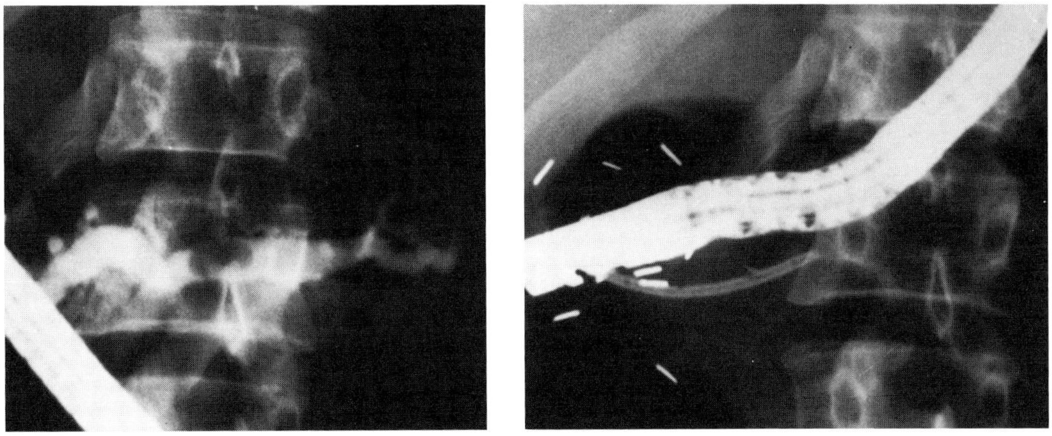

FIG. 12.147. Left: A dilated dorsal pancreatic duct with ectatic branches. **Right:** During the process of placing a prosthesis into the dorsal duct, the entire duct drained spontaneously through the prosthesis.

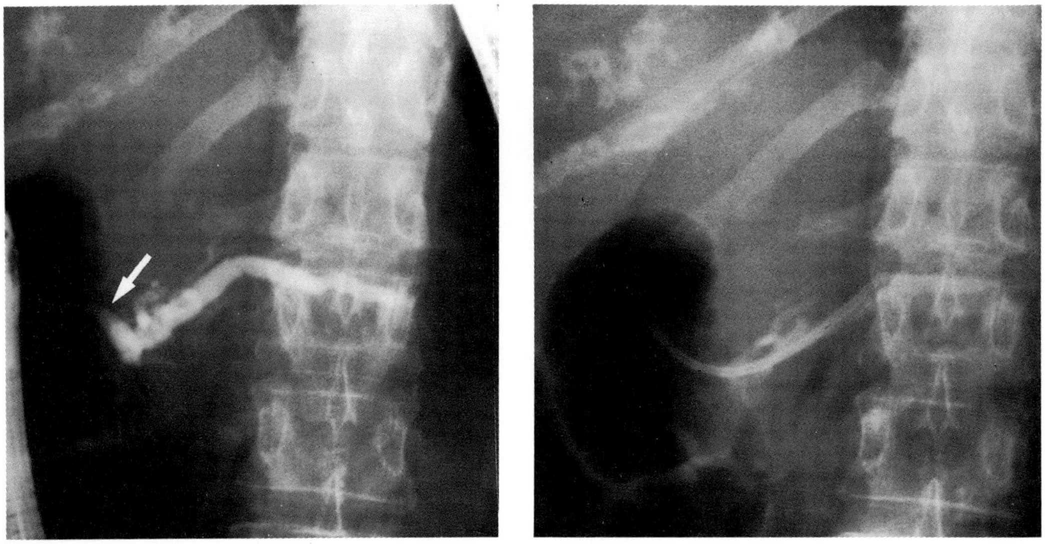

FIG. 12.148. Left: Blunting and dilatation of this dorsal duct of pancreas divisum. Note the tapering of the duct at the sphincter (*arrow*). **Right:** Symptoms were relieved after placing this prosthesis into the dorsal duct.

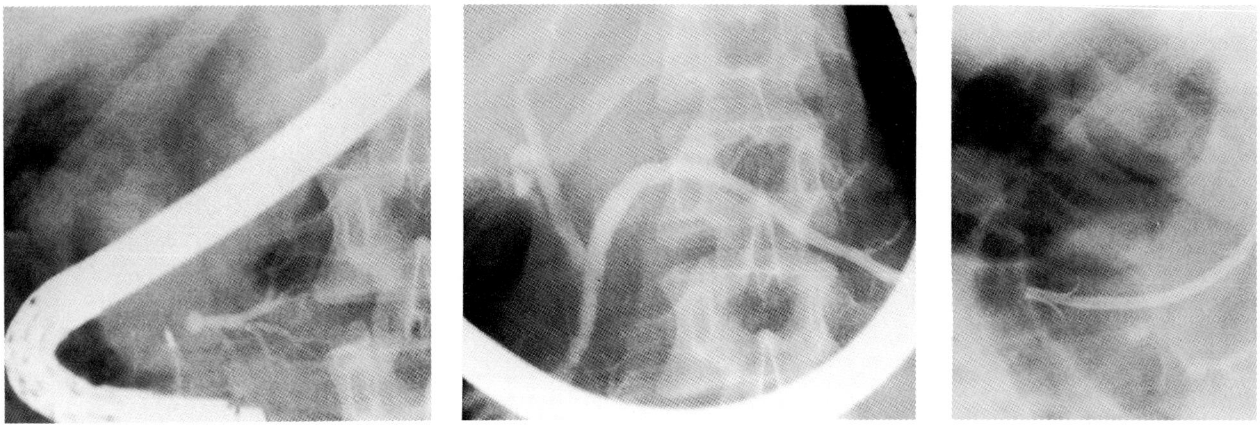

FIG. 12.149. Left: Opacification of the ventral duct of pancreas divisum. **Middle:** Opacification of the dorsal duct. **Right:** A prosthesis has been placed into the dorsal duct for decompression. This radiograph shows the complete configuration of the stent, which has extra side flaps.

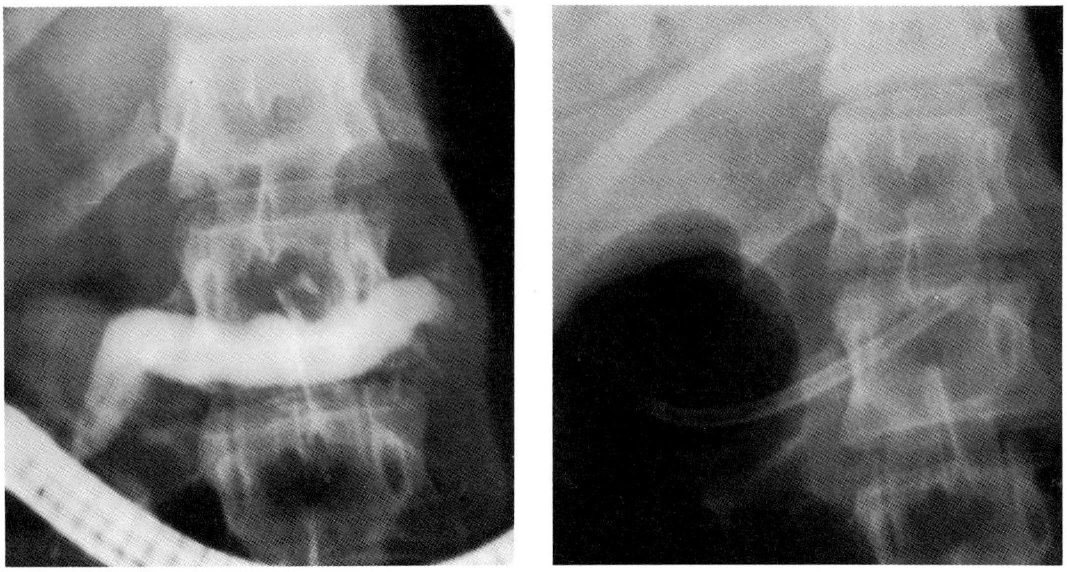

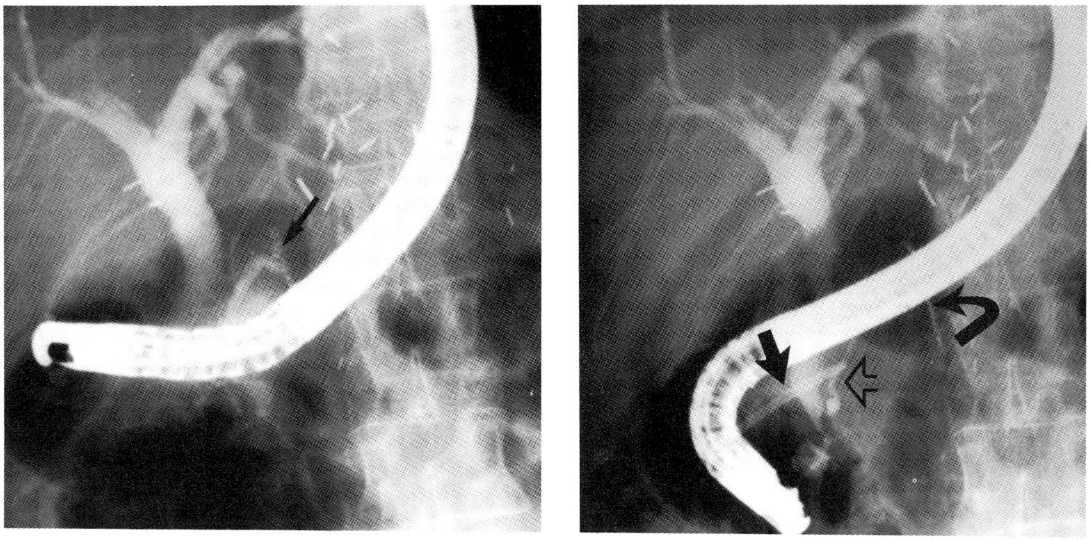

FIG. 12.151. Left: A radiograph taken during an ERCP examination of a patient with pancreatitis and pancreas divisum who had previously undergone resection of the tail. Note the row of staples (*arrow*) at the level of opacification of the remaining duct. **Right:** A prosthesis (*closed straight arrow*) was placed into the remaining segment of the dorsal duct with resolution of symptoms. Part of the ventral duct is being opacified (*open arrow*). The row of staples is visible near the spine (*curved arrow*).

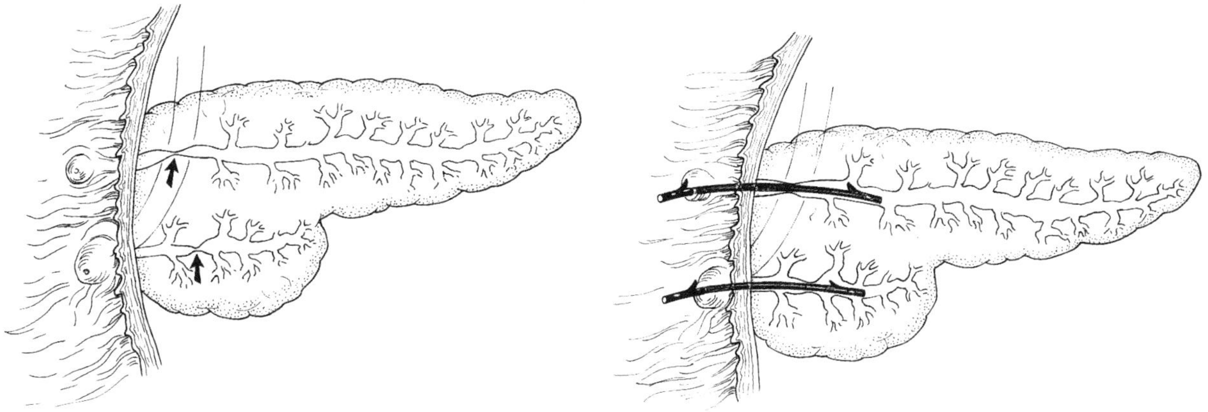

A B

FIG. 12.152. A: An illustration demonstrating evidence of pancreatitis (*arrows*) that involves both the dorsal and ventral ducts of pancreas divisum. **B:** Stents have been placed into both ducts through the strictures.

←

FIG. 12.150. Left: A dilated dorsal pancreatic duct is noted after opacification of the duct. **Right:** A 10Fr prosthesis was placed into this duct. Note complete emptying of the duct after placement of the large-caliber prosthesis.

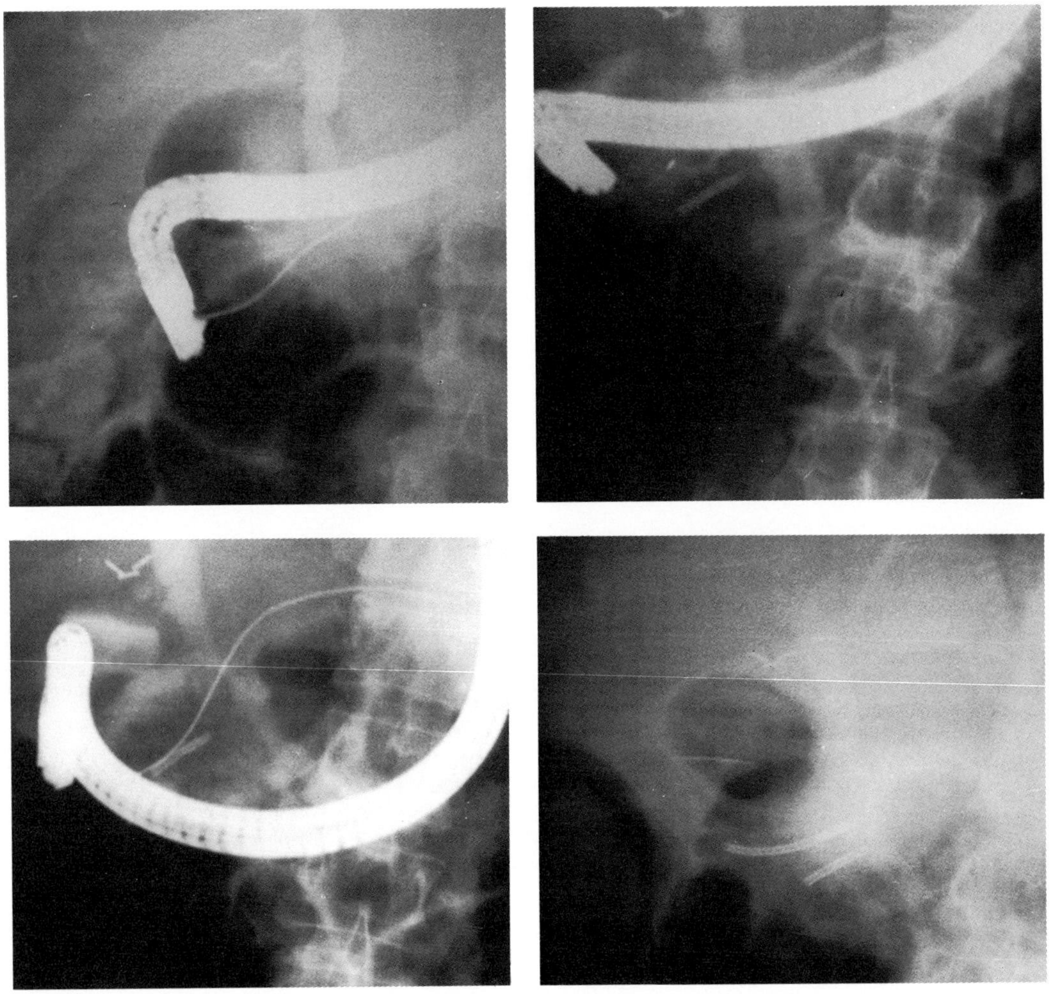

FIG. 12.153. Top left: A guidewire being placed into the ventral segment of pancreas divisum. **Top right:** A short stent is noted in the ventral duct. A needle-tip catheter is shown at the minor papilla, opacifying the dorsal duct. **Bottom left:** A guidewire is shown in place in the dorsal duct. **Bottom right:** Two stents are shown in place, one in the ventral duct and one in the dorsal duct.

Text continued from page 343.

in patients with symptomatic pancreatitis secondary to pancreas divisum. Figures 12.154 and 12.155 are videoimages of prostheses placed into the dorsal duct during ERCP, and Tables 12.18 through 12.22 summarize my experience in managing patients with pancreas divisum.

TABLE 12.18. *Pancreas divisum*

Demographics		
Patients		65
Women		45
Men		20
Mean age		35 yrs
Treatment distribution		
Group 1	15 patients (stents and surgery)	
Group 2	20 patient (stents)	
Group 3	30 patients (20 controls, 10 surgery)	

From ref. 124.

As reported in the latest follow-up of 65 patients with pancreas divisum, 35 stented, most did well with drainage of the dorsal duct provided by endoprostheses (124). My colleagues and I found from an earlier report

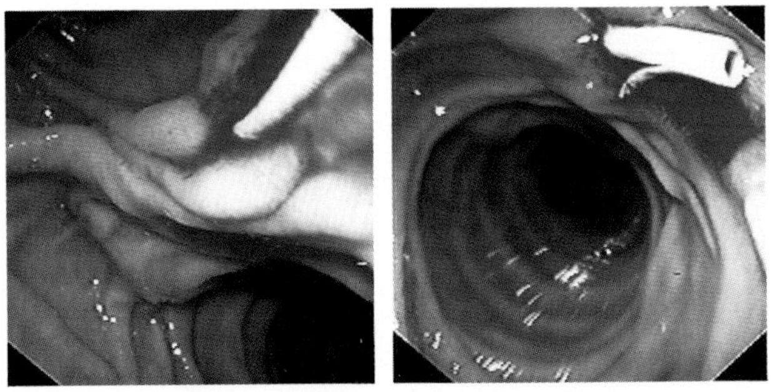

FIG. 12.154. Left: A guidewire in place in the minor papilla in preparation for placement of a prosthesis. **Right:** A 7Fr prosthesis has been placed into the minor papilla.

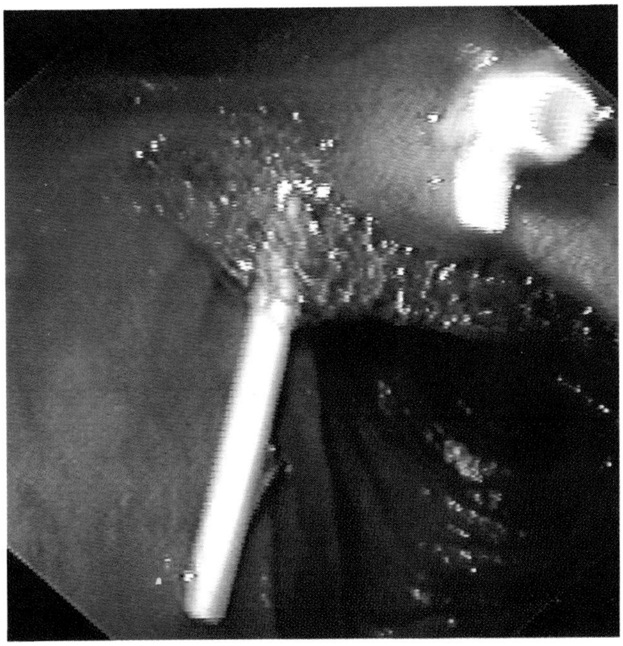

FIG. 12.155. A videoimage of a 5Fr pancreatic prosthesis (*green*) in place in the minor papilla and a 7Fr prosthesis (*blue*), which was placed into the ventral duct through the minor papilla.

of 31 patients who were stented that endoprostheses placed into the dorsal duct (70% success rate for insertion) provided relief of symptoms in 84% of the group (125). The patient served as his/her own control so that the endoscopist could determine whether the stent occluded or migrated as symptoms recurred. Exchanging the prosthesis resulted in improvement of symptoms.

Many of these patients ultimately underwent one or more of several types of surgical procedures, and the majority achieved long-term relief of symptoms (126). Thus, using the stent results as a guide, my colleagues and I embarked on an extended, prospective trial of endotherapy alone (as previously described), performing a sphincterotomy with the stent as a guide for the

TABLE 12.19. *Pancreas divisum—treatment of Group 1, stents and surgery (15 patients, 23 operations)*

Surgery	Follow-up: No. patients, years	Results
13 Sphincteroplasty, minor papilla	3 < 1	
	2 < 2	5 Asymptomatic
1 Whipple	3 < 4	8 Improved
3 Limited distal pancreatectomy, mucosal anastamoses, plus stents	1 < 5	2 No better
	2 < 6	
	4 > 6	
2 Puestow		
2 Distal resection		
2 Laparotomy		

From ref. 124.

TABLE 12.20. *Endotherapy—pancreas divisum (N = 20)*

Results	Follow-up: No. patients, years
17 Asymptomatic	7 < 1
	5 < 2
1 No better	1 < 3
	4 < 4
2 Lost to followup	1 > 4

TABLE 12.22. *Pancreas divisum—treatment of Group 3 (Controls)*

Results	Follow-up: No. patients, years
12 Improved—few or no dietary restrictions	2 < 1
	3 < 2
4 Unchanged	2 < 3
2 Difficult to evaluate	3 < 4
	5 < 5
2 Lost to follow-up	3 < 5

From ref. 124.

needle knife. We are currently tabulating our data from this trial and will hopefully report them soon.

Other groups are using similar techniques (127–132) and reporting favorable results. Because objective confirmation of pancreatitis is needed to support the diagnosis, more data will be available to assist us in managing these patients endoscopically. It is my belief that endoscopic treatment will be as effective as surgery but will offer greater benefits because it will eliminate the need for laparotomy and eradicate the frustration of repeat surgical procedures (133). This new frontier is evolving and promises to be exciting.

The only serious consequence of placement of endoprostheses into either pancreatic duct, major or minor, *may be* occlusion of the secondary radicals, leading to changes that simulate chronic pancreatitis (134). Kozarek, in his elegant article, reported reversible changes that occurred in the pancreatic duct subsequent to stent placement. Most investigators who have become involved in the management of pancreatitis, including endoscopic stent placement, have observed changes similar to those reported by Kozarek and have questioned the efficacy of this form of therapy. We reported similar changes that occurred in our series of patients with pancreas divisum who received endoprostheses (125). The effect was observed in one patient in the divisum series and has been seen in three of 40 patients in our series of idiopathic pancreatitis. Are the changes related to stent, occlusion and obstruction, progression of disease, or a combination of problems? I do not wish to ignore these changes but wonder if they are related to occlusion of the stent or to the presence of the stents. In patients undergoing surgery, the affected area was focal and was confined to the head of the gland. The surgeon did not observe diffuse disease, as one would expect with chronic pancreatitis. Therefore, as Kozarek observed, the changes, which are reversible, must be due to focal pancreatitis or stent occlusion and do not contribute to gland destruction. Sections of the gland obtained at surgery support this hypothesis (124–126).

Because we introduced the concept of stenting the pancreas, we share the concern of Kozarek and others and are embarking on a randomized trial comparing different stents and their configurations and the incidence of duct dilatation. If pancreatic stenting is contrary to our precepts, we will report it. If pancreatic stenting remains viable, however, we certainly will report this with shared enthusiasm.

TABLE 12.21. *Pancreas divisum—treatment of Group 3 (10 surgical patients)*

Operations	Results	Follow-up: No. patients, years
7 Sphincteroplasty	7 Asymptomatic	2 < 1
2 Puestow	2 unchanged	4 < 3
1 Biliary bypass	1 worse	2 < 4
(unsuspected cancer)		2 < 5

From ref. 124.

REMOVAL OF ENDOPROSTHESES

An endoprosthesis is removed using a simple technique employing either a polyp snare or a stone basket. The portion of the prosthesis that extends into the duodenum from the orifice of the appropriate duct is entrapped with a snare or basket, and the prosthesis, basket, and endoscope are removed simultaneously (Figs. 12.156–12.159). Occasionally, a small prosthesis

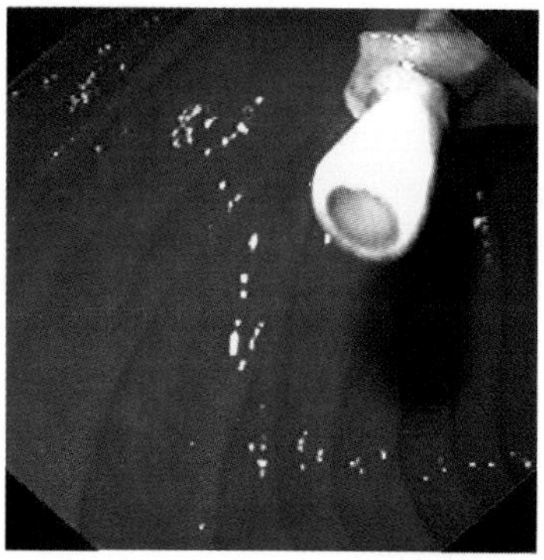

FIG. 12.156. An occluded prosthesis. Note the material adherent to the outer surface near the flap and the solid material present in the lumen of the stent.

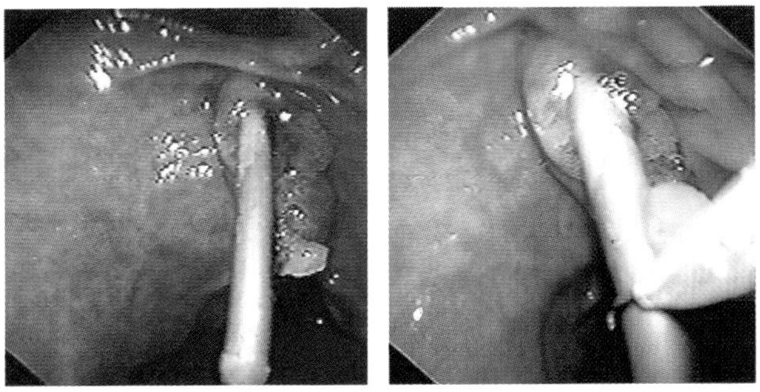

FIG. 12.157. **Left:** An occluded large-caliber biliary prosthesis. **Right:** The technique for snaring a stent for removal. The basket or snare is closed tightly, and the stent is pulled close to the endoscope. The basket or snare catheter is held firmly while pulling it with the stent against the tip of the endoscope. The stent, basket, snare, and endoscope are removed simultaneously.

can be removed through the endoscope while it is entrapped (5Fr through a 3.2 mm channel, 7Fr through a 4.2 mm channel). Some endoscopists have suggested removing the prosthesis from the duct and leaving it in the stomach while completing the study, therapeutic procedure, and/or stent exchange to avoid repeat intubation with the endoscope. After the diagnostic and therapeutic procedure, the discarded stent is retrieved and removed with the endoscope. This procedure may be obviated with the introduction of a new stent-removing device. I have found the former technique, removing the stent and entubating the patient again, more acceptable because the patient, who is consciously sedated, rarely recalls that the endoscope was introduced more than once. Also, I have occasionally found it difficult to entrap a free-floating prosthesis in

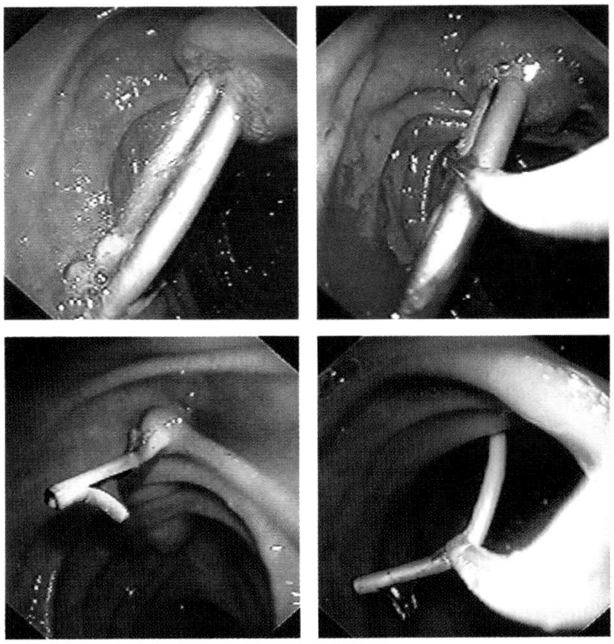

A

B

FIG. 12.158. A: Left: A videoimage showing two occluded stents exiting from the papilla. Note that they have become embedded in the opposing wall of the duodenum. If stents are embedded or the proximal ends extend too far into the duodenum, prohibiting placement of a basket or snare, one has to use either a biopsy forcep or special alligator–rat tooth forceps, especially when trying to ensnare a large-caliber prosthesis. **Right:** Both stents were ensnared simultaneously with a basket/snare, facilitating removal and avoiding repeat intubation. **B: Left:** This 5Fr prosthesis, which is located in the minor papilla, has occluded. Its removal is being planned on this examination. **Right:** The same prosthesis is entrapped with a basket and is being removed.

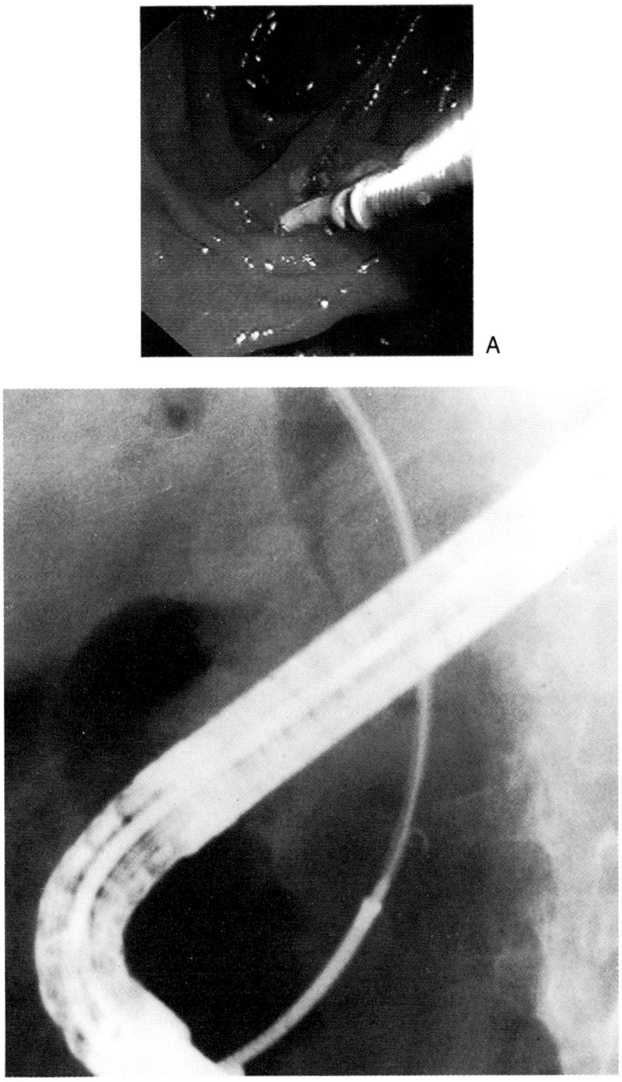

A

B

FIG. 12.159. A: A videodenoscopic image showing a stent that has been engaged by the stent remover. The tip of the coil-spring cable has engaged the stent by screwing into the stent. The device is turned in a clockwise direction, engaging the stent. The device and stent are removed over an indwelling guidewire, which is used for the replacement stent. **B:** The radiograph shows the stent remover engaging the stent, facilitated by passage over a guidewire. Once the stent remover has engaged the stent by screwing into it, the prosthesis can be removed through the endoscope, facilitated by the wire.

the stomach using the lateral-viewing endoscope, whereas a prosthesis that is in position in the appropriate sphincter is fixed and can be entrapped relatively easily. Newer devices (Soehendra-Wilson-Cook) that enable the endoscopist to capture and remove a stent of any size through the endoscope without having to remove the endoscope are now available (Fig. 12–159). Because the procedure is performed over a wire, the replacement prosthesis can be inserted during the same procedure. This modification saves time and will likely improve results for stent exchange.

MIGRATION OF PROSTHESES

Biliary Prostheses

If a prosthesis migrates from either duct into the intestinal tract, symptoms of cholestasis or pancreatitis recur, especially if obstruction to that duct system persists. The presence of a prosthesis in the intestinal tract, whether small or large, has not been associated with gastrointestinal symptoms in my experience. The stents usually pass out with the stool without producing symptoms of intestinal obstruction. To my knowledge, no migrated stent has perforated the bowel.

Should a prosthesis migrate proximally into the bile duct, there are several methods for removing it. The first method incorporates using either a basket or a snare to entrap the migrated stent. The snare or basket is advanced proximal to the prosthesis, the apparatus is opened, and the accessory is maneuvered in an attempt to entrap the prosthesis or, occasionally, the side flap. A pigtail prosthesis can also be retrieved in this manner, using a basket or snare. It may sometimes be easier to retrieve a migrated pigtail catheter because of the prominent end of the pigtail, which may be entrapped while maneuvering a basket or a snare above it. Occasionally, a biopsy forcep can be used to capture the more distal end of the prosthesis (that portion in the distal duct or duodenum) to withdraw it into the duodenum. A snare or basket can then be used for the routine removal of stents.

A large-caliber prosthesis that has migrated may be retrieved in a different manner, as follows: A catheter-guidewire assembly is introduced through the sphincterotomy and maneuvered in an attempt to place the guidewire through the more distal end of the prosthesis. Should the guidewire enter the prosthesis, it can be advanced more deeply through the prosthesis into the bile duct. The guiding catheter is removed from the guidewire, and a balloon catheter is then advanced over the guidewire and into the stent. The balloon catheter may occasionally advance completely through the stent. If so, the balloon can be inflated and the stent withdrawn into the duodenum and ultimately removed (Fig. 12.160). If the balloon catheter cannot be advanced through the prosthesis but has been introduced several centimeters, the balloon can still be inflated while in the stent, and the stent and balloon catheter can be withdrawn into the duodenum and removed.

Alternatively, once a guidewire is placed into the

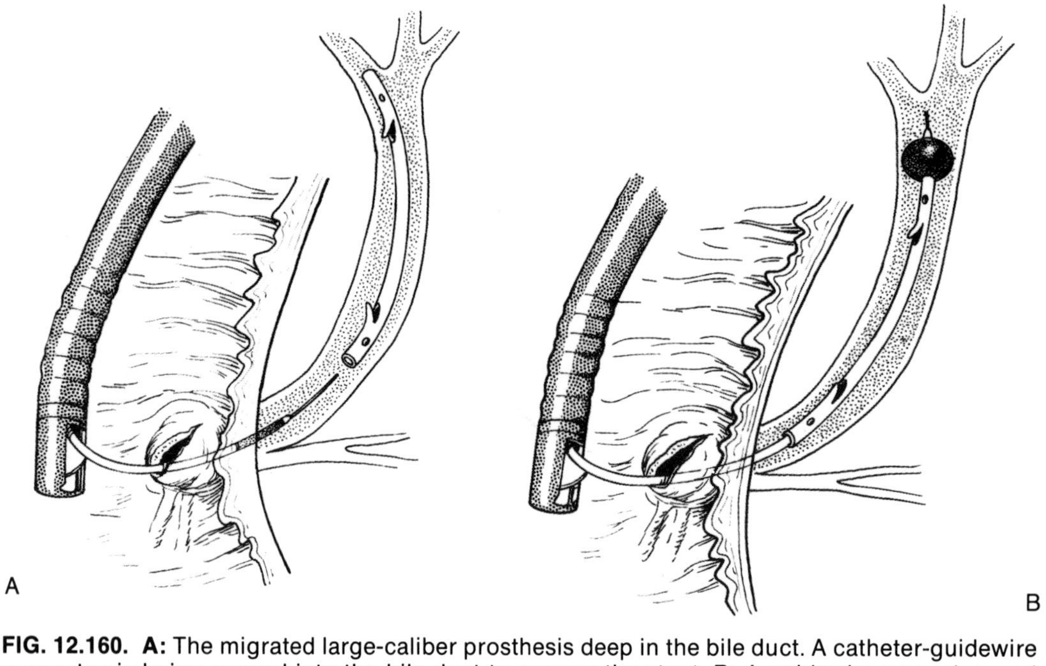

FIG. 12.160. A: The migrated large-caliber prosthesis deep in the bile duct. A catheter-guidewire apparatus is being passed into the bile duct to engage the stent. **B:** A guidewire was advanced through the stent, and a balloon catheter was passed over the wire into the stent. The balloon is inflated, and the stent can be pulled out of the duct.

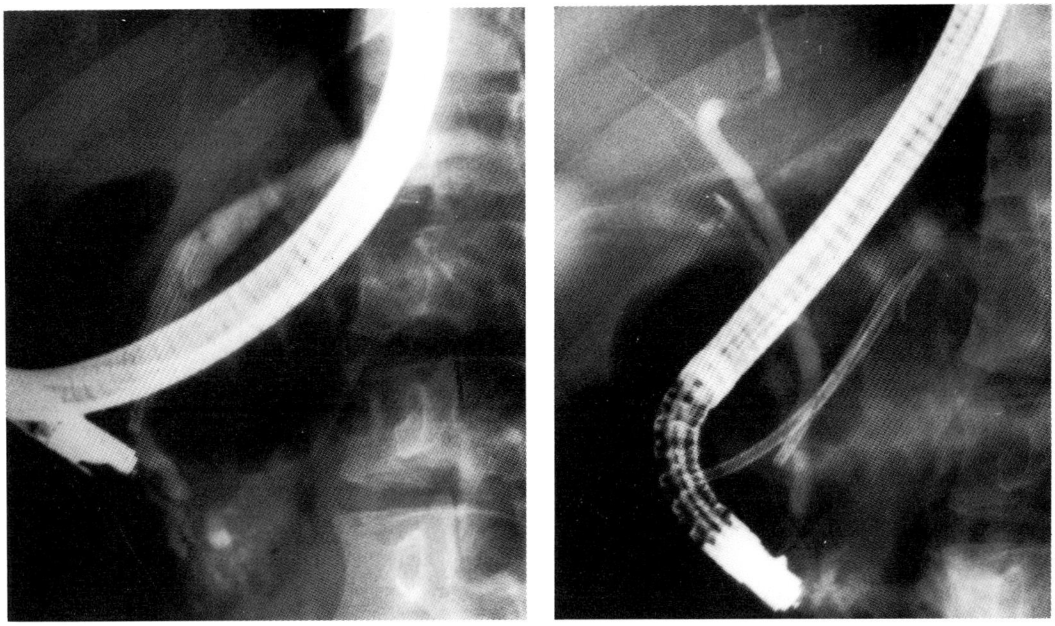

FIG. 12.161. Left: This radiograph shows a prosthesis that has migrated into the dorsal duct of a pancreas divisum. **Right:** The prosthesis could not be removed on this attempt, so another prosthesis was placed to permit decompression. The patent will return for another attempt to remove the stent.

migrated stent, the new retriever device can be advanced over the wire up to the stent. The retriever handle is turned in a clockwise fashion, attaching itself to the stent, and, with the wire left in place, the stent and retriever may be removed through the endoscope channel. A replacement prosthesis can be inserted because the guidewire is already in the proper position.

Pancreatic Prostheses

Migrated pancreatic prostheses (Figs. 12.161–12.163) are more difficult to retrieve because the pancreatic duct is usually not as dilated as the biliary tree and restricts the maneuverability of the accessories. Because most prostheses today are straight with side

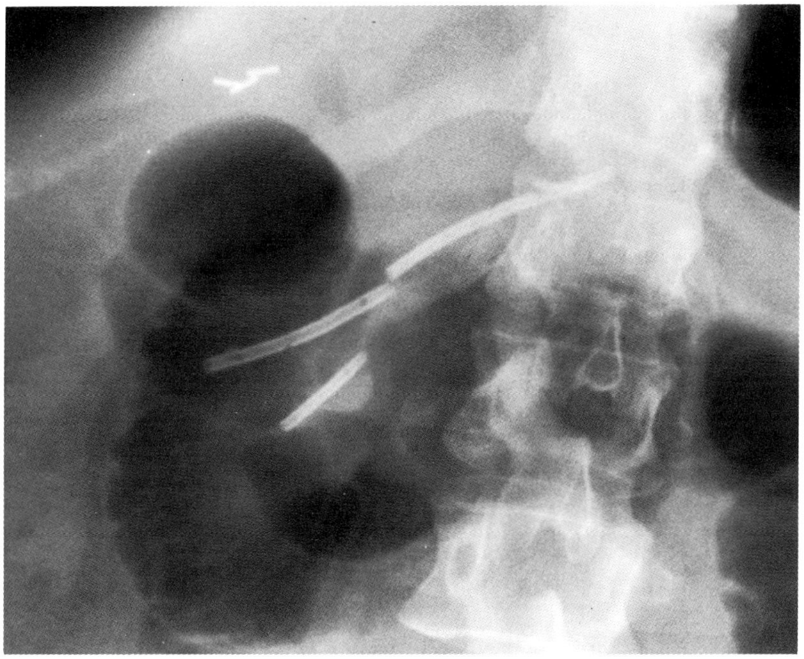

FIG. 12.162. A single prosthesis in the ventral duct of a pancreas divisum. Two stents are visible in the dorsal duct. One of these prostheses migrated into the duct, resulting in recurrent symptoms. After the placement of second stent, symptoms were relieved. The patient will return for another attempt to remove the migrated stent.

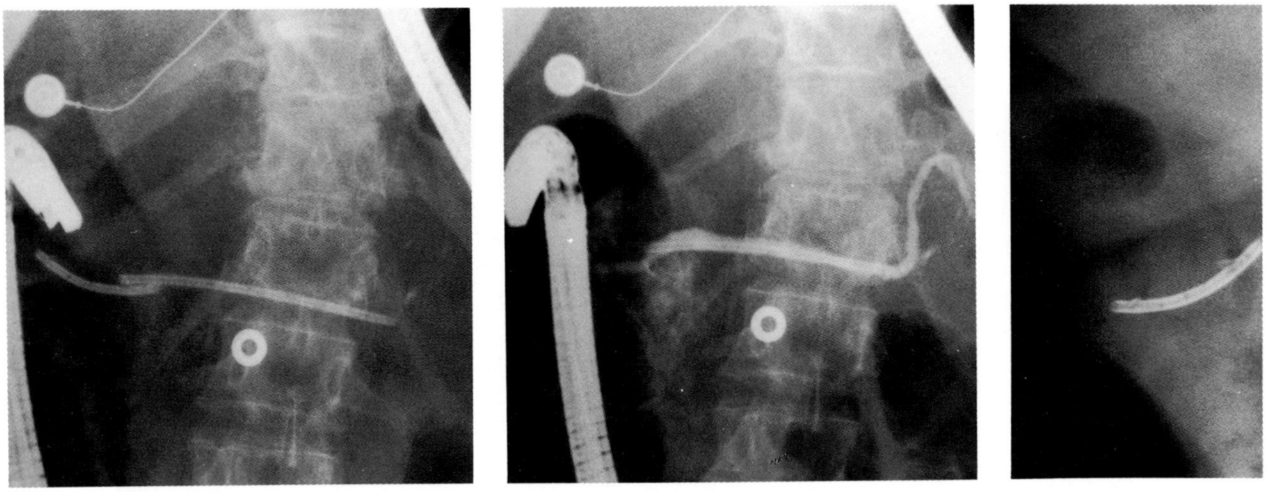

FIG. 12.163. Left: A migrated stent and a second stent in the dorsal duct of a pancreas divisum. **Middle:** The proximal stent has been removed, and attempts will be made to remove the migrated stent. **Right:** A single stent was placed into the duct after the migrated stent was removed.

flaps, a snare or basket can be used in an attempt to entrap the side flap or ultimately to encircle the prosthesis itself. A special device for retrieval of pancreatic prostheses (Geenen Pancreatic Retrieval Snare, Wilson-Cook) has been used very effectively in my experience. This device is simply a small loop snare that can be manipulated more readily in restricted areas to entrap the side flap for removal. It is very difficult to remove a prosthesis from the pancreatic duct without having performed a sphincterotomy, because the prosthesis will abut the sphincter and may become entrapped at the sphincter, denying retrieval. If the pancreatic sphincter has been dilated by the presence of a prosthesis, the prosthesis may be retrieved more easily than anticipated. More often, however, the prosthesis engages the sphincter and will not pass through.

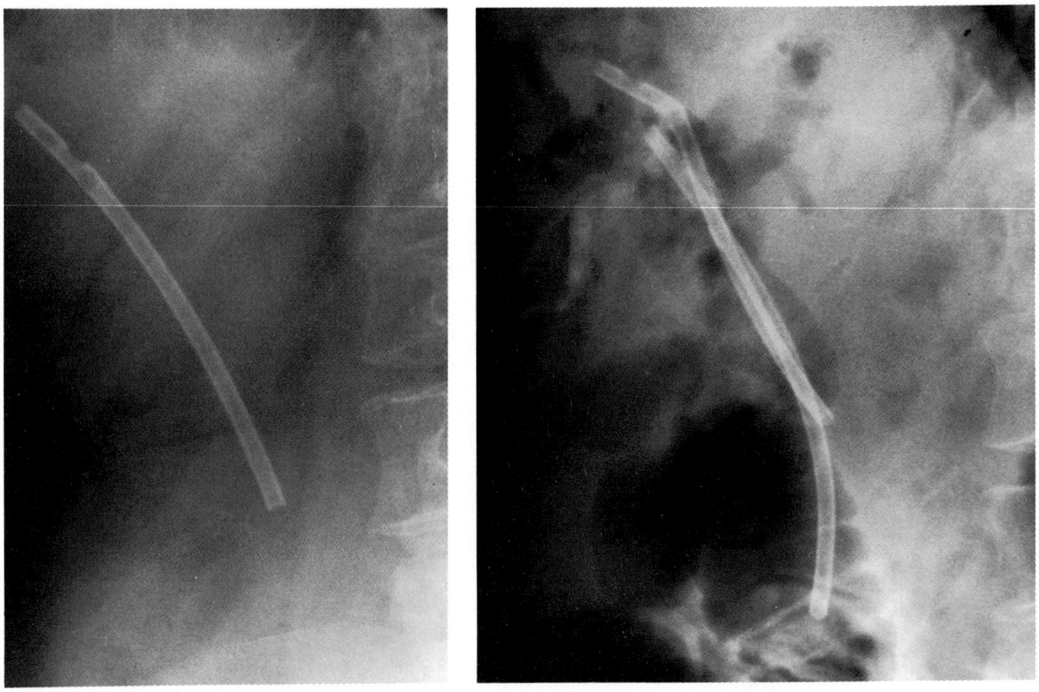

FIG. 12.164. Left: A migrated large-caliber biliary prosthesis. The patient returned with recurrent cholestasis. **Right:** The prosthesis could not be retrieved, so a second large-caliber prosthesis was placed for decompression. The migrated stent, although a foreign body and nidus of infection, will not complicate the clinical picture if drainage is reestablished using another stent.

I have used another technique for removing a migrated pancreatic prosthesis that utilizes a balloon catheter once again. The balloon catheter can be advanced beyond the prosthesis, and the balloon can be inflated and withdrawn toward the duodenum, engaging the prosthesis. Hopefully, the prosthesis will pass through the sphincter zone without becoming engaged and can then be retrieved.

Summary of Migrated Prostheses

In my experience, six biliary prostheses migrated, and all but one were successfully retrieved. In a patient with carcinoma of the pancreas, the prosthesis could not negotiate the stricture when being retrieved in an antegrade fashion. Therefore, another large-caliber prosthesis was inserted to provide drainage and decompression (Fig. 12.164). With drainage established, cholestasis improved, and the biliary infection also responded favorably. It is not absolutely necessary to remove a migrated prosthesis because the presence of another functioning large-caliber prosthesis provides decompression while ameliorating any problem related to migration and infection (Figs. 12.165, 12.166).

As reported (125), three pancreatic prostheses migrated into the dorsal duct of patients with pancreas divisum. Additionally, three migrated into the main pancreatic duct of patients treated for idiopathic pancreatitis. At surgery, one prosthesis was found to have penetrated the capsule of the pancreas, but the occurrence was benign, asymptomatic, and unsuspected. The stents were removed during a definitive surgical procedure.

Three other pancreatic stents that migrated were removed, and two others were left with a second stent placed alongside them. After the insertion of the additional stent, symptoms (which were much milder than those before the original procedure) were again ameliorated. Subsequently, the migrated stent and replacement stent have been removed in all but one patient, who, incidently, is asymptomatic because the additional stent provides decompression. Despite the presence of a foreign body in the pancreas, symptoms are minimal if present at all.

The incidence of sepsis occurring from an occluded pancreatic stent is almost nonexistent. Of more than 130 stents placed into either pancreatic duct system, only one patient presented with sepsis, and purulent material was found on the stent, which had been placed into the dorsal duct of pancreas divisum.

Usually, when a pancreatic stent occludes, the patient presents with mild recurrent symptoms of dyspepsia, indigestion, food intolerance, or pain. I stress *mild* recurrent symptoms: None have presented with severe pancreatitis associated with occlusion.

The usual scenario associated with occlusion is one of surprise. If the patient has found relief with the stent, the former symptoms have become unfamiliar. With occlusion and mild recurrence, patients can't un-

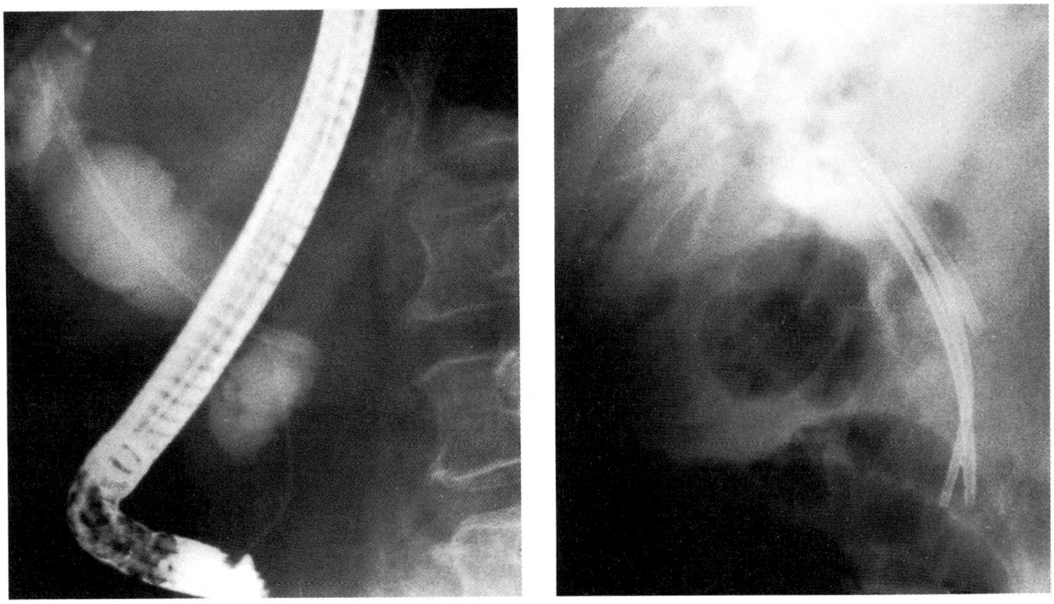

FIG. 12.165. Left: A migrated large-caliber biliary stent. A guidewire is placed to insert another prosthesis because the migrated prosthesis could not be retrieved. **Right:** Two medium-sized prostheses were placed for decompression, with immediate resolution of cholestatic symptoms.

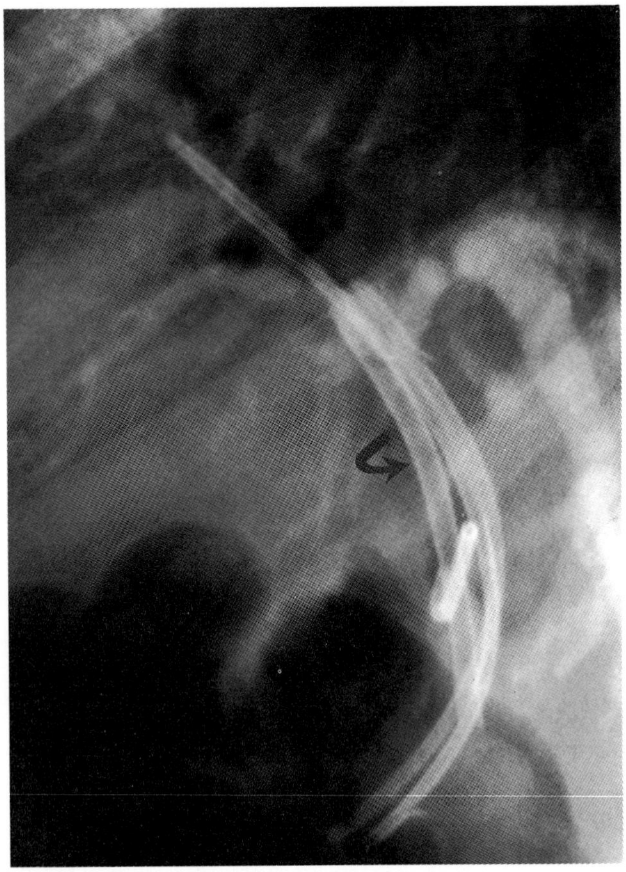

FIG. 12.166. A migrated large-caliber prosthesis (*arrow*), a fragmented pigtail, and two medium-sized prostheses of different lengths that were inserted into this bile duct to decompress the obstruction that recurred following migration. Cholestatic symptoms resolved immediately after insertion of the two smaller stents, which reestablished drainage. The fractured pigtail and migrated larger stent were subsequently removed, leaving the two medium-sized stents in place.

derstand why they are experiencing food intolerance. When they finally realize that the symptoms are reminiscent of the past, they call and return for a stent exchange.

STENT OCCLUSION (Table 12.23)

A number of investigators have reported the significance of biofilm, which is a composite of bacteria and proteinaceous material that forms in the stent lumen, adheres to the walls of the prosthesis, continues to accumulate, and ultimately occludes it (135–139). The biofilm of larger prostheses may also contain vegetable fibers and other digestive products that refluxed into the lumen of the larger stent. Despite the presence of debris, the larger prostheses remain patent longer than the smaller ones (44–48).

In addition to the internal diameter of the prostheses, other factors contribute to their patency or longevity.

TABLE 12.23. *Factors affecting stent patency*

Tube configuration
Tapered
Curved
Side holes
Tube diameter
Internal surface
Flow rate
Infecton
Benign disease
Malignant disease
Lithogenicity?

The configuration of the prosthesis has been shown to be important in maintaining patency (140). Leung et al. have shown that the straight prostheses last longer than curved or pigtail-configured stents, and I have observed that fewer side holes and flaps extend the patency rate by maintaining a steadier flow of bile. Side holes diffuse the flow rate affecting the pressure within the system and thus permitting biofilm to accumulate. I have tabulated the factors affecting patency (Table 12.23) and have suggested characteristics that should comprise an ideal stent (Table 12.24).

Although the expandable mesh stent promises to prolong patency, tumor growth within or superior to this stent has produced obstruction requiring unique methods to unplug it because it cannot be removed (50, 51). This stent will not be as universally accepted as our current polyethylene stents because of its higher cost and the fact that it cannot be exchanged or removed. Therefore, I believe that more work should be done to improve the polyethylene, polyurethane, teflon, and nylon stents.

Patient selection is certainly the most important factor in determining the type of stent to be inserted. The endoscopist will usually select the largest stent that can be safely inserted. If the patient is in poor condition and is terminally ill, the stent size is not important because the patient will not survive long enough for the stent to occlude. However, a healthier patient with

TABLE 12.24. *Prolonging stent patency*

Tube configuration
No taper
No acute curve (pigtail)
Fewer side holes and flaps
Larger tube diameter
Cholorrhetic agent
Antibiotics (doxycycline)
Aspirin
Ursodeoxycholic acid?
Smooth internal surface
Tube impregnated with antibiotics
Tube impregnated with hydromer
Tube impregnated with elemental substance (electron field)

an unresectable malignancy may live longer, and a larger stent is recommended.

Prevention of Occlusion (Table 12.24)

The Amsterdam researchers reported an interesting study in which they compared the effects of aspirin and doxycycline to placebo in reducing biofilm formation (141). They found that doxyclycline reduced the bacterial component of biofilm and that aspirin reduced the proteinaceous component. Both drugs can then contribute to prolonging patency of prostheses. The two drugs were not tried in combination, which should be studied to confirm whether they potentiate their single effects and prolong patency even more than individually.

We are currently inserting stents coated with a hydromer that is designed to decrease the stickiness of the wall to retard biofilm and bacterial attachment (Biosearch Medical Products). These stents look promising, but more work is needed in order to draw significant conclusions.

It has also been suggested that stents impregnated with antibiotics may retard bacterial attachment, but these prostheses are not yet available for study. Additional issues must be addressed, such as drug sensitivity and reactions.

Other ideas for prolonging patency of prostheses have been entertained. One novel and ingenius idea postulates that establishing an electron field within the stent wall by incorporating an element such as silver into the stent material would prevent bacterial attachment. The thought that an "electric" field would prevent the bacteria from clinging to the wall seems reasonable, and we are awaiting production of such prototypes to begin controlled trials.

Increasing the flow of bile by using a cholorrhetic agent has been proposed. The idea that increasing the flow of bile to create a "current" against which the bacteria would attempt to lay down a biofilm is intriguing. However, is it prudent or judicious to stimulate the liver continuously to produce and excrete bile, electrolytes, and essential nutrients? We don't know what deleterious effects would result from this form of treatment and suggest that animal studies be conducted before human trials.

ENDOSCOPIC EVALUATION AND MANAGEMENT OF COMPLICATIONS ASSOCIATED WITH LAPAROSCOPIC CHOLECYSTECTOMY (Tables 12.25, 12.26)

In spite of the less invasive nature of the new technique of laparoscopic cholecystectomy (lap chole), complications have occurred and will occur with unskilled or inexperienced surgeons as well as with surgeons who have extensive experience (142,143). Visualization of the biliary anatomy is excellent with this new technique but may not be absolute, and complications can result from inexact placement of clamps or dissection using electrocautery or laser technology.

We have assisted in the management of four patients who experienced complications after lap chole (Table 12.25). Two patients experienced jaundice and cholestasis secondary to complete obstruction of the common hepatic duct owing to placement of staples or clamps across the hepatic duct, and they both developed intraperitoneal fistulas and required drainage (144). Despite the successful placement of a prosthesis through the obstruction (Fig. 12.167), the fistula in one of these two patients, which originated from an injury to the right hepatic duct, continued to leak. This patient required open surgical repair, a hepaticojejunostomy. The second patient presented with biliary colic, and the ERCP cholangiogram revealed retained stones in the cystic duct remnant. This patient elected an open surgical procedure. The third patient presented with jaundice and ascites (draining bilious material through a percutaneous drain) and was found to have complete obstruction of the common hepatic duct caused by staple-clamp placement across the duct. Endoscopic drainage was unsuccessful, and the patient underwent a hepaticojejunostomy. The fourth patient presented with pain after a lap chole and was found to have a small hepatic duct fistula (Fig. 12.168) that was successfully treated with endoscopic stent placement. No surgery was necessary.

Complications associated with lap chole are potentially the same as those occurring with open cholecystectomy. Despite the fact that the clamps placed endoscopically are not placed with as much force or strength as those placed at open cholecystectomy, we

TABLE 12.25. *Complications of laparoscopic cholecystectomy evaluated by ERCP (N = 4)*

Stricture/staple obstruction	2
Common hepatic duct	
Fistula alone	1
Retained cystic duct stones	1

TABLE 12.26. *Subsequent management of complications of laparoscopic cholecystectomy*

Hepaticojejunostomy	2
1 stent failed	
1 unable to place stent	
Open removal cystic duct remnant and stones	1
Endoscopic management of fistula	1

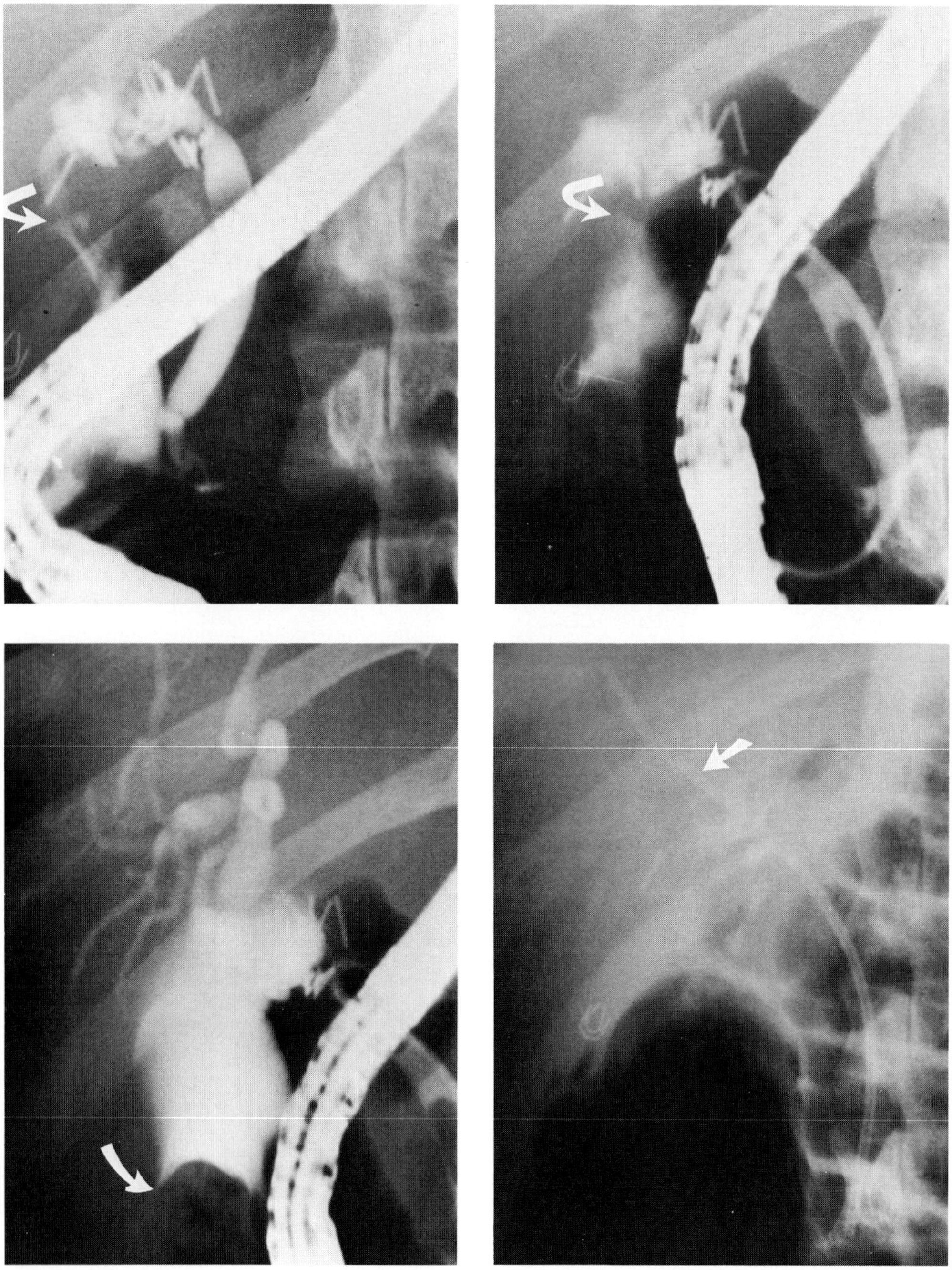

FIG. 12.167. Top left: A cholangiogram showing contrast filling the common bile duct. The retrograde flow stops abruptly at the area where staples were placed across the common hepatic duct. Note a fistulous tract filling with contrast (*arrow*). **Top right:** After performance of a sphincterotomy, attempts to place a guidewire were unsuccessful. Again, the fistulous tract is opacified (*arrow*). **Bottom left:** An occlusion balloon is placed at the stricture, and contrast is forcefully injected, opacifying a dilated proximal biliary tree. Note the collection of contrast in the fistulous tract spilling over a bowel loop (*arrow*). **Bottom right:** A prosthesis is placed through the stricture into the proximal biliary tree (*arrow*). Decompression was inadequate, and surgery was necessary because of a persistent leak from the right hepatic duct.

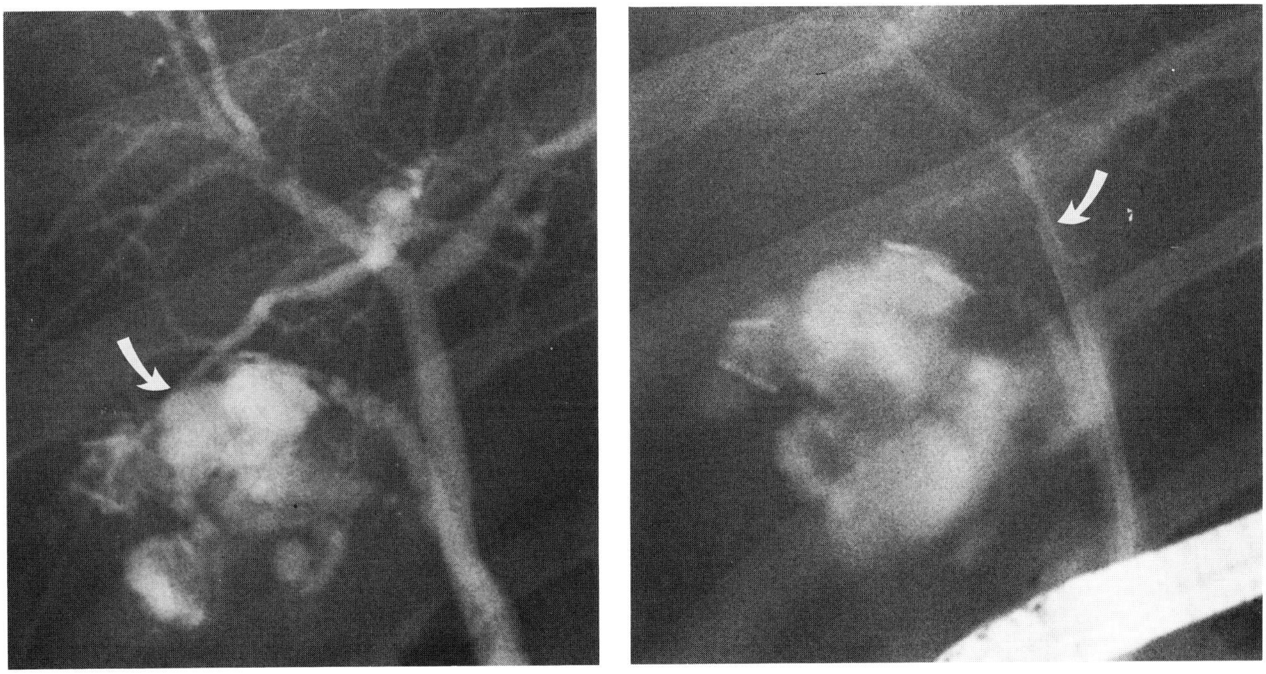

FIG. 12.168. Left: A cholangiogram obtained in a patient who experienced pain following laparoscopic cholecystectomy. Note the fistulous tract filling with contrast (*arrow*). **Right:** A prosthesis placed into the proximal biliary tree (*arrow*) provided adequate drainage and closure of the fistula. Surgery was not necessary.

have found it difficult to traverse the strictures, even with the new "slick" Terumo guidewire (Microvasive) (Table 12.26). This has been disappointing to us and to the patient, because open surgery is the only alternative.

The new procedure, lap chole, is becoming the cholecystectomy of choice. Unfortunately, not all surgeons are experienced with this procedure, but patients demand that this technique be universally available and not restricted to regional hospitals. Training programs for surgeons are available, but is every surgeon capable of learning this procedure and performing it skillfully? This book is not the proper forum to discuss surgical endoscopy training because therapeutic endoscopists are concerned about adequate training for medical endoscopists embarking upon endoscopic surgery. Neither pressure from the public nor personal economic loss should compromise this training. Not all physicians and surgeons are equal, and more selective certification criteria are needed to avoid unnecessary misadventure.

CONCLUSIONS

Ten years have passed since endoscopists began to insert indwelling prostheses for the treatment of obstructive jaundice, stone disease, cholangitis, and pancreatic diseases. The approach to the management of these diseases has become possible, ostensibly because of the proven safety and cost effectiveness of these modalities. Excellent randomized trials have proved the efficacy of endoscopic stents. It is imperative, however, to compare multiple parameters for each discipline (surgical, radiologic, and endoscopic) (Table 12.27) to determine the optimal palliative treatment modality. Table 12.28, which was compiled in our index article (65) comparing these three disciplines, summarizes a review of more than 200 articles from the literature.

In summary, the endoscopic stents are safer and associated with fewer complications than other techniques. The survival is the same for all modalities, but the quality of life and shortened hospital stay favor the

TABLE 12.27. *Evaluation and comparisons of biliary decompression techniques*

Technical success
Therapeutic failures
Thirty-day mortality
Complication rate
Occlusion rate
Hospital days
Mean survival

TABLE 12.28. *Summary of the results of decompression of biliary obstruction as estimated from medical and surgical literature*[a]

	Surgical bypass	Precutaneous stents	Endoscopic stents
30-day mortality	22%	22%	20%
	(4–44)[b]	(15–32)	(12–31%)
Hospital days	28	14	5
	(15–44)	(7–28)	(3–7)
Technical success rate	75%(?)	90%	90%
	(55–94)	(85–94)	(87–91)
Therapeutic failures	5%(?)	15%	11%
	(1–11)	(8–19)	(8–13)
Complication rate			
Major	(15–30%)	(5–15%)	(4–10%)
Total	50%	25%	21%
Occlusion rate	(1–5%)	10%/3 mos	25%/3 mos
	(reoperation rate 2–50%)	50%/6 mos	50%/6 mos
Mean survival	(3–6 mos)	(3–5 mos)	(2–9 mos)

[a] Conclusions: (1) The advantages of endoscopic biliary drainage are the low procedure-related mortality, the low incidence of major complications, and the short hospital stay. (2) Given the short mean survival of patients with unresectable malignant biliary obstruction, nonsurgical decompression should be given primary consideration for treatment; subsequent surgical treatment should depend on the response to decompression or indications of impending gastrointestinal obstruction. (3) The primary late complication of endoscopic prostheses is their occlusion, a problem that may resolve as optimal stent material, size, and configuration are determined.

[b] All values in parentheses represent the range of the means quoted in the references reviewed with other values representing an estimate of the mean of the range.

endoscopic group. As we continue our progress, we are reminded that more work lies ahead in order to improve these established techniques. More importantly, earlier detection of cancer and a cure rather than palliation will be a reality in the future.

REFERENCES

1. Wurbs D, Classen M. Transpapillary long standing tube for hepatobiliary drainage. *Endoscopy* 1977;9:192–3.
2. Cotton PB, Burney PGJ, Mason RR. Transnasal bile duct catheterisation after endoscopic sphincterotomy. *Gut* 1979;20:285–7.
3. Siegel JH, Yatto RP. Approach to cholestasis: an update. *Arch Intern Med* 1982;142:1877–9.
4. Siegel JH, Harding GT, Chateau F. Endoscopic decompression of benign and malignant biliary obstruction. *Gastrointest Endosc* 1982;28:77–82.
5. Huibregtse K, Tytgat GNJ. Endoscopic drainage of biliary tract obstructions. In: Kawai K, ed. *Frontiers of GI Endoscopy.* 1982;39–42.
6. Kozarek RA, Sanowski RA. Nonsurgical management of extrahepatic obstructive jaundice. *Ann Intern Med* 1982;96:743–5.
7. Zimmon DS, Clemett AR. Endoscopic stents and drains in the management of pancreatic and bile duct obstruction. *Surg Clin North Am* 1982;62:837–44.
8. Burcharth F, Hagenmuller F, Wurbs D. Non operative drainage of the bile ducts. Round table. *Internist (Berlin)* 1982;23:269–72.
9. Geenen JE. New diagnostic and treatment modalities involving endoscopic retrograde cholangiopancreatography and esophagogastroduodenoscopy. *Scand J Gastroenterol* 1982;77:93–106.
10. Safrany L, Schott B. Endoscopic bile duct drainage in malignant obstructive jaundice–an alternative procedure to palliative surgery. *Zentralbl Chir* 1983;108:1017–22.
11. Hagenmuller F, Classen M. Therapeutic endoscopic and percutaneous procedures. In: Popper H, Schaffner F, eds. *Progress in liver diseases,* vol III. New York: Grune and Stratton, 1982:229–317.
12. Kozarek RA. Transnasal pancreaticobiliary drains. Indications and insertion technique. *Am J Surg* 1983;146:250–3.
13. Huibregtse K. Techniques of Endoscopic Bile Drainage. In: Classen M, Geenen J, Kawai K, eds. *Nonsurgical biliary drainage.* Berlin: Springer, 1984;69–74.
14. Witzel L, Wiederholt J, Wolbergs E. Dissolution of retained duct stones by perfusion with monoctanoin via a Teflon catheter introduced endoscopically. *Gastrointest Endosc* 1981; 27:63.
15. Martin DF, McGregor JC, Lambert ME, Tweedle DEF. Pernasal catheter perfusion without dissolution agents following endoscopic sphincterotomy for common duct stones. *Br J Surg* 1989;76:410–1.
16. Leung JWC, Chung SCS, Sung JJY, Banez VP, Li AKC. Urgent endoscopic drainage for acute suppurative cholangitis. *Lancet* 1989;2:1307–9.
17. Cairns SR, Dias I, Cotton PB, Salmon PR, Russell RCG. Additional endoscopic procedures instead of urgent surgery for retained common bile duct stones. *Gut* 1989;30:535–40.
18. Venu RP, Geenen JE, Toouli J, Hogan WD, Kozlov N, Stewart ET. Gallstone dissolution using monoctanoin infusion through an endoscopically placed nasobiliary catheter. *Am J Gastroenterol* 1982;77:227–30.
19. Siegel JH, Pullano W, Ramsey WH. Sclerosing cholangitis, benign bile duct strictures, and biliary cutaneous/peritoneal fistulas: room at the top for endoscopic management. *Gastrointest Endosc* 1986;32:166 (abst).
20. Grijm R, Huibregtse K, Bartelsman J, et al. Therapeutic problems in primary sclerosing cholangitis. *Dig Dis Sci* 1986;31: 792–8.
21. Johnson GK, Geenen JE, Venu RP, Hogan WJ. Endoscopic treatment of biliary duct strictures in sclerosing cholangitis: follow-up assessment of a new therapeutic approach. *Gastrointest Endosc* 1987;33:9–12.
22. Soehendra N, Reynders-Frederiz V. Palliative bile duct drainage—a new endoscopic method of introducing a transpapillary drain. *Endoscopy* 1980;12:8.

23. Siegel JH, Harding GT, Chateau F. Endoscopic decompression of the obstructed biliary tree: transduodenal placement of stents. *Gastroenterology* 1981;80:1285.
24. Burchanth F. A new endoprosthesis for non-operative intubation of the biliary tract in malignant obstructive jaundice. *Surg Gynecol Obstet* 1978;146:78.
25. Nakayama T, Ikeda A, Okuda K. Percutaneous transhepatic drainage of the biliary tract: technique and results in 104 cases. *Gastroenterology* 1978;74:554.
26. Perieras RV Jr, Rheingold OJ, Hutson D, et al. Relief of malignant obstructive jaundice by percutaneous insertion of a permanent prosthesis in the biliary tree. *Ann Intern Med* 1978;69:589.
27. Ring EJ, Oleaga JA, Feinman DB, Husted JW, Lunderquist A. Therapeutic application of catheter cholangiography. *Radiology* 1978;128:333.
28. Kreek MJ, Balint JA. Skinny needle cholangiography. *Gastroenterology* 1980;78:598–604.
29. Dooley JS, Olney J, Dick R, Sherlock S. Non-surgical treatment of biliary obstruction. *Lancet* 1979;2:1040–3.
30. Cotton PB. Duodenoscopic placement of biliary prostheses to relieve malignant obstructive jaundice. *Br Surg* 1982;69: 501–3.
31. Lawrence BH, Cotton PB. Decompression of malignant biliary obstruction by duodenoscope intubation of bile duct. *Br Med J* 1980;280:522–3.
32. Siegel JH. Inteventional endoscopy in diseases of the biliary tree and pancreas. *Mt Sinai J Med* 1984;51:535–42.
33. Boey JH, Way LW. Acute cholangitis. *Ann Surg* 1980;191:264.
34. Welch JP, Donaldson GA. The urgency of diagnosis and surgical treatment of acute suppurative cholangitis. *Am J Surg* 1976;131:527.
35. Nunez D Jr, Guerra JJ Jr, Al-Sheikh WA, Russell E, Mendez G Jr. Percutaneous biliary drainage in acute suppurative cholangitis. *Gastrointest Radiol* 1986;11:85.
36. Pessa ME, Hawkins IF, Vogel SB. The treatment of acute cholangitis. Percutaneous transhepatic biliary drainage before definitive therapy. *Ann Surg* 1987;205:389.
37. Lois JF, Gomes AS, Grace PA, Deutsch LS, Pitt HA. Risks of percutaneous transhepatic drainage in patients with cholangitis. *AJR* 1987;148:367.
38. Leese T, Neoptolemos JP, Baker AR, Carr-Locke DL. Management of acute cholangitis and the impact of endoscopic sphincterotomy. *Br J Surg* 1986;73:988.
39. Yin TP, Frost RA, Goodacre RL. The benefit of emergency nasobiliary drain in cholelithiasis with ascending cholangitis, coagulopathy, and thrombocytopenia. *Surgery* 1986;100:105.
40. Siegel JH, Yatto RP. Biliary endoprostheses for the management of retained common bile duct stones. *Am J Gastroenterol* 1984;79:50–4.
41. Siegel JH, Pullano WE. Two new methods for selective bile duct cannulation and sphincterotomy. *Gastrointest Endosc* 1987;33:438–40.
42. Seldinger SI. Catheter replacement of the needle in percutaneous arteriography. A new technique. *Acta Radiol* 1953; 39:368–76.
43. Wurbs D, Phillip J, Classen M. Experience with the long standing nasobiliary tube in biliary diseases. *Endoscopy* 1980; 12:219–23.
44. Siegel JH. Improved biliary decompression with large caliber endoscopic prostheses. *Gastrointest Endosc* 1984;30:21.
45. Speer AG, Cotton PB, MacRae KD. Endoscopic management of malignant biliary obstruction: stents of 10 French gauge are preferable to stents of 8 French gauge. *Gastrointest Endosc* 1988;34:412–7.
46. Huibregtse K, Haverkamp HJ, Tytgat GNJ. Transpapillary positioning of a large 3.2 mm biliary endoprostheses. *Endoscopy* 1981;13:217–9.
47. Huibregtse K, Tytgat GNJ. Palliative treatment of obstructive jaundice by transpapillary introduction of a large bore bile duct endoprosthesis. *Gut* 1982;23:371–5.
48. Siegel JH, Pullano WE, Kodsi B, Cooperman A, Ramsey W. Optimal palliation of malignant bile duct obstruction: experience with endoscopic 12 French prostheses. *Endoscopy* 1988;20:137–41.
49. Cotton PB. Endoscopic management of biliary strictures. *Ann Gastrointest Endosc* 1990;94.
50. Huibregtse K, Cheng J, Coene PPLO, Fockens P, Tytgat GNJ. Endoscopic placement of expandable metal stents for biliary strictures—a preliminary report on experience with 33 patients. *Endoscopy* 1989;21:280–2.
51. Neuhaus H, Hagenmuller F, Classen M. Self-expanding biliary stents: preliminary clinical experience. *Endoscopy* 1989;21:225–8.
52. Brams HJ, Billmann P, Pausch J, Hostege A, Salm R. Nonsurgical biliary drainage: endoscopic conversion of percutaneous transhepatic into endoprosthetic drainage. *Endoscopy* 1986;18:52–4.
53. Tsang T, Crampton AR, Bernstein JR, Ramos SR, Willard JM. Percutaneous endoscopic biliary stent placement—a preliminary report. *Ann Intern Med* 1987;106:389–93.
54. Chespak LW, Ring EJ, Shapiro HA, Gordon RL, Ostroff JW. Multidisciplinary approach to complex endoscopic biliary intervention. *Radiology* 1989;170:995–8.
55. Dowsett JF, Vaira D, Hatfield ARW, et al. Endoscopic biliary therapy using the combined percutaneous and endoscopic drainage technique. *Gastroenterology* 1989;96:1180–6.
56. Kautz G. Transpillary bile duct drainage with a large caliber endoprosthesis. *Endoscopy* 1983;15:312–5.
57. Siegel JH, Daniel SJ. Endoscopic and fluoroscopic transpapillary placement of a large caliber biliary endoprosthesis. *Am J Gastroenterol* 1984;79:461–5.
58. Nakao NL, Siegel JH, Stenger RJ, Gelb AM. Tumors of the ampulla of Vater: early diagnosis by intra-ampullary biopsy during endoscopic cannulation. *Gastroenterology* 1982;83:459–64.
59. Langer B, Lipson R, McHattie JD, et al. Periampullary tumors: advances in diagnosis and surgical treatment. *Can J Surg* 1979;22:34–7.
60. Siegel JH, Yatto RP. Endoscopic evaluation and therapy of periampullary adenoma. *Am J Gastroenterol* 1983;78:225–6.
61. Huibregtse K, Tytgat GNJ. Carcinoma of the ampulla of Vater: the endoscopic approach. *Endoscopy* 1988;20:223–6.
62. Ponchon T, Berger F, Chavaillon A, Bory R, Lambert R. Contribution of endoscopy to diagnosis and treatment of tumors of the ampulla of Vater. *Cancer* 1989;64:161–7.
63. Shemesh E, Nass S, Czerniak A. Endoscopic sphincterotomy and endoscopic fulguration in the management of adenoma of the papilla of Vater. *Surg Gynecol Obstet* 1989;169:445–8.
64. Bickerstaff KI, Berry AR, Chapman RW, Britton BJ. Endoscopic sphincterotomy for the palliation of ampullary carcinoma. *Br J Surg* 1990;77:160–2.
65. Siegel JH, Snady H. The significance of endoscopically placed prostheses in the management of biliary obstruction due to carcinoma of the pancreas: results of non-operative decompression in 227 patients. *Am J Gastroenterol* 1986;81:634–41.
66. Neff RA, Fankuchen EL, Cooperman AM, et al. The radiological management of malignant biliary obstruction. *Clin Radiol* 1984;34:143–6.
67. Bowman PC, Harries-Jones R, Van Stiegman G, Terblanche J. Prospective controlled trial of transhepatic biliary endoprosthesis versus bypass surgery for incurable carcinoma of the head of the pancreas. *Lancet* 1986;69–71.
68. Speer A, Russell HCG, Hatfield A, et al. Randomised trial of endoscopic vs percutaneous stent insertion for malignant obstructive jaundice. *Lancet* 1987;2:57–61.
69. Sonnenfeld T, Gabrielsson N, Granquist S, Perbeck I. Non resectable malignant bile duct obstruction. Surgical bypass or endoprosthesis? *Acta Chir Scand* 1986;152:297–300.
70. Shephard HA, Royle G, Ross APR, Diba A, Arthur M, Colin-Jones D. Endoscopic biliary endoprosthesis in the palliation of malignant obstruction of the distal common bile duct: a randomized trial. *Br J Surg* 1988;75:1166–8.
71. McLean GK, Burke DR. Role of endoprostheses in the management of malignant biliary obstruction. *Radiology* 1989; 170:961–7.

72. Soehendra N, Grimm H, Berger B, Nam VC. Malignant jaundice: results of diagnostic and therapeutic endoscopy. *World J Surg* 1989;13:171–7.
73. Bengmark S, Ekberg H, Evander A, Klofver-Stahl B, Tranberg KG. The approach to carcinoma of the proximal hepatic ducts: more radical or more conservative. *Hepato Pancreato Biliary Surg* 1989;1:173–84.
74. Little JM. Hilar biliary cancer: are we getting it right? *Hepato Pancreato Biliary Surg* 1989;1:93–6.
75. Deviere J, Baize M, Busset G, Cremer M. Complications of internal endoscopic biliary drainage. *Acta Endosc* 1986;16:19–29.
76. Deviere J, Baize M, de Toeuf J, Cremer M. Long-term follow up of patients with hilar malignant stricture treated by endoscopic internal biliary drainage. *Gastrointest Endosc* 1988; 34:95–101.
77. Speer AG, Cotton PB. Endoscopic stents for biliary obstruction due to malignancy. In: Jacobson IM, ed. *ERCP—diagnostic and therapeutic applications*. New York: Elsevier Science Publishing, 1989;203–24.
78. Speer AG, Cotton PB, Dineen LP. Endoscopic stents in malignant hilar strictures, results in 70 patients. Proceedings of the 87th meeting of the American Gastroenterology Association. San Francisco, 1986.
79. Summerfield JA. Biliary obstruction is best managed by endoscopists. *Gut* 1988;29:741–5.
80. Kramer T, Max M. Carcinoma of the gallbladder. *Surg Gynecol Obstet* 1983;56:641–5.
81. Lameris JS, Stoker J, Dees J, Nix GAJJ. Non surgical palliative treatment of patients with malignant biliary obstruction—the place of endoscopic and percutaneous drainage. *Clin Radiol* 1987;38:603–8.
82. Robertson DAF, Hacking LN, Birch S, Ayres R, Shepherd H, Wright W. Experience with a combined percutaneous and endoscopic approach to stent insertion in malignant obstructive jaundice. *Lancet* 1987;2:1449–52.
83. Blumgart LH, Benjamin IS, Hadjis NS, Beazley R. Surgical approaches to cholangiocarcinoma at confluence of hepatic ducts. *Lancet* 1984;1:66–9.
84. Huibregtse K. Endoscopic biliary and pancreatic drainage. Stuttgart: George Thieme Verlag, 1989.
85. Polydorou AA, Chisholm EM, Romanos AA, Dowsett JF, Cotton PB, Hatfield ARW. A comparison of right versus left hepatic duct endoprosthesis insertion in malignant hilar biliary obstruction. *Endoscopy* 1989;21:266–71.
85a. Venu RP, Rolny P, Geenen JE, Hogan WJ, Johnson GK, Schmalz M. Is there a need for multiple stents in hilar strictures? *Gastrointest Endosc* 1990;36:197 (abst).
86. Glenn F. Iatrogenic injury to the biliary ductal system. *Surg Gynecol Obstet* 1978;146:430–4.
87. Warren KW, Jefferson MF. Prevention and repair of strictures of the intrahepatic ducts. *Surg Clin North Am* 1978;53:1169–90.
88. Way LW, Bernhoft RA, Thomas MJ. Biliary strictures. *Surg Clin North Am* 1981;61:963–72.
89. Pellegrini CA, Thomas MJ, Way LW. Recurrent biliary stricture. Patterns of recurrence and outcome of surgical therapy. *Am J Surg* 1984;147:175–80.
90. Pitt HA, Kaufman KL, Coleman J, White RJ, Cameron JL. Benign postoperative biliary strictures: operate or dilate? *Ann Surg* 1989;210:417–27.
91. Martin EC, Fankuchen EI, Laffey KJ, Sibley RE. Percutaneous management of benign biliary disease. *Gastrointest Radiol* 1984;9:207–12.
92. Vogel SB, Howard RJ, Caridi J, Hawkins EF. Evaluation of percutaneous transhepatic balloon dilatation of benign biliary strictures in high-risk patients. *Am J Surg* 1985;149:73–8.
93. Gallacher DJ, Kadir S, Kaufman SL, et al. Nonoperative management of benign postoperative biliary strictures. *Radiology* 1985;156:625–9.
94. Vallon AG, Mason RR, Laurence BH, Cotton PB. Endoscopic retrograde cholangiography in postoperative bile duct strictures. *Br J Radiol* 1982;55:32–5.
95. Siegel JH, Geulrud M. Endoscopic cholangiopancreatoplasty: hydrostatic balloon dilation in the bile duct and pancreas. *Gastroint Endosc* 1983;29:99–103.
96. Geenen JE. Balloon dilatation of bile duct strictures. In: Classen M, Geenen J, Kawai K, eds. *Nonsurgical biliary drainage*. New York: Springer-Verlag, 1984;105–8.
97. Foutch PG, Sivak MV Jr. Therapeutic endoscopic balloon dilatation of the extrahepatic biliary ducts. *Am J Gastroenterol* 1985;80:575–80.
98. Huibregtse K, Katon RM, Tytgat GNJ. Endoscopic treatment of postoperative biliary strictures. *Endoscopy* 1986;18:133–7.
99. Siegel JH. Endoscopic management of benign biliary strictures, biliary tract fistulae and sclerosing cholangitis. In: Jacobson IM, ed. *ERCP—diagnostic and therapeutic applications*. New York: Elsevier Scientific Publishers, 1989.
100. Berkelhammer C, Kortan P, Haber GB. Endoscopic biliary prostheses as treatment for benign postoperative bile duct strictures. *Gastrointest Endosc* 1989;35:95–101.
101. Geenen DJ, Geenen JE, Hogan WJ, et al. Endoscopic therapy for benign bile duct strictures. *Gastrointest Endosc* 1989;35:367–71.
102. Sauerbruch T, Weinzierl M, Holl J, Pratschke E. Treatment of postoperative bile fistulas by internal endoscopic biliary drainage. *Gastroenterology* 1986;90:1998–2003.
103. Smith AC, Schapiro RH, Kelsey PB, Warshaw AL. Successful treatment of nonhealing biliary-cutaneous fistulas with biliary stents. *Gastroenterology* 1986;90:765–9.
104. Ponchon T, Gallez JF, Valette PJ, Chavaillon A, Bory R. Endoscopic treatment of biliary tract fistula. *Gastrointest Endosc* 1989;35:490–8.
105. Siegel JH. Endoscopic approach to management of hepatico-pancreatico-biliary disorders. In: Bengmark S, ed. *Progress in surgery of the liver, pancreas and biliary system*. Denmark: Martinus Nijhoff, 1988.
106. Siegel J, Halpern G. A possible role for endoscopic therapy in the treatment of sclerosing cholangitis. *Gastrointest Endosc* 1984;30:161 (abst).
107. Wood RAB, Cuschieri A. Is sclerosing cholangitis complicating ulcerative colitis a reversible condition? *Lancet* 1984;2:716–8.
108. Allison MC, Buroughs AK, Noone P, Summerfield JA. Biliary lavage with corticosteroids in primary sclerosing cholangitis. A clinical cholangiographic and bacteriological study. *J Hepatol* 1986;3:118–22.
109. Johnson GK, Geenen JE, Venu RP, Schmalz MJ, Hogan WJ. Endoscopic treatment of biliary tract strictures in sclerosing cholangitis: a larger series and recommendations for treatment. *Gastrointest Endosc* 1991;37:38–43.
110. Fuji T, Amano H, Ohmura R, Akiyama T, Aibe T, Takemoto T. Endoscopic pancreatic sphincterotomy: technique and evaluation. *Endoscopy* 1989, 21:27–30.
111. Grimm H, Meyer WH, Nam VC, Soehendra N. New modalities for treating chronic pancreatitis. *Endoscopy* 1989;21:70–4.
112. Cremer M, Toussaint J, Dunham F. Endoscopic management of chronic pancreatitis. *Gastrointest Endosc* 1980;26:65–9.
113. Siegel JH, Yatto RP. Endoscopic management of chronic pancreatitis. *Gastrointest Endosc* 1981;27:240–1.
114. Veerappan A, Kothur R, Patel N, Pullano W, Siegel JH. A safer technique for performing endoscopic sphincterotomy (ES) in high risk situations: Bilroth II (BII), periampullary diverticulum (PAD), Wirsung sphincter (WS), and Santorini sphincter (SS). *Am J Gastroenterol* 1990;8:1259 (abst).
115. Provansal-Cheyland M, Bernard JP, Mariani A, et al. Occluded pancreatic endoprostheses—analysis of the clogging material. *Endoscopy* 1989;21:63–9.
116. McCarthy J, Geenen JE, Hogan WJ. Preliminary experience with endoscopic stent placement in benign pancreatic diseases. *Gastrointest Endosc* 1988;34:16–8.
117. Huibregtse K, Schneider B, Vrij AA, Tytgat GNJ. Endoscopic pancreatic drainage in chronic pancreatitis. *Gastrointest Endosc* 1988;34:9–15.
118. Kozarek RA, Patterson DJ, Ball TJ, Traverso LW. Endoscopic placement of pancreatic stents and drains in the management of pancreatitis. *Ann Surg* 1989;209:261–6.

119. Siegel JH. Endoscopic management of pancreatic strictures: catheter dilatation and insertion of pancreatic endoprostheses (PEP). *Gastrointest Endosc* 1983;29:174 (abst).
120. Cotton PB. Congenital anomaly of pancreas divisum as cause of obstructive pain and pancreatitis. *Gut* 1980;21:105–14.
121. Lowes JR, Lees WR, Cotton PB. Pancreatic duct dilatation after secretin stimulation in patients with pancreas divisum. *Pancreas* 1989;4:371–4.
122. Warshaw AL, Richter JM, Schapiro RH. The cause and treatment of pancreatitis associated with pancreas divisum. *Ann Surg* 1983;198:443–52.
123. Keith RG, Shapero TF, Saibil FG, Moore TL. Dorsal duct sphincterotomy is effective long-term treatment of acute pancreatitis associated with pancreas divisum. *Surgery* 1989;106:660–7.
124. Siegel JH, Cooperman AM, Pullano W, Hammerman H. Pancreas divisum: observation, endoscopic drainage, and surgical treatment. Results in 65 patients. *Hepatogastroenterology* (In press).
125. Siegel JH, Pullano W, Ben-Zvi JS, Cooperman AM. Effectiveness of endoscopic drainage for pancreas divisum. *Endoscopy* 1990;20:129–32.
126. Cooperman AM, Siegel JH, Hammerman H. Editorial: pancreas divisum—advocates and agnostics. *J Clin Gastroenterol* 1989;11:1–3.
127. Sherman S, Lehman GA, Nisi R, Hawes RH, Benage D. Results of endoscopic sphincterotomy of the minor papilla for pancreas divisum. *Gastrointest Endosc* 1990;36:198 (abst).
128. Benage D, McHenry R, Hawes RH, O'Connor KW, Lehman GA. Minor papilla cannulation and dorsal ductography in pancreas divisum. *Gastrointest Endosc* 1990;36:553–7.
129. Geenen JE. ASGE distinguished lecture—endoscopic therapy of pancreatic diseases; a new horizon. *Gastrointest Endosc* 1988;34:386.
130. Lehman G, O'Connor K, Troiano F, Benage D. Endoscopic papillotomy and stenting of the minor papilla in pancreas divisum. *Gastrointest Endosc* 1989;35:167 (abst).
131. Prabhu M, Geenen JE, Hogan WJ, et al. Role of endoscopic stent placement in the treatment of acute recurrent pancreatitis associated with pancreas divisum: a prospective assessment. *Gastrointest Endosc* 1989;35:165.
132. Barkun AN, Jones S, Putnam WS, Baillie J, Barker S, Cotton PB. Endoscopic treatment of patients with pancreas divisum and pancreatitis. *Gastrointest Endosc* 1990;36:206 (abst).
133. Warshaw AL, Simeone JF, Schapiro RH, Flavin-Warshaw B. Evaluation and treatment of the dominant dorsal duct syndrome (pancreas divisum revisited). *Am J Surg* 1990;159:59.
134. Kozarek RA. Pancreatic stents can induce ductal changes consistent with chronic pancreatitis. *Gastrointest Endosc* 1990; 36:93–5.
135. Leung JWC. Mechanism of biliary prosthesis blockage: scanning electron microscopy evidence. *Gut* 1986;27:602 (abst).
136. Groen AK, Out T, Huibregtse K, Delzenne B, Hoek FJ, Tytgat GNJ. Characterization of the content of occluded biliary endoprostheses. *Endoscopy* 1987;19:57–9.
137. Speer AG, Cotton PB, Rode J, et al. Biliary stent blockage with bacterial biofilm. *Ann Intern Med* 1988;108:546–53.
138. Leung JWC, Ling TKW, Kung JLS, Vellance-Owen J. The role of bacteria in the blockage of biliary stents. *Gastrointest Endosc* 1988;34:19–22.
139. Wosiewitz U, Schrameyer B, Safrany L. Biliary sludge: its role during bile duct drainage with an endoprosthesis. *Gastroenterology* 1985;88:1706.
140. Leung JWC, del Favero G, Cotton PB. Endoscopic biliary prostheses. A comparison of materials. *Gastrointest Endosc* 1985;31:93–5.
141. Smit JM, Out MMJ, Groen AK, et al. A placebo-contracted study on the efficacy of aspirin and doxycycline in preventing clogging of biliary endoprostheses. *Gastrointest Endosc* 1989;35:485–9.
142. Perissat J, Collet DR, Belliard R. Gallstones: laparoscopic treatment, intracorporeal lithotripsy followed by cholecystostomy or cholecystectomy—a personal technique. *Endoscopy* 1989;21:373–4.
143. Reddick EJ, Olsen DO. Laparoscopic laser cholecystectomy—a comparison with mini-lap cholecystectomy. *Surg Endosc* 1989;3:131–3.
144. Kozarek RA, Traverso LW. Endoscopic stent placement for cystic duct leak after laparoscopic cholecystectomy. *Gastrointest Endosc* 1991;37:71–3.

CHAPTER 13

Cholangiopancreatoplasty: Hydrostatic Dilatation of Strictures of the Biliary Tree and Pancreas

With the advent of interventional endoscopy, the use of catheters and guidewires became apparent and routine. Once a guidewire is inserted, the duct is assessed, which facilitates control for insertion and advancement of accessories. As mentioned earlier, many accessories can be advanced over the guidewire to ease therapeutic maneuvers. In earlier chapters, I described the techniques for insertion of sphincterotomes, prostheses, occlusion balloons, dilating catheters, and dilating balloons to complete the therapeutic manuevers that utilize guide catheters and guidewires. The approach to hydrostatic dilatation of biliary and pancreatic strictures is similar to that of the other endoscopic interventional procedures. After performance of an ERCP and identification of the area in the specific duct system that requires dilatation, a sphincterotomy is routinely performed unless contraindicated. After the sphincterotomy, a catheter-guidewire assembly is inserted through the stricture. Using a 7 French dilating catheter (Van Andel catheter, Wilson-Cook) may enable the endoscopist to determine the caliber and rigidity of the stricture. This sizing maneuver determines the balloon catheter size that can be advanced through the stricture. If the 7Fr dilating catheter meets little resistance, a balloon catheter (a 7Fr catheter containing a 6 mm balloon) should slide into the stricture with little difficulty (Fig. 13.1).

The dilatation procedure is performed under fluoroscopic control. For example, the catheter-guidewire assembly is advanced through the stricture into the proximal biliary tree. The guidewire is left in place as the guiding catheter or dilating catheter is removed and exchanged for the balloon catheter in a fashion described previously as the Seldinger technique (Chapter 12) (1). Once the guidewire is in place, the balloon catheter is advanced over it through the endoscope into the duodenum, sphincterotomy, and bile duct.

The balloon, which is polyethylene, is not elastic and is not flat against the catheter as are the latex occlusion balloons. Dilating balloons must be thoroughly aspirated and flattened against the shaft of the catheter to reduce friction. After aspiration of the balloon (applying steady, negative pressure using a syringe), the balloon is molded and twisted around the catheter to reduce the excess material, which, if not flattened maximally, will produce friction and interfere with the advancement of its catheter. To soften it and make it more pliable, the balloon is initially placed in warm or hot water so that it can be easily flattened and twisted about the shaft. After this maneuver, a compression sleeve is placed over the balloon to maintain compression and the flattened configuration. The balloon and sleeve are then placed in ice water to fix this preformed configuration of the balloon against the shaft. The sleeve is removed immediately prior to placement of the balloon catheter onto the wire and insertion into the biopsy channel of the endoscope. Adhering to these steps allows the balloon to remain as flat as possible against the shaft and to offer the least amount of resistance. This flattening procedure is recommended for balloon catheters that pass over a guidewire and through the endoscope and works for biliary and pancreatic balloons, which, when inflated, measure 4 mm, 6 mm, 8 mm, and 10 mm (2). Newer high-pressure balloons with different fabric (C.R. Bard) are presently being investigated (Fig. 13.2). The material is thinner, and the fabric is softer, returns to a tighter configuration after being inflated, and offers less friction and resistance when passed into the endoscope. In addition, with the new balloons, greater pressures can be

A

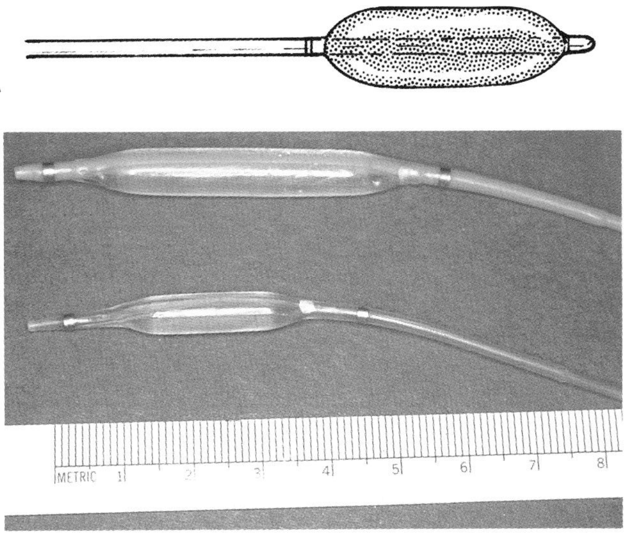

B

FIG. 13.1. A: A dilating balloon that has been inflated to its full diameter. Balloons for use in the biliary tree and pancreas are manufactured in several diameters varying from 4 mm to 10 mm. The 4 mm and 6 mm balloons are 2 cm long and are contained on a double-lumen catheter, which is 7Fr in diameter and can be passed through a standard duodenoscope with a 2.8 mm channel. The 8 mm and 10 mm balloons are contained on an 8Fr catheter and must be used in a larger channel instrument, channel size 3.2 mm or larger. These latter balloons are 3 cm in length. All balloons contain radiopaque markers at each end so that the balloon can be identified on fluoroscopy and can be placed exactly in the stricture. Syringes and injection guns attach to a gauge so that exact injection pressures may be generated in the balloon as dilatation is carried out. The most effective medium for dilatation is liquid, and contrast material, which opacifies the balloon, enables one to appreciate the diameter and configuration of the balloon on fluoroscopy during dilatation. **B:** Two dilating balloons (Microvasive) measuring 6 mm (lower) and 8 mm (upper) when inflated.

generated, facilitating dilatation of more resistant strictures.

The stricture to be dilated is negotiated with the catheter-guidewire assembly, and this assembly is advanced into the proximal bile duct or pancreatic duct (proximal referring to that part of the duct away from the sphincter). With the guidewire in place, access to the duct of intention is established. One has the option of using a series of dilating catheters, currently available to 12Fr (3) (the larger balloons and dilating catheters require the TJF therapeutic endoscope, which has a 4.2 mm channel), to prepare the stricture for insertion of the balloon catheter. After sequential dilatation of the stricture using dilating catheters over the guidewire, the endoscopist has the option of removing the catheters, leaving the guidewire in place, and advancing the balloon catheter.

If the stricture is dilated to 10Fr or 12Fr with the catheter, there should be little or no difficulty in advancing the 8 mm balloon catheter over the guidewire and into the stricture; the 8 mm balloon is contained on an 8Fr catheter, and if little resistance is encountered using the larger dilating catheter, the balloon catheter can be inserted.

Once the balloon catheter is in place within the stricture, its self-contained radiopaque markers, which define the length of the balloon, may be seen on the fluoroscope. The apparatus is then placed into the appropriate and optimal location within the stricture using fluoroscopic guidance. Once the balloon is in place, saline or a mixture of saline and contrast material is injected using a special injection gun or syringe attached to a pressure gauge that measures the maximum pressure exerted on the strictures. The balloon is usually inflated to approximately 5 ATMS and held

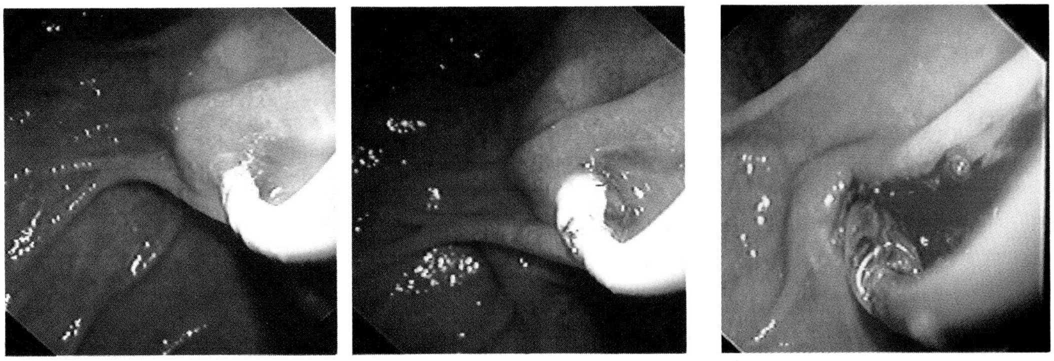

A B

FIG. 13.2. A: Left: This videoendoscopic picture shows the new, high-pressure balloon catheter being advanced into the minor papilla, facilitated by a guidewire placed earlier. **Right:** This 4 mm balloon is fully inflated in the minor papilla. After dilatation of the minor papilla, a 7Fr prosthesis was placed to maintain the effect of dilatation and provide decompression. The patient was discharged the same day. The major papilla can be seen below (inferior to) the balloon. **B:** A balloon catheter being inflated in the major papilla.

TABLE 13.1. *Endoscopic hydrostatic dilatation (EHD) (N = 193)*

Bile duct strictures	51
Hepatic duct	24
Bile duct (including anastomoses)	27
Papillary stenosis (dyskinesia or dysfunction of sphincter)	101
Pancreatic duct strictures	41
Main pancreatic duct	19
Pancreas divisum	22

TABLE 13.3. *Endoscopic hydrostatic dilatation (EHD): Complications*

Fever	23 (12%)
Septicemia	2 (1%)
Pancreatitis	29 (15%)
Surgery	0
Deaths	0
Perforation	0

for at least 30 seconds, deflated, and inflated at least once or twice more. The newer, high-pressure balloons are inflated to 150 PSI (lb/in^2). The advantages of the newer balloons include a more flexible and pliable fabric that inflates and deflates more rapidly and more readily than the old balloons.

After adequate dilatation of the stricture, a repeat cholangiogram or pancreatogram can be performed to confirm the effects of the dilatation procedure. Table 13.1 summarizes my experience in dilating strictures of the biliary tree and pancreatic duct, and the location of these strictures is identified in the table. The results of the dilatation procedures and the complications associated with the procedures are listed in Tables 13.2 and 13.3.

Because the cicatrix (stricture), or scar, is composed of fibrous tissue, the dilatation procedure, in simple terms, tears the fibrils of this tissue and relieves the obstructive process. Recurrent cicatrix and stricture formation following dilatation depends on two factors: tissue composition (i.e., inflammatory or collagen fibrils) and the age of the stricture being dilated. The time required for reformation of a stricture after treatment is not known but is critical to the success or failure of treatment. If a stricture is present for more than 4 to 6 months, the likelihood of the stricture recurring or reforming after dilatation is relatively high because the stricture subsequently becomes composed of fibrous tissue, which may not be permanently interrupted by dilating techniques. On the other hand, a recently formed stricture resulting from trauma at surgery (less than 2 months old) is mostly composed of inflammatory infiltrate and edema and is less likely to recur, or more likely to remain open, if treated early in the patient's course (4–22). Obviously appreciating the stricture and initiating treatment early reduces the likelihood that the stricture will recur or become chronic. Strictures formed in sclerosing cholangitis are different from those secondary to inflammation and trauma; that is, their composition may differ. However, balloon dilatation and stent placement have been effective palliative procedures for postponing liver transplantation while providing efficacious drainage and contributing to an improved quality of life (12–16,22).

To reduce the incidence of recurrent stricture reformation following dilatation, other groups and I began inserting prostheses through the stricture immediately after the dilatation procedure. This technique bridges the injured area while maintaining the integrity of the lumen and thus reduces the probability of restricturing (12–16,22,23). Chapter 12 includes details and descriptions of the endoscopic procedures used in the management of biliary and pancreatic strictures. Since our index article on cholangiopancreatoplasty in 1983, this technique has been employed and described by other groups and has been accepted as a treatment option in the management of strictures not only of the pancreaticobiliary system but also of the entire gastrointestinal tract (2,6).

Balloon dilators offer certain safety features that are not applicable to bougies or similar rigid dilating devices (Table 13.4). Balloons utilize a radial force that is evenly distributed, but they are effective only when a circumferential or complete stricture is present. If, for example, a tumor creates a stricture and the defect is elliptical rather than circumferential, the balloon will expand within the normal segment of tissue and incompletely dilate the tumor. This action may create a perforation in small tubular structures such as the bile duct or pancreatic duct if a large (8 mm or 10 mm) balloon is used. However, whether or not it is fortunate, strictures involving the pancreaticobiliary tree, unlike those of the esophagus or other intestinal luminal strictures, are generally circumferential and di-

TABLE 13.2. *Endoscopic hydrostatic dilation (EHD): Results*

Biliary tree: improved	119 (78%)
Pancreatic ducts: improved	28 (68%)

TABLE 13.4. *Hydrostatic dilating balloon*

Radial force
Evenly applied
Safety
Fixed diameter
Low compliance
Overinflation—balloon rupture

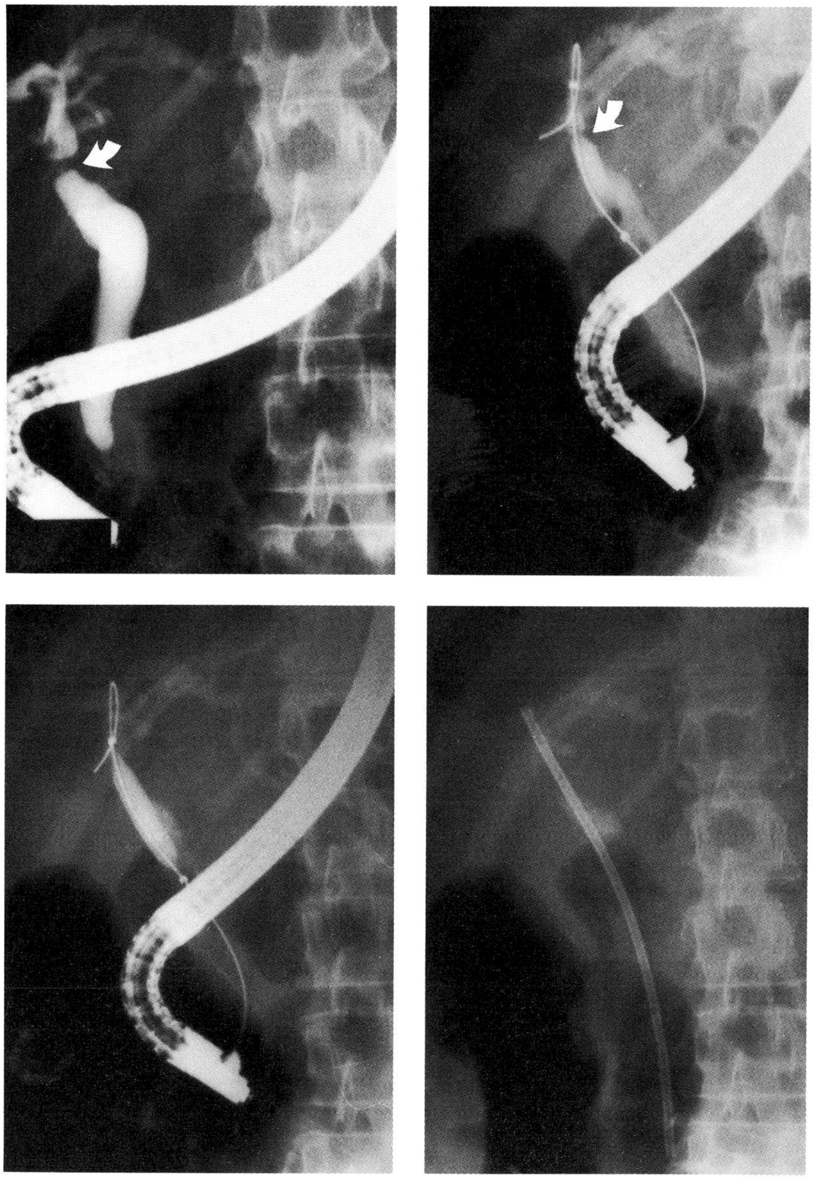

FIG. 13.3. Top left: A stricture in the common hepatic duct (*arrow*). **Top right:** A balloon catheter has been advanced over the guidewire into the stricture, and inflation with contrast material is beginning. Note the waist on the balloon in the stricture (*arrow*). **Bottom left:** The balloon is fully inflated. **Bottom right:** A stent has been placed through the stricture to maintain the integrity of the duct lumen.

late evenly with a balloon. Because these balloons have a fixed diameter and polyethylene is a low-compliance material, perforation of the duct is unlikely and has not occurred in our extensive experience. In fact, the balloon usually ruptures, commonly at its seal, before the duct perforates, which again emphasizes the safety features of balloons.

Figures 13.1 through 13.44 illustrate the technique of balloon dilatation of the pancreaticobiliary duct systems. Each figure is accompanied by a description of the procedure and should be clear to the reader. These are examples of balloon dilatation performed in patients with bile duct strictures (benign and malignant), including strictures secondary to arterial perfusion with chemotherapeutic agents and pancreatic strictures present in idiopathic pancreatitis and pancreas divisum.

As a prerequisite essential to the safe performance of therapeutic procedures, the endoscopist and his or her assistants must be completely familiar with all the available endoscopic accessories and their functions before embarking on these potentially dangerous procedures. Familiarity, preparation, and experience prevent misadventure.

(*References for this chapter follow on page 395*).

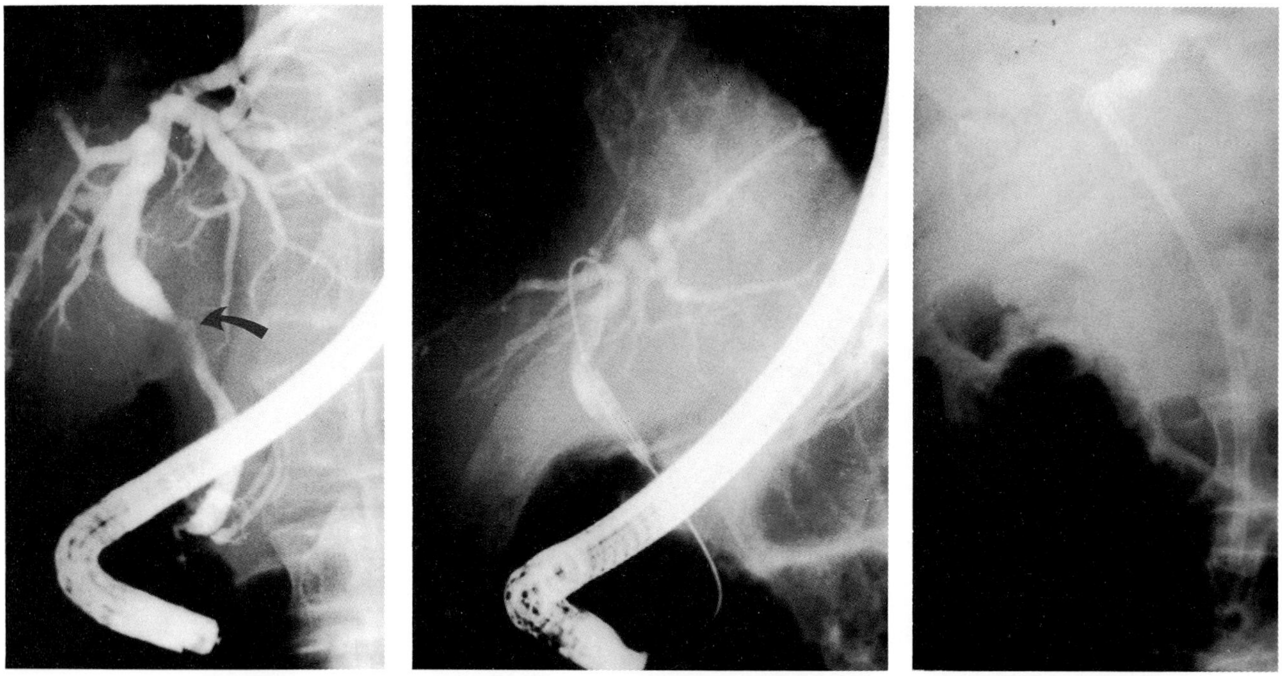

FIG. 13.4. Left: A high-grade stricture is shown in the mid common bile duct (*arrow*). **Middle:** The balloon catheter is dilated to maximum diameter in the stricture. **Right:** A large-caliber prosthesis is placed through the stricture to maintain the integrity of the lumen.

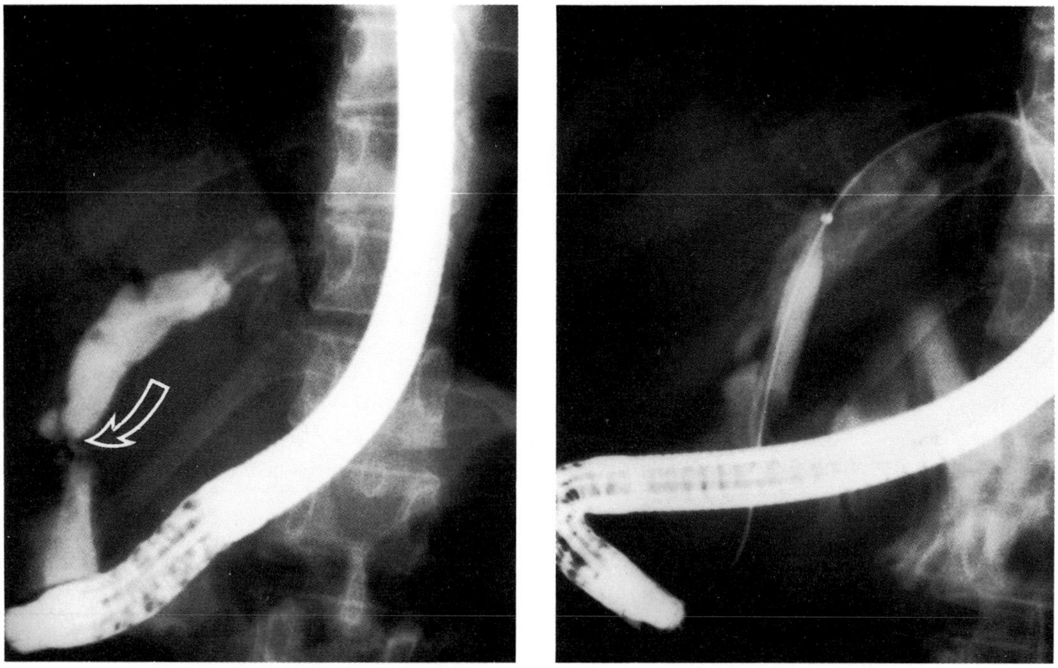

FIG. 13.5. Left: A stricture in the distal third of the bile duct (*arrow*). **Right:** An 8 mm balloon is inflated in the stricture to dilate it.

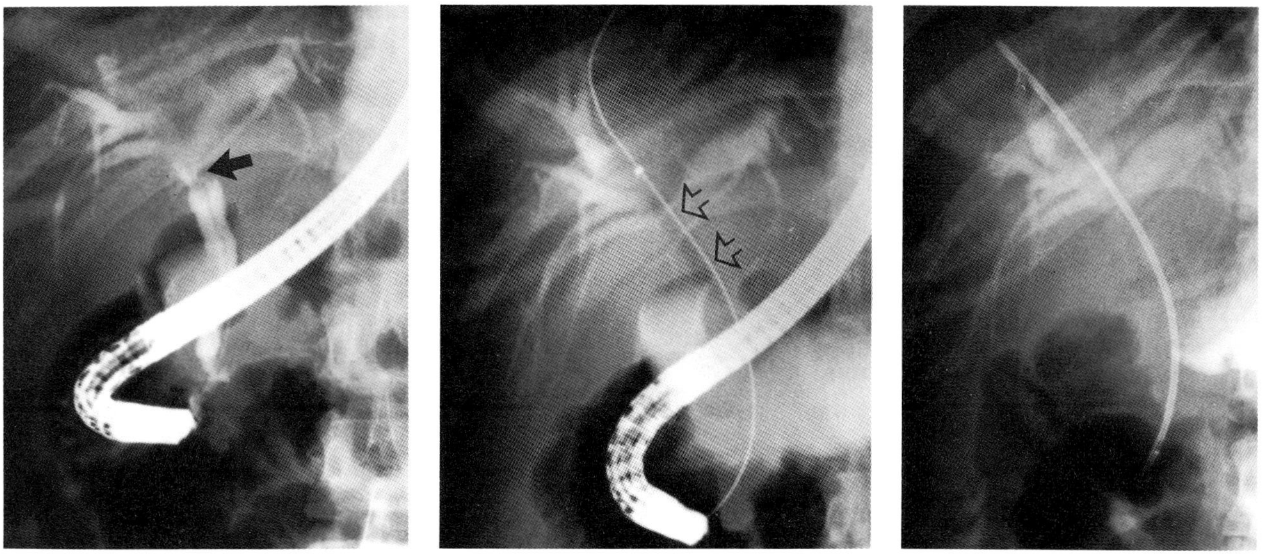

FIG. 13.6. Left: A high-grade stricture of the common hepatic duct (*arrow*). **Middle:** A balloon catheter has been inserted into the stricture and inflated with air (*arrows*). **Right:** After dilation of the stricture, a prosthesis is placed to maintain the integrity of the lumen.

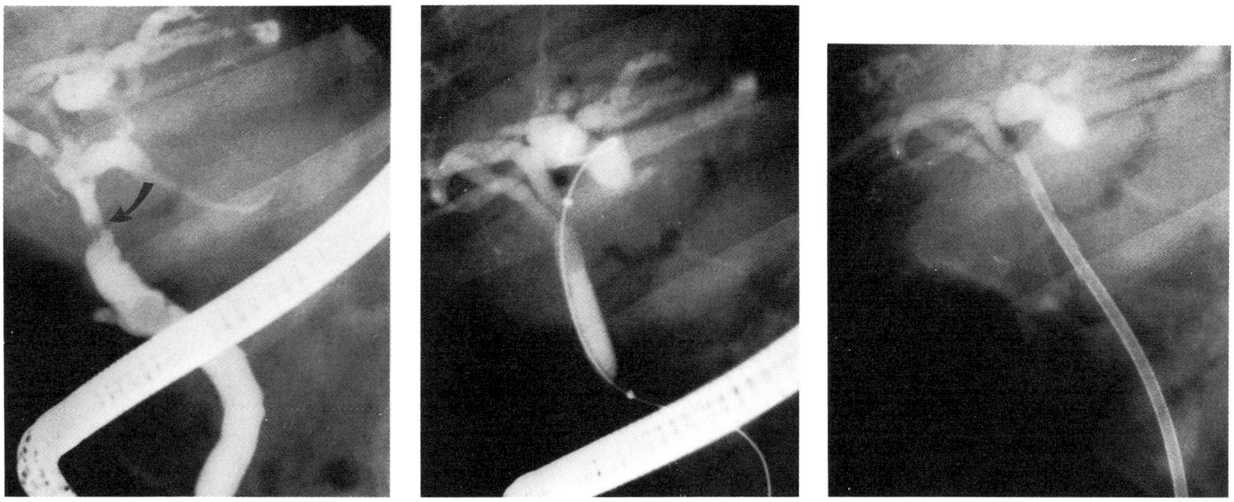

FIG. 13.7. Left: A high-grade stricture of the common hepatic duct (*arrow*). **Middle:** An 8 mm balloon is inflated with contrast to dilate the stricture. **Right:** A large-caliber prosthesis has been placed into the stricture to maintain the integrity of the lumen.

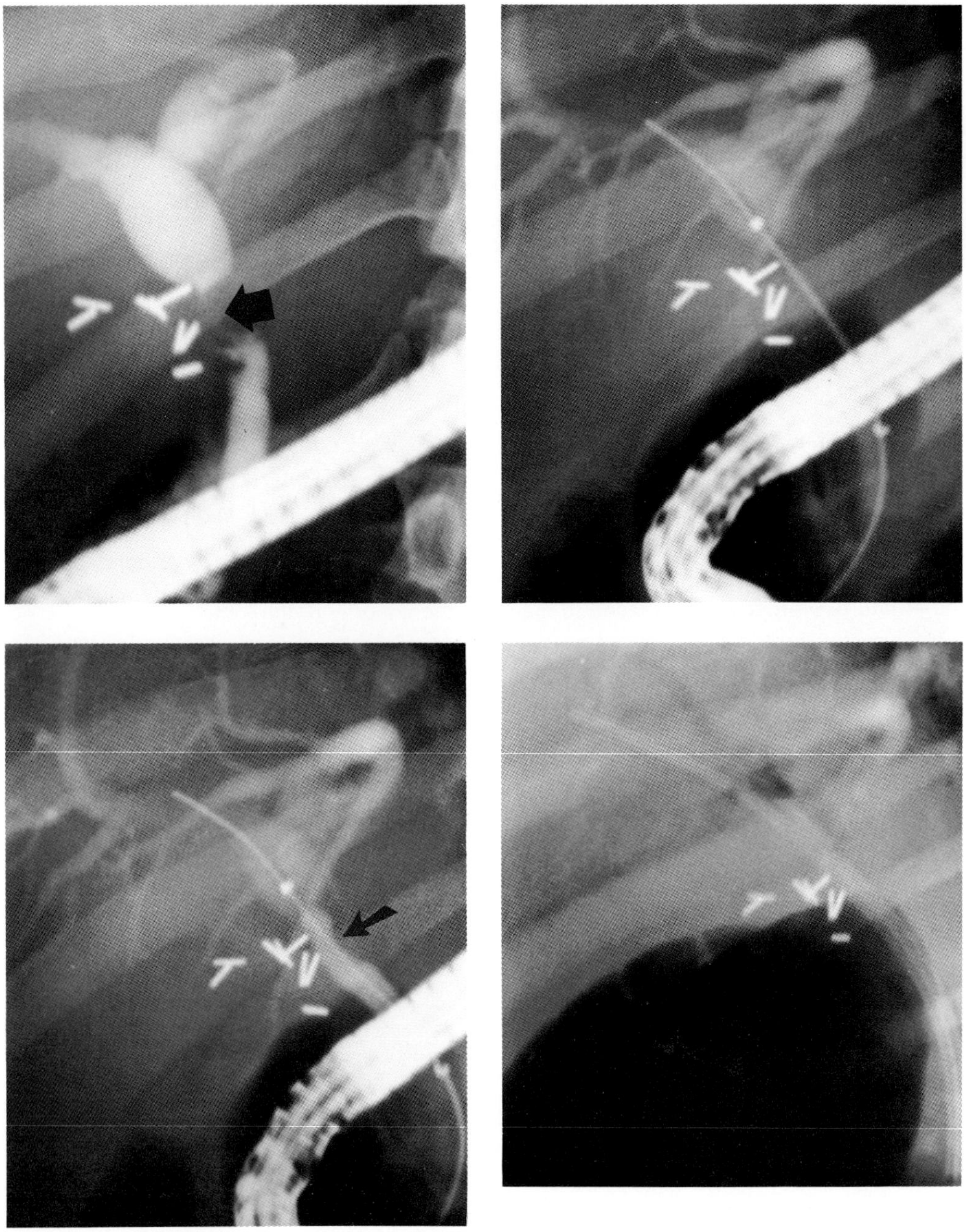

FIG. 13.8. Top left: A high-grade postoperative stricture of the common hepatic duct (*arrow*). **Top right:** A guidewire has been inserted through the stricture, and a balloon catheter has been advanced over the wire into the stricture. **Bottom left:** The balloon is shown being inflated. Note the indentation created on the balloon wall (*arrow*) as it is inflated with contrast material. **Bottom right:** Two prostheses have been placed into the stricture to maintain the integrity of the lumen.

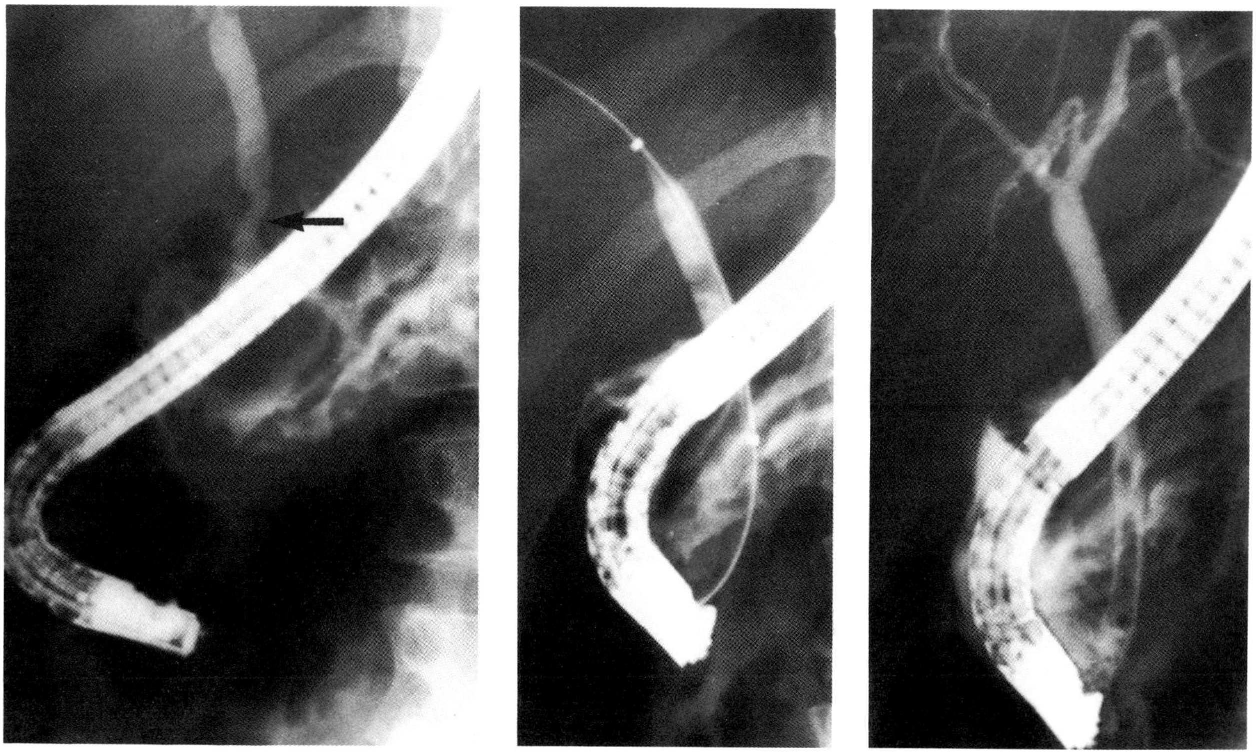

FIG. 13.9. Left: In this sequence, a stricture is demonstrated in the distal common bile duct (*arrow*). **Middle:** An 8 mm balloon is inflated with contrast. **Right:** The stricture has been completely dilated as evidenced by the appearance of the bile duct after removal of the balloon.

Dilalation of clipped duct

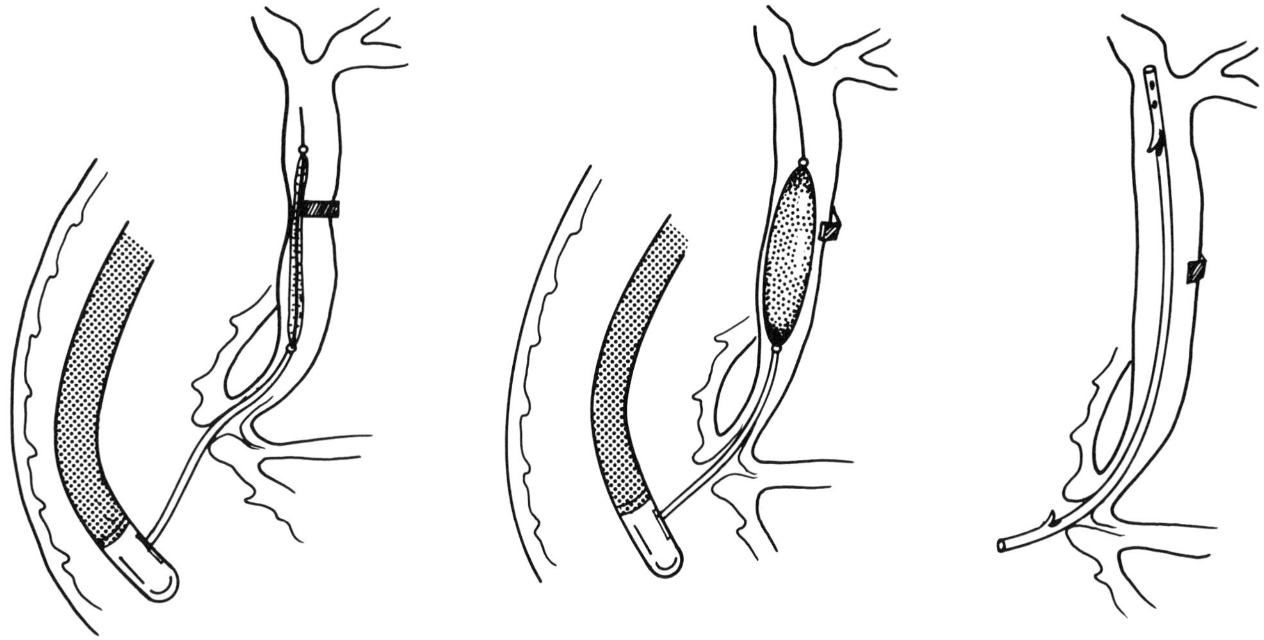

FIG. 13.10. Left: The formation of a stricture secondary to an inflammatory reaction caused by the placement of staples used during surgery for the removal of a long cystic duct remnant. **Middle:** A balloon has been successfully used to dilate the inflammatory stricture. **Right:** A prosthesis has been inserted.

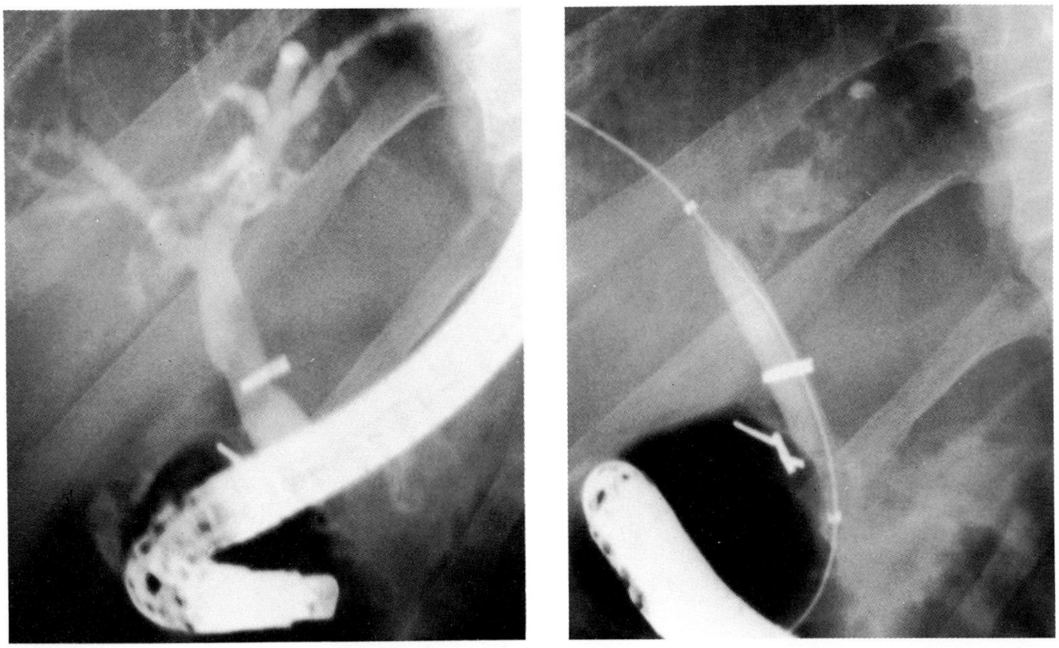

FIG. 13.11. Left: A bile duct stricture secondary to an inflammatory reaction from staples. **Right:** A balloon catheter is shown dilating the stricture.

FIG. 13.12. A: Top left: A high-grade stricture (*arrows*) is shown affecting the common hepatic duct. Note the close proximity of the metal staples. **Top right:** A guidewire has been placed through the stricture, and a balloon catheter is advanced into the stricture. **Bottom left:** The balloon has been fully inflated in the stricture, effectively dilating it. **Bottom right:** A large-caliber prosthesis has been placed to maintain the integrity of the lumen. **B: Left to Right:** A bile duct stricture near surgical clips; A balloon catheter being inserted; The balloon is fully inflated in the stricture, dilating it; A prosthesis is placed after the dilatation procedure.

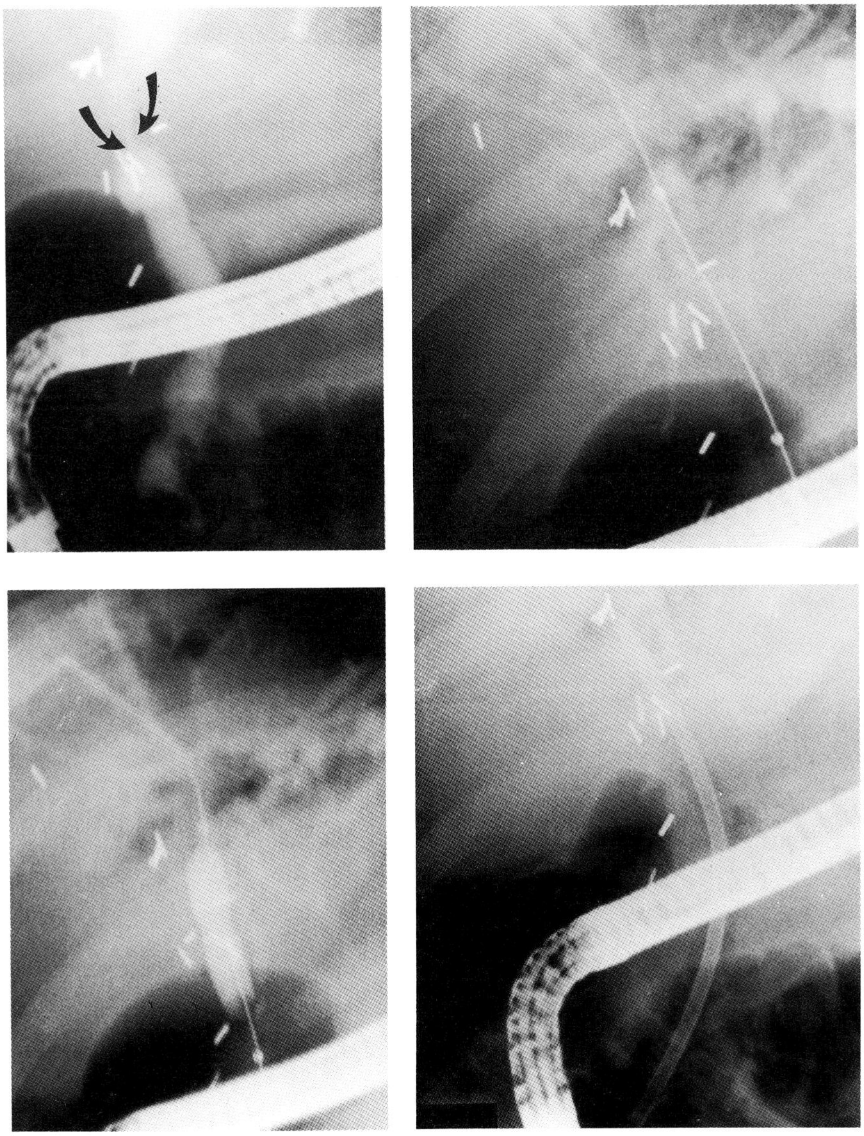

A

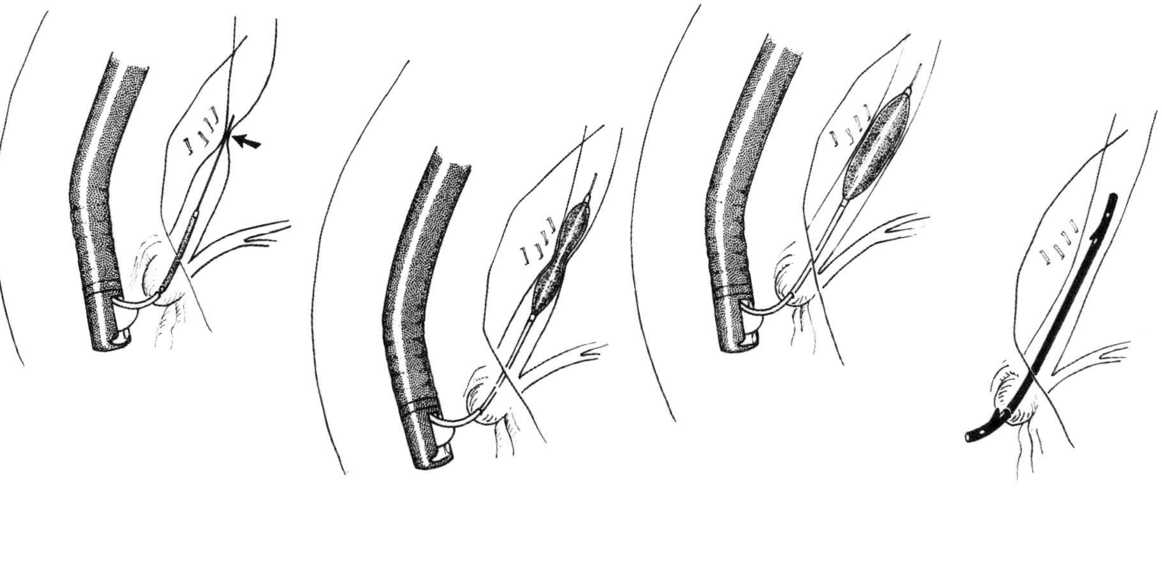

B

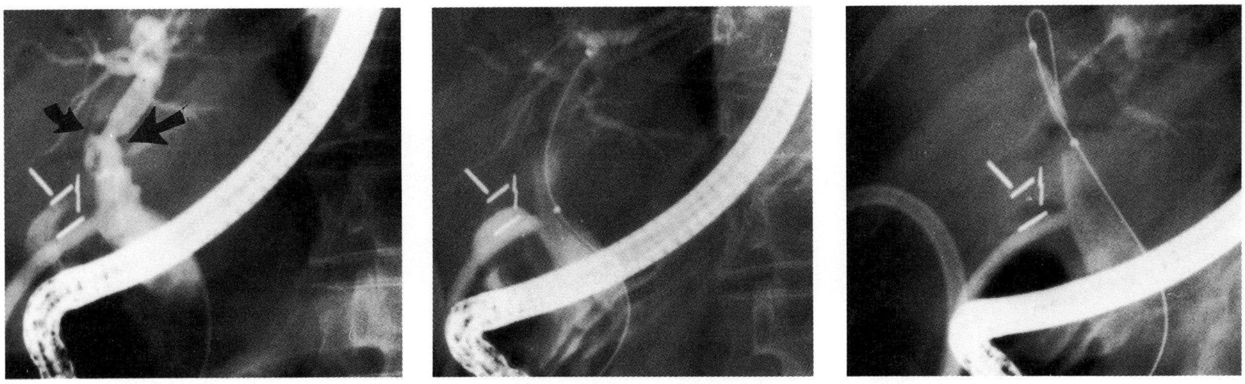

FIG. 13.13. Left: A stricture affecting the common hepatic duct at its bifurcation. A T-tube is in place, but filling of the right hepatic system is not complete (*arrows*). **Middle:** A balloon catheter is visible in the left hepatic duct. **Right:** A balloon catheter has also been placed into the right hepatic duct and inflated at the origin of the stricture.

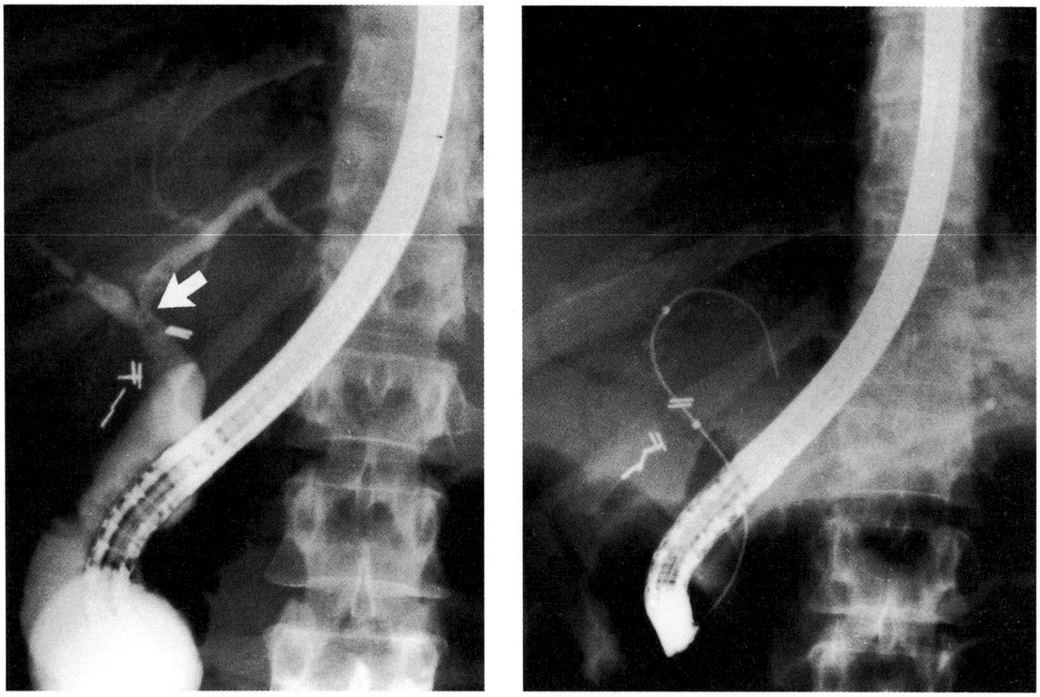

FIG. 13.14. Left: A stricture affecting the left hepatic duct at its origin (*arrow*). **Right:** A balloon catheter is selectively passed into the left hepatic duct.

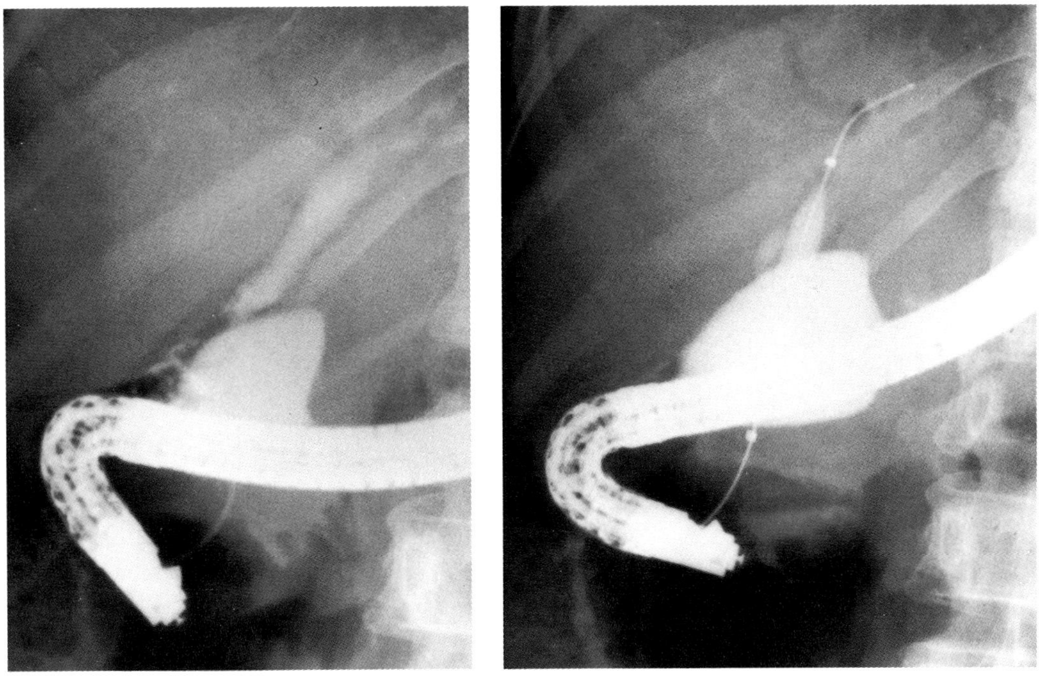

FIG. 13.15. Left: This radiograph shows a stricture formed at the anastomosis of a choledochoduodenostomy. The distal common bile duct has been cannulated through the papilla. **Right:** A large-caliber balloon is placed into the stricture and inflated. The collection of contrast in the duodenum, which is seen in both radiographs, resulted from reflux of contrast through the enterostomy stoma.

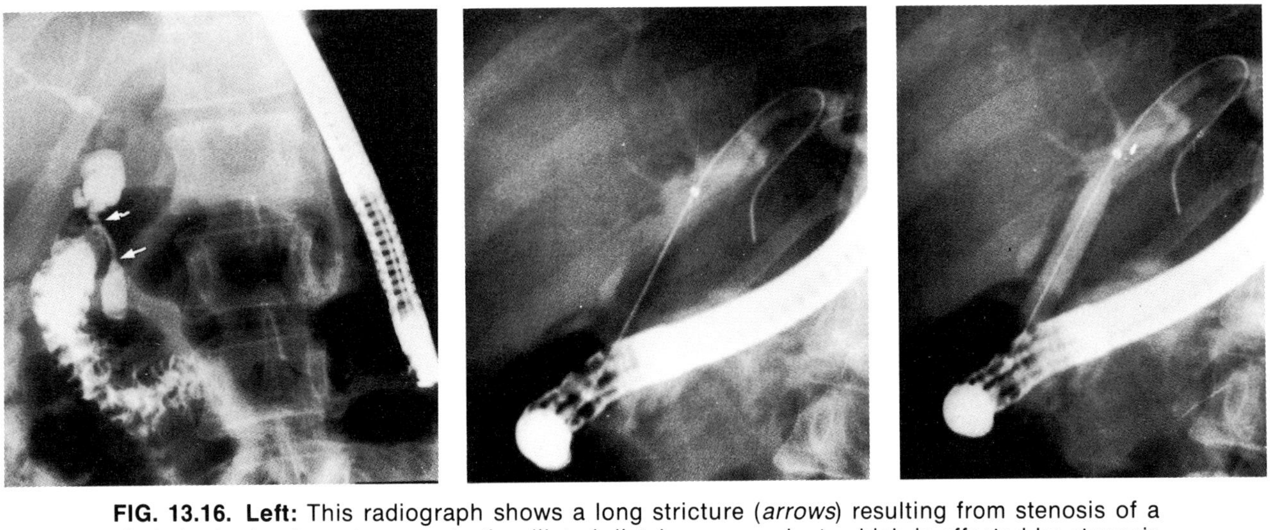

FIG. 13.16. Left: This radiograph shows a long stricture (*arrows*) resulting from stenosis of a choledochoduodenostomy; note the dilated distal common duct, which is affected by stenosis of the papilla. **Middle:** A guidewire has been advanced through the enterostomy, and a balloon has been passed over the wire. **Right:** The balloon is inflated to the maximum, 8 mm. (From ref. 2, with permission.)

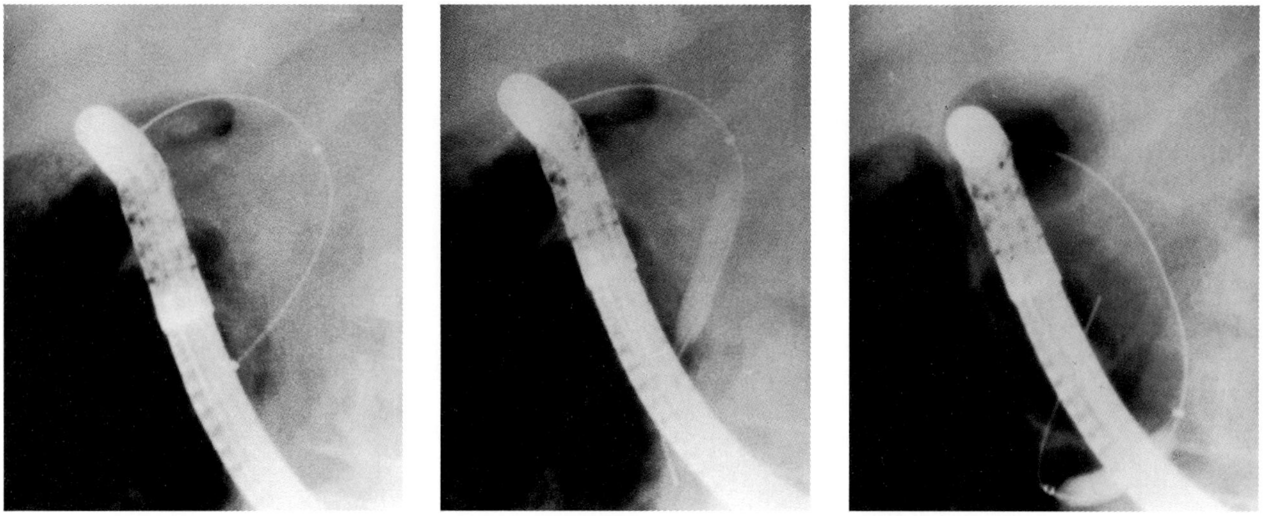

FIG. 13.17. The dilatation procedure of the distal common bile duct stricture and papilla shown in Fig. 13.16. **Left:** The guidewire is passed through the enterostomy, the distal common duct, and the papilla into the duodenum. **Middle:** The balloon is inflated in the distal bile duct. **Right:** The balloon is dilated in the papilla.

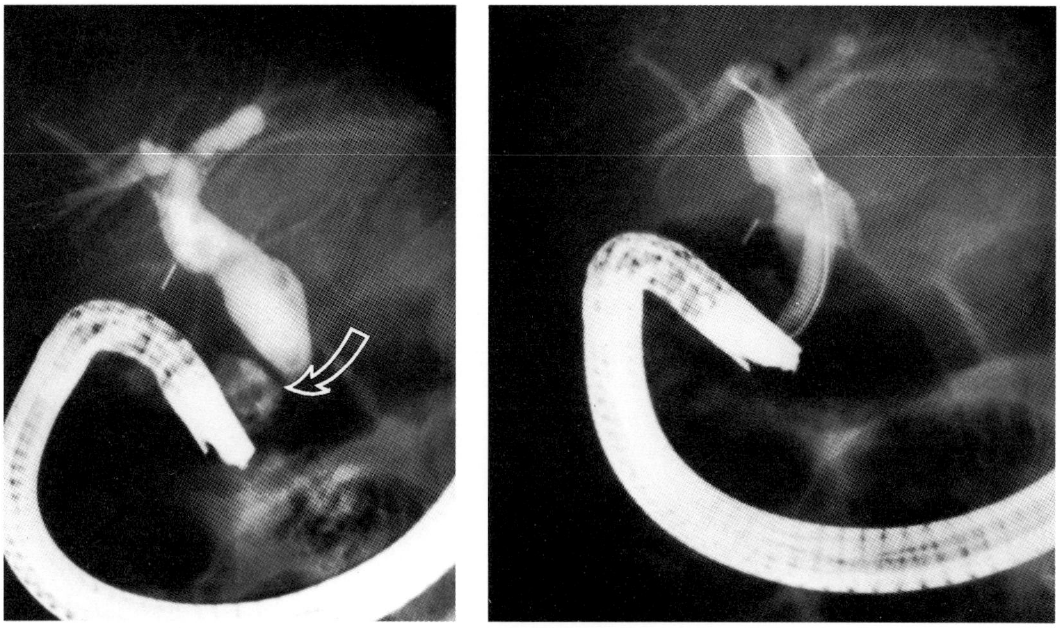

FIG. 13.18. Left: An anastomotic stricture (*arrow*) that occurred following a choledochoduodenostomy. **Right:** An 8 mm balloon is inflated in the anastomotic stricture.

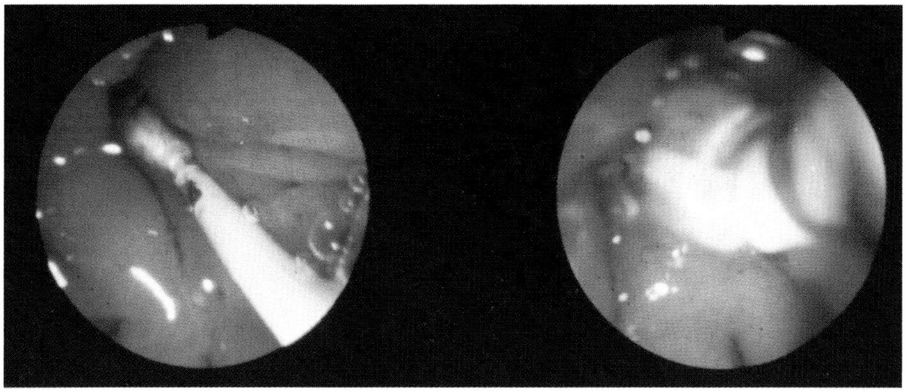

FIG. 13.19. Left: This endoscopic picture shows a prototype balloon catheter (Microvasive) being inserted into the stenotic biliary-enteric anastomosis. **Right:** The balloon being inflated.

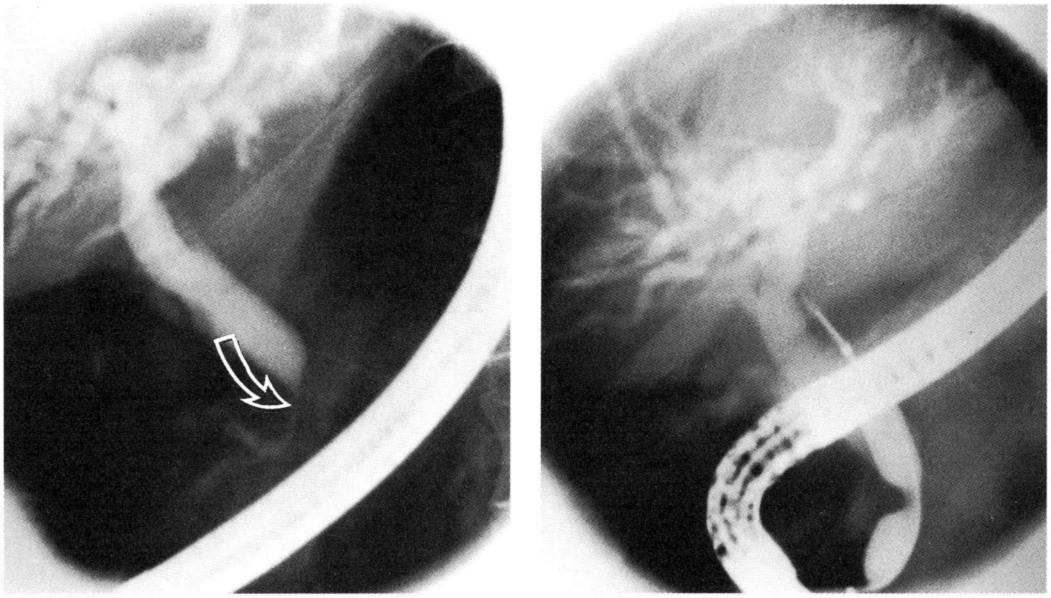

FIG. 13.20. Left: This distal common bile duct stricture (*arrow*) occurred following surgery for chronic pancreatitis. **Right:** A 10 mm balloon is being dilated in this very tight stricture. The balloon could not dilate the stricture more than 5 mm. The waist on the balloon is located within the stricture.

A

B

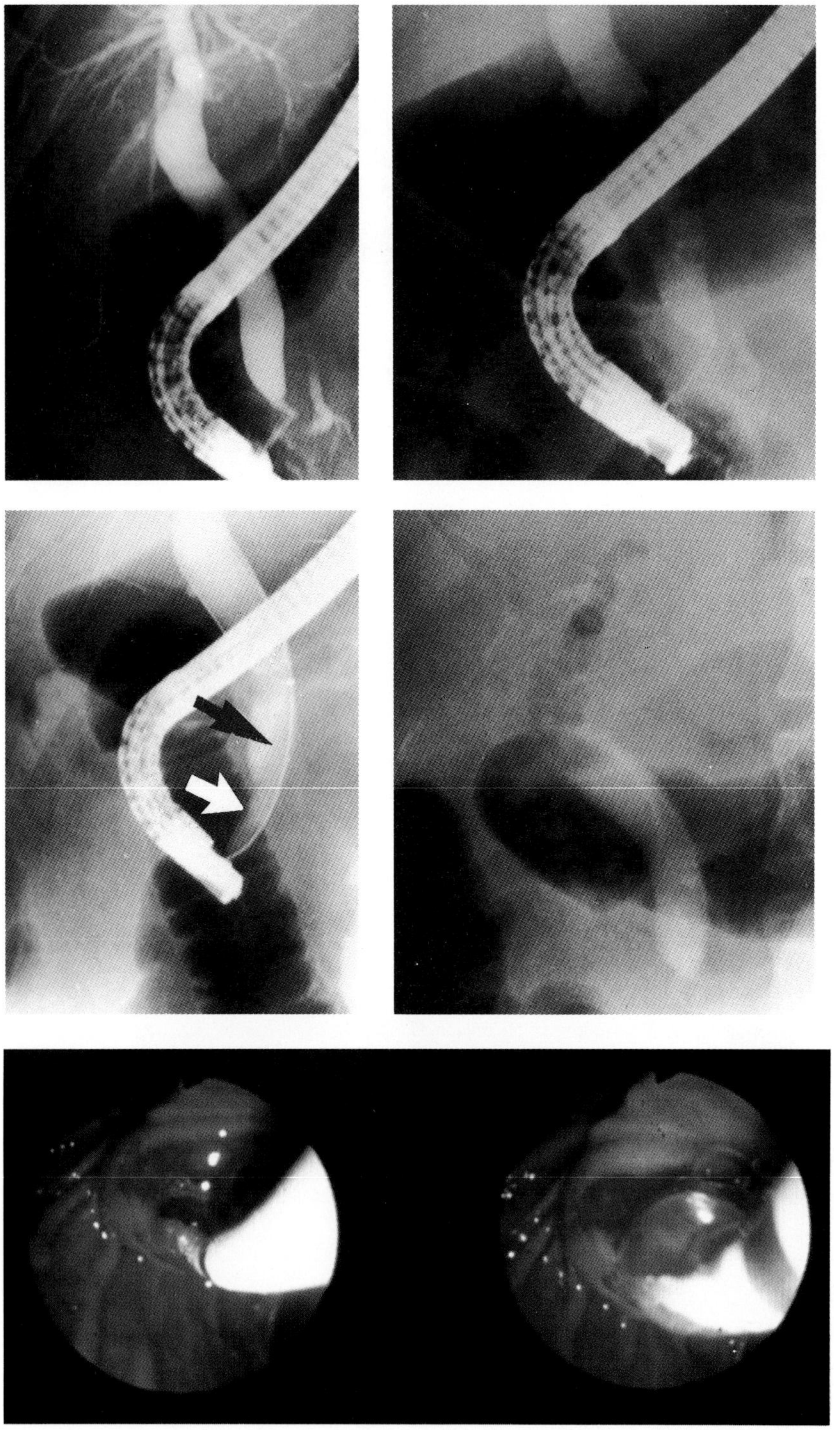

FIG. 13.21. A: Top left: A diagnosis of papillary stenosis was confirmed on this cholangiogram. **Top right:** A catheter-guidewire assembly is being passed into the bile duct through the stricture. **Bottom left:** An 8 mm balloon is being inflated in the stricture (*arrows*), dilating it. **Bottom right:** The bile duct is draining spontaneously after dilatation. Note the air in the biliary tree after the dilatation, indicating that the sphincter was successfully dilated, ostensibly creating a sphincterotomy. **B: Left:** A balloon catheter being inserted into the papilla before dilatation. **Right:** The balloon being inflated.

FIG. 13.23. Top left: Note the stricture in the mid common bile duct (*arrow*) in a patient who has previously undergone a cholecystectomy and who presented with fever, chills, and jaundice. **Top right:** A guidewire and balloon catheter have been advanced through the stricture. **Bottom left:** The balloon is being inflated with contrast material. **Bottom right:** The dilating balloon is used to inject contrast after dilating the stricture (note radiopaque marking superior to the endoscope). No evidence of the stricture remains.

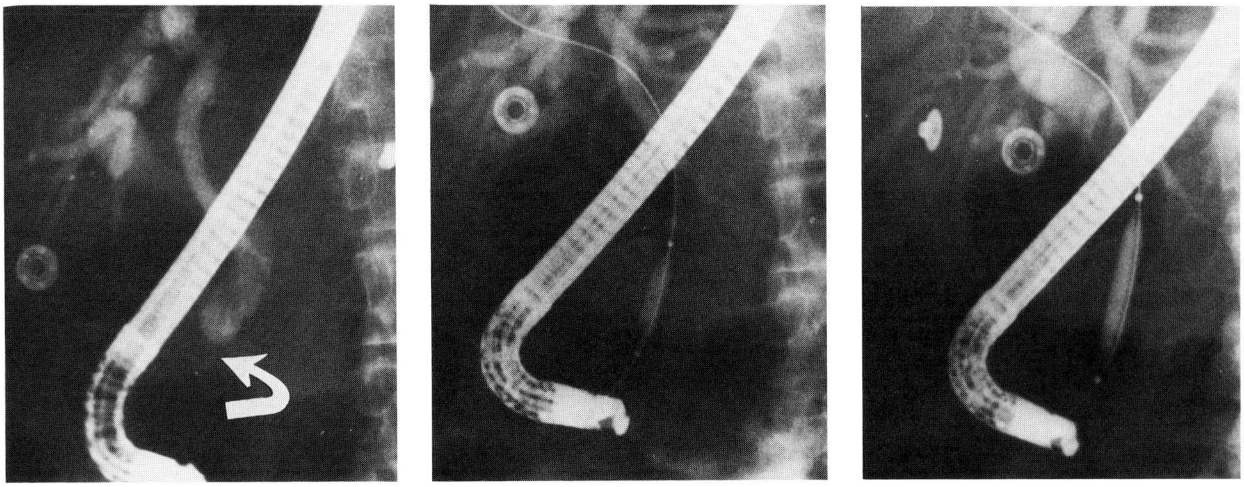

FIG. 13.22. Left: This radiograph confirms the presence of papillary stenosis as illustrated by the rounded and blunted distal common bile duct. Note that the stenotic segment extends beyond the duodenal wall (*arrow*). Therefore, sphincterotomy is not a consideration because perforation would likely occur. Balloon dilatation of the involved area, however, is plausible. **Middle:** A 6 mm balloon being inflated in the stricture. **Right:** An 8 mm balloon being inflated in the stricture to provide the maximum safe dilatation.

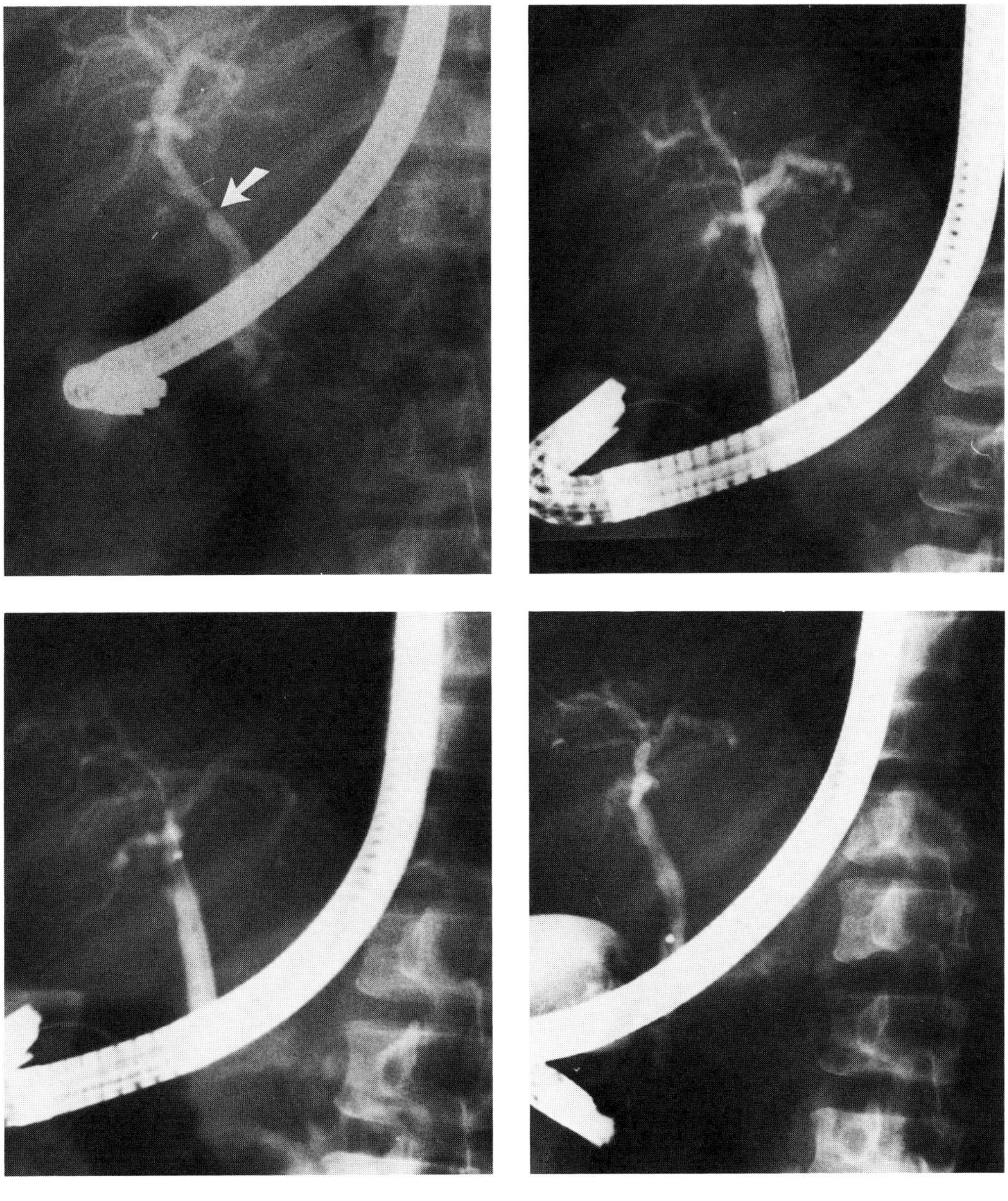

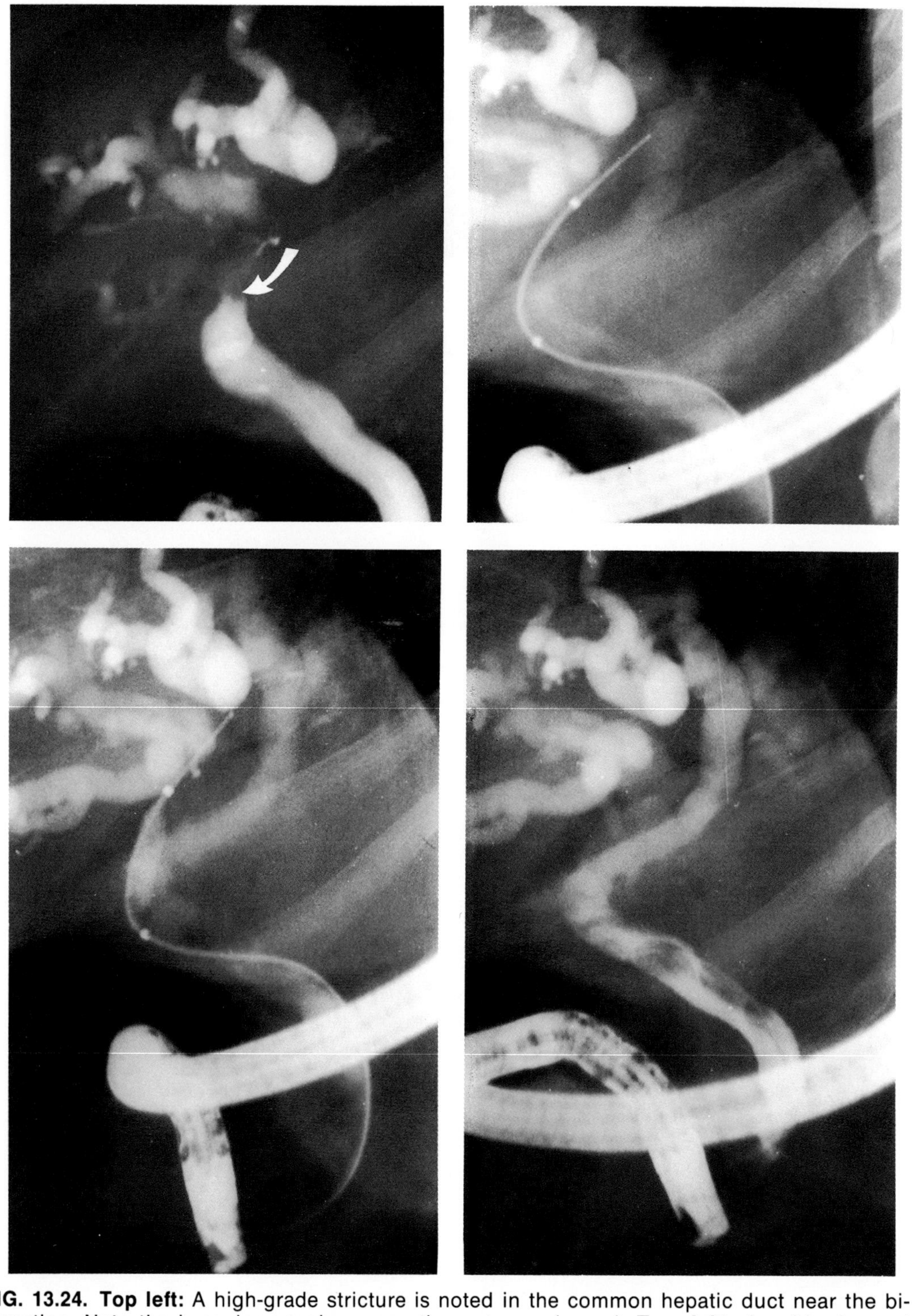

FIG. 13.24. Top left: A high-grade stricture is noted in the common hepatic duct near the bifurcation. Note the irregular margin, suggesting a tumor (*arrow*). **Top right:** A guidewire and balloon catheter are advanced into the left hepatic duct (note radiopaque markers of balloon). **Bottom left:** The balloon is inflated within the stricture. **Bottom right:** Complete recanalization of the duct is shown on this cholangiogram. The lucencies in the common bile duct are probably blood clots. (From ref. 6, with permission.)

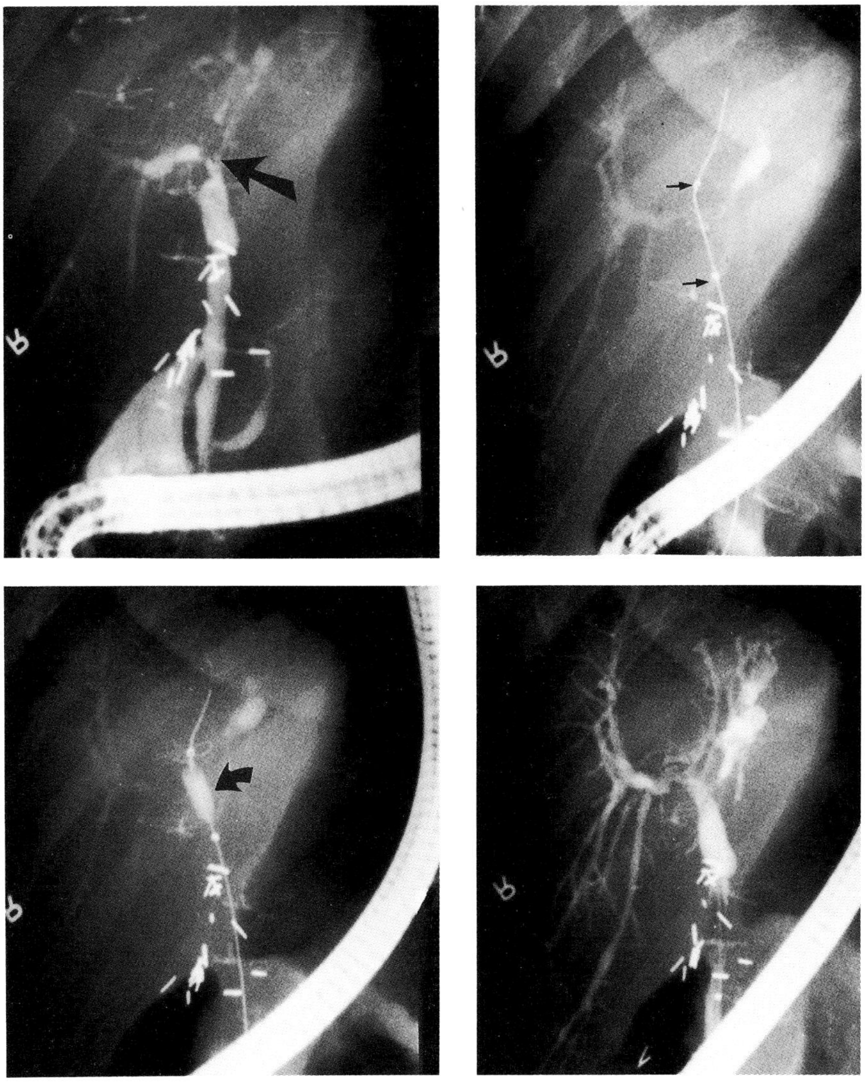

FIG. 13.25. Top left: This radiograph illustrating sclerosing cholangitis demonstrates severe intrahepatic changes and a dominant stricture at the bifurcation (*arrow*). **Top right:** A guidewire is visible in the left hepatic duct, and the balloon catheter has been placed in the stricture. The radiopaque markers of the balloon are identified by the arrows. **Bottom left:** A 6 mm balloon is being inflated with contrast medium (*arrow*). **Bottom right:** This postdilatation cholangiogram shows greater filling of both hepatic ducts, resulting from effective dilatation.

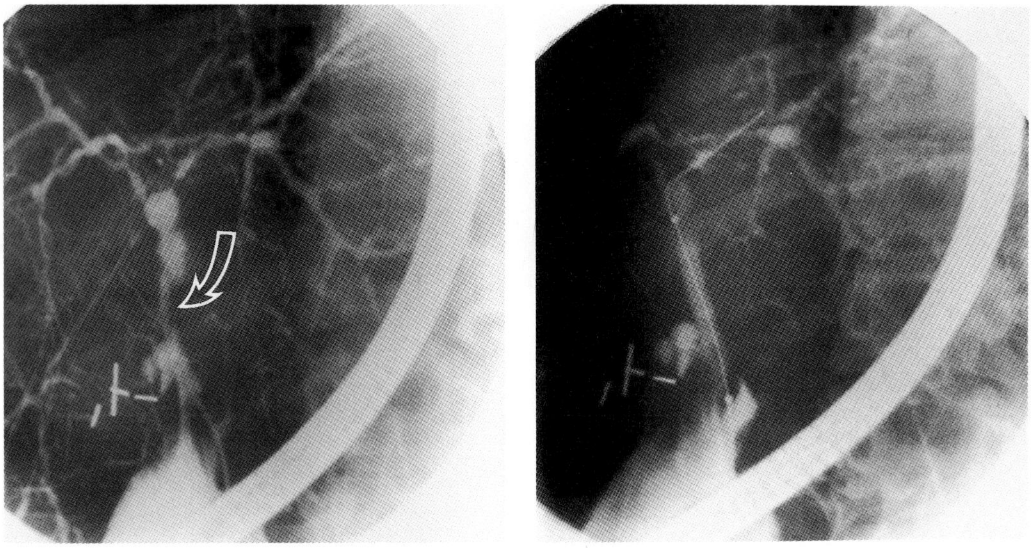

FIG. 13.26. **Left:** The characteristic findings of sclerosing cholangitis with stricturing more apparent at the mid common bile duct (*arrow*). **Right:** A 6 mm balloon is being inflated within the stricture.

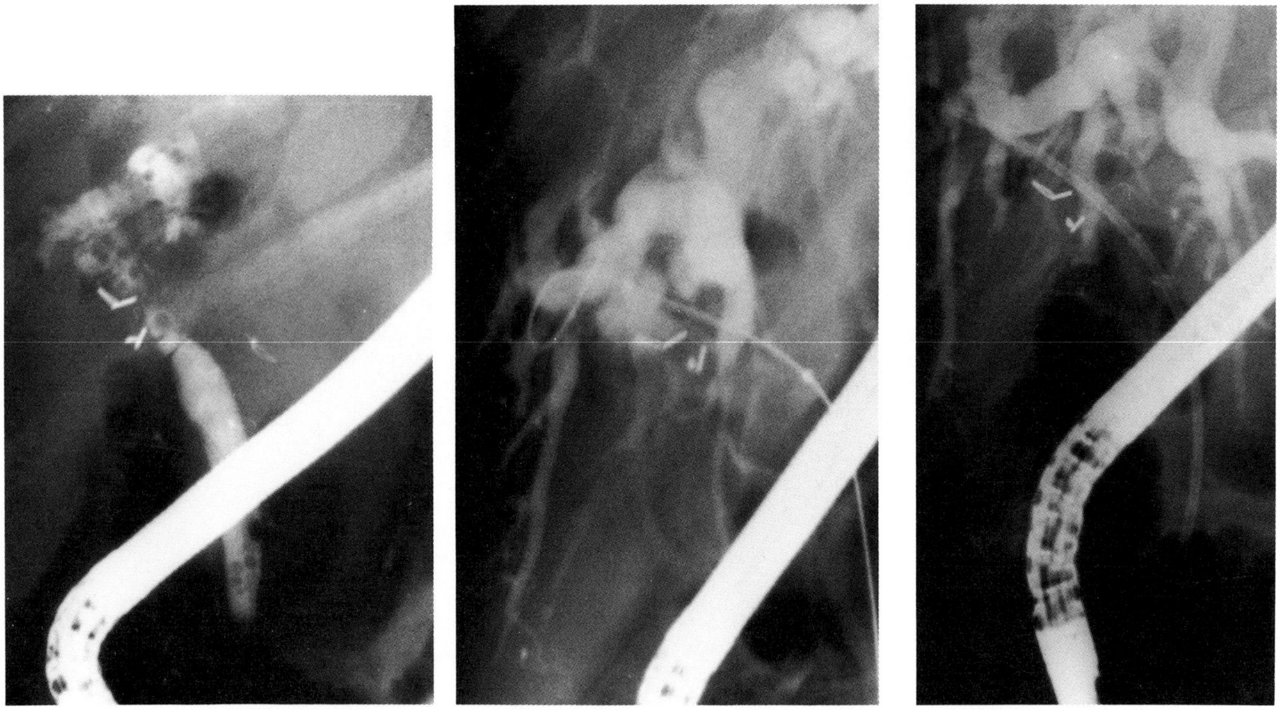

FIG. 13.27. **Left:** A dominant stricture of sclerosing cholangitis at the porta hepatis. Only a small amount of contrast entered the intrahepatic ducts. **Middle:** A balloon catheter has been placed through the stricture, and the balloon is filled with air instead of contrast. The intrahepatic ducts were opacified after using an occlusion balloon. **Right:** A medium-sized prosthesis has been placed through the stricture. Note filling of the intrahepatic ducts, which was accomplished after placing a dilating catheter through the stricture and injecting contrast medium.

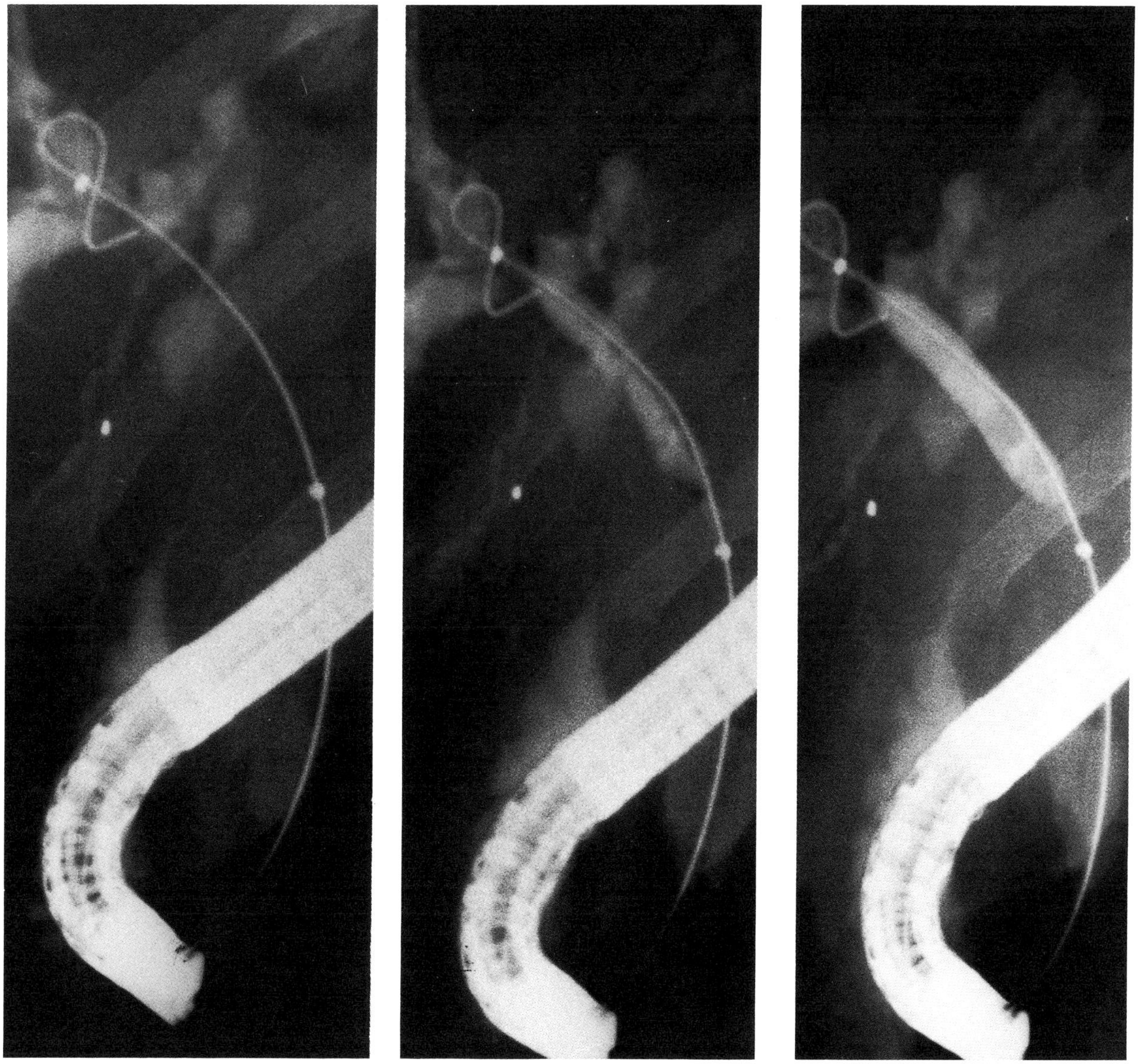

FIG. 13.28. Left: This series of radiographs demonstrates the technique of placing a guidewire and balloon catheter. **Middle:** Partial inflation of an 8 mm balloon in a dominant stricture. **Right:** Complete inflation of the balloon.

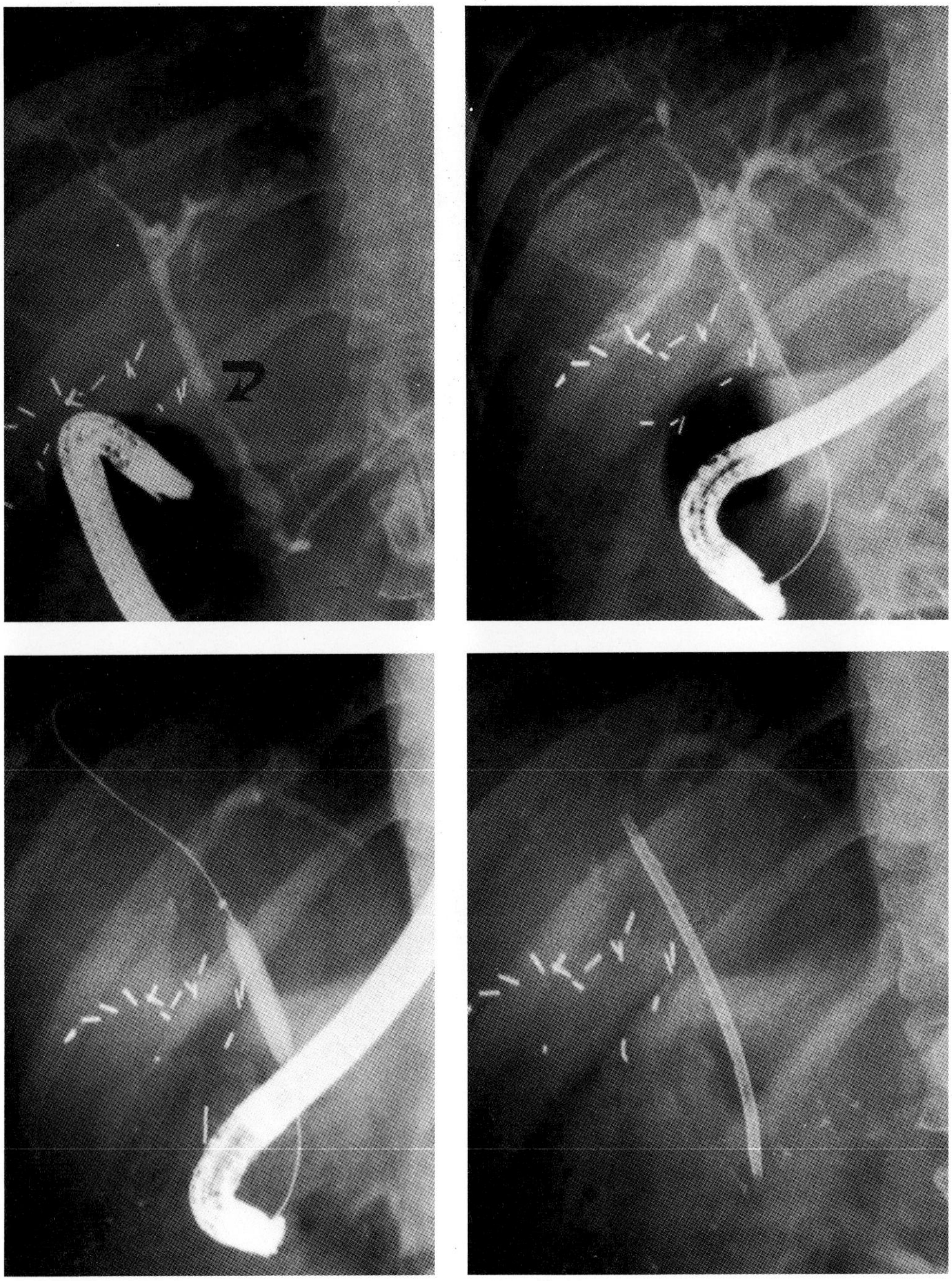

FIG. 13.29. Top left: A dominant stricture (*arrow*) is shown in the distal common bile duct in this patient with diffuse changes of sclerosing cholangitis. **Top right:** A small balloon is inflated in the bile duct stricture. **Bottom left:** A larger balloon is shown fully inflated. **Bottom right:** A large-caliber prosthesis is shown inserted into the bile duct. (From ref. 22, with permission.)

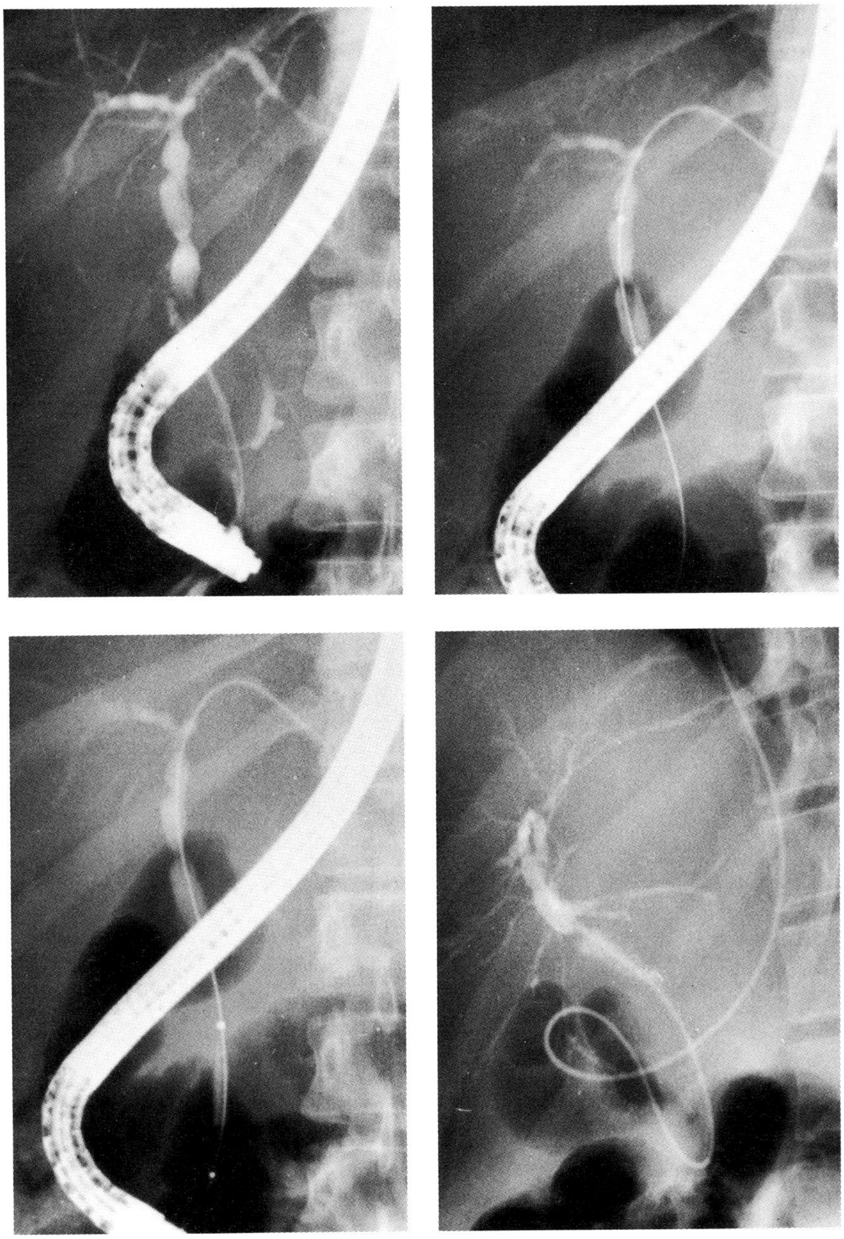

FIG. 13.30. Top left: A dominant stricture is visible in the mid common and distal common bile duct in this patient with sclerosing cholangitis. **Top right:** A balloon is inflated in the mid common bile duct. **Bottom left:** The balloon is being inflated in the distal common bile duct stricture. **Bottom right:** A nasobiliary tube has been placed for perfusion therapy. (From ref. 22, with permission.)

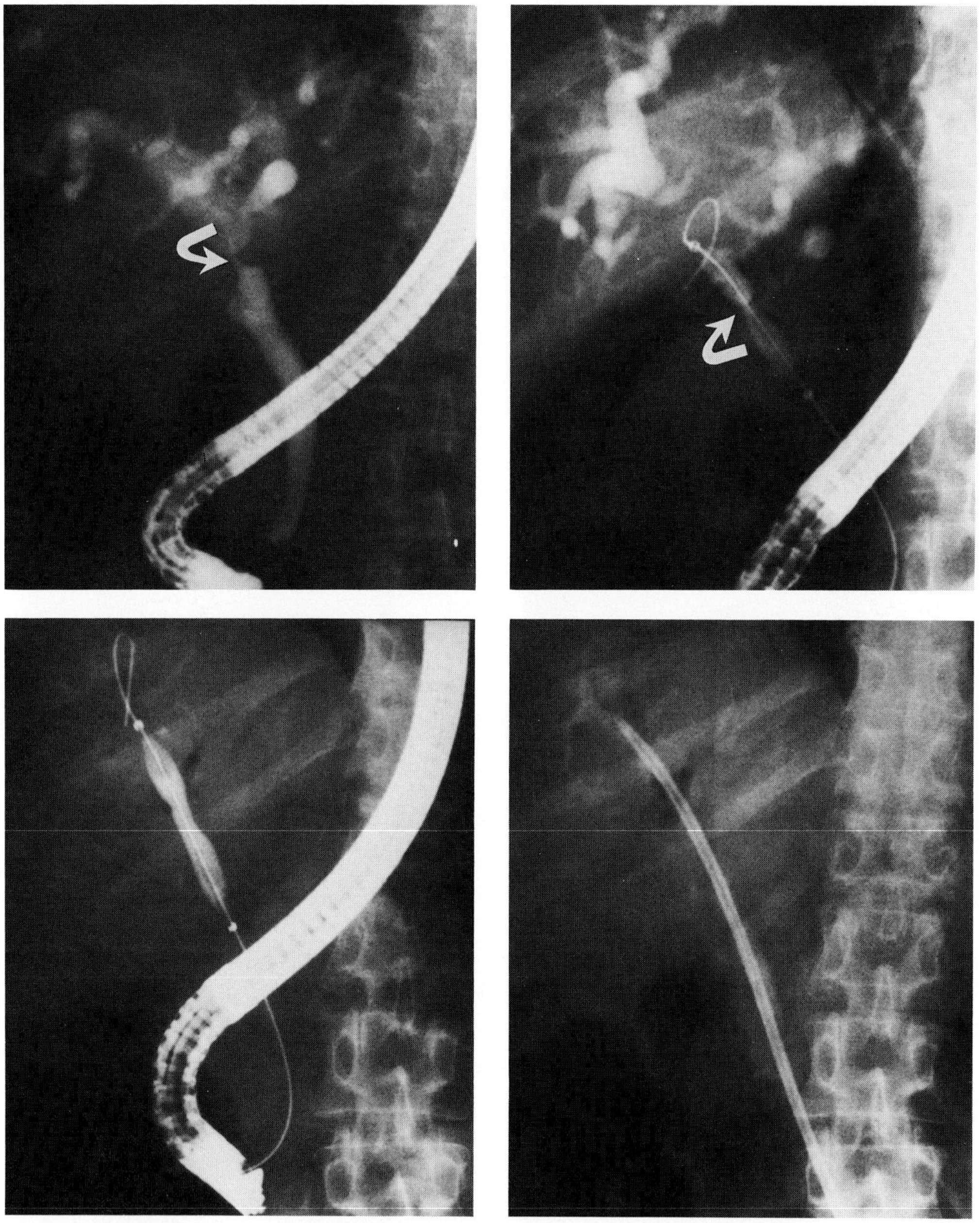

FIG. 13.31. Top left: This cholangiogram demonstrates a high-grade stricture at the porta hepatis (*arrow*). **Top right:** A balloon catheter is placed into the stricture, and the balloon is being inflated. Note the waist (*arrow*) on the balloon created by the stricture. **Bottom left:** The 6 mm balloon is nearly completely distended, dilating the stricture. **Bottom right:** A large-caliber prosthesis has been placed through the stricture to maintain the integrity of the lumen.

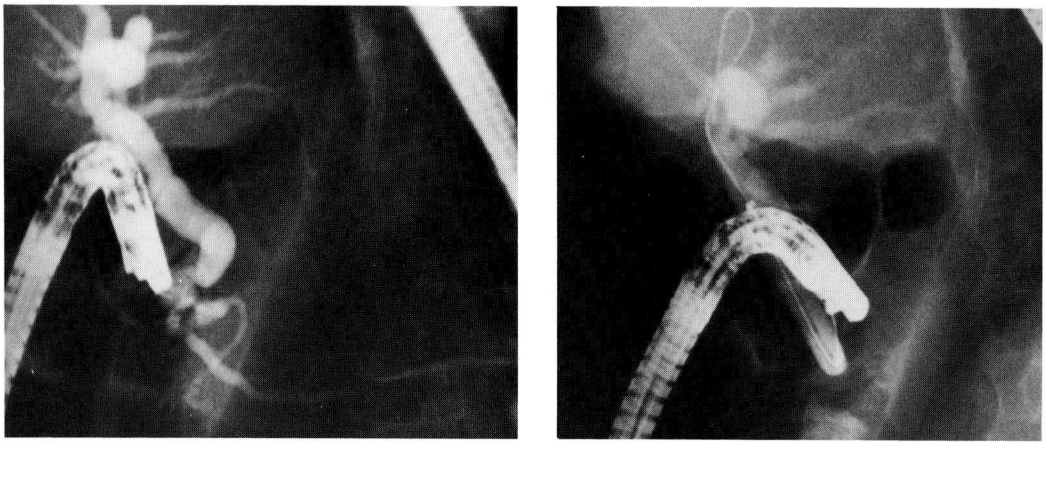

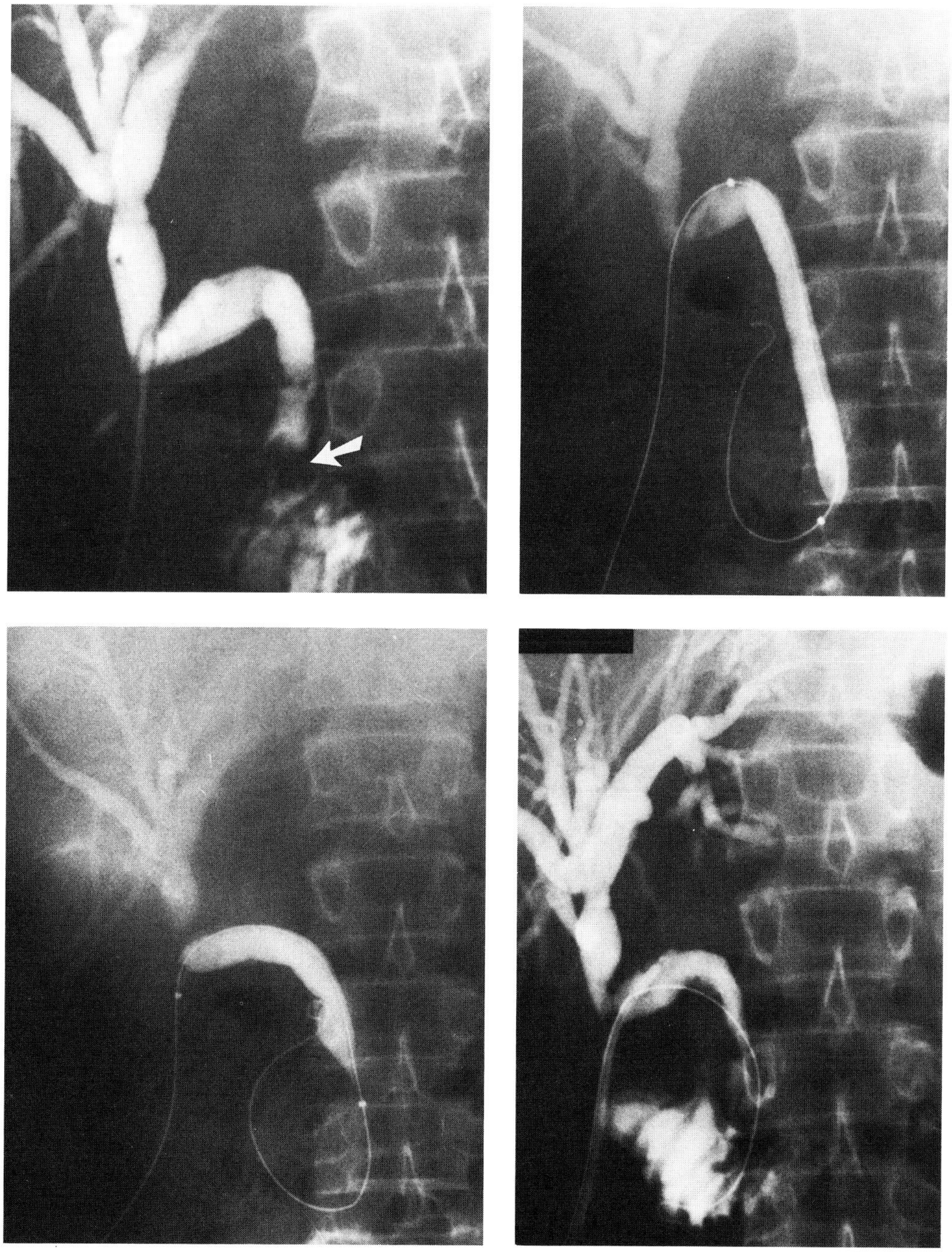

FIG. 13.33. This series of radiographs demonstrates a percutaneous approach to the management of a retained stone and distal bile duct stricture in a patient who had previously undergone a hemigastrectomy. **Top left:** This radiograph, obtained through a T-tube, shows a lucency in the distal common bile duct (*arrow*). **Top right:** With the T-tube tract, a large balloon catheter is advanced over the guidewire; the balloon is fully distended, dilating the stricture. **Bottom left:** A large balloon is being utilized, dilating the stricture and papilla to 1.5 cm. **Bottom right:** A repeat cholangiogram demonstrates free flow of contrast into the duodenum. No stone is visible in this picture, and the bile duct is less distended now that obstruction to flow has been relieved.

FIG. 13.32. Left: A stricture of the distal common bile duct is visible on this ERCP in a patient with pancreas divisum. **Right:** With a large-caliber endoscope, a 1 cm balloon is used to dilate the area of stenosis. Note that in order to place a 1 cm balloon on this catheter, the length of the balloon was also extended to more than 3 cm. This length is acceptable for a distal stricture, but it is not appropriate for a proximal stricture because part of the balloon would have to be placed into either hepatic duct, which could induce injury.

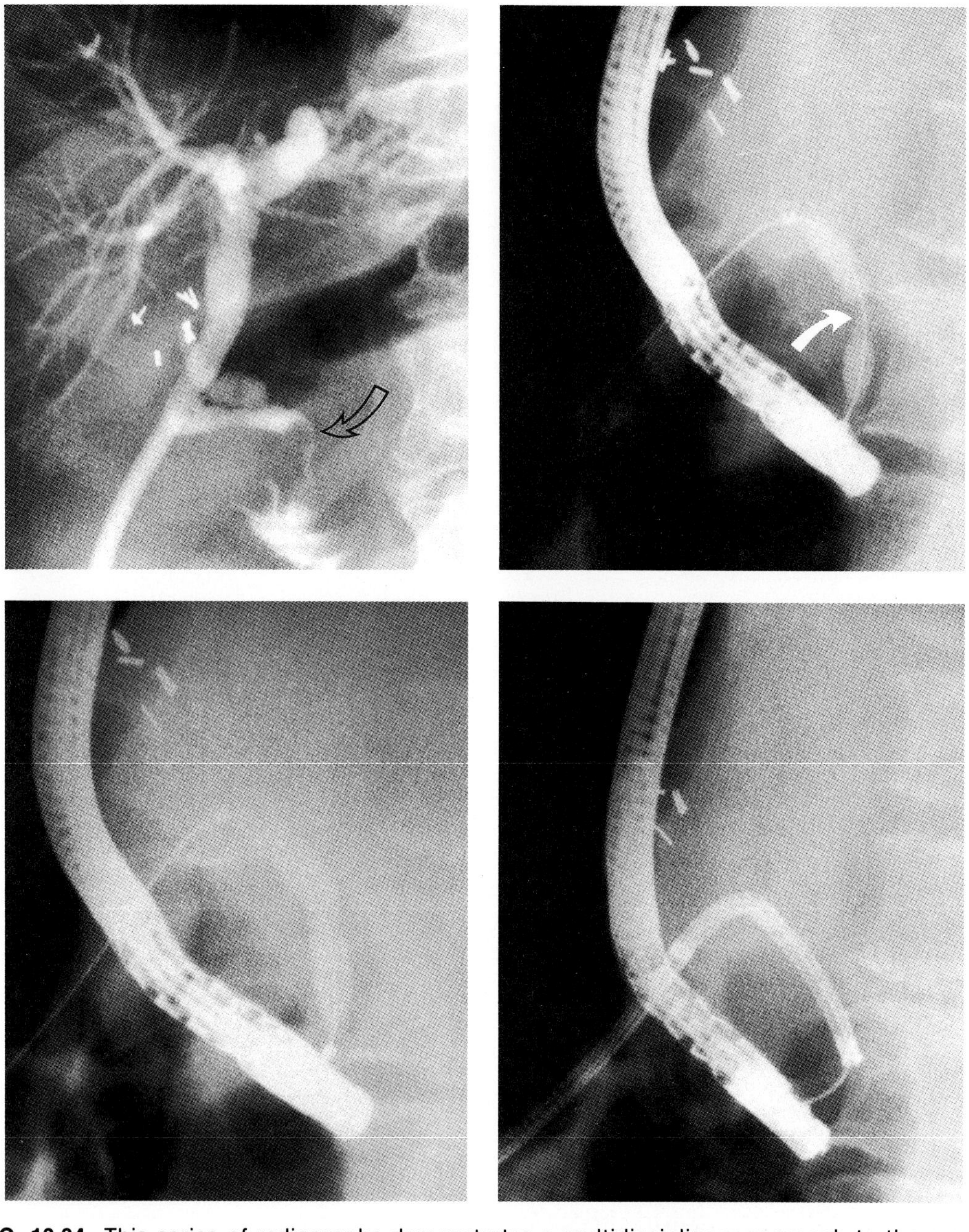

FIG. 13.34. This series of radiographs demonstrates a multidisciplinary approach to the management of a distal common bile duct stricture. **Top left:** A radiograph obtained through a T-tube showing a stricture in the distal common bile duct (*arrow*). **Top right, bottom left:** Inflation of a dilating balloon. A waist is evident in the balloon (*arrow*), and the balloon is nearly fully distended in the lower bottom left. Note that the T-tube was removed and that an ERCP was performed. A guidewire was advanced through the endoscope and out the T-tube tract. This guidewire was utilized to advance the balloon catheter: Traction on it facilitated advancement of the balloon. **Bottom right:** A choledochoscope was then advanced over the guidewire into the bile duct and duodenum, providing endoscopic evaluation of the stricture. (From ref. 25, with permission.)

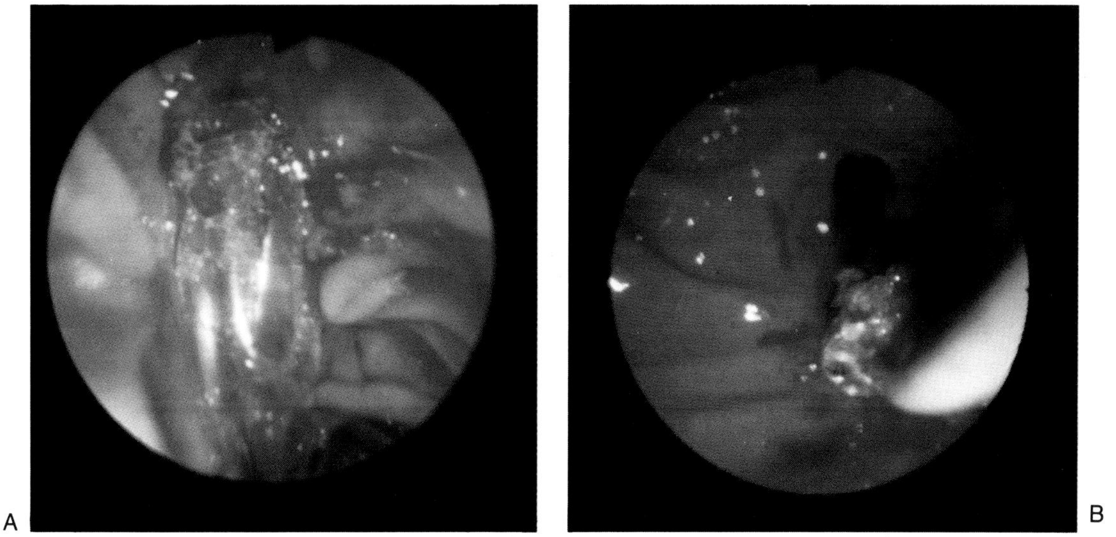

FIG. 13.35. A: This endoscopic picture shows a large balloon exiting from the papilla into the duodenum. The balloon was advanced over a guidewire, which was placed through the T-tube tract. **B:** The choledochoscope is seen exiting the sphincterotomy, passing over the guidewire. Stone material was pushed through the dilated stricture into the duodenum.

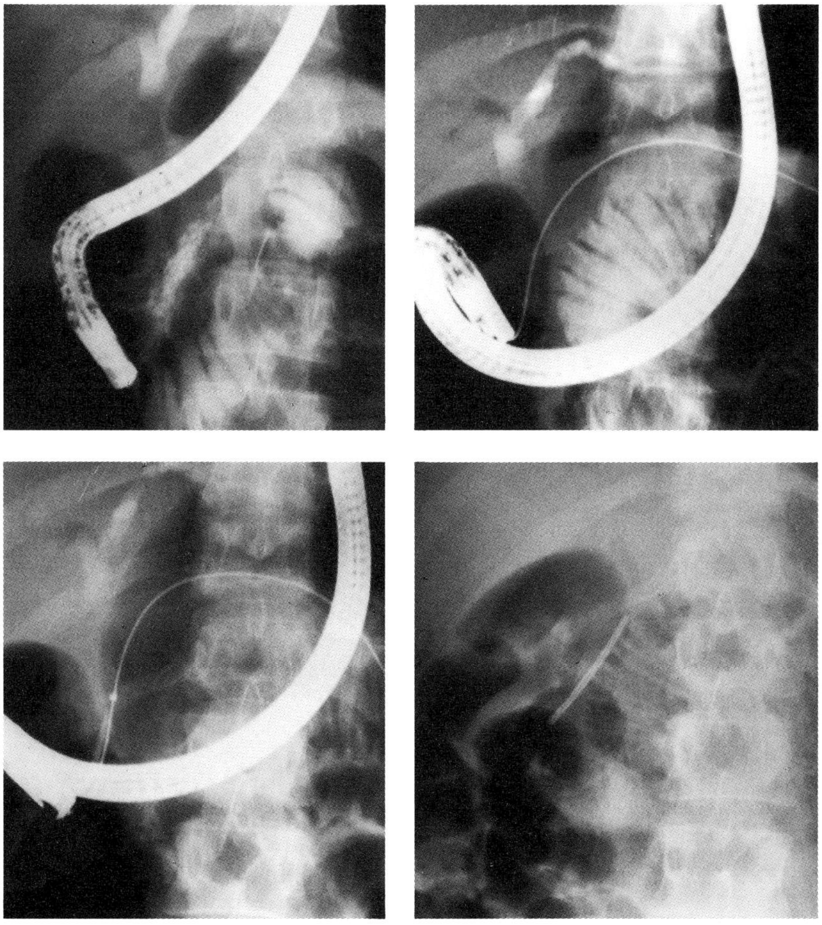

FIG. 13.36. Top left: Extravasation of contrast into the parenchyma of the ventral pancreas of pancreas divisum. **Top right:** A guidewire has been advanced through the minor papilla into the dorsal duct. **Bottom left:** A balloon is being inflated in the minor papilla to facilitate placement of a prosthesis. **Bottom right:** The prosthesis is shown in position in the dorsal duct.

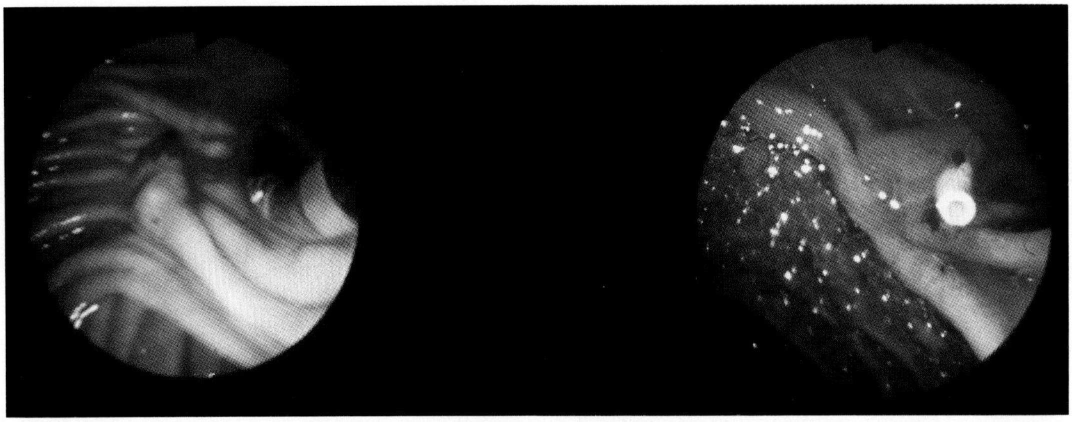

FIG. 13.37. Left: This endoscopic photograph demonstrates the placement of a balloon catheter into the minor papilla. The major papilla and sphincterotomy of that papilla are shown inferior to the balloon catheter. **Right:** A prosthesis is in place in the minor papilla.

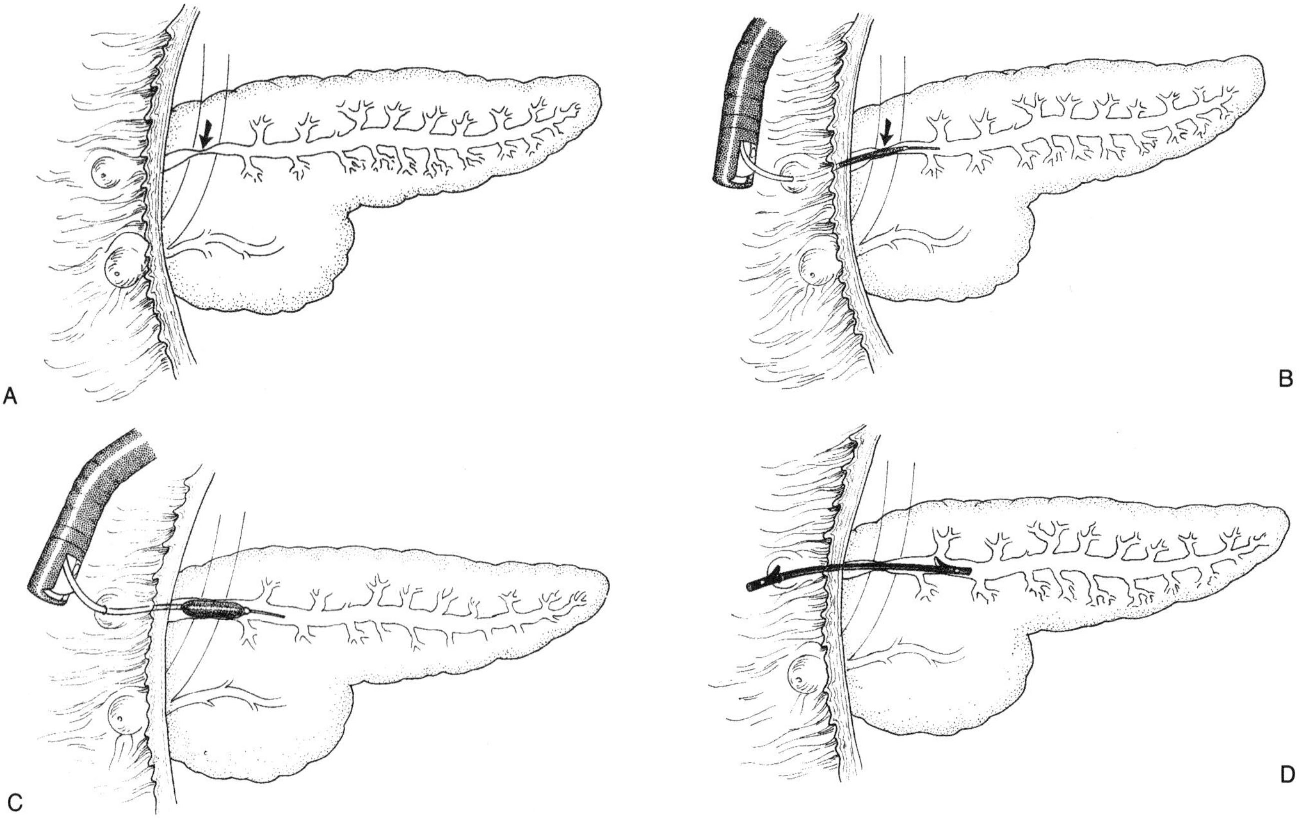

FIG. 13.38. A: A stricture in the dorsal duct of pancreas divisum (*arrow*). **B:** A balloon catheter is being inserted through a stricture (*arrow*) of the dorsal pancreatic duct. **C:** The balloon is fully inflated, facilitating insertion of a prosthesis. **D:** A prosthesis has been inserted.

FIG. 13.40. Top left: This ERCP shows evidence of pancreatitis with a stricture at the papilla and extravasation of contrast into the head of the gland. **Top right:** A balloon is being inflated in the pancreatic sphincter. **Bottom left:** A pancreatic prosthesis is being placed into the pancreatic duct. The endoscope remains in place. **Bottom right:** The prosthesis is in place in the pancreatic duct. The direction of the stent is correct because the pancreatic duct in this case deviates laterally, as shown in the radiograph in the top left.

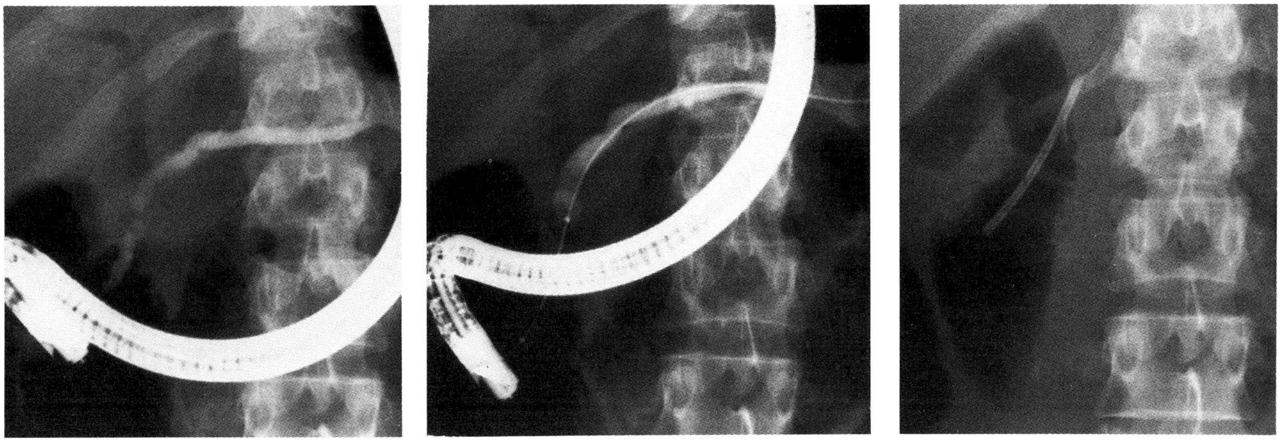

FIG. 13.39. Left: Cannulation of the dorsal duct of pancreas divisum shows beading and irregularity of the duct secondary to inflammation. **Middle:** A balloon catheter is inserted into the dorsal duct over a guidewire in preparation for inflation. **Right:** A prosthesis is visible in the dorsal duct after dilatation. (From ref. 24, with permission.)

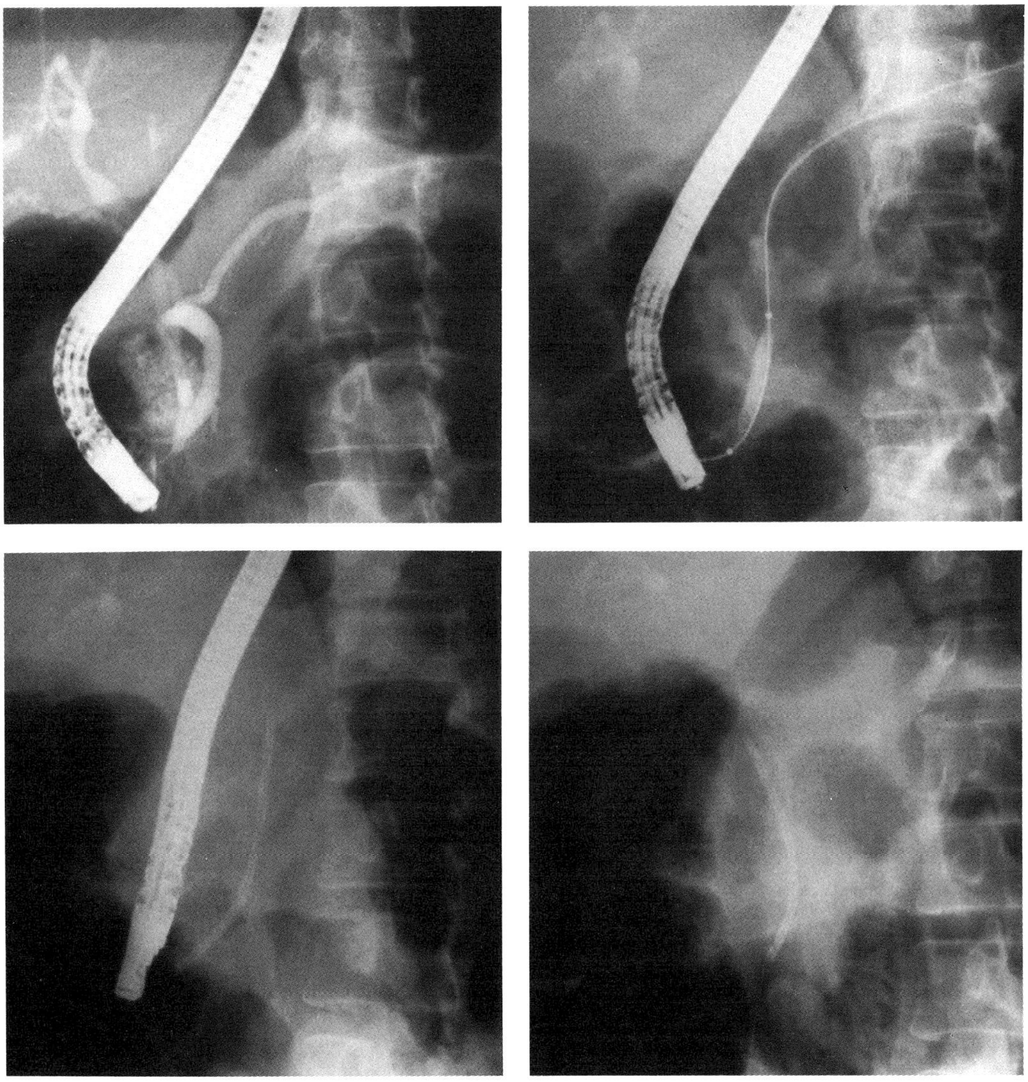

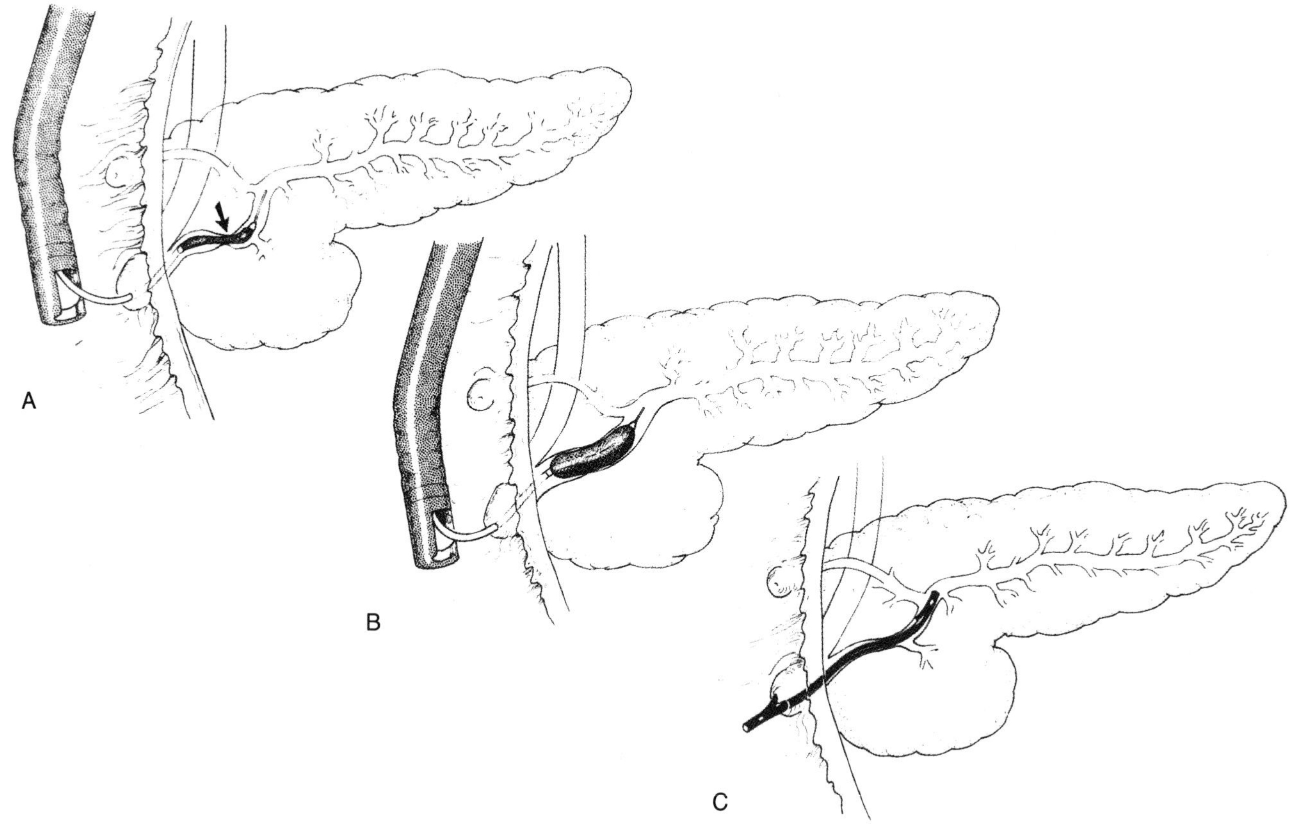

FIG. 13.41. A: A balloon catheter being placed into a stricture (*arrow*) in the main pancreatic duct. **B:** The balloon is fully inflated. **C:** A prosthesis has been advanced through the stricture.

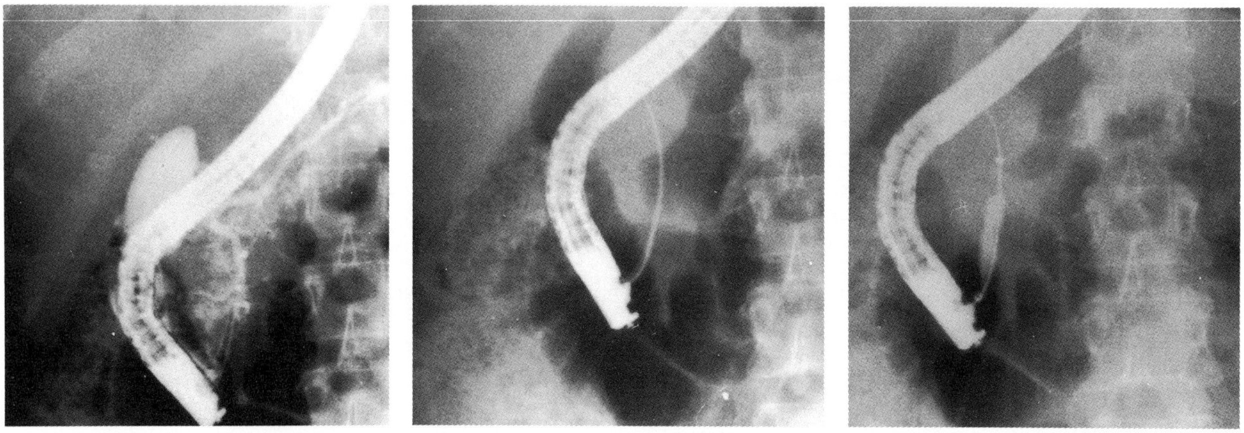

FIG. 13.42. Left: Extravasation of contrast is noted on this pancreatogram obtained in a patient with pancreatitis secondary to a hypertensive sphincter. **Middle:** A guidewire and dilating catheter are advanced into the duct. The guidewire is not visible at the genu because it is being concealed by the endoscope. **Right:** A balloon is being inflated in the sphincter.

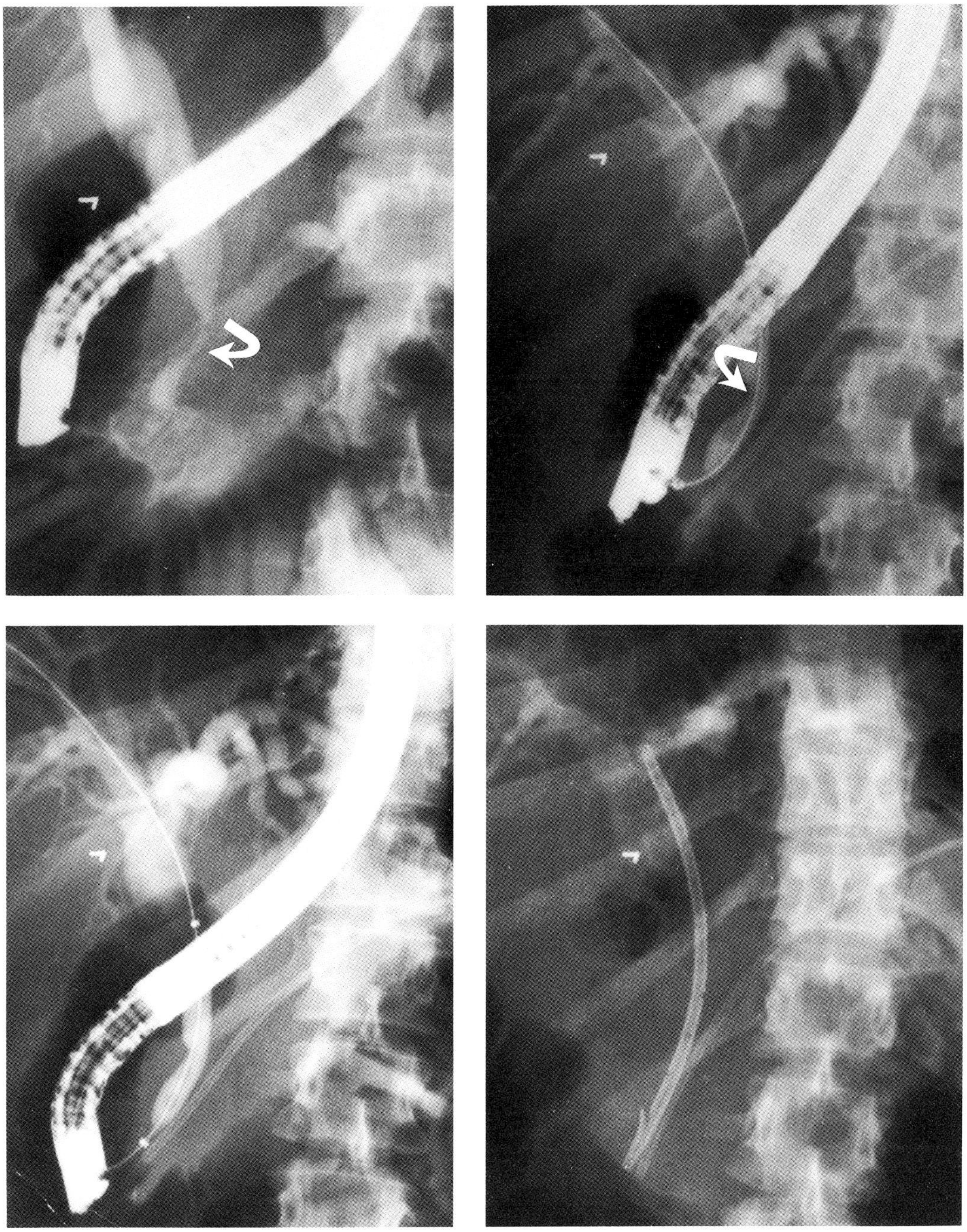

FIG. 13.43. Top left: A stricture (*arrow*) is visible in the distal common bile duct in this patient with chronic pancreatitis. **Top right:** A prosthesis has been placed into the pancreatic duct, and a balloon catheter is evident in the bile duct. The balloon is being inflated. Note the waist on the balloon (*arrow*). **Bottom left:** The balloon is being inflated to its maximum diameter. **Bottom right:** A large-caliber prosthesis is placed into the bile duct to maintain the integrity of the dilated lumen.

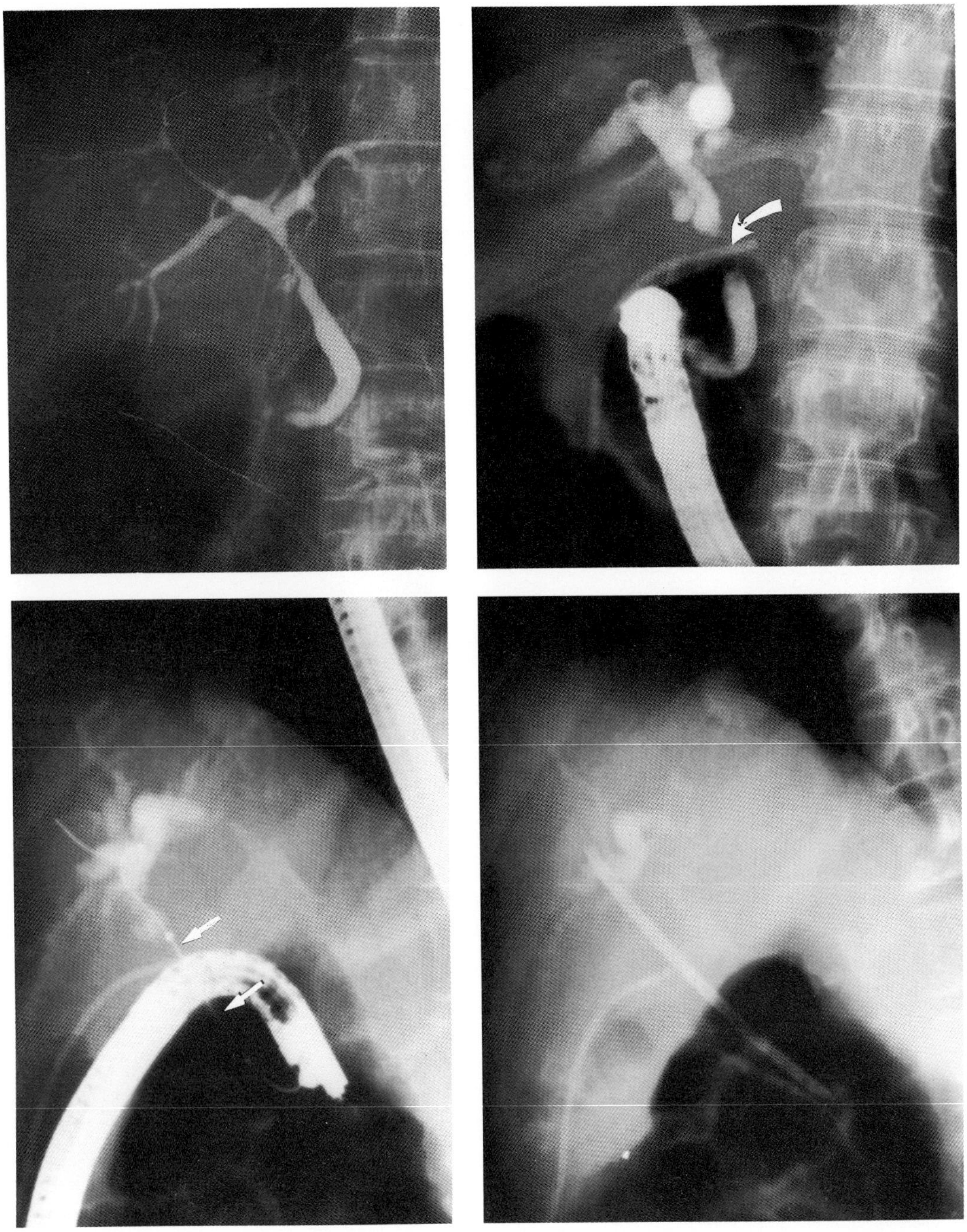

FIG. 13.44. Top left: A cholangiogram reveals evidence of diffuse intrahepatic disease simulating sclerosing cholangitis in a patient receiving hepatic artery perfusion of 5-FUDR. **Top right:** A mid common bile duct stricture has developed from injury and perforation of the duct by the catheter. The catheter is opacified (*arrow*) on this study because of communication with the bile duct. Note the dilated ducts on this study done 3 months after the first initial cholangiogram. **Bottom left:** A balloon catheter is placed into the duct to dilate the stricture. The length of the balloon is outlined by arrows. **Bottom right:** A large-caliber prosthesis is placed for decompression.

REFERENCES

1. Seldinger SI. Catheter replacement of the needle in percutaneous arteriography. A new technique. *Acta Radiol* 1953; 39:368–76.
2. Siegel JH, Guelrud M. Endoscopic cholangiopancreatoplasty: hydrostatic balloon dilatation in the bile duct and pancreas. *Gastrointest Endosc* 1983;29:99.
3. Siegel JH. Combined endoscopic dilatation and insertion of large diameter endoprostheses for bile duct obstruction. *Gastrointest Endosc* 1984;30:91–2.
4. Geenen JE. Balloon dilatation of bile duct strictures. In: Classen M, Geenen J, Kawai K, eds. *Nonsurgical biliary drainage*. Berlin: Springer, 1984;105–8.
5. Geenen JE, Derfus D, Welch JM. Biliary balloon dilatation. *Endosc Rev* 1985;2:10–6.
6. Siegel JH, Yatto RP. Hydrostatic balloon catheters: a new dimension of therapeutic endoscopy. *Endoscopy* 1984;16:231–6.
7. Foutch PG, Sivak MV Jr. Therapeutic endoscopic balloon dilatation of the extrahepatic biliary ducts. *Am J Gastroenterol* 1985;80:575–80.
8. Willett IR, McCutcheon AD, Dudley FJ. Endoscopic balloon dilatation of biliary strictures. *Med J Aust* 1985;143:208–10.
9. Guelrud M, Siegel JH. Hypertensive pancreatic duct sphincter as cause of recurrent pancreatitis: successful treatment with hydrostatic balloon dilatation. *Dig Dis Sci* 1984;29:225–31.
10. Shemesh E, Brook O, Bat L. Endoscopic Gruntzig balloon dilatation of benign strictures in the biliary system. *Isr J Med Sci* 1985;21:889–91.
11. Kozarek RA. Hydrostatic balloon dilatation of gastrointestinal stenoses: a national survey. *Gastrointest Endosc* 1986;32:9–15.
12. Johnson GK, Geenen JE, Venu RP, Hogan WJ. Endoscopic treatment of biliary duct strictures in sclerosing cholangitis: follow-up assessment of a new therapeutic approach. *Gastrointest Endosc* 1987;33:9–12.
13. May GR, Bender CE, LaRusso NF, Wiesner RH. Nonoperative dilatation of dominant strictures in primary sclerosing cholangitis. *AJR* 1985;145:1061–4.
14. Skolkin MD, Alspaugh JP, Casarella WJ. Sclerosing cholangitis: palliation with percutaneous cholangioplasty. *Radiology* 1989;170:199–206.
15. Johnson GK, Geenen JE, Venu RP, Schmalz MJ, Hogan WJ. Endoscopic treatment of biliary tract strictures in sclerosing cholangitis: a larger series and recommendations for treatment. *Gastrointest Endosc* 1991;37:38–43.
16. Huibregtse K, Katon RM, Tytgat GNJ. Endoscopic treatment of post operative biliary strictures. *Endoscopy* 1986;18:133–7.
17. Berkelhammer C, Kortan P, Haber GB. Endoscopic biliary prostheses as treatment for benign bile duct strictures. *Gastrointest Endosc* 1989;35:95–101.
18. Geenen DJ, Geenen JE, Hogan WJ, et al. Endoscopic therapy for benign bile duct strictures. *Gastrointest Endosc* 1989;35:367–71.
19. Vogel SB, Howard RJ, Caridi J, Hawkins EF. Evaluation of percutaneous transhepatic balloon dilatation of benign biliary stricture in high-risk patients. *Am J Surg* 1985;149:73–8.
20. Martin EG, Fankuchen EI, Laffey KJ, Sibley RE. Percutaneous management of benign biliary disease. *Gastrointest Radiol* 1984;9:207–12.
21. Gallacher DJ, Kadir S, Kaufman SL, et al. Nonoperative management of benign postoperative biliary strictures. *Radiology* 1985;156:625–9.
22. Siegel JH. Endoscopic management of benign biliary strictures, biliary tract fistula, and sclerosing cholangitis. In: *ERCP: diagnostic and therapeutic applications*. Jacobson IM, ed. New York: Elsevier Scientific Publishers, 1989.
23. Siegel JH, Ramsey WH. Endoscopic biliary stent placement for bile duct stricture after hepatic artery infusion of 5 FUDR. *J Clin Gastroenterol* 1986;8:673–6.
24. Siegel JH, Ben-Zvi JS, Pullano W, Cooperman AM. Effectiveness of endoscopic drainage for pancreas divisum: endoscopic and surgical results in 31 patients. *Endoscopy* 1990;22:129–33.
25. Siegel JH. Endoscopic decompression of the biliary tree. In: Silvis S, ed. *Therapeutic gastrointestinal endoscopy*. New York: Igaku-Shoin, 1984.

CHAPTER 14

New Horizons

The diagnostic and therapeutic modalities employed with ERCP are listed in Table 14.1. This list of therapeutic procedures continues to grow, entrenching the endoscopist as a key player in the management of pancreaticobiliary disorders. Most of these modalities have already been described in detail in preceding chapters. New procedures that are being investigated are listed in Table 14.2 and include insertion of radioactive material into the biliary tree or pancreas for the treatment of malignant disease, laser therapy of malignant strictures, selective cannulation of the cystic duct and gallbladder, and choledochoscopy. I also include my experience using a bipolar sphincterotome for the performance of sphincterotomy, another area of interest and current research.

INTRALUMINAL IRRADIATION

Since reporting the preloading technique of inserting iridium 192 into a special double-lumen prosthesis to provide intraluminal irradiation to malignant strictures (Figs. 14.1, 14.2) (1), my colleagues and I have modified the technique in order to reduce unnecessary exposure to radiation, for the patient, the endoscopist, the assistant, and the other team members. We are currently using an after-loading technique, a technique somewhat similar to other techniques (2–4). But, rather than using iridium 192, which still exposes personnel to radiation hazards, we utilize a high-dose-rate remote delivery system (Nucleotron) to treat bile duct tumors, which does not expose personnel to harmful radiation (5). This new technique requires the use of a 10Fr nasobiliary tube, which is inserted through the stricture and is left in place for as long as needed for calculations and treatment. A smaller catheter containing a dummy wire is inserted into and advanced through the 10 French catheter. Radiopaque markings placed onto the dummy wire are used to identify its

TABLE 14.1. *Endoscopic interventional techniques for the management of pancreaticobiliary disorders*

ERCP	Drains
Sphincterotomy	Nasobiliary
Choledocholithotomy	Nasopancreatic
Occlusion balloons	Nasocystic
Baskets	Endoprostheses
PEERS[a]	Bile duct
T-tube tract	Pancreatic duct
De novo	Pancreatic cysts
Lithotripsy	Hydrostatic balloon dilatation
Mechanical	Intraluminal irradiation
Electrohydraulic	Iridium
Ultrasound	High-dose-rate generator
Pulsed-dye laser	

[a] Percutaneous endoscopic extraction of retained stones

TABLE 14.2. *Endoscopic interventional techniques under investigation*

Bipolar sphincterotomy
Cystic duct cannulation
  Perfusion of dissolution agents
  Extraction of stones
  Placement of prostheses
Choledochoscopy
  Peroral
    Choledochoduodenostomy
    Transpapillary
      Mother-daughter system
  Percutaneous
    De novo
    T-tube tract
Pancreatoscopy
  Transpapillary
    Mother-daughter system
Laser therapy bile duct tumors
  Percutaneous
    De novo
  Mother-daughter system
    Transpapillary

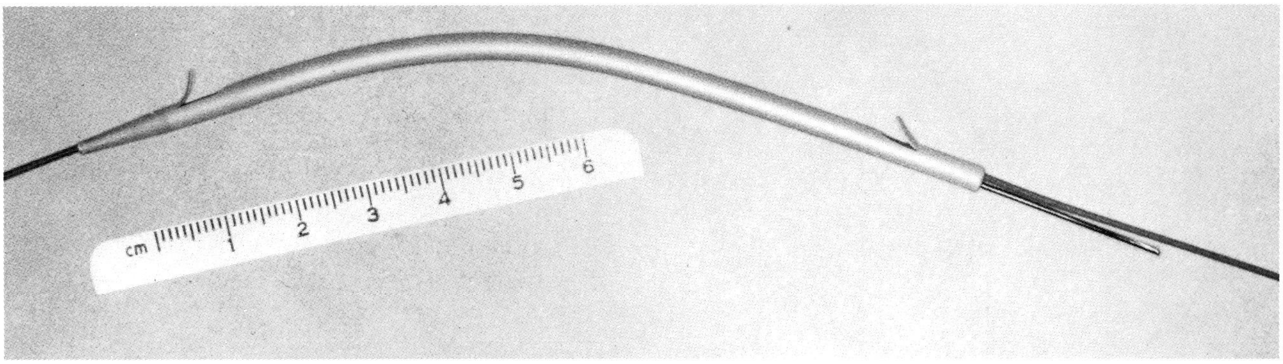

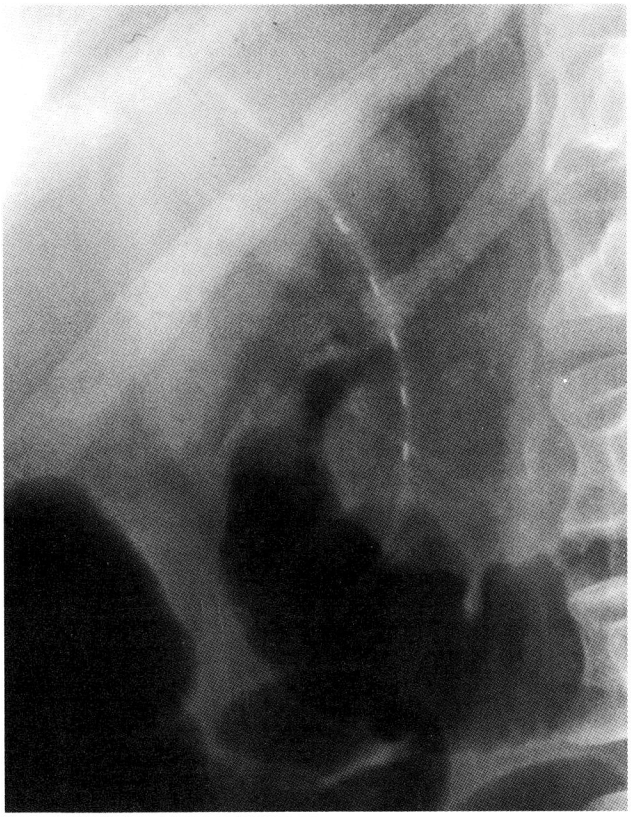

FIG. 14.1. Top: The 11Fr double-lumen prosthesis used for implantation of iridium 192. One lumen accommodates the guidewire over which the stent is inserted. The other lumen is used to insert the iridium. The latter lumen is sealed at the proximal end, and, after the iridium is placed into the lumen, a metal plug is placed to contain the iridium and to prevent dislocation. **Bottom:** The iridium stent in place in the bile duct of a patient being treated. The iridium seeds are radiopaque and are lined up in the stent.

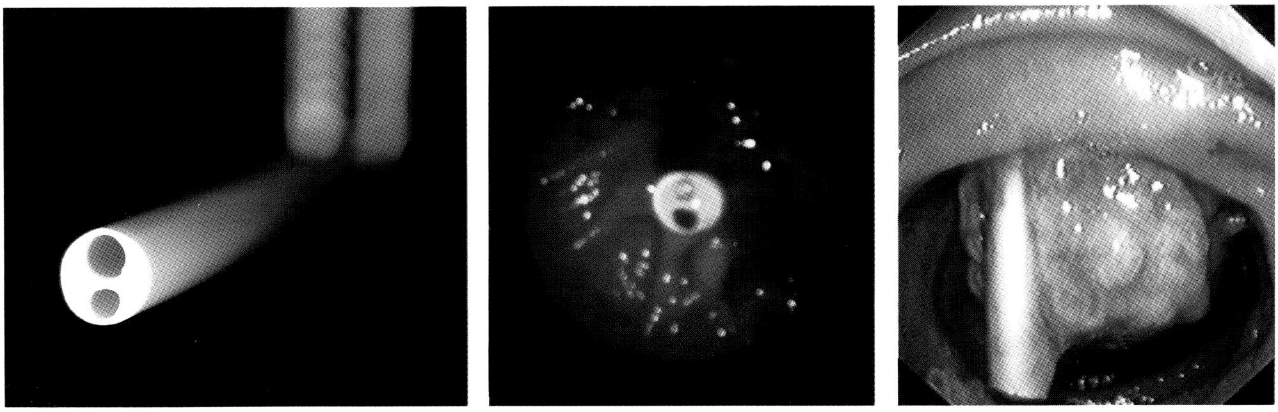

FIG. 14.2. Left: The double-lumen stent on end to identify the two lumen. **Middle:** The double-lumen stent in place in the duodenum. The open lumen provides drainage and maintains decompression during the 48 hours of treatment. A metal plug is visible in the other lumen and contains the iridium. **Right:** A videoimage of a double-lumen prosthesis in place in a patient with an ampullary tumor.

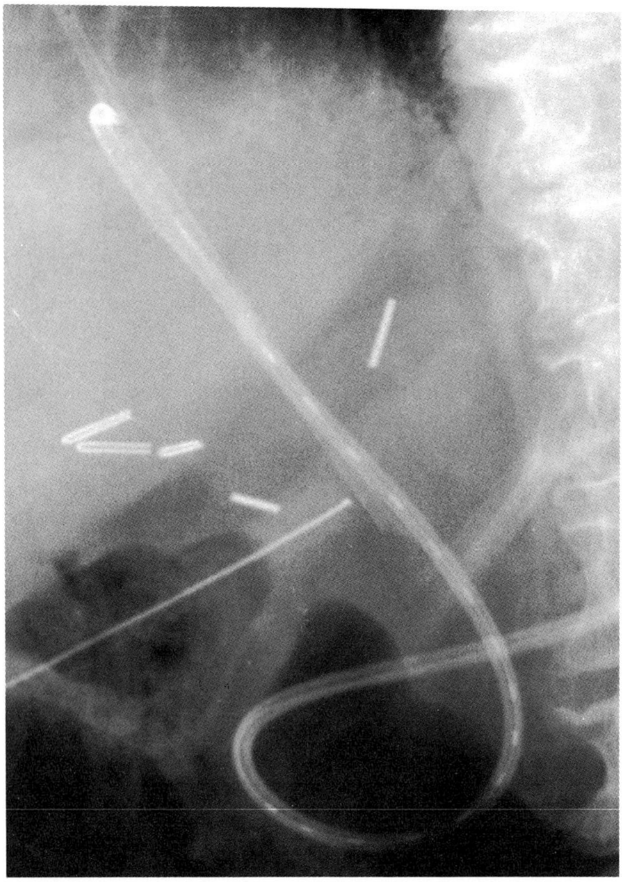

FIG. 14.3. This radiograph shows a 10Fr nasobiliary tube in place in a stricture of the bile duct caused by gallbladder carcinoma. The vertical opaque markers are part of a dummy wire that will be used to calculate the dosage to be transmitted down the wire by the high-voltage generator (Nucleotron). The horizontal opaque wire is part of an abdominal drain (Jackson-Pratt) to accommodate drainage following surgery.

position in the bile duct in relation to the stricture. Special attention is directed to the stricture and the position of the wire and markings by utilizing biplane fluoroscopy, which is essential for spatial orientation. Anterior-posterior and lateral radiographs are taken as hard copy to confirm and localize the catheter (Fig. 14.3). These data are then compiled and tabulated to prepare an isodose chart and to calibrate the irradiation dosage (Fig. 14.4). With a high-dose-rate remote system, a tumor dose is delivered in minutes rather than days, and subsequent sessions can be scheduled during the same period of hospitalization. During treatment, the patient is placed in an isolated chamber, and irradiation is delivered to the lesion without exposing others. Unlike the after-loading iridium delivery system reported by others, which provides irradiation in a linear fashion with rapid fall-off after 1 cm, the high-dose-rate generator can be programmed to deliver radiation in different configurations that conform more specifically to the shape of the tumor (Fig. 14.4).

We have treated only six patients to date using this technique, and the results are not significant enough to propose it for general use. However, a trial using combined internal and external irradiation is currently under way at our institution, and we are anxiously awating the results. If this form of therapy provides effective palliation and is possibly curative, it offers promise to patients with cholangiocarcinomas and, possibly, tumors of the pancreas (5).

LASER AND ELECTOCAUTERY THERAPY FOR BILE DUCT TUMORS AND STRICTURES

Utilizing the mother-daughter endoscope system for performing direct cholangiopancreatoscopy, the endoscopist should be able to deliver thermal energy to obstructing lesions of the biliary tree and pancreas. Fibers small enough to be inserted through the baby scope (daughter scope) (channel size 1.5 mm) are available and can deliver laser energy. The major physical problem, however, is the same for all lasers; surmounting the problem of delivering energy around curves and bends. Because looping of the endoscope occurs when the instrument, by necessity, conforms to the configuration of the stomach and intestines, delivery of laser energy may be impossible. Experience is accummulating for laser lithotripsy (6–8), but the wavelength for this function is different, thermal versus mechanical. Laser tumor therapy can be provided

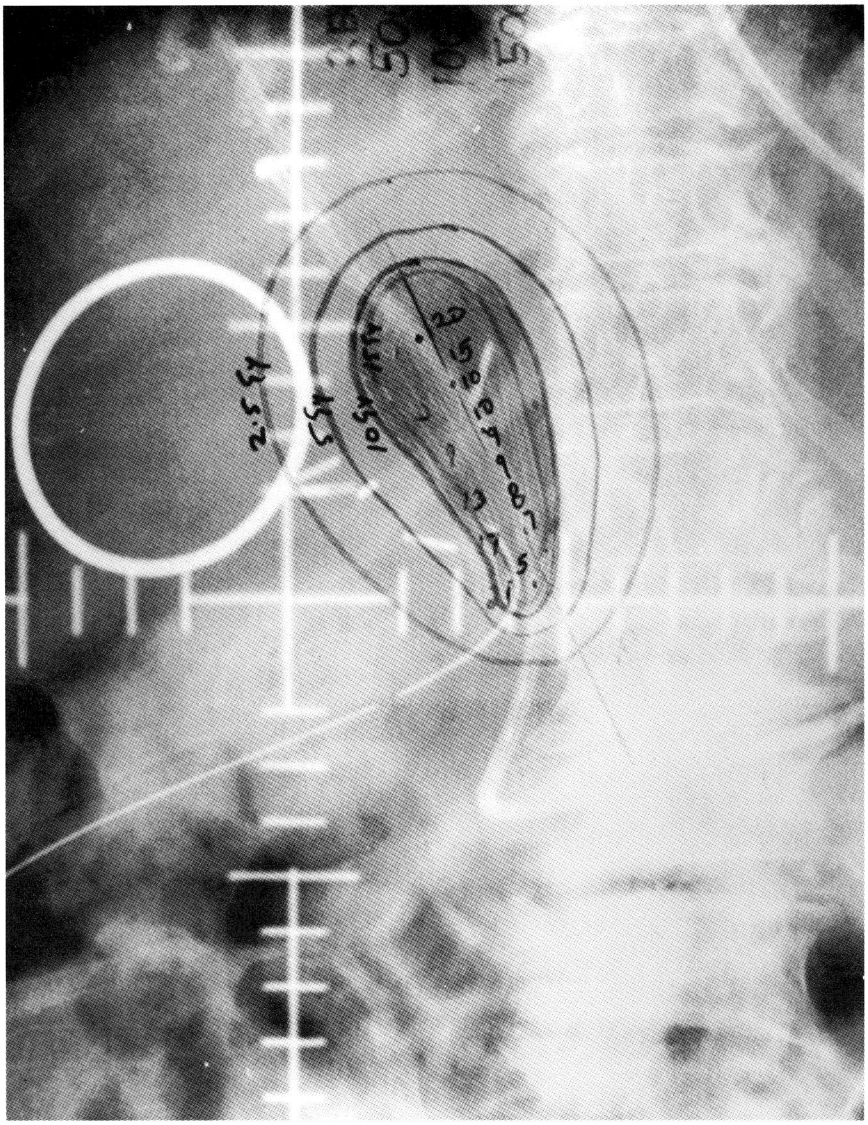

FIG. 14.4. An isodose chart superimposed onto the area of treatment. The high-voltage irradiation can be programmed into any shape and can be transmitted deeper and further than iridium because the drop-off is less than that with the isotope.

through the percutaneous route (9), so it is only a matter of time until the routine delivery of thermal lasers will be possible using a duodenoscope delivery system.

The possibility does exist that electrocautery energy can be used for treatment of bile duct tumors, again delivered directly through the daughter endoscope. Emphasis must be placed on safety because direct application of electrocautery current to any lesion requires visualization to control treatment. Relying on one-dimensional fluoroscopy rather than direct visualization could lead to misadventure and danger. I discourage the application of electrocautery (and laser) unless monitoring is possible by direct vision through a daughter endoscope per orally or through a choledochoscope placed either through a mature T-tube tract or through a percutaneous tract established de novo through the liver. More work is needed in this area, but it will be restricted to centers equipped with the mother-daughter endoscope system and laser technology. Again, I look forward to reports from investigators currently using this technology.

CHOLEDOCHOSCOPY—PANCREATOSCOPY

Percutaneous Routes

Direct endoscopic examination of the biliary tree and pancreas has always been an intriguing challenge for endoscopists. Other researchers, as well as my colleagues and I, have reported using a flexible endoscope—initially a modified bronchoscope (Fig. 14.5) and subsequently a flexible choledochoscope—which is inserted percutaneously through a mature T-tube tract (10–14). Additionally, percutaneous choledochoscopy is possible de novo through an established

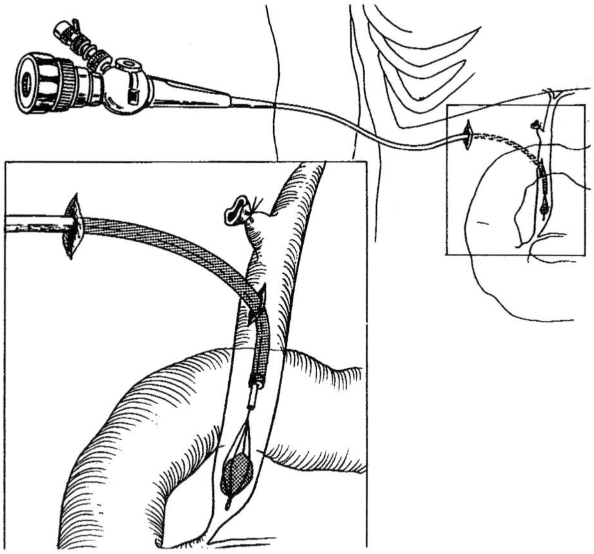

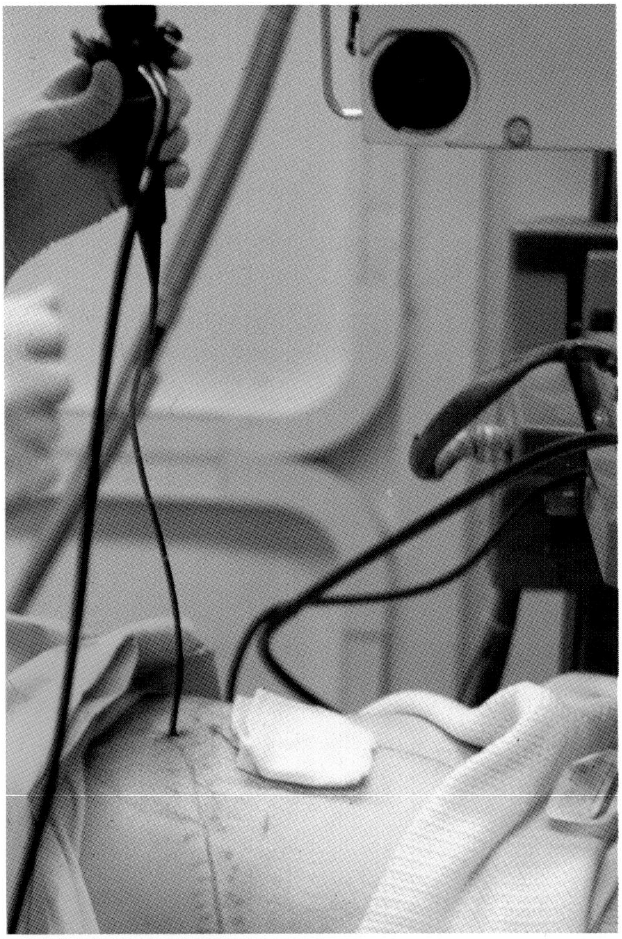

FIG. 14.5. Left: The technique for inserting a choledochoscope (a bronoscope and special valve, which were initially used) through a mature T-tube tract to identify and capture a stone with a basket. **Right:** The choledochoscope being inserted into the T-tube tract. The T-tube was placed anteriorly in this obese patient.

tract. In fact, Yamakawa (15,16) has extracted and crushed stones, placed prostheses, and treated strictures with laser through de novo established tracts. Whichever route is used, the direct visualization technique enables the endoscopist to examine the bile duct adequately, inspect suspicious areas found on cholangiography, obtain tissue (Fig. 14.6), remove stones (Fig. 14.7), and access the duct for stent insertion or laser therapy. Other choledochoscopic pictures are shown (Figs. 14.8–14.15) to present a spectrum of findings.

The advantages of percutaneous endoscopic extraction of retained stones (PEERS) are listed in Table 14.3. When evaluating a patient's bile duct or gallbladder through a mature, percutaneous tract, one can provide direct examination of the duct (or gallbladder) and eliminate false-positive findings seen on contrast

TABLE 14.3. *Percutaneous endoscopic extraction of retained stones (PEERS)*

Direct examination of bile ducts
No false-positive or false-negative results
Little exposure to x-rays
Decrease procedure time

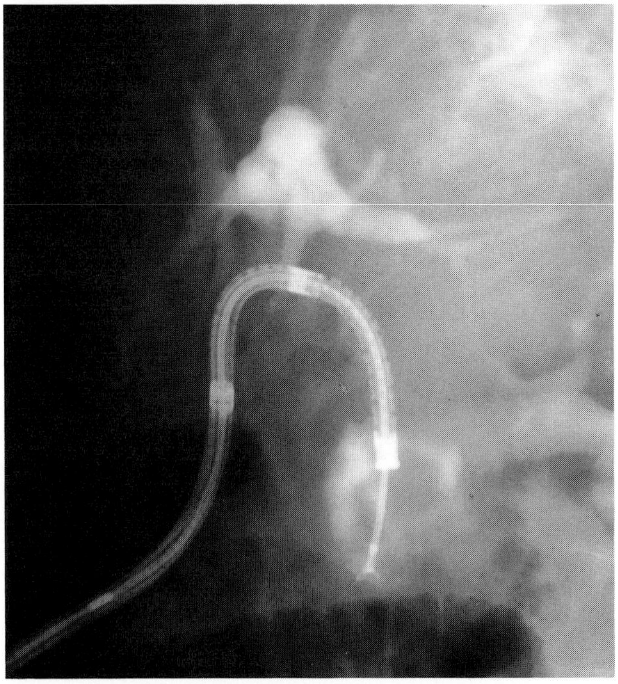

FIG. 14.6. This radiograph shows a choledochoscope being advanced through a percutaneous tract into the distal common bile duct. Biopsy forceps are opened to obtain a direct biopsy.

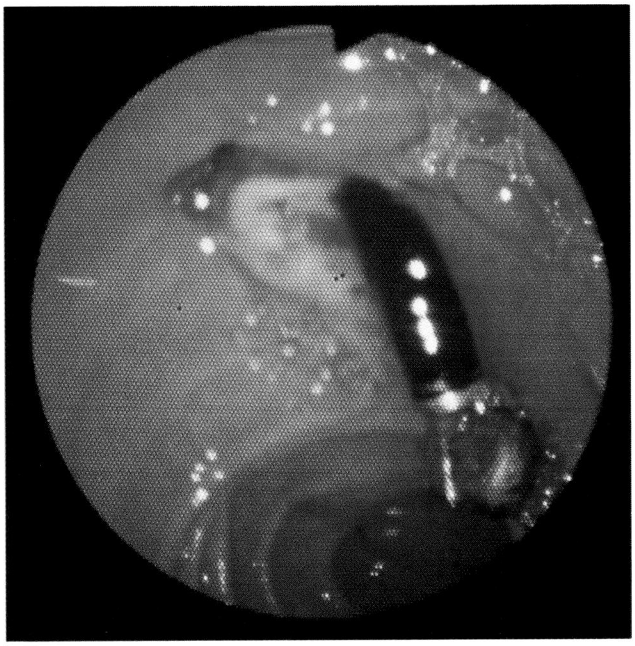

A

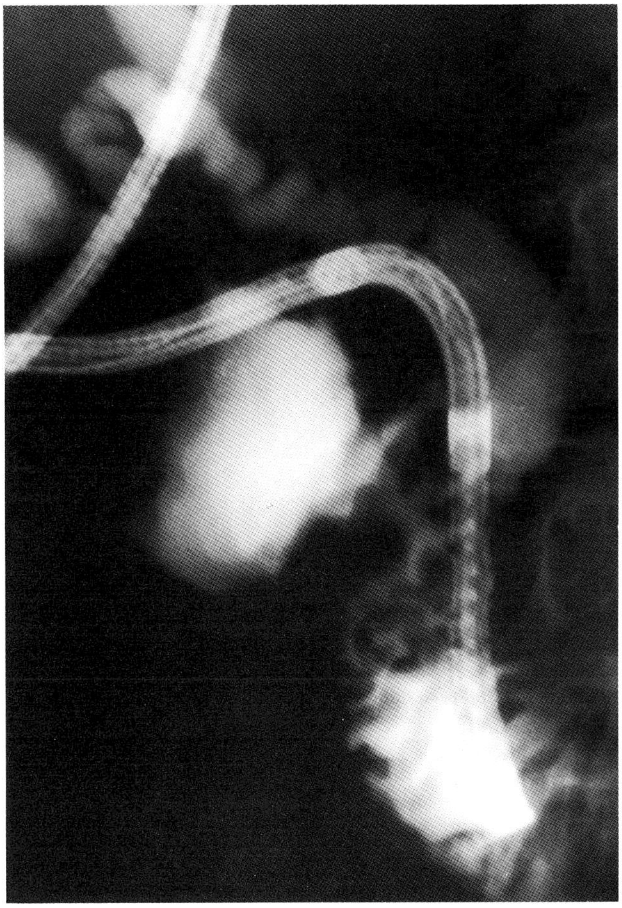

B

FIG. 14.7. A: This endoscopic picture was obtained with a duodenoscope that was left in place after performing a sphincterotomy. The sphincterotomy was performed to facilitate passage of the choledochoscope, which was used to entrap a stone and push it into the duodenum. **B:** A choledochoscope being advanced from the T-tube tract, down the bile duct, through the sphincterotomy, and into the duodenum.

studies. Air bubbles contained within the T-tube or cholecystostomy tube often appear as lucencies or false-positive stones: Direct visualization confirms stones or air bubbles.

One concern of physicians utilizing a T-tube tract for catheter extraction of a stone is exposure to fluoroscopic radiation. The entire radiographic technique of basket extraction (17) is performed under the fluoroscope, exposing not only the patient but also the physician and assistants to ionizing radiation. The endoscopic technique, alhtough it is performed in the fluoroscopic room, utilizes x-ray intermittently to assist in guiding the endoscope. The remainder of the

Text continues on page 404.

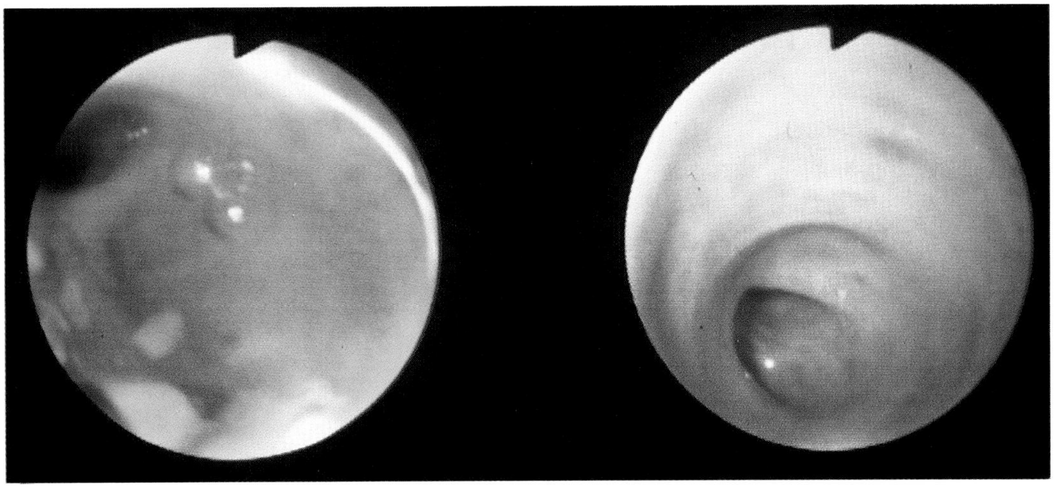

FIG. 14.8. Left: The proximal biliary tree with bifurcations of the ducts. Note cholesterol stone material. **Right:** A choledochoscopic picture of the distal common bile duct.

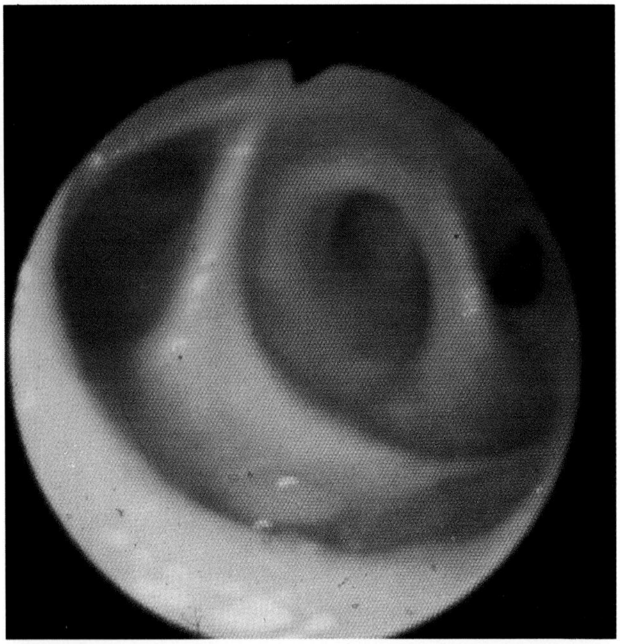

FIG. 14.9. A choledochoscopic picture of the proximal biliary tree showing three branches of the ducts.

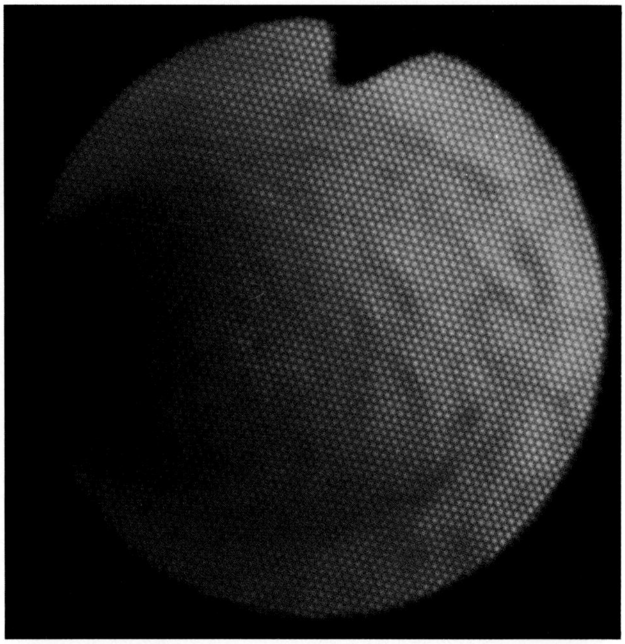

FIG. 14.10. The distal common bile duct and its typical mucosal pattern.

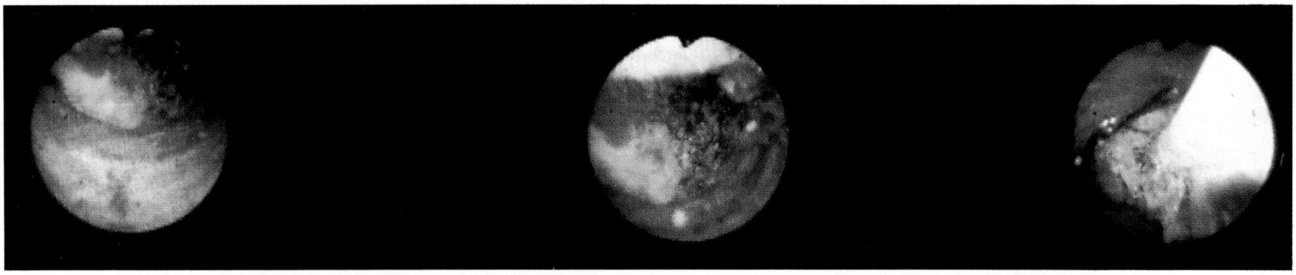

FIG. 14.11. **Left:** A stone in the bile duct. **Middle:** A basket catheter being advanced to entrap the stone. **Right:** The entrapped stone ready to be removed through the T-tube tract.

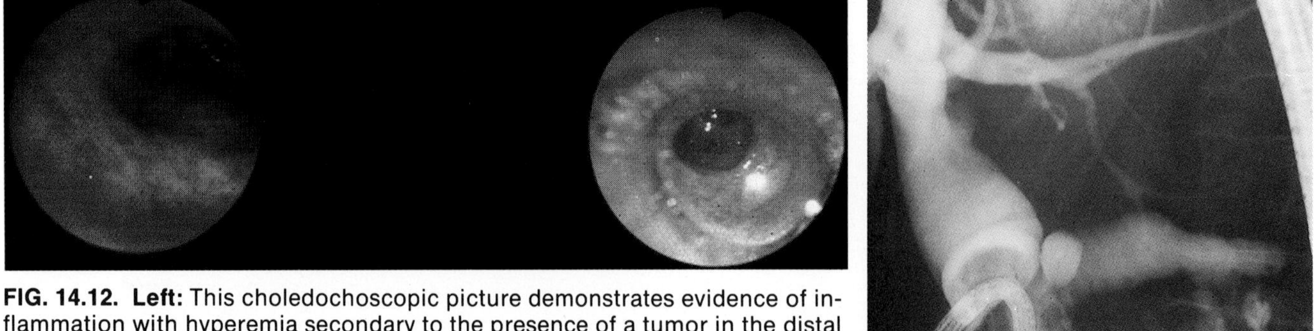

FIG. 14.12. **Left:** This choledochoscopic picture demonstrates evidence of inflammation with hyperemia secondary to the presence of a tumor in the distal common bile duct. **Middle:** The normal appearance of the distal common bile duct. A sphincterotomy is visible in the distance. **Right:** The choledochoscope in the distal common bile duct within the mass. Note the dilated bile duct and pancreatic duct secondary to tumor obstruction.

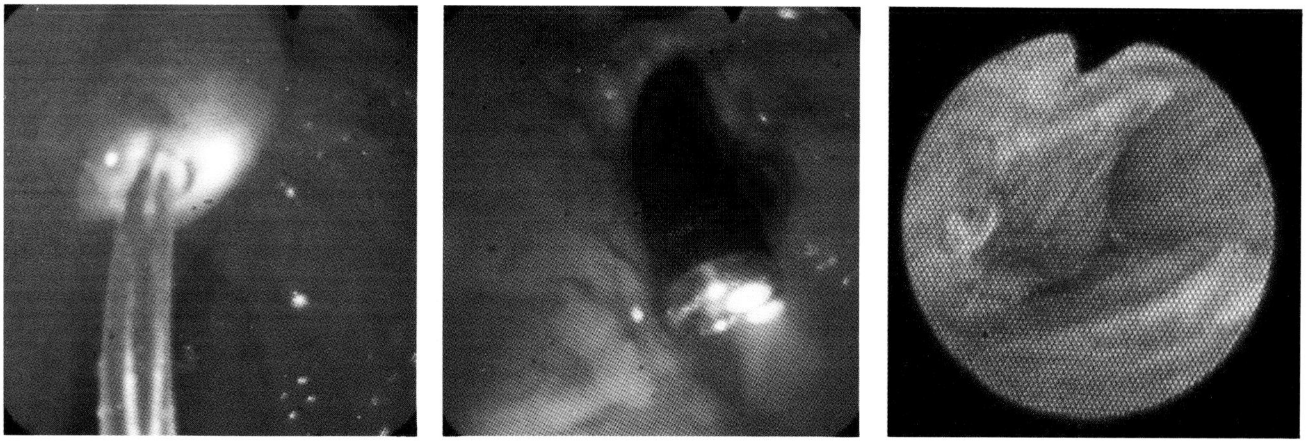

FIG. 14.13. Left: A catheter protruding through the intact papilla, being advanced through a choledochoscope. The papilla is transilluminated by the light from the choledochoscope. **Middle:** The choledochoscope protruding through the sphincterotomy into the duodenum. **Right:** The distal common bile duct and a fresh sphincterotomy with a basket catheter passed through the sphincterotomy into the duodenum.

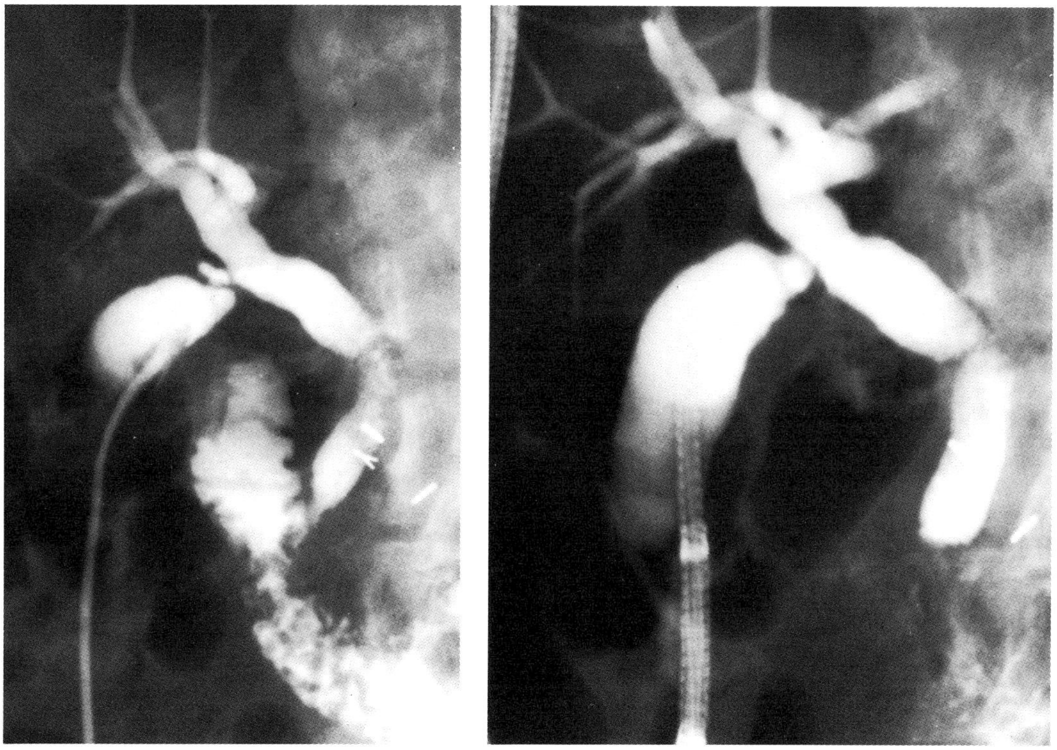

FIG. 14.14. Left: A cholecystocholangiogram through a catheter left in place in the gallbladder. **Right:** A choledochoscope is passed through the mature cholecystostomy tract into the gallbladder.

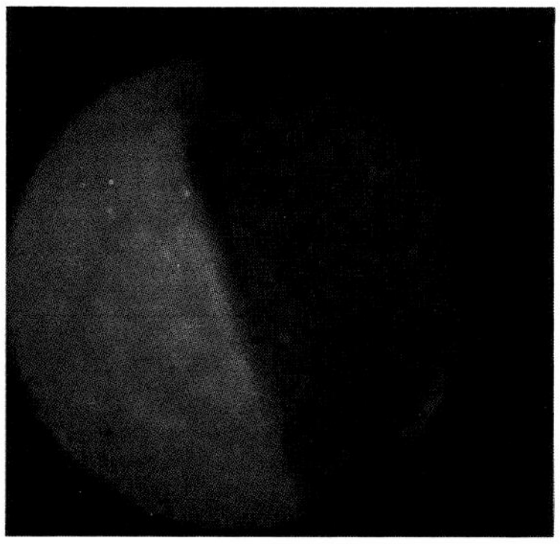

FIG. 14.15. An endoscopic picture of the gallbladder demonstrating an inflamed gallbladder wall and bile, which is layered to the right of the picture.

Text continued from page 401.
procedure is performed endoscopically. And, because of direct visualization, the procedure time is reduced.

CHOLEDOCHOSCOPY—PER ORAL

Choledochoduodenoscopy

I have referred to per oral choledochoscopy techniques in conjunction with studies used to establish or confirm the sump syndrome (see Chapter 10). Per orally a standard or pediatric instrument can be used to enter the enterostomy so that both the proximal common hepatic duct and the distal common bile duct (the sump) can be examined (18,19). The endoscope can be utilized to extract stones or bezoar material or to perform a sphincterotomy. If the enterostomy stoma is stenosed and will not admit the endoscope, I do not advise using a sphincterotome to extend the opening further because perforation or hemorrhage may ensue. Instead, I recommend either balloon dilating the stoma (Chapter 13) or performing a transpapillary sphincterotomy for the sump syndrome (20,21).

Mother-daughter System; Ultrathin Fiberscopes

A mother-daughter endoscope prototype has been available for years, but until recently it was not uni-

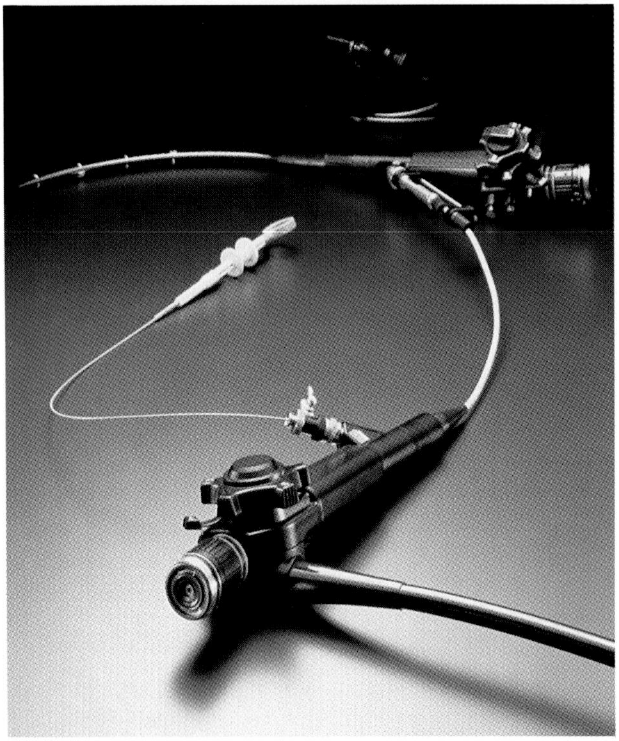

FIG. 14.16. The mother-daughter system. The daughter endoscope is in the foreground, and a biopsy forceps is shown inserted through its channel.

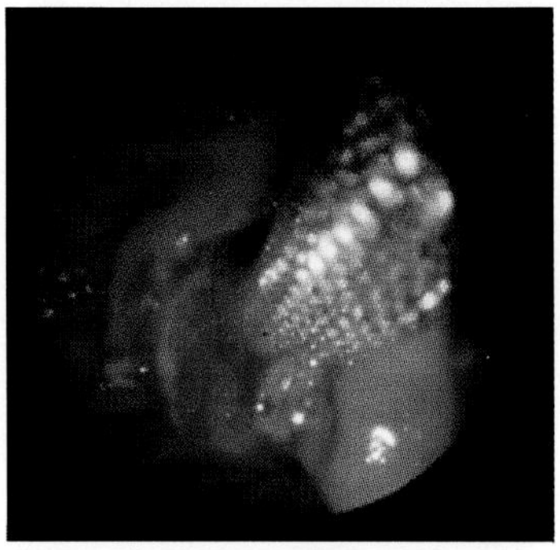

FIG. 14.17. A daughter endoscope inserted through a sphincterotomy incision into the bile duct.

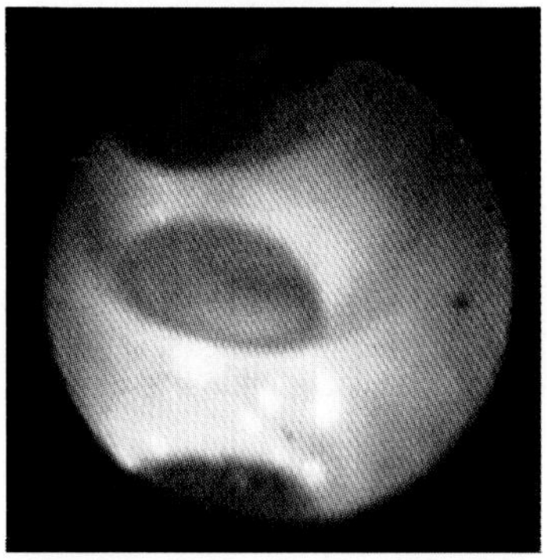

FIG. 14.18. This enlarged endoscopic picture shows the bifurcation of the biliary radicals.

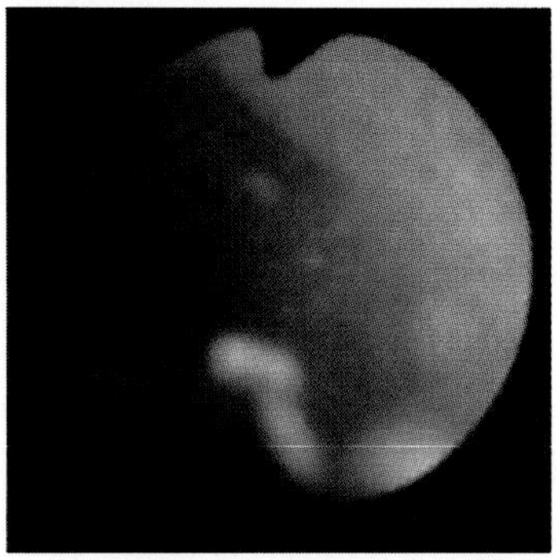

FIG. 14.19. An endoscopic picture of a pigmented stone seen through the daughter endoscope.

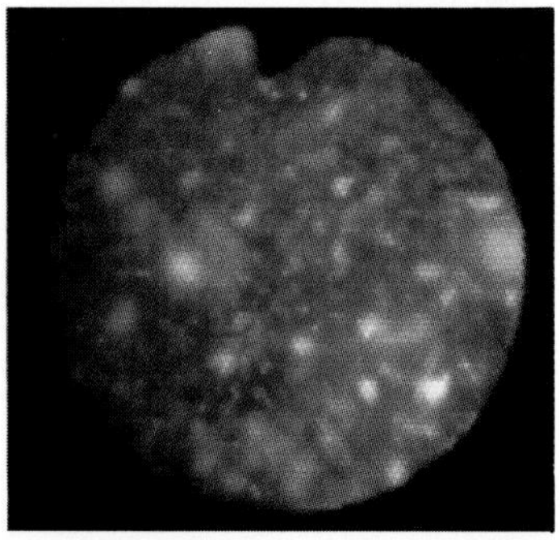

FIG. 14.20. This endoscopic photograph shows bile in the duct and cholesterol stone material following lithotripsy.

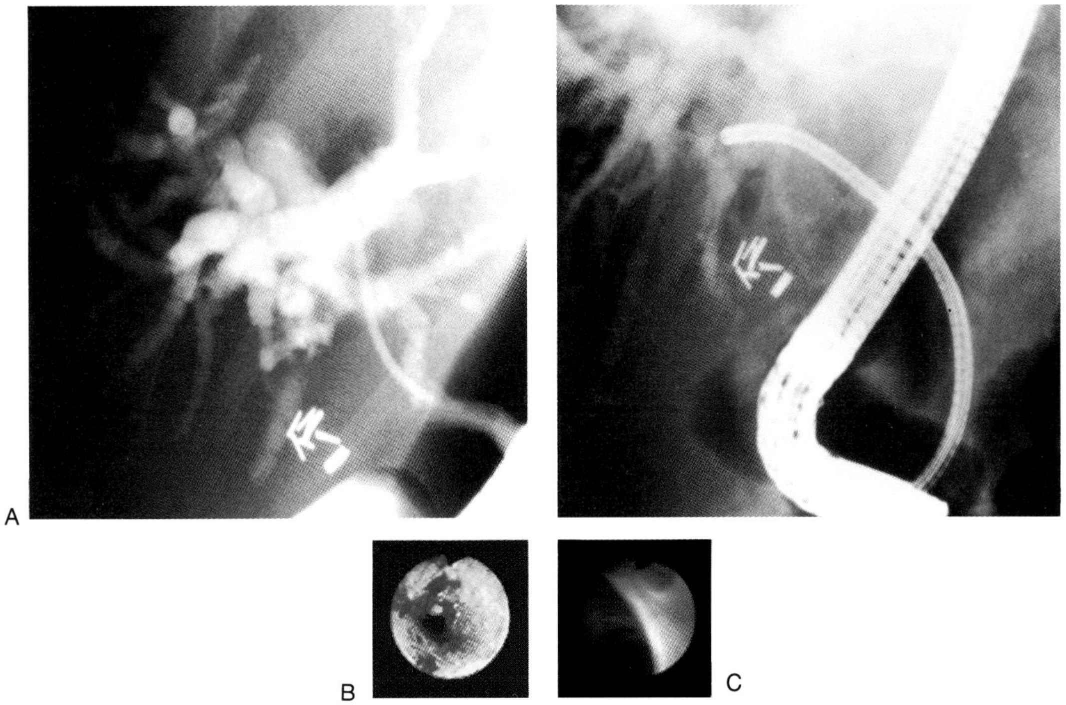

FIG. 14.21. **A: Left:** This ERCP cholangiogram reveals a high-grade stricture at the bifurcation, probably a Klatskin II lesion. **Right:** The daughter endoscope inserted through the stricture. **B:** A videoendoscopic picture taken with the daughter endoscope that shows a friable, scirrhous lesion consistent with a cholangiocarcinoma. **C:** This endoscopic picture taken with the daughter endoscope shows the bile duct and the opening of the cystic duct, which is visible under the endoscope arrow.

versally available or frequently utilized because of its fragility. In selective cases, the system was used as a curiosity. I have recently had the opportunity to use a newer, more durable system (Olympus Corporation) that incorporates a larger mother endoscope, channel size 5.5 mm, and a larger daughter endoscope (Figs. 14.16, 14.17). The resolution of the baby instrument is improved and clear (Figs. 14.18–14.21). Its larger channel permits biopsies (see Fig. 6.16); stone extraction; and insertion of laser fibers for lithotripsy or tumor treatment or insertion of an electrohydraulic probe for lithotripsy (22–25). Mother-daughter endoscopy requires two light sources and suction units, and two endoscopists are required to perform the procedure. Videoadaptors are available so that choledochoscopy can be witnessed by others and so that both video and hard copy can be obtained for documentation of the findings.

Similarly, pancreatoscopy can be performed (26,27) using the mother-daughter system. Again, video documentation is available, and biopsy capability under direct visualization offers an additional advantage. This type of examination of the pancreas would certainly be more definitive, and those of us with this endoscopic system look forward to the development of new and unusual atlases of cholangioscopy and pancreatoscopy.

CYSTIC DUCT CANNULATION

I have selectively cannulated the cystic duct, and occasionally the gallbladder, most often unintentionally during bile duct exploration. Stents have been placed into the gallbladder for direct drainage, and stones have been extracted from that organ as well (Chapters 10 and 12). Extraction of gallbladder stones cannot always be performed and does not always have to be attempted. Selective cannulation of the cystic duct may become more predictable and realistic using newer accessories such as steerable catheters and the Terumo guidewire (Microvasive). I am keenly interested in embarking on a study to assess the success of

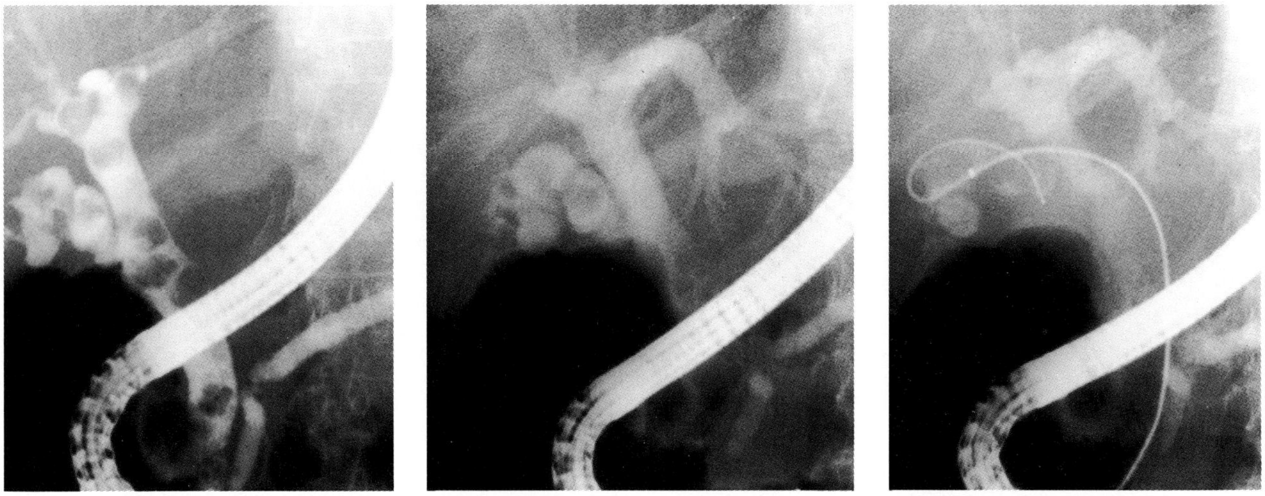

FIG. 14.22. Left: Multiple stones in the bile duct and cystic duct. **Middle:** After performance of a sphincterotomy and clearing of the bile duct, some cystic duct stones remain. **Right:** A guidewire was placed into the cystic duct, and an occlusion balloon (opaque marker) was used to extract the cystic duct stones. Following the procedure, a stent was placed into the the cystic duct to prevent occlusion. The patient has not exhibited evidence of cholecystitis despite the cystic duct-enteric communication.

selective cannulation of the cystic duct and gallbladder (Fig. 14.22) in order to dissolve or pulverize stones.

Dissolution techniques using an occlusion balloon have been tried (28). However, the major deterrent to this procedure is the fact that the dissolving agent, methy-ter-butyl ether, dissolves latex. In order to dissolve gallbladder stones via direct cannulation of the cystic duct, occlusion balloons have to contain the ether within the gallbladder to enhance dissolution and to retard absorption of the substance and prevent toxicity. Unfortunately, the occlusion balloons we are now using are made of latex, which is dissolved by the agent (ether). Therefore, in order to dissolve gallstones via selective intubation of the cystic duct and gallbladder, occlusion balloons must be made of material resistant to ether, and these are not yet available for general use.

As we endoscopists develop our skills, I predict that more of us will be selectively entering the gallbladder in an attempt to treat cholelithiasis directly. This prospect is exciting, but radiologic percutaneous dissolution techniques and laparoscopic surgery are more practical today. However, endoscopists should develop newer skills, and cannulating the cystic duct provides the skill and associated challenges that will allow our subspeciality to continue its outstanding progress.

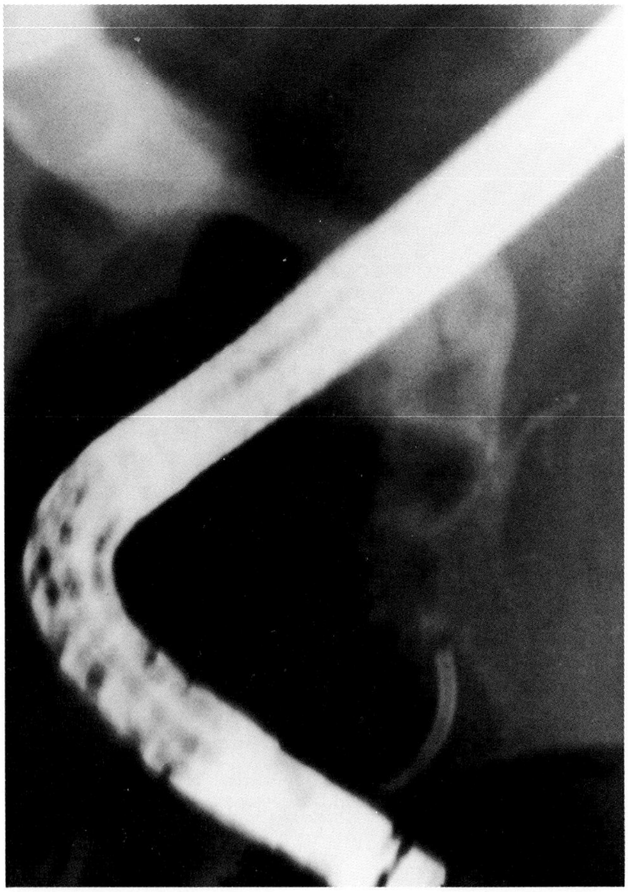

FIG. 14.23. A dilated bile duct with several stones within it. The metal-tipped catheter seen extending from the endoscope is a bipolar sphincterotome. The metallic portion of this accessory functions as a ground.

BIPOLAR SPHINCTEROTOMY

Finally, my colleagues and I have been investigating a bipolar cautery system (Everest Medical) with the

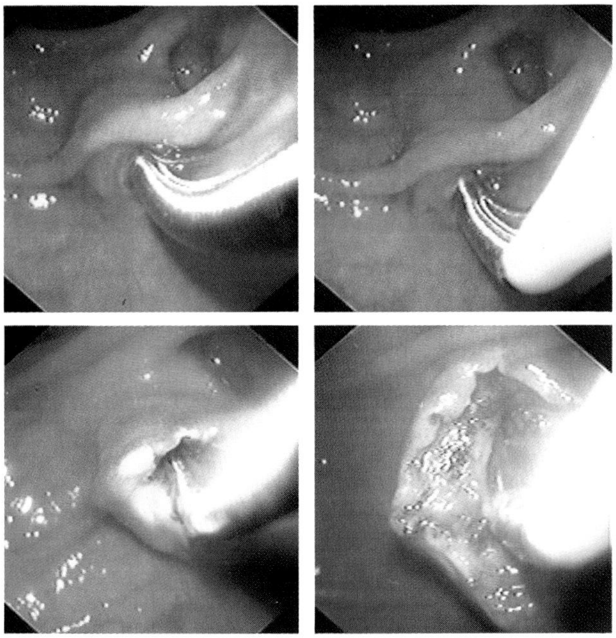

FIG. 14.24. Top left: This videoendoscopic picture shows the bipolar sphincterotome being placed into the papilla. A periampullary diverticulum is present. **Top right:** The sphincterotome is inserted to the proper depth before application of cautery current. **Bottom left:** The sphincterotomy has commenced. **Bottom right:** A maximum incision has been completed. No bleeding is present.

intention of performing a safer sphincterotomy. It is thought that bipolar energy reduces the transmission of thermal energy to the pancreas and bowel wall, thus reducing complications. No ground pad is necessary with the bipolar system because it is built into the sphincterotome (Figs. 14.23, 14.24). The ground is contained on the sphincterotome and is in apposition to the active or cutting wire completing the circuit. We have used this sphincterotome more than 50 times and have experienced success without complications. No patient has developed pancreatitis, and no bowel wall injuries or bleeding have occurred.

Despite this optimistic report, I have found the bipolar sphincterotome difficult to insert because of stiffness and the necessary extension of the nose of the catheter. Ordinarily, the length of the catheter's leading edge should not make a difference (some monopolar systems have a 3 cm leading edge), but because of material used in the bipolar catheter system and its diameter, it cannot always be inserted into the duct. Occasionally, a wire-guided bipolar sphincterotome is necessary to enter the duct and complete the incision. Once a guidewire is inserted, the sphincterotomy can be completed routinely.

More trials are needed to determine if the bipolar is safer than monopolar current. Randomized trials are certainly essential to establish the efficacy of this system, and we are presently engaged in such a study.

THE FUTURE

Having been witness to the evolution of endoscopy for the past 30 years and having been directly involved with research and development for the past 16 years, I can attest to the progress achieved in this field. Not only have we witnessed the evolution from incandescent lights to fiberoptic illumination and images, but we have now entered the electronic era of microprocessors, chips, hard copy, videotaping, word and image processors, and even voice-activated simulation. Our images are stored on large-capacity, space efficient disks, and these images can be instantly recalled and incorporated into an official report. With this modern age of teletransmissions and modems, images can be transmitted anywhere in the world to be interpreted or reviewed by others. The primary endoscopist can be connected to an encyclopedic database at any given time. What a far cry from our initial ventures into 16 mm movies or 35 mm stills (½ frame), which required days of processing before they could be viewed and incorporated into the permanent record.

Since the incorporation of therapeutic modalities into our armamentarium, the endoscopist has become an endoscopic surgeon despite the fact that the overwhelming majority of endoscopists were trained in a medical, not surgical, discipline. The endoscopist must be aware of the array of therapeutic modalities and should attend courses and visit centers especially proficient with ERCP techniques. Not all procedures are successful, and most are associated with risks to the patient. It is incumbent upon the endoscopist to explain these risks in detail to patients and their relatives or accompanying persons, because morbidity and mortality are associated with ERCP, sphincterotomy, and their interventional techniques. The interventional endoscopist must therefore be thoroughly prepared, thoroughly trained, and willing to accept a great moral and ethical responsibility.

I endorse additional training for therapeutic procedures, especially ERCP, and encourage program directors to open their programs to an additional year of training, not only to allow trainees to become more proficient with difficult therapeutic procedures, but also to expose them to mature, experienced endoscopists who can impart this real sense of responsibility.

I have been a witness to our past, when "show and tell" were the mainstays of endoscopy. This book is intended to demonstrate more than show and tell and to impress upon the endoscopist the significance of maintaining accurate records and databases. I have presented large series of patients included in open (prospective) trials of several therapeutic modalities, and data from such series have often been corroborated by randomized trials. Data presented here should not be considered circumspect, and I call for randomized trials to substantiate their validity and more importantly to verify the effectiveness and safety of the proposed procedures. I offer encouragement to those beginning ERCP and hope that this book will be helpful in establishing a firm foundation. I trust that experienced endoscopists will find this book important to their continued success in performing complex therapeutic procedures.

REFERENCES

1. Siegel JH, Lichtenstein JL, Pullano WE, et al. Treatment of malignant biliary obstruction by endoscopic implantation of iridium 192 using a new double lumen endoprosthesis. *Gastrointest Endosc* 1988;34:301–6.
2. Lawrence BH. Iridium 192. Irradiation of biliary tract malignancy. In: Jacobson IM, ed. *ERCP: diagnostic and therapeutic applications*. New York: Elsevier Scientific, 1989.
3. Venu RP, Geenen JE, Hogan WJ, Johnson GK, Klein K, Stone J. Intraluminal radiation therapy for biliary tract malignancy: an endoscopic approach. *Gastrointest Endosc* 1987;33:236–8.
4. Levitt MD, Laurence BH, Cameron F, Klemp PF. Transpapillary iridium 192 wire in the treatment of malignant bile duct obstruction. *Gut* 1988;29:149–52.
5. Urban MS, Siegel JH, Pavlou W, et al. Treatment of malignant biliary obstruction with a high-dose rate remote afterloading device using a 10Fr nasobiliary tube. *Gastrointest Endosc* 1990;36:292–6.
6. Ell CH, Lux G, Hochberger J, Muller D, Demling L. Laser lithotripsy of common bile duct stone. *Gut* 1988;29:746–51.
7. Kozarek RA, Lov DE, Ball TT. Tunable dye laser lithotripsy: in-vitro studies and in-vivo treatment of choledocholithiasis. *Gastrointest Endosc* 1988;34:418–21.
8. Cotton PB, Kozarek RA, Schapiro RH, et al. Endoscopic laser lithotripsy of large bile duct stones. *Gastroenterology* 1990; 1128–33.
9. Classen M, Hagenmuller W, Gossner T, et al. Laser treatment of bile duct cancer via percutaneous choledochoscopy. *Endoscopy* 1987;19:74–5.
10. Yamakawa T, Mieno K, Nognchi T, et al. An improved choledochofiberscope and non surgical removal of retained biliary calcul under direct visual control. *Gastrointest Endosc* 1976; 22:160–4.
11. Moss JP, Whelan JG, Powel RW, et al. Postoperative choledochoscopy via the T-tube tract. *JAMA* 1976;236:2781–2.
12. Yamakawa T, Komaki F, Shikata J. Experience with routine postoperative choledochoscopy via the T-tube sinus tract. *World J Surg* 1985;2:379–85.
13. Siegel JH, Sherman HI, Davis RC Jr, Webb A. Modification of a bronchoscope for percutaneous choledochoscopy. *Gastrointest Endosc* 1981;27:179–81.
14. Siegel JH, Harding GT, Chateau F, Sherman HI, Davis RC Jr, Webb WA. Percutaneous endoscopic extraction of retained stones (PEERS). *N Y State J Med* 1981;81:327–30.
15. Yamakawa T. Percutaneous transhepatic stone extraction technique for management of retained biliary tract stones. In: Okuda K, Nakayama F, Wand J, eds. *Intrahepatic calculi*. New York, 1984.
16. Yamakawa T. Cholangioscopy. In: Silvis S, ed. *Therapeutic gastrointestinal endoscopy*. New York: Igaku-Shoin, 1989.
17. Burhenne JH. The technique of biliary duct stone extraction. Experience with 126 cases. *Radiology* 1974;113:567.
18. Siegel JH. Per oral choledochoduodenoscopy. *Gastrointest Endosc* 1982;28:192–3.
19. Siegel JH. Biliary bezoar: the sump syndrome and choledochoenterostomy. *Endoscopy* 1982;14:238–40.
20. Siegel JH, Guelrud M. Endoscopic cholangiopancreatoplasty: hydrostatic balloon dilatation in the bile duct and pancreas. *Gastrointest Endosc* 1983;29:99–103.
21. Siegel JH. Duodenoscopic sphincterotomy in the treatment of the sump syndrome. *Dig Dis Sci* 1981;26:922–8.
22. Kozarek RA. Direct cholangioscopy and pancreatoscopy at the time of endoscopic retrograde cholangiopancreatography. *Am J Gastroenterol* 1988;83:55–7.
23. Ponchon T, Charaillon A, Ayela P, Lambert R. Retrograde biliary ultrathin endoscopy enhances biopsy of stenoses and lithotripsy. *Gastrointest Endosc* 1989;35:292–7.
24. Kozarek RA. Direct cholangiopancreatoscopy. In: Jacobson IM, ed. *ERCP: diagnostic and therapeutic applications*. New York: Elsevier Scientific, 1989.
25. Riemann JF, Kohler B, Harloff M, Weber J. Peroral cholangioscopy—an improved method in the diagnosis of common bile duct diseases. *Gastrointest Endosc* 1989;35:435–7.
26. Kohler B, Kohler G, Riemann JF. Pancreoscopic diagnosis of intraductal cystadenoma of the pancreas. *Dig Dis Sci* 1990; 35:382–4.
27. Fujita R, Hirata N, Fujita Y. Peroral cholecystoscopy. *Endoscopy* 1989;21:378–80.
28. Miller GI, Lawrence BH, McCarthy JH. Cannulation of the cystic duct and gallbladder. *Endoscopy* 1989;21:223–4.

Subject Index

1st edit by 101 (bc)

C